HEALTH ASSESSMENT

HEALTH ASSESSMENT

Lois Malasanos, R.N., Ph.D.

Professor and Dean, College of Nursing, University of Florida,
Gainesville, Florida

Violet Barkauskas, R.N., C.N.M., M.P.H., Ph.D.

Associate Professor, School of Nursing, University of Michigan,
Ann Arbor, Michigan

Muriel Moss, R.N., M.A.

Public Health Nurse, South Central District Health Department,
Twin Falls, Idaho; formerly Assistant Professor, Department
of Public Health Nursing, College of Nursing,
University of Illinois at the Medical Center,
Chicago, Illinois

Kathryn Stoltenberg-Allen, R.N., M.S.N.

Formerly Assistant Professor, Department of Public Health Nursing,
College of Nursing, University of Illinois at the Medical Center,
Chicago, Illinois

THIRD EDITION

with **1029** illustrations and **6** color plates

The C. V. Mosby Company

ST. LOUIS • TORONTO • PRINCETON   1986

MOSBY

A TRADITION OF PUBLISHING EXCELLENCE

Editor: Barbara Ellen Norwitz
Developmental editor: Sally Adkisson
Editing supervisor: Judi Wolken
Manuscript editor: Melissa Neves
Book design: Nancy Steinmeyer
Cover design: John Rokusek
Production: Susan Trail

THIRD EDITION

Previous editions copyrighted 1977, 1981
Printed in the United States of America

The C.V. Mosby Company
11830 Westline Industrial Drive, St. Louis, Missouri 63146

Library of Congress Cataloging in Publication Data

Main entry under title:

Health assessment.

    Includes bibliographies and index.
    1. Nursing.   2. Medical history taking.
3. Physical diagnosis.   I. Malasanos, Lois, 1928-
[DNLM: 1. Medical History Taking.   2. Physical
Examination.   WB 205 H434]
RT48.H4   1986   616.07′5   85-7272
ISBN 0-8016-3094-0

TS/VH/VH 9 8 7 6 5 4 3 2 1   03/C/320

To our families and friends—
who encouraged and sustained us, and

To our students—
*who persisted in their efforts to find knowledge
enabling them to provide better health care to their clients*

PREFACE

This text is designed for students and beginning practitioners who are learning skills that will enable them to assess the health status of the client by obtaining a health history and performing a physical examination. Clinical skills are best acquired when learning experiences are organized and the learner is provided with opportunities to gain knowledge and to practice with experienced preceptors in settings that enhance learning (for example, a laboratory where learners can practice their new skills with each other or a clinical setting where the clients have been informed of the learner's purpose and have agreed to participate). Therefore, this text is intended for use in conjunction with structured learning experiences that enable the learner to acquire the theory and skills of health assessment.

This book contains substantive detail regarding examination procedures and findings. Thus, the student is not expected to "outgrow" the book after the health assessment course. The book is also designed to be a valuable reference for the practitioner.

Health assessment skills are useful to the practitioner in any clinical setting. However, this text is especially aimed at helping the student or practitioner who is preparing for a role in primary care, where the health maintenance of the client is a priority. The focus is on wellness, and the parameters of normal health are incorporated into the process of obtaining a health history and performing a physical examination. The discussion of selected problems is also included in the text as a way of demonstrating differences or deviations from the parameters of normal health. Within the framework of health maintenance, emphasis is placed on the early detection of changes in the health status of the client for the purpose of preventing a more serious problem or disability. This is compatible with the plan to assist the learner in defining the parameters of wellness and subtle or gross deviations that occur in illness.

The consumer of health care is referred to as the *client* in this text because the term implies the ability of a person, whether well or sick, to contract for health care as a responsible participant with the providers of health care. The label *patient* has been avoided because it has traditionally been used to describe someone who is ill and/or a dependent receiver of care. Health care providers can no longer expect consumers of care to accept health advice or treatment plans unless they have been included in the decision-making process. Thus, the use of the term *client* is more appropriate in today's health care milieu.

This text is intended as a guide to assist the learner in conceptualizing the assessment of the whole person, taking into account the parameters of good health practices and the factors that impinge on health. The assessment that incorporates these components provides a basis for the development of an optimum plan for health care and health teaching that is reasonable in terms of the individual client's life situation.

The chapters on the integrative components of the assessment, including the history, nutritional assessment, and assessment of sleep-wakefulness patterns, are organized in the beginning portion of the text so that the practitioner can gain an appreciation of the whole person and some aspects of individual life-styles before proceeding to the more specific assessment of the body systems.

A discussion of the purposes and techniques of interviewing precedes the chapter on the health history so that the learner may become more sensitive to the process of obtaining information within the framework of a beginning or continuing relationship with the client. Since communication is the basis for obtaining this information, the possession of keen communication skills distinguishes effective information gathering from haphazard data collection. Therefore, within the chapter on interviews, renewed emphasis is placed on respect for empathy with the client.

Finally, the learner is encouraged to consider specific ways of organizing the assessment and of recording the data obtained. There is little value in obtaining information that is unclear to the practitioner or other members of the health team at a future time when it may be of critical importance as part of an overall data base from which problems are identified and actions planned.

Responses to the first and second editions of this book have been very positive. The book has served as an introductory health assessment text for thousands of health professional students in the United States and around the world. The content and format of this book have been scrutinized and found to be accurate, relevant, and clearly presented. In this third edition of *Health Assessment* we have strived to make the product even better.

The major goal for this revision was the strengthening of the content throughout the book through clarification, elaboration, and updating of information. Substantive changes were made in the chapters on developmental assessment, assessment of the pediatric client, and assessment of the aging client. Also, a new color plate of the eye and one of skin changes in the elderly have been included. Changes in the printed presentation of material were designed to enhance the book's readability and appearance.

Many people have contributed to the development of this text. Without their support and assistance it would not have been possible. Carrie Schopf, M.D., was our reviewer, supporter, and teacher for the first edition. The excellent photography of Patricia Urbanus, M.S.N., R.N., C.N.M., continues to serve this book well. Additional photographers for the third edition include Jerry Hadam and James Stoltenberg. Our thanks is also extended to Scott Thorn Barrows, William R. Schwarz, Robert Parshall, Christo Popoff, Marion Howard, and Mary Ann Olson for their outstanding artwork. In addition, we would like to express our appreciation to those colleagues, students, and practitioners who have suggested changes that are included in the revision.

Lois Malasanos
Violet Barkauskas
Muriel Moss
Kathryn Stoltenberg-Allen

CONTENTS

Color plates

CHAPTER 1

INTRODUCTION

RECOGNITION OF THE NEED FOR HEALTH ASSESSMENT AND UNIVERSAL HEALTH CARE

As long ago as the beginning of the Civil War an article was published recommending periodic health examinations in the interest of the early detection of disease (Dobell, 1861). This concept was adopted by the American Medical Association in 1922 in the form of a resolution advocating periodic health assessment. In 1925 the procedure was formalized in a manual published by this organization.

In 1956 the declaration that health care is a basic human right was made at a White House Conference on Aging. The general public has expressed with increasing frequency the expectation that preventive health care constitutes a fundamental part of this care. Leavell and Clark have defined preventive health care in three categories: primary, secondary, and tertiary prevention. Primary prevention involves those aspects of health care that are aimed at avoiding the contraction of a disease. Secondary prevention is aimed at stopping or attenuating the process of disease, and tertiary prevention deals with rehabilitative processes. The objective of tertiary prevention is the restoration of optimum function to a person after the disease process has been arrested.

Each level of prevention is based on a thorough assessment of the client's health status. Preventive health care can be planned only from a complete data base of both the client and his family.

Government leaders emphasize the need for provision of adequate and accessible health care for all Americans regardless of their ability to pay and regardless of where they live. The two words that frequently appear in discussions relevent to this issue are *equity* and *access*.

The need to establish facilities for health care in the communities where people live is receiving more attention among legislators. The negative aspects of asking the client to travel long distances for preventive care are increasingly clear. In many cases the distance to the physician or hospital is the major determinant of whether a client seeks care. The famous anecdote among the people of Watts makes the point well. In this community in the early 1970s the cost of a taxi to the hospital was $10. These people often had to be quite sick before they sought medical help. When they did go to the hospital, they referred to themselves as being "$10 sick."

One way in which the government of the United States has recognized the universal need for comprehensive health care has been through the encouragement of health maintenance organizations. These institutions are designed to provide preventive health care that is community based.

On the other side of the coin, physicians control health care in the United States as a result of both legislative action and tradition. Although the number of physicians has increased to 170 per 100,000 population, a number greater than at any other time in the history of this country, there are wide gaps between the consumer, the health care demands, and the capabilities of the available physicians to meet them. The major deficit is in the number of primary care physicians prepared to provide the degree of preventive health care known to be needed. Several British writers have taken the position that it is the primary care practitioner who can give preventive care most effectively.

The process of specialization in medical practice makes it increasingly more difficult for physicians to obtain salient family and community information. At this time the majority of preventive care is performed in physicians' offices and in emergency rooms. Care essentially involves providing prescriptions and treatment for symptomatic clients.

Thus, most health care treatment in this country is oriented toward dealing with crisis situations. Health maintenance efforts are directed toward large industrial groups, antenatal women, well babies, school children, and military groups but remain on the whole a matter of individual responsibility. The periodic health examination for adults usually represents an attempt to screen an individual for disease. The depth and quality of the screening examination vary widely. For example, the executive checkup includes a vast battery of laboratory tests, a treadmill ECG, and contrast and fiberoptic studies of the gastrointestinal tract, but the examination of a woman by a gynecologist may be limited to the breasts and pelvis.

ADVANTAGES OF ASSESSMENT

The value of periodic health examinations has been attested to in several studies. As early as 1921 the Metropolitan Life Insurance Company reported a 28% reduction in mortality as a result of early disease detection incurred through periodic health examinations. Studies related to disability reported in the 1960s showed a savings in employee disability payments that amounted to four times more than the cost of the examinations; the studies also showed that as much as 13% of the disease that produces disability in executives could be detected in the periodic health examination before the disability was incurred. Although later studies have failed to substantiate the wide margins suggested in these early studies, there is little doubt that the general public would benefit not only from the early detection of disease but also from the provision of a constantly updated baseline of relevant data. This information would benefit the individual by allowing a comparison of parameters obtained during a well visit with those observed during a suspected illness; this comparison would potentially afford a more accurate diagnosis. Furthermore, significant epidemiological data obtained during these examinations would be a secondary gain.

INCREASING ACCESSIBILITY TO ASSESSMENT

The health examination is frequently the mechanism of entry into the health care system. Since accessibility has been shown to be an important factor in determining whether a client will seek health care, alternate modes of providing health care to greater numbers of people have been explored.

Recent studies have indicated that although periodic health examinations have proved beneficial, they may not necessarily need to be performed by a physician. Controlled studies comparing physicians' and nurses' problem lists after they have examined the same client show no appreciable differences. At least one author has suggested that as many as three fourths of the clients who visit a primary care physician for health care could be safely monitored by an allied health professional. It is reasonably clear that making health services available to the entire population in an effective manner will include both medical and nurse practitioners.

That there is a need to develop a core of individuals skilled in assessing the health status of persons seeking such care has been attested to by the Russians' use of Feldsher and by the use of public health nurses, nurse practitioners, and physicians' assistants in the United States. These nonphysician practitioners have helped to make preventive care an actuality by increasing accessibility to the system, both through increasing the number of people able to give this care and by providing care in communities that had previously been underserved. The provision of these services is evidence of sensitivity to the public's need and an effort to make health care more convenient.

These groups of health care workers have entered into situations involving varying degrees of responsibility for patient care. In all cases they are involved in the assessment of health status; there are some differences in expectations of their abilities to identify normal versus abnormal traits. In many cases standardized treatment schedules or protocols allow these individuals to render treatment and follow-up care. This can be a workable reality in those cases where the medical community has achieved consensus as to appropriate care for specific problems.

OBJECTIVES AND TYPES OF ASSESSMENT

The purposes of health assessment include surveillance of health status, identification of latent or occult disease, screening for specific type of disease (called *case finding*), and follow-up care.

The public has been educated and often required to seek certain health examinations, such as well baby, preschool, premarital, precollege, prenatal, preemployment, and preinsurance examinations. Both men and women in their middle years have been educated to their increased vulnerability to disease and thus seek care at this time.

Many words have developed to describe the act of health assessment. Some of these are *physical examination, health appraisal, checkup,* and *screening examination.* These types of assessment generally include a history, a physical examination, and a routine battery of clinical laboratory tests. Such appraisals are often thought of as isolated incidents. The *periodic health examination,* on the other hand, is regarded as occurring at regular intervals. A return or follow-up visit is one that is scheduled to assess the progress or abatement of diagnosed dysfunction.

Examinations performed for the purpose of case

finding are directed at significant diseases for which there is a recognized treatment. Furthermore, definitive tests or examinations should be recognized as being specific to the condition and the population tested. In addition, there should be an early symptomatic or latent stage of the disease, so that intervention will prevent progress of the disease.

INCREASING CLIENT PARTICIPATION IN HEALTH CARE

The health assessment should accurately define the health and sick care needs for the individual at that specific point in time.

The information obtained in the interview and physical examination is used to formulate the exchanges of responsibility in defining the contract. The client should be apprised of the services available that will be useful in dealing with his problems.

The findings of the health assessment are shared with the client in a clearly understandable manner. In many cases this may mean educating him to the anatomy and physiology of his diseased tissues so that he can fully understand the meaning and level of his dysfunction.

Only with a clear definition of his problem is the client capable of assuming active involvement in decision making for his own care.

The World Health Organization (WHO) has defined health education as the active mechanism of facilitating an optimum state of social, emotional, and physical functioning that should be available to all people. Patient education is implicit in preventive care.

The concept of normality has not been extensively studied. Normal ranges are defined for technological tests such as pulmonary function tests. The major focus of traditional medical education has been to eliminate signs and symptoms of disease and thereby restore the client to health. Thus, the physician's attention has been directed to the abnormal or pathological behaviors. Almost by default, those individuals with no signs or symptoms and who need no medical treatment are considered normal or healthy. The descriptions of homeostasis by Cannon emphasized the body's total functioning and the complex interactions of multiple body systems in maintaining the internal milieu. The body was viewed as being in dynamic equilibrium. Persons who have disease may have minimum dysfunction and may be viewed as having good health. Ryle studied variability within normal range. He emphasized the importance of determining borderline states and suggested that persons with values in extremes of normal range might play a role in explaining individual susceptibility to disease. Other approaches have been to study associations between genetic constitution, early life experiences, stressors, and the interplay between body systems. This multiple approach has been helpful in reducing the absolute dichotomy between health and illness.

Primary prevention may be facilitated through teaching the client the general tenets of a healthful lifestyle. Some of the topics that may be explained are the optimum nutritional habits, sleep-activity patterns, exercise regimens, and recreational patterns. The client may also be warned against such potentially dangerous health patterns as smoking and diets typified by high sugar content.

The adolescent may particularly benefit by educational efforts concerning alcohol, drugs, and sexuality.

Genetic counseling may be considered one form of primary prevention, the need for which may become apparent during the course of the health assessment.

Several authors contend that individuals should be educated to the most common problems experienced by the general public in their particular geographical locale to take care of themselves more effectively. Moreover, the public needs sufficient information to make responsible use of the health services available to them.

In many situations clients may be taught to monitor their own disease process. More common examples are the hypertensive client who checks his own blood pressure and the diabetic client who tests for the presence of sugar and acetone in his urine. Many assessment techniques may be easily taught to clients, particularly those involving inspection and palpation.

Another form of increasing the participation of the client in the management of his health problems is one of teaching him the untoward side effects that commonly occur with medications that are prescribed for him and the steps he should take in the event these side effects happen to him.

An exploration with the client should be planned that will allow the practitioner to understand the attitudes and feelings of the client toward the health care system. Questions may be formulated that will reveal the nature of the client's earlier experiences with physicians, nurses, and allied personnel and health care agencies. This discussion may also bring out an appreciation of the kind of problems the client feels would warrant a visit to a health care agency. This information may be used in planning the mechanisms that will help the individual to continue in the system.

Several studies have been done that contribute to the knowledge of the client's attitudes and values toward health care. Some of the findings are useful. The client imparts to the health professional a faith in the fact that technical competence is a given, that the professional's educational preparation has guaranteed this aspect. The client further expects that all the equipment necessary for his examination is available and in working order and that all the tests necessary to explore his problems will be ordered, performed, and interpreted correctly. The health professional is expected by the client to show a genuine interest in his general welfare, that the client is worth the time required to evaluate and intervene in the disease processes the professional may find. The client frequently correlates the competence of the health professional with the amount of time the professional is willing to spend with the client, the professional's demonstrated willingness to allow the client to fully discuss his problems, and the degree to which the professional answers questions lucidly and honestly. The client is not loath to visit several health professionals if the opinion of specialists is needed in reaching a diagnosis. He is, however, better satisfied if the health professional he visits actively intervenes in his disease process.

The prospect of an individual seeking health care in relation to a specific illness corresponds directly with his perception of (1) the dangers of the disease (disability, death), (2) his own susceptibility to the disease, and (3) the possibility that the illness can be cured by the intervention of health professionals.

The levels of income and education are positively correlated with those populations who seek health care. Furthermore, those with education regarding hygiene are more prone to ensure their well-being by attaining health surveillance. They are also more likely to secure verification of symptoms that they feel may connote disease.

The aged, the poorly educated, and the socioeconomically disadvantaged are less likely to feel that health care is meeting their needs. It has been shown that women, poorly educated individuals, and elderly individuals are less likely to demonstrate compliance in health care. Thus, these groups are less likely to seek a health examination to follow the therapeutic regimen established for them, and to return for further help.

Studies have shown that women with family respon-

sibilities only are less likely to seek health care than those with family responsibilities who have career commitments as well.

Conditions for which health care is needed and for which case finding may be necessary include self-destructive behavior leading to early death, sickness, and debility. Such conditions may be drug dependency, alcoholism, venereal disease, and obesity. Because of the stigma attached to many of these states, the affected individuals may not seek health care. Frequently, inadequate services are available for those who do. The individual feels devalued in his own estimation and is hesitant to reveal what he considers a weakness, an aberration, over which he feels he "should" have control. It has been shown that return visits of such individuals are increased by encouraging them to assume responsibility for planning.

FREQUENCY OF ASSESSMENT

There is considerable controversy surrounding the issue of how often the periodic health examination should be performed on the ostensibly healthy client. Early recommendations suggested that the health examination should be done each year. More recent evaluation of the findings of examinations by age groups suggests that younger individuals need not be assessed as frequently as older people. One recommendation is that persons under 35 years of age be assessed every 4 to 5 years, that persons 35 to 45 years of age be assessed every 2 to 3 years, and that only persons over 45 years of age undergo a thorough health assessment every year (Table 1-1).

LIFETIME HEALTH MONITORING PLAN (LHMP)

An emphasis on preventive health care has led to the development of a proposal for a Lifetime Health Monitoring Program (LHMP) by Breslow and Somers. This plan for preventive health care provides a definition of health care for the entire life of the individual and is organized around ten periods in the person's life. The goals for health care and the criteria for the health care provider activities and patient participation are defined for each age group. The divisions adopted include the pregnancy-perinatal period, infancy (the first year), preschool child, school age child, adolescence, adult entry, young adult years, middle adult years, older adult years, and old age. A summary of these recommendations follows:

Table 1-1
Recommendation for the frequency of health assessment

Client's age	Frequency of health assessment
< 35	Every 4-5 years
35-45	Every 2-3 years
> 45	Every year

A. Pregnancy-perinatal age group
1. Goals
   a. To improve the quality of life of this and future generations by improving the outcome of every pregnancy
   b. To make available a single standard of optimum care—including specialized care where needed—for every obstetrical client regardless of her economical and social standing
   c. To ensure the mother the best chance of a healthy, full-term pregnancy and rapid recovery after a normal delivery
   d. To identify and categorize high- and low-risk patients and their newborns
   e. To facilitate the live birth of a normal baby, free of congenital or developmental damage
   f. To help both mother and father achieve the knowledge and capacity to provide for the physical, emotional, and social needs of the baby

2. Recommended assessment periods for the normal pregnant woman
   a. First visit—early in the first trimester (ideally, about 2 to 4 weeks after the first missed period)
   b. During the initial 28 to 32 weeks of gestation—every 2 to 4 weeks
   c. 28 to 32 to 36 weeks of gestation—every 2 weeks
   d. 36 weeks of gestation to delivery—weekly

Ideally, counseling is initiated before the pregnancy, and in early childhood the need for a program for exercising and maintaining normal weight should be emphasized. For the woman who is assessed to be obese in the childbearing years, a program of weight reduction should be accomplished before pregnancy. If it is determined by history that the individual smokes, the smoker is counseled to quit before conception. Birth control pills are generally discontinued 2 to 3 months before attempts to conceive.

Recommended professional services for the pregnancy-perinatal age group

Education and counseling

Anatomical, physiological, and psychological changes
Nutrition and weight gain
Exercise
Cigarette, alcohol, and drug use and avoidance
Unnecessary x-ray examinations
Exposure to infection
Signs and symptoms of abnormalities
Travel, clothing, employment
Labor and delivery
Infant care and parenthood preparation
Contraception
Abortion and adoption

High-risk patients

Amniocentesis
Gonorrhea culture
Sonogram

Medical evaluation

Comprehensive history and physical examination
Dental examination
Weight*
Blood pressure*
Urinalysis (sugar, albumin, bacteriuria)*
Hematocrit, hemoglobin†
Blood sugar‡
Urine culture and colony count‡
Blood grouping, Rh determination, Rh antibody,† irregular antibody screen†
VDRL
Rubella, toxoplasmosis, cytomegalic inclusion virus, herpes simplex titer (if available as single test; otherwise, rubella and, possibly, toxoplasmosis)
Pap smear
Tuberculin test†
Abdominal examination*
Fetal heart tones*
Pelvic examination (near term)

Adapted from Somers, A.R.: Lifetime health monitoring: preventive care for the child in utero, Patient Care 13(3):162-178, 1979. Copyright © 1979, Patient Care Publications, Inc., Darien, Conn.
*Repeat every visit.
†Repeat in third trimester.
‡Not recommended for all patients by all physicians.

B. Infancy (birth to age 1 year)
   1. Goals
      a. To enter the child in an ongoing system of primary health care
      b. To establish immunity against specified infectious disease
      c. To detect and prevent certain other diseases and problems, including precursors of adult diseases before irreparable damage occurs
      d. To facilitate emotional, intellectual, and physical growth and development to the infant's optimum potential
      e. To provide a basis for a lifetime of emotional stability, especially through a loving relationship with mother, father, and other family members
   2. Four to six visits for preventive health care are recommended in the first year of life. Somers recommends a visit with a nurse at 10 days of age and visits with a physician at 6 weeks, 4½ months, and 9 months.

Overall goals for children in the growing period include (1) facilitating the child's optimum physical, mental, emotional, and social growth and development; (2)

Recommended preventive procedures for the first year of life

Before discharge		After discharge	
Condition	**Procedure**	**Condition**	**Procedure**
Growth retardation	Height and weight, at birth and at discharge	Diphtheria	Immunization
		Pertussis	Immunization
Congenital abnormalities	Physical examination	Tetanus	Immunization
Strabismus	Eye examination	Poliomyelitis	Immunization
Parenting disorders	Observation, counseling	Phenylketonuria	Blood test
Neonatal gonococcal ophthalmia	Silver nitrate eye drops	Hypothyroidism	Blood test
		Tuberculosis	Skin test
Hemorrhagic disease of the newborn	Vitamin K	Anemia	Hematocrit, hemoglobin
		Growth disorders	Height, weight, head circumference
Phenylketonuria	Blood test		
Hypothyroidism	Blood test	Nutritional problems	History and parent counseling
Accidental injury or death	Parent counseling		
		Congenital disorders	Physical examination
Inadequate preparation for infant care	History and parent counseling	Strabismus	Eye examination
		Developmental disorders	Observation
Parent failure to bring baby for immunizations and wellbaby checks	Parent counseling		Denver Developmental Screening Test
		Hearing defects	Observation and noise-maker test
		Accidental death or injury	Parent counseling
		Sudden infant death syndrome	Parent counseling
		Inadequate preparation for infant care	History and parent counseling
		Acquiring a life-style that may adversely affect health and longevity	History and parent counseling
		Dental caries	Fluoride and parent counseling

Adapted from Somers, A.R.: Lifetime health monitoring: preventive care, Patient Care 13(3):162-178, 1979. Copyright © 1979, Patient Care Publications, Inc., Darien, Conn.

establishing and maintaining a healthy, effective parent-child relationship (This goal is expanded as the child grows to include other family members, peers, and others outside his home.); and (3) establishing healthy behavioral patterns for nutrition, exercise, study, and recreation as a basis for a healthy life-style.

C. Preschool child (ages 1 to 5)
  1. Goals
    a. To facilitate the child's optimum physical, emotional, and social growth and development
    b. To begin the child's process of socialization through happy and effective relations with parents and other family members and gradually to introduce the child to school and other aspects of life outside the home
    c. To identify possible precursors of adult disease such as obesity or high blood pressure
  2. Generally two visits are recommended for preventive care in the second year of life. After this, the visits are spaced at every 12 or 18 months until age 5.

Recommended preventive procedures for the preschool child

The following chart summarizes the recommendations for preventive health care for the child age 1 to 5.

Condition	Procedure	When
Developmental abnormalities	History, observation	Each visit
Problems with parent-child relationship	History, observation, counseling	Each visit
Discipline or behavior problems	History, observation, counseling	Each visit
Nutritional problems	History, counseling, height and weight measurement	Each visit
Accidental death or injury	Counseling	Each visit
Poisoning	Counseling about syrup of ipecac	Age 15-18 months
Dental caries	Examination, counseling	Each visit
	Fluoride supplementation	Throughout tooth development years
Congenital anomalies and growth abnormalities	Height and weight	Each visit
	Head circumference	Age 15-18 months
Eye defects, strabismus	Examination	Age 15-18 months and age 24 months or each visit*
Visual acuity	Examination	Each visit, age 3 and older
Hypertension	Blood pressure determination	Each visit, age 3 and older
Hearing defects	Audiometry	Each visit, age 3 and older
Measles, mumps, rubella	Immunization	Age 15 months
Diphtheria, tetanus, pertussis	Immunization	Age 18-24 months and age 5
Poliomyelitis	Immunization	Age 18-24 months and age 5
Tuberculosis	Skin test	Every 1-2 years or only at age 5*
Anemia	Hematocrit or hemoglobin†, sickle cell screen	Age 15-18 months, if not done at 9-12 months, and age 5
Bacteriuria	Urinalysis†	Each visit, age 2 and older, or only age 5*
	Urine culture (girls)†	Age 5
Toileting	—	—

Adapted from Somers, A.R.: Lifetime health monitoring: preventive care age 1 through adolescence, Patient Care **13**(8):201-216, 1979. Copyright © 1979, Patient Care Publications, Inc., Darien, Conn.
*Authorities disagree over the frequency of this procedure.
†Some authorities question whether this procedure should be included.

D. School age child (ages 6 to 11)
   1. Goals
      a. To facilitate the child's optimum physical, mental, emotional, and social growth and development, including a positive self-image
      b. To establish and maintain a healthy, effective parent-child relationship
      c. To establish healthy behavioral patterns for nutrition, exercise, study, and recreation as a foundation for a healthy lifestyle
   2. Although some recommend only one visit for this age span, others believe that the child should receive preventive care every 1 to 2 years.

Recommended preventive procedures for the school age child

The following chart summarizes the recommendations for preventive health care for the child age 6 to 11.

Condition	Procedure	When
Developmental abnormalities	History, observation	Each visit
Problems with parent-child relationship	History, observation, counseling	Each visit
Nutritional problems	History, counseling, height and weight	Each visit
Accidental death or injury	Counseling	Each visit
Dental caries	Counseling	Each visit
Growth	Height and weight	Each visit
Vision	Examination	Each visit
Hearing defects	Examination	Each visit
Hypertension	Blood pressure determination	Each visit
Scoliosis	Examination	Each visit, starting at age 8-9
Tuberculosis	Skin test*	Every 2 years
Enlarged thyroid	Examination	Each visit
Bacteriuria	Urinalysis* Urine culture (girls)*	Each visit
Smoking, drug abuse, lack of sex education	Counseling	Each visit
School performance	Counseling	Each visit

Adapted from Somers, A.R.: Lifetime health monitoring: preventive care age 1 through adolescence, Patient Care **13**(8):201-216,1979. Copyright © 1979, Patient Care Publications, Inc., Darien, Conn.
*There is disagreement whether this procedure should be included.

E. Adolescence (ages 12 to 17)
  1. Goals
     a. To continue optimum physical, mental, emotional, and social growth and development
     b. To reinforce healthy behavior patterns and discourage negative ones in physical fitness, nutrition, exercise, study, work, recreation, sex, individual relations, driving, smoking, alcohol, and drugs as a foundation for a healthy life-style
  2. Recommendations for the timing of preventive care in this age span range from one visit at age 14 to 15 to a yearly session.

Recommended preventive procedures for the adolescent

The following chart summarizes the recommendations for preventive health care for the child age 12 to 17.

Condition	Procedure	When
Accidental death or injury	Counseling	Each visit
Family problems	History, counseling	Each visit
School problems	History, counseling	Each visit
Negative behavior patterns	History, counseling	Each visit
Unwanted pregnancy	History, counseling	Each visit
Growth abnormalities	Height and weight	Each visit
Developmental abnormalities	Observation	Each visit
Nutritional abnormalities	History, height and weight, counseling	Each visit
Vision	Examination	Each visit
Hypertension	Blood pressure determination	Each visit
Acne	Observation	Each visit
Scoliosis	Examination	Each visit to age 15
Tetanus and diphtheria	Immunization booster	Age 15 or 10 years since previous booster
Rubella titer	Blood test	Age 15 or 10 years since previous booster
Bacteriuria	Urinalysis*	Each visit
	Urine culture (girls)*	Each visit
Tuberculosis	Skin test	Age 15 or every 2 years†
Cervical cancer	Pap smear	Every 2 years for girls who are sexually active or who were exposed to DES in utero
Testicular cancer	Examination	Each visit
Dental caries and periodontal disease	Counseling	Each visit
Smoking, drug abuse, sex education, and contraception	Counseling	Each visit

Adapted from Somers, A.R.: Lifetime health monitoring: preventive care age 1 through adolescence, Patient Care **13**(8):201-216, 1979.
Copyright © 1979, Patient Care Publications, Inc., Darien, Conn.
*There is disagreement whether this procedure should be included.
†There is disagreement over the frequency of this procedure.

F. Entering adulthood (ages 18 to 24)
  1. Goals
    a. To facilitate transition from dependent adolescent to mature independent adult with maximum physical, mental, and emotional resources
    b. To achieve useful employment and maximum capacity for a healthy marriage, parenthood, and social relations
  2. It is recommended that the 18- to 24-year-old adult undergo health appraisal once. After the initial health assessment, the client is asked to return every 1 to 2 years.

Recommended preventive procedures for the adult age 18 to 24

The following chart summarizes the recommendations for preventive health care for the patient entering adulthood. The column on the left lists the condition to be prevented or detected, the column in the middle lists the procedure to be used, and the column on the right lists how frequently the procedure should be repeated between ages 18 and 24.

Condition	Procedure	Frequency
Smoking	History and counseling	At least once
Unwanted pregnancy	Counseling	At least once
Problem drinking, alcoholism	History and counseling	At least once
Drug abuse	History and counseling	At least once
Accidents	History and counseling	At least once
Obesity	History and weight, counseling	Every 2-4 years
Lack of exercise	History and counseling	At least once
Hypertension	Blood pressure measurement	Every 2 years
Breast cancer	Breast examination, counseling about self-examination	Every 1-2 years
Refractive errors	Eye screen*	Once
Tetanus and diphtheria	Booster	Once if 10 years since last one
Cervical cancer	Pap smear	Every 2-3 years
Diabetes	Urinalysis*	Once
Proteinuria	Urinalysis*	Once
Bacteriuria	Urinalysis*	Once
Birth defects	Rubella titer	Once in unimmunized women
Tuberculosis	Skin test	Once
Anemia	Hematocrit or hemoglobin*	Once
Syphilis	Blood test*	Once
High cholesterol and/or triglyceride levels	Serum cholesterol,* serum triglyceride*	Once
Dental caries and periodontal disease	Dental examination and cleaning	Every 1-2 years
Contraception	History and counseling	Each visit

Adapted from Somers, A.R.: Lifetime health monitoring: a whole life plan for well patient care, Patient Care 13(11):83-153, 1979. Copyright © 1979, Patient Care Publications, Inc., Darien, Conn.
*There is debate on whether this procedure should be included.

G. Young adult (ages 25 to 39)
  1. Goals—see goals of entering adulthood.
  2. The individual in this age group should receive preventive health care every 1 to 2 years.

Recommended preventive procedures for the adult age 25 to 39

The following chart summarizes the recommendations for preventive health care for the young adult. The column on the left lists the condition to be prevented or detected, the column in the middle lists the procedure to be used, and the column on the right lists how frequently the procedure should be repeated between ages 25 and 39.

Condition	Procedure	Frequency
Smoking	History and counseling	Every 2 years
Obesity or poor eating habits	History and counseling	Every 2 years
	Weight	Every 2-4 years
Lack of exercise	History and counseling	Every 2 years
Accidental injury or death	History and counseling	Every 2 years
Problem drinking, alcoholism	History and counseling	Every 2-4 years
Drug abuse	History and counseling	Every 2-4 years
Unwanted pregnancy	History and counseling	Every 2 years
Hypertension	Blood pressure measurement	Every 2 years
Breast cancer	Breast examination, counseling about self-examination	Every 1-2 years
Tetanus and diphtheria	Immunization	Every 10 years
Cervical cancer	Pap smear	Every 2-3 years
Tuberculosis	Skin test	
Diabetes	Urinalysis*	Every 4 years
Bacteriuria	Urinalysis*	Every 4 years
Proteinuria	Urinalysis*	Every 4 years
Coronary artery disease	Serum cholesterol determination*	Every 4 years
Vision defects	Examination*	Every 4 years
Anemia	Hematocrit or hemoglobin*	Every 4 years
Syphilis	Blood test*	Every 4 years
Dental caries and periodontal disease	Dental examination and cleaning	Every 1-2 years
Contraception	History and counseling	At least once

Adapted from Somers, A.R.: Lifetime health monitoring: a whole life plan for well patient care, Patient Care **13**(11):83-153, 1979. Copyright © 1979, Patient Care Publications, Inc., Darien, Conn.
*There is debate on whether this procedure should be included.

H. Middle adult (ages 40 to 59)
  1. Goals—to prolong the period of maximum physical energy and optimum mental and social activity, including adjusting to menopause
  2. Preventive health care is recommended every 2 years for those 40 to 50 years of age. However, it is recommended that individuals receive health care every year after age 50.

Recommended preventive procedures for the middle adult years (age 40 to 59)

The following chart summarizes the recommendations for preventive health care for those 40 to 59 years of age. The left-hand column lists the condition to be detected or prevented, the middle column indicates the recommended screening procedure, and the right-hand column indicates how frequently to repeat the procedure.

Condition	Procedure	Frequency
Smoking	History and counseling	At least once
Problem drinking, alcoholism	History and counseling	At least once
Accidents	History and counseling	At least once
Problems related to job, family, menopause, retirement planning, etc.	History and counseling	At least once
Lack of exercise	History and counseling	At least once
Colonic cancer	History, test of stool for occult blood*	Every 2 years (annually after age 50)
Obesity	Height and weight	Every 4-5 years
Hearing problems	Screening*	Every 4-5 years
Visual impairment	Screening*	Every 4-5 years
Hypertension	Blood pressure determination	Every year
Breast cancer	Physician examination	Every 1-2 years (annually after age 50)
	Counseling about self-examination	Every 1-2 years (annually after age 50)
	Mammography*	Every 1-2 years after age 50
Cervical cancer	Pap smear	Every 2 years
Anemia	Hematocrit, hemoglobin*	Every 4-5 years
Syphilis	Blood test*	Once
Tuberculosis	Skin test*	Once
Diabetes	Urinalysis*	Every 4-5 years
Renal disease	Urinalysis*	Every 4-5 years
Bacteriuria	Urinalysis*	Every 4-5 years
Tetanus and diphtheria	Immunization	Every 10 years
Dental caries, periodontal disease	Dental examination and cleaning	Every 1-2 years
High cholesterol and triglyceride levels	Serum cholesterol,* serum triglyceride*	Every 4-5 years

Adapted from Somers, A.R.: Lifetime health monitoring: a whole life plan for well patient care, Patient Care 13(11):83-153, 1979.
Copyright © 1979, Patient Care Publications, Inc., Darien, Conn.
*There is debate on whether this procedure should be included.

I. Older adult (ages 60 to 74)
   1. Goals
      a. To prolong the period of optimum physical, mental, and social activity
      b. To minimize handicapping and discomfort from the onset of chronic conditions
      c. To prepare, in advance, for retirement years
   2. Preventive health care is recommended annually.

Recommended preventive procedures for the older adult years (age 60 to 74)

The following chart summarizes the recommendations for preventive health care for those 60 to 74 years of age. The left-hand column lists the condition to be detected, the middle column indicates the recommended screening procedure, and the right-hand column indicates how frequently to repeat the procedure.

Condition	Procedure	Frequency
Accidental injury or death, particularly from falls	History and counseling	Every 2 years
Lack of preparation for retirement	History and counseling	Every 2 years
Nutritional problems	History and counseling	Every 2 years
	Height and weight	Every 2-4 years
Colonic cancer	History	Annually
	Test of stool for occult blood*	Annually
Hearing defects	Screening*	Every 2 years
Visual impairment	Screening*	Every 2 years
Hypertension	Blood pressure determination	Every year
Breast cancer	Physician examination	Annually
	Counseling about self-examination	Annually
	Mammography*	Every 1-2 years
Cervical cancer	Pap smear	Every 2 years
Anemia	Hematocrit, hemoglobin*	Every 4-5 years
Syphilis	Blood test*	Once in this age group
Tuberculosis	Skin test*	Once in this age group
Diabetes	Urinalysis*	Every 4-5 years
Bacteriuria	Urinalysis*	Every 4-5 years
Renal disease	Urinalysis	Every 4-5 years
Tetanus, diphtheria	Immunization	Every 10 years
Dental caries and periodontal disease	Dental examination and cleaning	Every 1-2 years
Poor fitting dentures	Dental examination	Every 2-3 years

Adapted from Somers, A.R.: Lifetime health monitoring: a whole life plan for well patient care, Patient Care 13(11):83-153, 1979. Copyright © 1979, Patient Care Publications, Inc., Darien, Conn.
*There is debate on whether this procedure should be included.

J. Old age (75 and older)
  1. Goals
     a. To prolong the period of effective activity and ability to live independently and avoid institutionalization as far as possible
     b. To minimize inactivity and discomfort from chronic conditions in terminal illness
     c. To assure as little physical and mental distress as possible
     d. To provide emotional support to patient and family
  2. Preventive health care is recommended annually.

Recommended preventive procedures for the patient over age 75

The following chart summarizes the recommendations for preventive health care for those over age 75. The left-hand column lists the conditions to be detected or prevented, the middle column indicates the recommended screening procedure, and the right-hand column indicates how frequently to repeat the procedure.

Condition	Procedure	Frequency
Accidental injury or death, particularly from falls	History and counseling	Annually
Loss of mental acuity	History and observation	Annually
Nutritional problems	History and counseling	Annually
	Height and weight	Annually
Colonic cancer	History	Annually
	Test of stool for occult blood*	Annually
Hearing defects	Screening	Annually
Hypertension	Blood pressure determination	Annually
Breast cancer	Physician examination	Annually
	Counseling about self-examination	Annually
	Mammography*	Every 1-2 years
Cervical cancer	Pap smear	Every 2 years
Tetanus and diphtheria	Immunization	Every 10 years
Dental caries and periodontal disease	Dental examination and cleaning	Every 1-2 years
Poor fitting dentures	Dental examination	Every 2-3 years

From Somers, A.R.: Lifetime health monitoring: a whole life plan for well patient care, Patient Care 13(11):83-153, 1979. Copyright © 1979, Patient Care Publications, Inc., Darien, Conn.
*There is debate on whether this procedure should be included.

PRINCIPLES FOR SCREENING DISEASE

The World Health Organization published the following principles for *Screening for Disease* in 1968:

1. *The condition being sought should be an important health problem for the individual and/or the community.* The screening for hypertension may be seen as a common problem that could lead to serious complications for the individual and may lead to great expense to the community in the case of stroke and end stage renal disease. Hypothyroidism in the newborn could lead to mental retardation and result in considerable anguish to the family and public expense.

2. *An acceptable form of treatment should be available.* This principle precludes interventions that are not curative.

3. *The natural history of the disease including the development from latent to declared disease should be adequately understood.* Since the pathophysiology of many diseases is incompletely developed, this principle precludes many conditions.

4. *The disease should have a recognizable latent or early symptomatic stage.* The early detection of a breast mass would be an example.

5. *A suitable screening test for detection of the disease in question should be available and acceptable to the population.* The performance of phlebotomy to obtain a blood sample is acceptable to most individuals whereas routine tissue biopsy would not be.

6. *There must be a shared policy about whom to treat.* That is, there is sufficient scientific data available so that most health care professionals could agree on a method of treatment.

7. *Early treatment should favorably influence the course and prognosis of the disease.* The detection of carcinoma of the cervix early in the course of the disease increases the likelihood of survival.

8. *The cost of case finding and treatment must be economically balanced against the cost of health care as a whole.* The providers of health care in the United States are only beginning to dialogue on this ethical issue.

9. *Case finding is a continuing process.* This is support for periodic health examinations.

AMERICAN CANCER SOCIETY RECOMMENDATIONS

In 1980 new guidelines were developed by the American Cancer Society for individuals *without signs or symptoms of cancer.* These recommendations would result in fewer annual examinations. The following specific recommendations were published:

1. Annual health assessment only for men and women past 40 and every 3 years for individuals between 20 and 40

2. A Pap test every 3 years for women following two negative tests a year apart

3. Proctosigmoidoscopic examinations every 3 to 5 years after age 50 following two negative examinations a year apart

4. Annual test for occult blood after age 50

5. Breast manual examination (a) by health professional every 3 years before age 40 and then annually; (b) self-performed each month after age 20

6. Breast mammography examination baseline check between ages 35 to 40 and annually after age 50

Annual lung and sputum examinations in the effort to detect lung cancer are *not recommended.* It should be borne in mind that those individuals who are members of high-risk groups may need more frequent examinations.

HUMAN VARIATION

Sequential multiple analysis of 12 variables of blood samples results in normal values for each variable in only 50% of healthy individuals. When the analysis includes 20 variables, 20% to 40% of healthy persons have all values in the normal range. Thus there is questionable value for apparently healthy persons.

It is refreshing to note that a Kaiser Permanente Study revealed that men who had undergone four annual checkups reported less self-rated disability, time lost from work, and use of medical care service.

ASSESSMENT TECHNIQUES

The history and review of systems that are obtained by interviewing the individual to be examined provide subjective information. The information obtained is the verbalized perceptions and interpretations of the client. Although the major emphasis of this volume is health assessment, there are certain physiological functions and perceptions that are considered to be integral to examination of the client; these are the skills that contribute to the art of physical diagnosis. These are the processes through which objective data are obtained. The four major procedures of physical diagnosis are inspection, palpation, percussion, and auscultation. These procedures are described here and are further developed in chapters dealing with their application for specific organs and systems.

Inspection

Inspection (L. *inspectio,* the act of beholding) is the act of concentrating attention to the thorough and unhurried visualization of the client. Inspection also involves listening to any sounds emanating from the client and being attuned to any odors that may be present.

Lighting must be adequate. Daylight or artificial light is suitable. The specific cues to which the examiner should be alert are discussed in Chapter 7 on general assessment.

Palpation

By palpation (L. *palpatio,* the act of touching), the examiner's hands may be used to augment the data gathered through inspection. The skilled examiner will use the most sensitive parts of the hand for each type of palpation. The pads of the fingers are thought to be most effective in those tasks requiring discrimination through touch. Vibration is detected most effectively with the palmar surface of the metacarpal phalangeal joints. Rough measures of temperature are best determined with the dorsum of the hand. The position and consistency of a structure may best be determined by employing the grasping fingers. The examiner may use touch to seek out and determine the extent of tenderness and tremor or spasm of muscle tissues or to elicit crepitus in bones and joints. Individual structures within body cavities, particularly the abdomen, may be palpated for position, size, shape, consistency, and mobility. The examining hand may be used to detect masses. Palpation may also serve to evaluate abnormal collections of fluid. Both light and deep palpation may be used in the examination. Light palpation is always performed first. In the case of superficial masses the fingers are moved in a circular motion in the region suspected of containing a mass. The skin and hair are examined for moisture and texture through the use of touch.

Percussion

Percussion (L. *percussio,* the act of striking) involves a cause-and-effect relationship. This summary term includes the act of striking or otherwise producing the impact of one object against another—this is the cause. The result of this rapping is the production of a shock wave that in some cases results in vibration. The vibration may produce sound waves that may reach the ear to be interpreted as sound. In the process of physical diagnosis, percussion means the striking or tapping of a body surface such as the back or the abdomen while listening with the unassisted ear or with the stethoscope.

Auenbrugger, the originator of the technique, described what has been termed *immediate percussion.* Immediate percussion means the striking of a finger or hand directly against the body. The term *mediate percussion* is used to describe the refinement in technique that was developed some time in the nine-

teenth century. Instruments called the *pleximeter* and *plexor* were devised. The plexor was a small rubber hammer, much like the reflex hammers used today. This plexor was used to strike a blow against the pleximeter, a small, flat, solid object, often made of ivory, that was held firmly in place against the client's body.

Mediate percussion using the middle finger of one hand as the plexor that strikes against the middle finger (pleximeter) of the other hand is the method in use in current clinical practice.

The passive hand is placed gently against the body surface while the distal portion of the middle finger is placed firmly against the skin. The middle finger is dealt a blow at or immediately distal to the distal interphalangeal joint with the middle finger of the other hand. The blow must be delivered crisply, sharply, and with the plexor perpendicular to the pleximeter.

The speed and force of a blow by the plexor are made possible by wrist action. The hand is flexed back on the forearm and brought forward with a clean, snapping motion that allows a fast strike and rapid removal of the plexor (Fig. 1-1) in order not to dampen the vibration. Fingernails of the plexor finger should be cut sufficiently short to avoid cutting the skin of the pleximeter. Fatty tissue overlying the tissue to be percussed may dampen the blow. To overcome this, it has been suggested that more force can be brought to bear on the body surface by striking the lateral aspect of the thumb. Rapid pronation of the forearm is used to provide the quick, striking movement.

The vibration produced through percussion involves only the tissue closely adjacent to the pleximeter (approximately 3 to 5 cm). Percussion over bones is affected by lateral transmission of vibration.

The change from resonance to dullness is more easily perceived than the dull-to-resonant transition. Thus, the examiner organizes a percussion protocol to progress from more resonant regions to lesser ones.

Fist percussion is, as the name implies, striking with the hand in a fisted position. The blow is delivered with the lateral aspect of the hand. The purpose of this type of percussion is to elicit sensation by the vibration of the tissue. The most common applications are to stimulate pain or tenderness caused by hepatitis, cholecystitis, or kidney disease.

The sound waves that result from percussion are evaluated with reference to intensity, pitch, quality, and duration (Table 1-2).

Sound is produced by vibrating structures. The vibrations generate a series of compression waves in the medium that is capable of sound transmission. Solids, liquids, and gases that are sufficiently elastic to convert energy to motion may transmit sound. The compression waves initiate vibrations of the tympanic

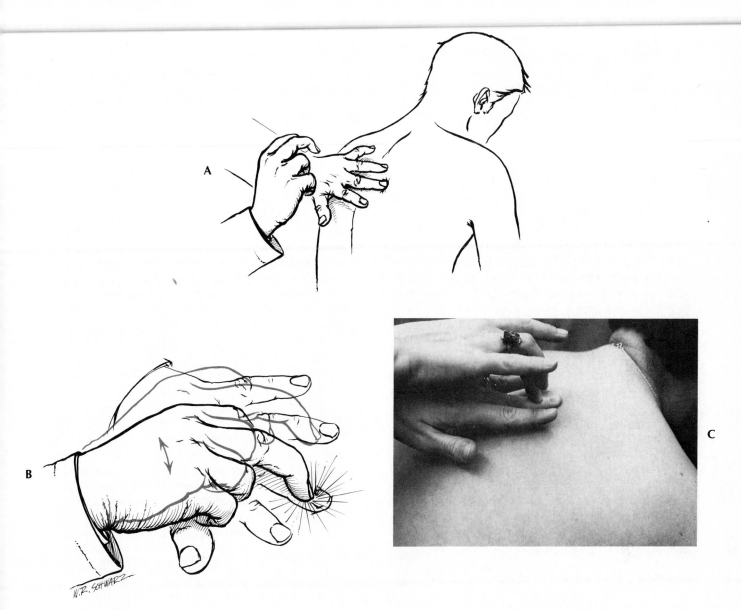

Fig. 1-1
Percussion. **A,** Positioning of the hands. **B,** Hand movement. **C,** Percussion of the posterior thorax.

Table 1-2
Sounds produced by percussion

Record of finding	Intensity	Pitch	Duration	Quality	Anatomical region where sounds may be encountered
Tympany	Loud	High	Moderate	Drumlike	Air in closed structure vibrates in concert with tissue surrounding it; the gastric air bubble; air in intestine
Hyperresonance	Very loud	Very low	Long	Booming	Air-filled lungs, as in emphysema
Resonance	Moderate to loud	Low	Long	Hollow	Normal lung
Dullness	Soft to moderate	High	Moderate	Thudlike	Liver
Flatness	Soft	High	Short	Flat	Muscle

membrane, which moves in and out with the frequency of the sound waves. The mechanical energy of the compression waves is transduced into neural signals by receptor structures of the middle ear. These neural signals are transmitted to the temporal cortex and perceived as sound.

Intensity, loudness. The physical property of sound called intensity produces the effect of loudness in the human auditory apparatus. As a sound wave travels through a point in the air, the air molecules are compressed and then expanded in the wake of the compression wave. The difference between maximum pressure and minimum pressure is the amplitude of the sound wave. The greater the displacement of air, the more movement during vibration of the tympanic membrane and the louder the perception of sound. Loudness is a psychological variable as well. The individual listener may be attentive to or selectively unaware of the many sounds in the environment. Also various alterations in the conduction apparatus of the ear or the sensory neural components of audition may produce alteration in the perception of sound.

Pitch, frequency. The frequency of sound is a physical property that corresponds to the number of vibrations of the sound source per second. Pitch is related to the frequency of sound.

The waveform of a sound of single frequency is sinusoidal, ⌒⌒⌒⌒ , with perfectly matched hills (peaks) and valleys (troughs). The distance from one peak to the next is 1 cycle. The recording of frequency is in cycles per second (cps), or hertz (Hz). The human ear is capable of detecting sounds in the frequency range of 15 to 30 cps to 20,000 cps. With advancing age, the human ear becomes progressively less sensitive to the higher sound frequencies. The sounds of speech and music (250 to 2,048 cps) are most frequently lost. However, most sounds of importance in physical diagnosis are in the frequency range below 1,000 cps and more particularly in the range of 40 to 500 cps. Thus, the ability to hear sounds that are important to health assessment is not compromised by aging.

Quality, harmonics. *Harmonic*, or *overtone*, refers to the physical property of sound that causes the psychological effect called quality or *timbre*. A sound of single frequency produces a pure tone. The lowest frequency at which a piano wire vibrates is called the *fundamental*. Most objects vibrate at more than one frequency. The piano wire may vibrate as a single unit or in halves or thirds that oscillate at their own frequency. These frequencies will be whole-number multiples of the single frequency. The fundamental and the multiples of the single frequency are the harmonics. Sound quality is produced by the sum of the harmonics present and their intensities. The quality is recorded in descriptive terms such as *humming, buzzing,* or *roaring*. The fundamental is the first harmonic. A musical sound is one wherein the mix of intensity and pitch is pleasing to the ear, whereas *noise* is the term given an unpleasant sensation. Most sounds heard in the course of the physical examination are perceived as noise.

An axiom of the physical examination is that, like the drum, the more air the tissue contains (the less dense the tissue), the deeper, louder, and longer the sound will be. The corollary is that the more compact the tissue, the higher, fainter, and shorter the sound will be. The sounds elicited in percussion are recorded in relation to the density of the tissue being vibrated. The least dense tissues produce tympany, whereas successively more dense tissue results in hyperresonance, resonance, dullness, and flatness.

The percussion hammer (see Fig. 23-48) is used to strike a blow to tendons that serves to stretch the tendon such that a deep tendon reflex is elicited. This will be described in greater detail in the neurological examination.

Auscultation

Auscultation (L. *auscultate*, to listen to) is the process of listening for the sounds produced by the human body. The sounds of particular importance are those produced by (1) the thoracic or abdominal viscera and (2) the movement of blood in the cardiovascular system. *Direct*, or *immediate*, *auscultation* is accomplished by the unassisted ear, that is, without any amplifying device. This form of auscultation often involves the application of the ear directly to a body surface where the sound is most prominent. The use of a sound augmentation device such as a stethoscope in the detection of body sounds is called *mediate auscultation*.

Hippocrates described chest sounds in his writings, and Harvey mentioned heart sounds in the early 1600s. Direct, or immediate, auscultation was practiced until 1816, when Laennec devised the first stethoscope, which consisted of a series of rolled up papers held in place with gummed paper. Laennec continued to improve the device and ultimately used a wooden tubing with an earpiece. Later, flexible ear trumpets were modified for use in auscultation. This monaural form of mediate auscultation was succeeded by a binaural instrument in the middle of the nineteenth century.

The three types of stethoscopes that enjoy clinical popularity today are the acoustical, magnetic, and electronic stethoscopes.

The *acoustical stethoscope* (Fig. 1-2) is essentially a

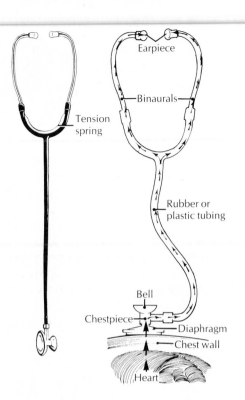

Tension spring

Earpiece

Binaurals

Rubber or plastic tubing

Bell

Chestpiece

Diaphragm

Chest wall

Heart

Fig. 1-2
Acoustical stethoscope. (Adapted from Patient Care, March 15, 1974. © Copyright 1974, Miller & Fink Corp., Darien, Conn. All rights reserved.)

closed cylinder, which serves to inhibit the dissipation of the compression waves produced by the sound source in the column. The diaphragm of the acoustical stethoscope screens out low-frequency sounds and is therefore most effective in assessing high-frequency sounds. The diaphragm is applied firmly to the skin so that it moves synchronously with the body wall. The bell-type head is most effective in detecting low-frequency sounds. Care is taken not to flatten the skin by pressing the bell too firmly, since the vibrations of the surface tissues in response to visceral vibration are the source of sound; stretching these tissues inhibits vibration, actually converting the tissue to a diaphragm. The bell chestpiece should be wide enough to span an intercostal space in an adult and deep enough so that it will not fill with tissue.

Several sizes of earpieces are supplied with better stethoscopes. The examiner should determine which size fits the external meatus most snugly. The earpieces should occlude the meatus, thus blocking extraneous sound. However, the earpieces should not be painful to the examiner. Earpieces that are too small will enter the ear canal, causing pain. The binaurals (metal tubing) are angled somewhat toward the nose of the wearer to project the sound onto the tympanic membrane. The direction of the angle may be adjusted by the tension spring. The tubing should not be longer than 12 to 14 inches to minimize sound distortion. It is more likely that with longer tubing the sound will be diminished.

An internal bore of ⅛ inch has been suggested for best sound transmission. The purpose of the stethoscope is to exclude environmental sound; the system does not magnify sound.

The Harvey stethoscope, a variation of the acoustical type, has three heads: a bell for low frequencies, a corrugated diaphragm for midrange, and a flat diaphragm for high frequencies. This stethoscope also has separate tubes leading to each head.

The *magnetic stethoscope* (Fig. 1-3) has a single head that is a diaphragm. Magnetic attraction is established between an iron disk on the interior surface of the diaphragm and a permanent magnet installed behind it in the head. A strong spring keeps the diaphragm bowed outward when not compressed against a body surface. Application of the diaphragm with the appropriate amount of pressure allows activation of the air column. A dial allows the user to adjust for high-, low-, and full-frequency sounds.

The *electronic stethoscope* (Fig. 1-4) functions as a result of vibration of a diaphragm or microphone occurring as a result of the body surface vibrations. These vibrations are transduced into electrical pulses, which are amplified and converted back to sound at a low speaker.

The use of the stethoscope is described in Chapter 15, "Assessment of the Respiratory System," and in Chapter 16, "Cardiovascular Assessment: the Heart and the Neck Vessels."

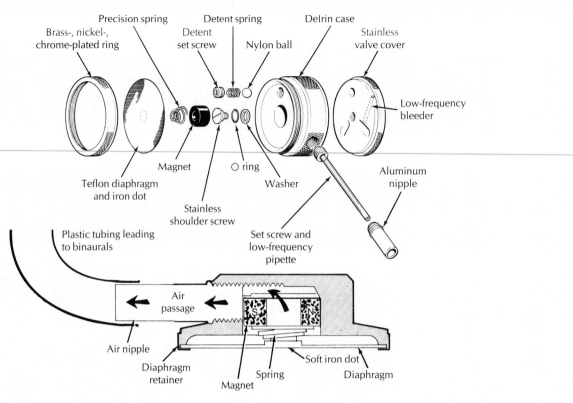

Precision spring
Detent spring
Delrin case
Brass-, nickel-, chrome-plated ring
Detent set screw
Nylon ball
Stainless valve cover
Low-frequency bleeder
Teflon diaphragm and iron dot
Magnet
O ring
Washer
Aluminum nipple
Stainless shoulder screw
Set screw and low-frequency pipette

Plastic tubing leading to binaurals
Air passage
Air nipple
Diaphragm retainer
Magnet
Spring
Soft iron dot
Diaphragm
S   N

Fig. 1-3

Magnetic stethoscope. (From Patient Care, March 15, 1974. © Copyright 1974, Miller & Fink Corp., Darien, Conn. All rights reserved.)

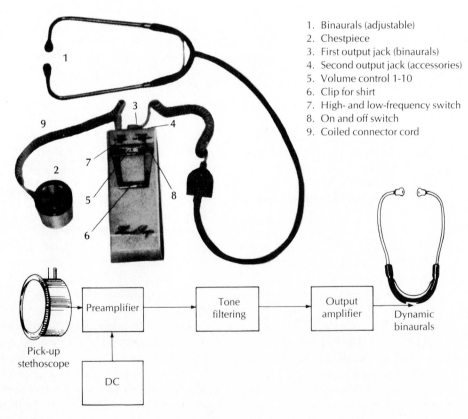

1. Binaurals (adjustable)
2. Chestpiece
3. First output jack (binaurals)
4. Second output jack (accessories)
5. Volume control 1-10
6. Clip for shirt
7. High- and low-frequency switch
8. On and off switch
9. Coiled connector cord

Pick-up stethoscope
Preamplifier
Tone filtering
Output amplifier
Dynamic binaurals
DC

Fig. 1-4

Electronic stethoscope. (From Patient Care, March 15, 1974. © Copyright 1974, Miller & Fink Corp., Darien, Conn. All rights reserved.)

EQUIPMENT USED FOR EYE AND EAR ASSESSMENT
The ophthalmoscope

The ophthalmoscope was first used by Von Helmholtz in 1850. It provides a method of illuminating the interior structures of the eye and of viewing these structures as a result of an arrangement of mirrors and lenses.

The instrument and its assembly. The head of an ophthalmoscope and the five apertures that may be available are shown in Fig. 1-5. The ophthalmoscope head is seated in the handle by fitting the male adapter end of the handle into the female receptacle of the ophthalmoscope head. The head is pushed in the direction of the handle while turning in a clockwise direction until the stop is felt.

The ophthalmoscope is turned on by depressing the button on the rheostat and turning the rheostat clockwise to the appropriate intensity of light. The instrument is turned off after use to prevent shortening the useful life of the bulb and the battery life in battery-operated ophthalmoscopes. The beginner may be-

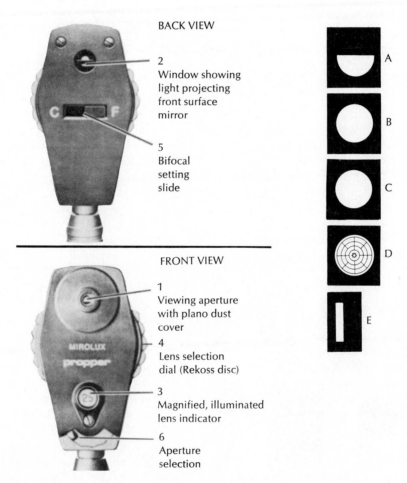

BACK VIEW

2
Window showing light projecting front surface mirror

5
Bifocal setting slide

FRONT VIEW

1
Viewing aperture with plano dust cover

4
Lens selection dial (Rekoss disc)

3
Magnified, illuminated lens indicator

6
Aperture selection

A

B

C

D

E

Fig. 1-5
The head and five apertures of an ophthalmoscope. **A,** Hemispot is used for small pupil examinations and to aid in eliminating the corneal light reflex. **B,** Full spot is provided in two different sizes. The small one is used for undilated pupils or to eliminate the corneal reflex in examination of the macula. The large one is used for dilated pupils. The large beam is the one most frequently used because it provides a wide field for the general fundus examination. **C,** Red free filter is a green beam used for examining the optic disc for pallor and the retina for hemorrhages. Hemorrhages appear black with the red free filter, whereas melanin deposits appear gray. **D,** Fixation star and polar coordinates (grid) are used to determine the fixation pattern and for relating the characteristics, size, and location of fundal lesions. **E,** Slit is used for examining the anterior segment of the eye and for determining the elevation or depression of fundal lesions.

come familiar with the apertures by projecting them onto a piece of paper. The aperture may be changed by moving the aperture selection lever.

The structure being examined is brought into focus by rotating the lens selector dial until the image becomes clear. The instrument may be held and focused with one hand. On the front of the ophthalmoscope head is an illuminated aperture displaying the number of the lens in position before the viewing aperture. The value of the lens is indicated in diopters. Black numbers are for positive values; red figures are for negative values.

When the lens selector is rotated clockwise beginning with zero (0) the positive numbers (+1, +2, +3, +4, +5, +6, +8, +10, +12, +15, +20, +40) appear, and when the selector is rotated counterclockwise from zero (0) the negative numbers (−1, −2, −3, −4, −5, −6, −8, −10, −15, −20, −25) are seen.

The lens system can compensate for hyperopia or myopia. However, there is no correction for astigmatism.

Examination with the ophthalmoscope. The examination with the ophthalmoscope is best accomplished in a semidarkened or darkened room. It is recommended that neither the examiner nor the client wear glasses during the examination. However, if the examiner is highly astigmatic or myopic, glasses should be worn. The lens selector is moved to the dioptric value that corrects the spherical refractive error of the examiner (for most normal individuals this setting is usually 0).

To examine the right eye the examiner sits or stands to the client's right side. The ophthalmoscope is held in the right hand with the viewing aperture as close as possible to the examiner's right eye. The right index finger is placed on the lens selection dial to be prepared to change lenses as necessary.

The examiner's head is placed about 1½ ft (45 cm) in front of and about 15 degrees temporal (to the right of the line of vision of the right eye). The client is instructed to look straight ahead at some fixed point at eye level. The light beam is then directed into the client's pupil. The examiner selects a strong lens with a high positive number (6 to 8 for an examiner with normal vision).

The fundus will be viewed as a red disk (the red reflex). While keeping the red reflex in view, the examiner moves slowly toward the client. The presence of cataracts or other opacities of the cornea or lens may partially or totally occlude the red reflex. Lens correction is made while moving; a strong negative lens is appropriate for viewing structures of the fundus.

The optic disc may be viewed when the examiner is approximately 3 to 5 cm from the eye. A helpful measure in sighting the optic disc is to focus on a vessel and follow it in a nasal direction to the disc. The appropriate lens is brought into the viewing aperture to provide clear definition of the structures of the fundus. The normal retina is magnified approximately 15 times. These structures are described in Chapter 11, "Assessment of the eyes." The optic disc is examined for clarity of outline and elevation. The blood vessels are followed from the disc to the periphery while the examiner appraises size and structural integrity. The client is then asked to look up so that the superior retina can be examined and down so that the inferior retina can be examined. The examiner looks toward the nose for examination of the nasal retina and laterally for examination of the temporal retina. The peripheral retina may be difficult to examine if the pupils are not dilated.

Examination of the left eye is made in a manner similar to that of the right eye but by standing on the left side of the client and by using the left eye and holding the ophthalmoscope in the left hand.

It is possible to determine the degree of elevation of the retinal disc using the ophthalmoscope. The examiner first focuses on a nonedematous area close to the retinal disc. The dioptric number is read in the lens indicator aperture. Then the crescent of the optic disc is brought into clear focus and the dioptric reading is again noted. The difference between the two dioptric values divided by three is equal to the elevation in millimeters.

The otoscope

The otoscope provides a source of illumination for examination of the external auditory canal and the tympanic membrane. The power source for the otoscope is the same as that for the ophthalmoscope. The otoscope head is seated in the same manner as the ophthalmoscope head. The speculum chosen by the examiner should be the largest one that will comfortably fit the external meatus of the client.

Examination with the otoscope. The otoscope is held in the dominant hand. The client is asked to tip his head to the side opposite from the ear being examined. The superior posterior auricle is grasped between thumb and index finger and in the adult pulled upward, backward, and slightly away from the body. This helps to straighten the external auditory canal, which is angled downward and is slightly forward in the adult. For infants, the posterior inferior auricle is grasped and pulled downward and slightly away from the body to accommodate for the external auditory canal, which is angled upward and forward. The remainder of the fingers are rested against the head to achieve pressure restraint or to move with the head, should the client move with the speculum in place. Before insertion of the otoscope the external ear is carefully inspected for the presence of a foreign body that could be removed. Cerumen may occlude the ear. When cerumen is wet, it is viscous, sticky, and a shade of orange-yellow or, with aging, dark brown or even black when it has been in the canal a long time. Cerumen may occlude the external meatus such that the otoscope may not be passed. A cerumen spoon may be used to remove this excess.

The otoscope is advanced carefully and slowly. The inner two thirds of the external meatus is thin and quite sensitive to pressure. Pain may be caused by too large a speculum or by sharply angling the speculum over the thin tissue covering the bone. The speculum is advanced until the tympanic membrane can be seen. It is necessary to vary the angle of the speculum to visualize the entire tympanic membrane. This examination is more fully explained in Chapter 10.

SUGGESTED EQUIPMENT FOR HEALTH ASSESSMENT

Sphygmomanometer
Stethoscope
Ophthalmoscope
Otoscope
Percussion hammer
Tuning fork
Cotton balls
Cotton-tipped applicators
Tongue blades
Ruler
Tape measure—metal or nonstretchable plastic
Safety pins
Vaginal speculum
Examination gloves
Flashlight

BIBLIOGRAPHY

American Cancer Society report on the cancer related health checkup, CA **50**(4):193, 1980.
Andreopoulos, S., editor: Primary care: where medicine fails, New York, 1974, John Wiley & Sons, Inc.
Breslow, L., and Somers, A.R.: The lifetime health monitoring program: a practical approach to preventive medicine, N. Engl. J. Med. **296**:601, 1977.
Canadian Task Force: Report on the periodic health examination, Can. Med. Assoc. J. **121**(9):1193, 1980.
Collen, M.F.: Periodic health examinations, Primary Care **3**:197, 1976.
Dales, L.G., Friedman, G.D., and Collen, M.F.: Evaluating periodic multiphasic health checkups: a controlled trial, J. Chronic Dis. **32**(5):385, 1979.
Garfield, S.R., and others: Evaluation of new ambulatory medical care delivery system, N. Engl. J. Med. **294**:426, 1976.
Hart, C.R.: Screening in general practice, Edinburgh, 1975, Churchill Livingstone.
Javits, J.: National health care policy for the future, J. Politics Policy Law **1**:5, 1976.
Leavell, H.R., and Clark, E.G.: Preventive medicine for the doctor in his community, ed. 3, New York, 1965, McGraw-Hill Book Co.
Mushkin, S.J., editor: Consumer incentives for health care, New York, 1974, Prodist.
Rappaport, M.D., and Sprague, H.B.: The effects of tubing bore on stethoscope efficiency, Am. Heart J. **42**:605, 1951.
Somers, A.R.: Lifetime health monitoring: preventive care for the child in utero, Patient Care **13**(3):162, 1979.
Somers, A.R.: Lifetime health monitoring: preventive care: age 1 through adolescence, Patient Care **13**(8):201, 1979.
Somers, A.R.: Lifetime health monitoring: a whole-life plan for well patient care, Patient Care **13**(11):83, 1979.
Spitzer, W.O., and others: The Burlington randomized trial of the nurse practitioner, N. Engl. J. Med. **290**:251, 1974.

CHAPTER 2

THE INTERVIEW

The major *purpose of the interview* conducted before the physical examination is to obtain a health history and to elicit symptoms and the time course of their development. The goal of an effective interview is to obtain a complete and accurate data base. However, although assessment may be the main emphasis of a given exchange, the primary care practitioner must bring to bear skillful communication techniques to establish the rapport necessary for a full sharing of the client's relevant life experiences. A climate of trust must be established that will allow a full expression of the client's needs. Furthermore, an analysis of the reactions of the client during the interview will allow the examiner to predict the ability and willingness of the client to comprehend and therefore carry out the directions given to him as part of the therapeutic plan.

The practitioner does not perform the first interview *tabula rasa*. The students of the health professions have had many years of interacting with fellow human beings and have practiced the establishment of relationships in many settings. Most students have learned which communication techniques work well for them, particularly in social settings. The focus of this discussion will be the characteristics of information exchange that will allow the client and health care professional to work toward the mutual goal of establishing a data base.

The mutual analysis of client and interviewer begins with introductions. The interviewer generally has the advantage of knowing the client's name and may greet him warmly, respectfully, and by name. A handshake is appropriate if the examiner is comfortable in reaching out in the initial encounter.

The communication skills and sensitivity of the practitioner during the interview process may well be the most important examiner skills making up the assess-

ment armamentarium. To this end, the practitioner must develop a flexible framework for obtaining the information or behavior needed in the assessment that will also facilitate the interaction necessary for a therapeutic relationship.

The most effective place to learn how to interview is at the bedside and in the clinic while dealing with actual clients. Initial interviews should be supervised by a skilled professional who will provide approbation or suggestions for modification immediately after leaving the client.

It is helpful to have videotapes of practice sessions made so that the learner may more objectively analyze his or her own interviewing skills and maximize those special talents made evident by direct viewing. The goal of the effective communicator is to demonstrate genuine warmth and the sincere desire to engage in tasks necessary to meeting the client's health care needs.

The use of a written record of the interview, called a process recording, may be helpful in identifying communication problems. However, a tape recording of a verbal interchange between the client and the practitioner may serve the same ends.

Particularly at the first interview, the client should be allowed to talk freely, to ramble on in his description of his health condition. One frequently observed error is the monopoly of the interview by the practitioner. Frequently clients report that they did not mention symptoms because they did not have an opportunity or were not encouraged to do so—"He asked so many questions that I didn't get a chance to say anything." When one of the participants does most of the talking during the interview, in essence delivers a monologue, the other may be silent for long periods or repeat certain phrases again and again. Thus, "uh huh" or "okay" said repeatedly by one person in the interview is characteristic of stifled communication. The practitioner should bear in mind that the perception of what is being said in conversation is often decreased when one is listening to a long presentation. The most effective communication exists when the client takes an active role in the interview. The interview might begin with a general invitation to the client to speak freely such as "Tell me how you see your state of health," or "What is the nature of the problem that brings you here?"

THE CONTRACT

The interview is a verbal and nonverbal exchange that provides for the beginning and development of a relationship. Initially, the participants are strangers, each presenting his own style of relating and adapting. Defining the terms of the relationship early in the interview obviates unnecessary stressors and provides goals for the participants. Common symbols—those that are consensually validated between examiner and client, that is, have the same meaning to both participants—must be achieved, since the quality of the communication will determine the value of the relationship. Unlike many others, the association between health professional and client has a mutual concern, the well-being of the client. This commonality of interest will facilitate progress toward the sharing of information, ideas, and emotions. A mutually understandable language and an understanding of the significance of body language, such as gestures and facial expressions, and somatic language (signs of autonomic nervous system reactions) will increase the exchange of information between the client and the practitioner and enrich the data obtained.

Facial expressions are the most widely used nonverbal communication and the message most frequently observed by the client. Eye contact is frequently used. Human beings invite communication with another person by looking directly at him. Generally speaking, this kind of open stare is regarded positively; the person who looks another in the eye while talking is generally considered open and honest. However, should the person being gazed upon decline the invitation, he generally does so by averting eye contact, most often looking downward. Although a short gaze may be interpreted as accessibility and interest on the part of examiner, it is important to avoid long periods of looking directly at the client because this may be interpreted as an invitation to deeper relationship by the client.

The client's perception of interviewer competence is determined by title (role), reputation, and behavior.

The contract, or basic operating agreement between the client and the practitioner, should include the following points:

1. Time and place that the interview and subsequent examinations will occur
2. Duration of time involved in the present and future examinations
3. Number of sessions required
4. Expectations for participation by the client in the assessment process
5. Confidentiality of shared information and findings—responsibilities of each member
6. Rules regarding the presence of other professionals or of the client's relatives or other advocates
7. Cost to the client where applicable
8. Therapeutic goals subsequent to the assessment process

The advantage of the contract to the practitioner is that the client is relieved of misconceptions, fears, or fantasies he may have had concerning what might happen during the interview and examination. Thus, the contract establishes norms and role behavior. A social system with definable, interdependent parts, so that a change in one part effects changes in other parts, has been identified. The practitioner and the client have expectations of each other. Abrogation of responsibility threatens the relationship.

The expectation that there will be shared decision making in the management of his health care should be made very clear to the client. To this end, the client is encouraged to learn more about himself to identify health needs and recognize he has an option in determining if and how his health needs are met.

In traditional health care relationships there is an inequity in that the health professional is in the authority role whereas the client is, at least to some degree, dependent. The client has initiated the interview by seeking help for his problems. In his efforts to obtain aid from the professional, the client must determine the kind of information and behavior expected. The professional is obligated to analyze the client's communication pattern to explain to the client what is needed for the professional to give the help that is needed. The interaction provides a kind of negotiation for the terms on which the relationship can continue, that is, a contract defining the roles of the participants. The verbal and nonverbal dialogue that occurs in the first few minutes of this social exchange may well determine not only the reliability and amount of information the client will furnish to the interviewer but also the character of the relationship that follows.

SETTING

To promote the most effective attention to communication and therefore to build rapport, the practitioner should carefully construct the interview environment to avoid interruption, distraction, or discomfort.

At the outset it should be determined if the time scheduled for the interview is mutually convenient to the client and interviewer. Although geographical privacy may not be a luxury that can be obtained in emergency rooms, large clinics, or in multiple bed units in the hospital, psychological protection may be provided. Some of the assurances important to the client are that (1) the client is not being heard by other clients or personnel not concerned in his care, (2) the practitioner is giving his highest level of attention to the client, and (3) the information the client is sharing will be regarded as confidential or that the conditions of sharing will be defined.

In the more ideal setting, the privacy of the client's thoughts and his comfort can be guaranteed by conducting the interview in a private room where optimum temperature and lighting can be controlled. Indirect lighting is preferred so that the patient is not looking into a bright light or exposed to glare from a window.

The physical position of the practitioner as related to the client can have implications in the control process. For a mutual sharing of the control of the interview or to suggest that the client has some option for control, the chairs or other furniture should be arranged so that a face-to-face alignment to ensure eye contact is possible. The commonly used position of standing over (looking down at) the client suggests that the practitioner has assumed leadership for the interchange. Leaning forward appropriately conveys alert attention. However, relaxed body posture should be maintained.

Excessively long interviews are tiring to the client. There may be a need to schedule more than one session to complete the data base, particularly if the health history is complex or the client is critically ill or debilitated.

It is important that the client obtain a sense of the interviewer's full involvement in the process. It is important to be aware of body language that could convey boredom or restlessness, such as shifting from one foot to another, sighing, or edging toward the door.

COMMUNICATION PROCESS

Anxiety is an anticipated element in an initial interview for both the health professional and the client. Some of the indications of acute anxiety that may be observed include a furrowed brow, squinting, dilated pupils, tensed facial muscles, distended neck vessels, rapid talk, a dry mouth, frequent hand gestures, a tense posture, an increased heart rate and blood pressure, sweaty palms and axillae, and a sweaty pubic area. Shuffling of feet may indicate a desire by the client to escape the interview. The client's anxieties may be associated with the symptoms of his illness,

with the practitioner's reaction to him, with fees, or with expectations of future appointments. The practitioner is concerned with the client's response to the interview, with his or her (the practitioner's) ability to get appropriate information, and with his or her ability to synthesize the data provided so that the problems can be correctly defined. The practitioner is further concerned that problem management is appropriate and that referral is properly instituted. Clues that interview items are anxiety producing are long pauses, nervous laughter, dry coughing, and sighing.

To facilitate the development of rapport, the health professional must use communication skills to project to the client that he or she is interested and concerned with providing the support needed by the client. The practitioner might convey support by assuring the client, "I'll do all I can to find out what is making you feel this way." To demonstrate interest and the willingness to listen, the practitioner must also be aware of the message conveyed nonverbally.

The practitioner must deal with both the information needed and given by the client and with the process of the interview. This process is the developing relationship and will include not ony what is said but those elements that are implied by words and gesture, that is, the manner in which data are supplied and withheld and the client's efforts to control the interview.

Particular attention is given the remarks made as the client is entering the room or as he is leaving, since these comments frequently have special significance. The client may reveal his chief complaint at these times and avoid mentioning it during the formal interview.

The amount of structure that is brought to bear in the interview is dependent on the level of organization of ego functioning exhibited by the client. In general, the client with the lesser degree of organization needs more structure in the interview to increase the amount of data obtained in a given period of time and to decrease anxiety.

The communication process involves feedback in that each message sent involves a response. This response affects the next message sent and its reaction. The skilled practitioner readily settles in the communication mode that is most effective for the individual client. This is particularly important in the choice of the type of questions used to obtain the health history.

A common communication error that occurs in this society is that of thinking of the next remark, thereby not fully perceiving what is being said. This is a particular hazard for the student who is not yet fully comfortable with the interview pattern. Such an individual may perceive little of valuable data being given by the client since that individual must concentrate on the format of questioning and on how best to word the next query.

Types of questions

Questions should be carefully designed to deal with one issue at a time. Questions should not demand two or more rejoinders, particularly conflicting answers.

Examples of questions to avoid are "Did you have measles, mumps, or whooping cough?" or "Did you have pain in your shoulder or not?" Avoid questions that suggest a possible answer to the client—"You don't have any blood in your urine, do you?"

Open-ended questions or suggestions. Although the interview is aimed at getting more or less specific answers concerning the events surrounding the client's signs and symptoms, each point should be developed by the client in his own words. An open-ended question or suggestion is one aimed at eliciting a response that is more than one or two words in length. This type of question is effective in stimulating descriptive or comparative responses. Observation of the client as he describes a symptom may give valuable information concerning his attitudes and beliefs. In addition, it allows the client to provide information when he is ready to disclose it; he is not forced to divulge information when sharing it may trouble him. This free description may also provide clues to the alertness, or level of mental abilities of the client and to the organization of his ego functioning, revealed through the organization of his thoughts and through his vocabulary. Furthermore, rapport is strengthened through the demonstration that the practitioner wants to invest time in hearing the thoughts of the client.

Examples of open-ended questions or suggestions are "How have you been feeling lately?" and "Tell me about your problem."

The disadvantage of this type of question is that it may result in responses that are not relevant to a specific point being assessed. The client may use the opportunity provided by an open-ended question to digress in order to avoid discussing relevant data because it is distressing to him. Although this technique might yield important information, there are times when the examiner needs data quickly and must sacrifice to get it. This is particularly true in emergency care. When the drug overdose victim rouses, the only piece of data of importance may be elicited by a closed question ("What did you take?")

Closed questions. The closed question is a type of inquiry that requires no more than a one- or two-word answer. This might be agreement or disagreement. The response may be a yes or no and may be answered nonverbally by a nod of the head. This is the kind of question most appropriate for eliciting age, sex, marital status, and other forced-choice responses.

Examples of closed questions are "What did you eat for dinner last night?" and "What medication did you take?"

The educationally impoverished or those who lack culturally enriching experiences are often more comfortable with this type of question because they know what is expected. The open-ended question may pose anxiety to the client with poor articulation, since he may be afraid that the display of his lack of verbal skill will disadvantage him with the practitioner. On the other hand, the closed question by its nature limits the amount of information that is obtained in the health history and may convey to the client that the practitioner is too busy or disinterested to listen to him. It has been observed that practitioners use more closed questions in initial interviews and when the process is stresssful, as well as when time constraints are marked.

Biased or leading questions. Questions that carry a suggestion of the kind of information that should be included in the response are called *leading* or *biased*. The client is presented with an expectation by the practitioner. This kind of question may seriously limit the value of the health history. For example, the question "You haven't *ever* had venereal disease, have you?" implies that the possibility that the client *has had* venereal disease would be outside the limits of reality for the practitioner. The client who has experienced the disease may not say so to avoid disappointing the questioner.

The presence of emotionally charged words in a given question may make the question a biased one. For example, there is one in the question, "You haven't been masturbating, have you?" Since the Judeo-Christian ethic defines masturbating as "bad," bias has been inflicted. In this case the practitioner has suggested that the answer should be no. The client may well avoid all matters dealing with sexuality to avoid the possible loss of the approval of the practitioner.

The practitioner must balance the goals of efficiency and effectiveness in the interviews. In obtaining a historical data base, the practitioner asks the client many questions, the object of which is to obtain thorough, relevant information. However, a comprehensive interview is a very time-consuming activity and practitioners often attempt to save time by asking closed questions. More information is gained by open-ended questions that may supply much relevant and extraneous data. Therefore, the interviewer needs to consider the relative importance of the interview questions in the gathering of the data base to obtain the most useful information within a reasonable time.

Use of silence

Periods of silence during the interview are helpful in making observations, such as is the client comfortable? Angry? Confused? Silence provides an opportunity to assess the level of anxiety in both the practitioner and the client. Also the client is provided with sufficient time to carefully organize his thoughts for a coherent explanation in response to questions. The rapid presentation of questions may not allow time for sufficient thought or reflection by the client. Silence is also useful as an indicator of the amount of anxiety the client is experiencing. The client's silence may indicate absorbing thought, boredom, deep affection, or grief. Silence encourages communication on the part of the client.

Facilitation. Facilitation is an act that stimulates the client to continue talking. However, the topic is not specified. Silence may be facilitative as are encouraging words—"Yes, I see," "Mm-hm," and "Go on."

Methods for assuring understanding

The practitioner must use validation maneuvers to determine if both participants understand what has been said. A clear understanding of what the client is trying to say is essential to the establishment of an accurate data base. The health history should not contain assumptions of what the client meant but a clear accounting of exactly what he said. There are many techniques that provide for encouragement of the client to expand on a description or to clarify the explanation that has been given. A workable example might be "Tell me more about it."

Use of a common language. The practitioner must carefully plan questions and give particular care in selecting the vocabulary to be used in order that the client perceive the question in the same sense that it is intended by the practitioner. The practitioner is aided in processing the language and behavior of the client for what is usual or "normal" by having an understanding of cultural and ethnic differences. Medical terminology or jargon should not be used excessively. When medical diagnoses are employed, the meaning should be explained to the client when the words are first used.

Frequently, the professional uses these terms to avoid communication altogether or to terminate conversations with clients. Should the client use a medical diagnosis, the practitioner should ascertain that the client's understanding of the word matches the practitioner's. For example, many lay people believe that *neoplasm* is synonymous with *cancer*.

Planning the questions. The client is asked one question at a time. In order for the client to give the information needed for the health history, the questions must be phrased in such a way that the client knows what kind of answers are expected. When the client's response is not appropriate, a reordering of the question or a more explicit choice of vocabulary may be indicated. It may be helpful to emphasize the key words in the question. In designing questions, one should avoid the use of ambiguous terms, medical language, or words with more than one meaning.

Use of an example. Comparison with a common experience, that is, a concrete happening, may help to clarify an abstract concept or hazy terminology. The practitioner may use an example as part of the questioning process when the meaning is not clear. For example, the practitioner may ask the client, "Was it as large as a cherry?"

Restatement. Restatement is the formulation of what the client has said in words that are more specific; it provides an opportunity for validation of the practitioner's conception. The client is cued that he is expected to give attention to the thought by phrases such as "Do you mean . . .," "In other words . . .," or "If I understand you correctly. . . ."

Reflection or echoing. Reflection, or echoing, means repeating a phrase or a sentence the client has just said. The suggestion to the client that the practitioner is still involved in that part of the communication may focus further attention or rumination on that thought. The strategy is aimed toward further elaboration in the form of the recall of facts or feeling states that surrounded the circumstance. The technique should allow clarification or expansion of the information just given by the client. Examples are as follows:

Client: My mother has been drinking a fifth a day for 6 years. She's an alcoholic.
Interviewer response: You say your mother is an alcoholic?

Client: The spot on my arm is painful, you know.
Interviewer response: Painful?

Clarification. Questions designed to obtain information to more clearly understand conflicting, abstract, vague, or ambiguous statements are requests for clarification.

"You say you felt depressed? Tell me what you mean."

"You had constant headaches? Tell me what you remember about them."

Encapsulation or summary. Encapsulation, or summary, is a technique that allows for the condensation of facts into a well-ordered review. It is particularly useful following a rambling, detailed description. The summary further signals the client that this particular segment of the interview is terminating and suggests to him that he should give further input immediately, since closure is imminent.

Confrontation. Telling the client something about himself is known as confrontation. This may be a helpful technique to use when inconsistencies are noticed, for example, "When you tell me how painful your arm is, I notice that you are smiling. Why is this?" Confrontation may also be of use in helping the client to discuss his emotions, for example, "You say you are not uncomfortable, but you are frowning and your muscles appear very tense." Confrontation is also used to seek further information when the client has presented unrealistic ideas.

Interpretation. The examiner may arrive at a conclusion from the data the client has given. Sharing the interpretation with the client allows the individual to confirm, deny, or offer an interpretation of his own. Making an interpretation involves the risk of being wrong, and the examiner should be prepared to deal with this eventuality. The interpretation may also constitute an act of empathy or confrontation.

> **Interviewer:** Since your mother and brother died in the same week, you must have felt very depressed.
> **Client:** Yes, I was somewhat upset, but I had lived with my grandmother since my brother was born and really was not as close as you might expect.

Filling in omitted data

Clinical impressions reached by the practitioner must be regarded as fluid in the sense that in further conversation with the client new information may be provided. The client may withhold information if he fears that sensitive information may be shared indiscriminately or if he has not been able to trust the practitioner. Furthermore, he may regard certain facts as unimportant or irrelevant to the focus of the interview. There are many instances when the client is so eager to comply with questions that he gives a hurried accounting and leaves out significant data. In ordering the data the practitioner may note that information is missing or that there are inconsistencies. Further interviews may be scheduled. The client may simply need to be given a summary of his previous conversation in order for him to detect the areas where he needs to interject information. These gaps may be filled by direct questioning. Another method of asking for the missing facts may be to suggest to the client that the practitioner is confused and needs to be told again a particular sequence of events. A remark such as the following would invite this input: "Now, tell me again all that you remember from the time you first vomited until you came here."

In addition, the possibility of past evaluation and treatment of symptoms should be investigated. The important facts are those obtained by asking when, where, and by whom. Were laboratory or other diagnostic tests performed? Are results available? What diagnosis was made? Was a treatment instituted? Was the treatment helpful?

Obtaining data from people other than the client

The client who is critically ill, confused, or intellectually impaired may be unable to give the information necessary to an adequate history. A close relative or a person who knows the client well may be able to provide the information necessary to understand the presence or nature of problems of the individual being examined. If an ineffective attempt has been made to obtain the history from the client, it may be psychologically prudent to ask permission to go over the details again with the second person. Such comments as "I want to be sure that I have what has happened to you correctly in my mind," or "I'd like to go over this one more time to make sure I've got the facts right and in the correct order," may help to gain the client's permission to interview relatives or friends. The parents may be the only reliable source of information for the young child.

Nonverbal communication—kinesis

Nonverbal communication is that which takes place in the form of behavior patterns that are expressive in the use of (1) *body movements,* (2) *space or territoriality,* (3) *voice tone,* (4) *time,* (5) *appearance,* (6) *acceptance,* (7) *empathy,* and (8) *termination.* The behaviors can convey emotional or feeling state messages or can be used to impart instruction or direction.

Communication through body movement

Some of the gestures to be observed are movements of the body, limbs, hands, or feet; facial expressions, particularly smiling and frowning; and eye behavior such as blinking, the direction of gaze, and the length of time of gaze. Posture is particularly expressive.

Extension of large muscles is associated with relaxation, whereas contraction of large muscles is associated with anxiety and fear. The individual who sits stretched out and gestures away from the body gives an aura of assurance.

Kinesis is the communication provided through body movement. The posture or movement of the client's body may provide valuable clues to his health status. The messages given by the client through his body language may provide additional and sometimes more reliable information than his words, since many persons employ less conscious control over this aspect of behavior. Thus, by his actions the client may convey thoughts that he cannot or refuses to commit to words. Interpretation of the full meaning of the gestures and action of the client must be performed against a comparison of their sociocultural meanings. For instance, the downcast eyes of the Muhammadan woman could be interpreted as the usual or normal response to the practitioner, whereas in the United States one might become alert to other indications of fear, withdrawal or depression, or lack of attentiveness. The use of eye contact assumes a good deal of meaning among Greek and Indian cultures, whereas torso messages are common in Africa.

Posture. A closed body posture is one in which the limbs are held in defensive positions, that is, close to the body, flexed, with muscles tense. The arms may be held very close to the body as though hugging oneself. The position is most often interpreted as distrustful. An open body posture is one that is more relaxed, that is, limbs extended, arms hanging loosely at sides.

Facial expression. Clenched teeth (strongly contracted masseter and temporal muscles) and contracted pupils provide a message of tension and may represent an effort to avoid saying something unpleasant to the listener. This expression is generally interpreted as one of anger.

An individual who smiles constantly may be using this expression as a mask to cover feelings of fear or depression. On the other hand, this may simply be the trademark of an individual with a strong desire to please.

The person who covers his mouth with his hands may be expressing a desire to avoid talking.

Oculesics. Oculesics is the communication that occurs through glances and eye movements. The practitioner may detect signals of disagreement, aversion, or disgust in the client through subtle eye movements. Dilation of the pupils of the eyes generally accompanies pleasurable experiences, whereas offensive or unpleasant circumstances generally result in contracted pupils.

Touch. The act of touching is one of the most intimate forms of nonverbal communication. Cultural traditions prescribe the ritual of touch or define the taboos. Touch is regulated by social-distancing techniques and is apparent in all living groups. Touch has special meaning among health professionals. Many professionals conceive of themselves reaching out in support of their clients. Touch, when used judiciously, conveys a message of closeness, encouragement, and caring and plays a prominent part in the health practitioner–client interaction.

Although in American culture a pat on the back, the handshake, a gentle squeeze of the hand, or a slap on the cheek may be well understood, the practitioner must bear in mind that this community of understanding does not exist for many touching processes. The physical contact of palpation may be misperceived as it is translated from stimulus received to perception. Touch as a form of communication precedes speech in the individual's life. Manners and mores involving

touch are given to the developing child through the actions of his significant others. In America there is a taboo against touching without permission to do so. So, we talk about the reassuring pat of the hand and the warm handshake and define who is permitted to do these acts. There is often confusion when the client opts to touch the health professional.

Effect of space or territoriality on communication

A good deal of symbolism has been attributed to one's position in a group. Definition of a cultural group's concern or rejection is provided by distancing. The distance between the practitioner and the client may determine the relationships developed.

The size of space allowed the client may be related to status or to the differential importance accorded him.

Hall has coined the word "proxemics" to describe the use of space by Americans as zones he calls intimate, personal, social, and public.

Intimate distance. Intimate distance is the distance used for physical lovemaking and intense verbal exchange and is defined as a distance up to 18 inches. This is the distance from which most of the clinical examination is performed. Body contact is expected during the physical examination and the practitioner must use the intimate space of the client and must be concerned with sensory overload. Thus, sensation may frequently be distorted. The presence of another body at this close distance intrudes on the senses and is sometimes overwhelming to the client.

At this close distance the odors of each body are prominent in the senses. The examiner is aware of diagnostic body odors and of the client's general hygiene. The examiner should also be aware of his or her own body smells; the use of pungent toiletries is often offensive to the client. Even the heat extruded by the bodies of participants may be a part of the interchange.

This close phase is also the distance used by the client for touch and intimate skin manipulation. This may be pleasurable and reassuring or threatening to the client. Muscular tension is heightened as though in preparation for movement.

Visual detail is sharpened. The eyes are pulled inward in accommodation, and the individual may appear to squint. Vocalization may be involuntary at the near point but become low and more frequent as the periphery of this zone is approached.

Since it would appear that it is a natural instinct to maintain and protect the space immediately around us, the intrusion on the client's intimate zone should be carefully planned. The client may be carefully assessing the practitioner's use of space. His perceptions may be largely determined by what he assesses of the practitioner in the visual domain.

Frequently, the use of social measures that allow the acceptance of a shortened distance for communications may be helpful; these include introductions, an explanation of the roles of the practitioner and the client, and an explanation of the benefits to be achieved by allowing the closer contact. The client should have each procedure communicated to him before its actualization with the full knowledge that he has the option to refuse. The practitioner should use simple sentences and a carefully chosen, nonthreatening vocabulary and speak in quiet, low tones.

The hospital room or clinic office visit seriously threatens the control of space by the client. He is told where and how he must cooperate in order that his body may be invaded by tactile, visual, auditory, and olfactory probing. The culture may permit this invasion of privacy by physicians and nurses, since they are given special status by the professional roles. The endowment of the role with technical skill, authority, and confidentiality protects the client from the shame that has been cultivated in him for exposure of the body to a stranger. It has been shown that when more evidence is given of the roles of health professionals and these roles are well understood, it is easier for the client to submit to the encroachment of privacy. To this end, the professional uniform of white coat, and so on, is effective, as is the health professional's careful adherence to the behaviors recognized to be part of that role.

The client needs time to adjust to the levels of the space provided for the physical examination. The interview allows a reordering of the perimeters defining the client's space bubble. The client should be allowed as much decision making as possible. He should be allowed to order the disposition of his personal belongings. Questions regarding the use of space should be seriously attended.

Personal distance. Personal distance limits physical contact and is defined as a distance of 1½ to 4 feet. Although holding and grasping are possible at the near point, touching is the form of physical contact most frequently used. Visual perception is less distorted, and there is a three-dimensional impression of the person involved. As the distance between participants lengthens, the gaze may encompass the entire face rather than a single part of it, such as the eye or the chin. Vocal volume is moderate, and body odors and heat are less intruding.

This is the ideal distance for viewing nonverbal behaviors and is the distance most frequently used for the interview. Trust is best developed from this distance.

Social distance. Social distance provides protection from others without one's having to declare or demand it and is defined as a distance of 4 to 12 feet. The visual image includes more of the total person, and the fine detail of the body is lost. Eye contact becomes more important. Body heat and odor are lost. Vocalization is louder and loses its aura of privacy because it can be overheard. Interaction becomes more ritualized or formal. The threat of domination is less from this distance. This distance allows a limited view of the physical aspects of the client, and his revelation of attitudes and feelings in general is censored from this distance.

Public distance. Public distance is defined as separation of communicants by more than 12 feet. Gait and general coordination may be analyzed at this distance while watching the client enter the examining room. Children may be more effectively observed at play when the distance between the child and examiner is increased.

Vocalics

Vocalics is the information that is transmitted through the delivery of speech. The individual who screeches "I'm not afraid of the operation!" reveals that he is terrified.

Chronemics

Chronemics is the term used to describe the information that is transmitted through the use of time. The health practitioner is generally perceived by the client to be the one of superior status in the health care visit. Thus, the client deems it appropriate to wait past the appointment time. On the other hand, the client may be revealing some of his opposing feelings by a pattern of lateness in meeting appointments.

Similarly, the person with perceived superior status is allowed to talk longer. Interruption of the practitioner by the client with an unrelated thought while the practitioner is explaining treatment requirements may signal that the client holds the advice at low value.

Effect of appearance on communication

Both clothing and cosmetics may be used to create an impression. In general, adults aim to reflect the current mode of "handsome" or "beautiful" and, in most cases, "young." Furthermore, financial status may be revealed by the cut of the garments or the label of the manufacturer.

Persons in the health professions, as well as the bulk of American society, are more generous and outgoing in their feelings toward the physically attractive individual. This is true of practitioners working with all age levels. The practitioner must frequently work through attitudes and emotions to touch the diseased individual without visible indications of restraint or repugnance, such as tensed musculature, frowns, or touching only with the fingertips.

Acceptance

Supportive remarks and actions should be a part of the interview process. Although it is not credible to attest to supportiveness, the practitioner should try to convey interest and understanding of the client's problem and the desire to help the client meet and work through problems.

Gestures that say "I like you; you're acceptable" include smiling and moving closer. The basic projection is pleasant, and the words that are chosen say nice things.

Clients have been shown to be more cooperative when they feel accepted and respected by the health care worker. Verbal or nonverbal messages expressing unfriendliness, tension, or punishment markedly inhibit the client's motivation for interaction with the interviewer.

Effective communication is best accomplished in a climate of warmth, empathy, and genuineness. The conveyance of a feeling of positive attitude toward the client may be initiated with a hospitable greeting while devoting full attention to him. Clients most frequently interpreted warmth from the behavior of health care personnel that included direct attention and appropriate eye contact by the examiner. Thus, it is important to read or write in the chart minimally while with the client. Other behaviors that have been shown to convey warmth include a relaxed posture while leaning slightly foward in an open arm position and appropriate smiling and nodding. Positive regard may be demonstrated by complimenting aspects of health care that the client is practicing appropriately.

The examiner should guard against communicating haste to the client because the client may believe the examiner has low regard for the interview. Some behaviors that convey impatience are frequent checking of the time, walking to the door, or standing with the hand on the doorknob.

Sincerity or genuineness on the examiner's part may be conveyed by assuring that there is congruence between the remarks made to the client and the nonverbal cues accompanying the messages. Body language that does not correspond with what is being said may be confusing or frightening to the client. The facial and body movements should correspond with what is said. The interviewer may have to spend some time learning to be aware of his or her own facial, body, and voice behaviors to effectively use them in communicating with clients. Although the practitioner may be frowning because of worry unrelated to the interview, the client in the process of revealing sensitive information may conclude that the information is unacceptable to the interviewer.

Body movements that may convey that the client is uncomfortable include avoidance of eye contact, stiff posture, nervous or inappropriate laughter, and tapping the foot against the floor. The examiner would do well to ask the client about his feelings when these behaviors are observed.

Empathy

Role taking has been suggested to be synonymous with empathy. More simply, it is voluntarily putting oneself in another person's place in one's imagination. The four phases of empathic experience include:

1. Identification—investing oneself in thinking about the person and what is happening to him
2. Incorporation—being aware and receptive of the person, rather than projecting one's own feelings and thoughts
3. Reverberation—an interaction between the feelings and experiences of the client and the examiner
4. Detachment—return to one's own identity

The insight that is a result of the experience is helpful in understanding and meeting the needs of the client. Empathy has been described by some as active listening; it is understanding and acceptance of the client's feelings. Empathic responses may be verbal, for example, "That must have made you feel very frightened" or "That must have been very painful to you." Understanding and acceptance may also be conveyed nonverbally, for example, a hand placed on the client's shoulder.

It is important that the interviewer be correct in responding to the client. Classic errors have been described such as sympathizing in the assumed painful loss the client felt on the death of his father when in fact the father had been a considerable financial and emotional burden to the client.

Empathy is thought to be necessary to the therapeutic relationship. It helps to establish rapport to show understanding and support.

Termination

The interviewer allows the client to terminate the session when the interviewer determines that there are no further questions that he or she feels would produce productive information in the session. He signals the client that the interview is in its final phase by saying something such as, "I have no more questions; is there anything more you would like to share with me?" or, "Is there anything we may have omitted?"

HEALTH HISTORY INTERVIEW

The first step in health assessment is the interview in which the information of the health history is obtained. This is a structured interview aimed at the collection of specific information. This type of interview may present some difficulty for the individual who has been accustomed to less structured methods, that is, more nondirective techniques. Although the client may give a good deal of the history—at least the description of the problem for which help is sought—without the benefit of direct questioning, the complete information of the health history may not be obtained. In that case the practitioner must ask direct questions that will provide the necessary information. In an emergency situation, the examiner may be forced to use only closed questions.

Encouraging a complete description of the symptom

The descriptions by the client of the changes he has perceived in the structure of his body or its functions are called symptoms. The interview should provide the most accurate and constructive picture of the symptom that can be obtained, since this is the base from which the client's problems can be defined.

The practitioner carefully avoids devaluing the client's symptoms by such remarks as, "You have nothing to be nervous about," or, "That's nothing; now, last week we had a really bad case."

There are eight criteria that can be used to provide this delineation: anatomical location, quality of the symptom, quantity of the symptom, time sequence of the symptom, geographical or environmental locale in which the symptom occurs, precipitating conditions that cause the symptom to be more severe, circumstances that alleviate the symptom, and other symptoms that occur in conjunction with the symptom.

Guideline	Interview items to elicit symptom description
1. Anatomical location Radiation of the symptom	"Tell me where it hurts." "Show me where it hurts."
2. Quality or character	"What does it feel like?" "Can you compare this to something you have felt in the past?"
3. Quantity	"How bad [intense] is the pain?" "How much does the pain immobilize you?" "What effect does the pain have on normal daily activities?"
4. Time sequence	"When did you first notice the pain?" "How long does it last?" "How often have you had it since that time?"
5. Geographical or environmental factors	"Where were you when the pain occurred?"
6. Precipitating conditions	"Do you find that the pain occurs at a certain time of day?" "Does heat or cold seem to affect the pain?" "What causes the pain?"
Conditions making the symptom more severe	"Have you noticed anything that makes the pain worse?"
7. Alleviating condition	"What seems to help you when you have the pain?"
8. Concomitant symptoms	"Have you noticed any other changes that are present when you have the pain?"

To clarify the use of these guidelines in the interview setting, consider a client who comes for treatment with a chief complaint of pain (see above column).

The accuracy of the diagnostic process is dependent on exploring the ramification of these eight areas for data collection.

Common problems in interviewing

McGuire determined that six problem areas were common in the interviewing procedures of senior medical students:

1. Omission of questions aimed to promote discussion of personal or affective matters
2. Failure to explain the purpose of the interviews
3. Inability to keep the patient focused on interview items
4. Emphasis on one or a few problems while failing to explore additional problem areas
5. Failure to seek clarification
6. Failure to be precise in reporting dates and times or chronological developments of illness or symptoms

Careful attention to these potential trouble spots in the interviewing process may obviate similar difficulties for the learner of interviewing skills.

BIBLIOGRAPHY

Argyle, M.: The psychology of interpersonal behavior, Baltimore, 1967, Penguin Books.

Benjamin, A.: The helping interview, ed. 3, Boston, 1981, Houghton Mifflin Co.

Bernstein, L., and Bernstein, R.S.: Interviewing: a guide for health professionals, ed. 3, New York, 1980, Appleton-Century-Crofts.

Bernstein, L., and Dana, R.S.: Interviewing and the health professions, New York, 1970, Appleton-Century-Crofts.

Bird, B.: Talking with patients, ed. 3, Philadelphia, 1973, J.B. Lippincott Co.

Cormier, L., Cormier, W., and Weiser, R., Jr.: Interviewing and helping skills for health professionals, Monterey, Calif., 1984, Wadsworth Health Sciences.

DiMatteo, M.R.: A social-psychological analysis of physician-patient rapport toward a science of the art of medicine, J. Soc. Issues **35**:12, 1979.

Ehmann, V.E.: Empathy: its origin, characteristics and process, Perspect. Psychiatr. Care **9**:72, 1971.

Enelow, A.J., and Swisher, S.N.: Interviewing and patient care, New York, 1979, Oxford University Press.

Engel, G.L., and Morgan, W.L., Jr.: Interviewing the patient, Philadelphia, 1973, W.B. Saunders Co.

Fast, J.: Body language, New York, 1970, M. Evans & Co., Inc.

Foley, Rand Sharf, B.: The five interviewing techniques most frequently overlooked by primary care physicians, Behav. Med. **26**:31, 1981.

Friedman, H.S.: Nonverbal communication between patients and medical practitioners, J. Soc. Issues. **35**:82, 1979.

Froehlich, R.E., and Bishop, F.M.: Clinical interviewing skills: a programmed manual for data gathering, evaluation, and patient management, ed. 3, St. Louis, 1977, The C.V. Mosby Co.

Gill, M., Newman, R., and Redlich, F.: The initial interview in psychiatric practice. New York, 1954, International Universities Press.

Gordon, R.: Interviewing: strategy, techniques and tactics, Homewood, Ill., 1969, Dorsey Press.

Hall, E.: The silent language, Greenwich, Conn., 1959, Fawcett.

Hall, E.: The hidden dimension, Garden City, N.Y., 1969, Doubleday & Co., Inc.

MacKinnon, R.A., and Michels, R.: The psychiatric interview in clinical practice, Philadelphia, 1971, W.B. Saunders Co.

McGuire, P.: Teaching essential interviewing skills to medical students. In Osborne, P.J., Gruneberg, M.M., and Eiser, J.R., editors: Research in psychology and medicine, London, 1979, Academic Press, Inc.

Morgan, W.L., Jr., and Engel, G.L.: The clinical approach to the patient, Philadelphia, 1969, W.B. Saunders Co.

Okun, B.: Effective helping: interviewing and counseling techniques, Monterey, Calif., 1982, Brooks/Cole Publishing Co.

Reiser, D., and Schoder, A.: Patient interviewing: the human dimension, Baltimore, 1980, Williams & Wilkins.

Richardson, S., Dohrenwend, B.S., and Klein, D.: Interviewing: its forms and functions, New York, 1965, Basic Books, Inc., Publishers.

Sullivan, H.: The psychiatric interview, New York, 1954, W.W. Norton & Co., Inc.

Ware, J.E., Jr., Davies, A.A., and Stewart, A.L.: The measurement and meaning of patient satisfaction, Health Med. Care Serv. Rev. **1**:1, 1978.

CHAPTER 3

THE HEALTH HISTORY

The health history is an extremely important part of the health assessment. Its performance is the primary vehicle by which rapport is established between the practitioner and the client. The information derived from the history-taking interview assists the practitioner in assessing and diagnosing the client's health problems and in obtaining knowledge of the client's problems and needs within the context of that particular client's life. The health history not only records the problems of the client but also describes the client as a whole and in relation to his social and physical environment. Thus, it records not only weaknesses and abnormalities but also the strengths that will support therapy and care.

Other important components of the history data base are the perceptions of the client regarding his health, his illness, and his past experiences with health delivery systems. These perceptions must be known if future care is to be relevant and, consequently, effective.

In practice, the taking of the health history is implemented in two phases: (1) the client interview phase, which elicits the information, and (2) the recording of data phase. The information as presented in this chapter is organized according to a systematic method for recording the history. The client interview may or may not proceed in the same sequence. Each portion of the health history discussed contains descriptions of processes for both eliciting and summarizing data. Examples of two recorded health histories are included at the end of this chapter.

Certain principles of the history-taking procedure should be emphasized. The importance of privacy seems obvious, but this principle is too often violated in actual practice. Another apparent principle is the maintenance of eye contact (Fig. 3-1), but what does one do about recording? The practitioner must immediately note specific information, such as dates, age, and so on, or it may be forgotten. Also, the client expects the practitioner to consider his information important

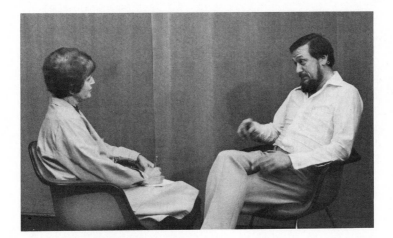

Fig. 3-1
Interview.

enough to have it recorded. It is a temptation to attempt to complete the recorded history during the interview, but it is not possible to do this and simultaneously observe the client and his responses. Thus, the interviewer must develop a routine that allows for eye contact with and observation of the client and for the taking of the notes that will serve as the outline for the recorded history.

FORMAT

The health history, as described in this chapter, is an extremely complete one. In many actual client care situations, it may not be possible, or even appropriate, to obtain the complete history at the first encounter or at all. For clients receiving continuous care, the history can be obtained in portions during several encounters.

For clients requiring episodic care, decisions regarding the data essential for immediate therapy guide the content of the history.

However, the beginning historian should practice obtaining the complete health history to develop skill in interviewing and in recording data and to establish priorities for focused interviews. During this practice process the learner will develop an appreciation for the client management implications of each portion of the health history.

The format used in this text for the complete health history is as follows:
A. Biographical information
B. Chief complaint or client's request for care
C. Present illness or present health status
D. Past history
E. Family history
F. Review of systems
　1. Physical
　2. Sociological
　3. Psychological
G. Developmental data
H. Nutritional data

Biographical information

At the beginning of any health record, there should be a place to record commonly used and sometimes critically important biographical information. This information should be obtained early during the client's first visit or admission; otherwise, it may be omitted, only to be needed in an emergency or at a time when the client is unavailable or unable to respond.

The following information is to be recorded in the introductory, biographical section of the history:
A. Full name
B. Address and telephone numbers
　1. Client's permanent
　2. Contact of client

C. Birthdate
D. Sex
E. Race
F. Religion
G. Marital status
H. Social Security number
I. Occupation
　1. Usual
　2. Present
J. Birthplace
K. Source of referral
L. Usual source of health care
M. Source and reliability of information
N. Date of interview

First, the client's name is recorded. Persons in an ethnically homogenous geographical area often have similar names. Precise identification, using first, middle, and last names, assists in assuring accurate information retrieval and coordination. If additional identifying information is needed, parents' names, including the mother's maiden name, can be recorded.

Next, the client's full mailing address and telephone number are recorded. Also recorded are the name, address, and telephone number of one of the client's friends or relatives, someone with whom he is in frequent contact and who would be willing and able to relay a message to the client in an emergency or if the client could not be located.

Birthplace, sex, race, marital status, and religion information are self-explanatory. Many health problems and needs are age, sex, race, or social situation related. This information might be correlated with problems discovered later in the history.

There are justifiable reasons for the notation of the client's Social Security number, including the precise identification of each client and a potential access to a large pool of health-related information. Potential violations of confidentiality are a disadvantage.

A significant difference may exist between the client's current and usual occupations. The nature of the difference may be indicative of the severity of the client's health problems and the level of disability resulting from them. In addition, knowledge of past occupations might provide clues to past or present environmental hazards contributing to the present illness. A mine worker with a respiratory system complaint is an example.

Knowledge of the client's birthplace provides geographical implications for the origin of problems and cultural implications for therapy and health maintenance.

If the current caregiver is not the usual and primary source of the client's care, the name and address of the individual or institution so identified should be recorded. In addition, the practitioner should record the reason for the client's entering a new health care system. The client may be in crisis, he may be dissatisfied with past care, or he may be "shopping." If the past source of care possesses significant data about the client's health and if the client intends to continue in the current health care system, the client should be asked to sign a permission for the transfer of information. Later in the health history, the practitioner will have the opportunity to record, in some detail, past patterns of health care.

The source of client payment for care is usually information included on administrative records. However, information here might be useful in guiding the choice of intervention.

Next, the practitioner makes a statement about the source of the information to follow. In most cases the source is the client, but this cannot be assumed unless the information is specifically identified. If the information is given by someone other than the client, the degree of the informant's contact with the client should be described. For example, in the case of a child, the practitioner would use the history given by a grandmother who resides with the child differently from one given by a grandmother who visits the child once a week.

Along with the statement of the informant, an evaluation of his reliability is made. For example, one of the following may be stated: "inconsistent," "unclear about recent events," "evasive," or "cooperative and reliable." These statements serve as simple criteria by which the remainder of the information in the history is judged by other health care providers and may indicate a need to retake or supplement the history at a future date or to consult with other informants to determine the accuracy of the data.

The history is dated. In a situation where the client's condition changes rapidly, events can be correlated only if their temporal relationships are known.

Chief complaint or client's request for care

The chief complaint (CC) statement is a short statement, in the client's own words and recorded in quotation marks, that indicates the client's purpose for requesting health care at this time. In the case of a client who is ill, the CC statement is of the acute or chronic problem (or problems) that is the client's priority for treatment. The CC statement, whenever relevant, includes a notation of the problem's duration. The duration, as stated by the client, may not be the actual duration of the symptoms. However, it is an indication of the time during which the complaint has become intolerable enough to motivate the client to seek help.

In the case of a well client, the CC statement may be a statement of the client's request for a health exami-

nation for health screening, health promotion, or disease case-finding purposes.

The CC statement is not a diagnostic statement. Actually, it is very hazardous to state a chief complaint in diagnostic terms. For example, a client who has frequent asthmatic attacks appears for treatment with respiratory system complaints and states that he is having an "asthmatic attack." This may or may not be the case. In this early portion of the history, client and interviewer bias must be avoided; otherwise the interview and the problem solving may be set in one, and potentially a wrong, direction.

The following are examples of adequately stated chief complaints.

> "Chest pain for 3 days."
> "Swollen ankles for 2 weeks."
> "Fever and headache for 24 hours."
> "Pap smear needed. Last Pap 9/8/83."
> "Physical examination needed for camp."

The following are examples of inadequately stated chief complaints:

> "Thinks she might be pregnant."
> "Sick."
> "Nausea and vomiting."
> "Hypertension."

The CC statement may seem superfluous, especially since the next section on the present illness describes the symptoms in detail. However, this is one of the few places in the recorded history of a client's encounter with the health care system where he has the opportunity to have recorded, in his own words, his needs. Too often, the practioner loses sight of the client's priorities for care. The consistent recording of a chief complaint or reason for the visit will assist in keeping the system responsive to the client's perceived needs.

In some instances the client may present several complaints. No more than three should be stated in this portion of the history and the client's stated priorities should be noted first. There is the opportunity to discuss all problems in the present illness portion of the health history.

Present illness or present health status

The present illness (PI) section describes the information relevant to the chief complaint. In the case of a client with a health problem, this portion of the health history challenges the interviewing, clinical knowledge, and written communication skills of the practitioner. The practitioner needs to learn the minute details of the chief complaint and its associated phenomena. Information must be comprehensive, it must be recorded concisely and comprehensively, and it must provide the practitioner with enough information to initiate additional assessment and the intervention measures.

The interviewing and recording for the present illness portion of the health history is especially difficult for beginning practitioners because the processes require both skill in interviewing and history taking, as well as clinical knowledge. Outlining the progression of the present illness before writing the narrative discussion is sometimes helpful. Although the student learning health assessment has probably not yet learned client care management, the student may find the referral to clinical management references for the system(s) discussed with the patient will often alert him or her to the most valuable pieces of data and highlight important omissions, which can be incorporated in future interviews.

In the case of a well client, the interviewer usually describes the client's usual health and briefly summarizes his health maintenance needs and activities.

The following are the components of the PI section:

I. Introduction
   A. Client's summary
   B. Usual health
II. Investigation of symptoms: chronological story
   A. Onset
   B. Date
   C. Manner (gradual or sudden)
   D. Duration
   E. Precipitating factors
   F. Course since onset
      1. Incidence (frequency)
      2. Manner
      3. Duration (longest, shortest, and average times)
      4. Patterns of remissions and exacerbations
   G. Location
   H. Quality
   I. Quantity
   J. Setting
   K. Associated phenomena
   L. Alleviating or aggravating factors
III. Negative information
IV. Relevant family information
V. Disability assessment

Introduction. The introduction to the PI section should be succinct; its major purpose is to provide the reader with a general orientation to the client.

The introduction indicates the client's previous admissions or visits, if any, to the institution or service. Next, there is a short summary of the client's biographical data. Age, race, marital status, employment status, and occupation are the items of information usually recorded. If the client is being hospitalized and has been hospitalized in the past, the client's total number of hospitalizations and the number of hospitalizations for complaints related to the current illness are noted.

The practitioner next describes the client's usual health and records any significant past diagnoses or past or current health problems that might have caused the client to enjoy anything other than good health.

Investigation of symptoms: chronological story. The practitioner usually initiates the PI description by asking the client: "Tell me about it [the problem mentioned in the CC statement]," or "How did it start and what has happened since it started?" The client will usually respond to this inquiry with a long but usually diagnostically incomplete discourse about his health problems and needs. The practitioner exercises skill in determining when to interrupt the client and more specifically direct his responses by asking additional, clarifying questions and when to allow the client to continue the narration of those events significant to him.

The practitioner needs a mental or actual list of the areas of symptom investigation as an aid in attaining comprehensive information. Regardless of the nature of a problem, each of the areas of investigation is relevant, and any health problem analysis would be incomplete without the description of all areas.

The practitioner also attempts to determine the chronological sequence of the client's problem. The client is apt to best remember his most recent episode of illness and in the case of a prolonged illness will need direction in tracing the problem back to its first symptomatic event. Once this first event is identified, it is investigated in detail and its date, manner of onset, duration, and precipitating factors are described in the recording.

Each symptom's course since onset is described. Frequency in a specific time interval is determined. Clients may state vaguely that they have a symptom "all the time." This may mean once a month to one client or ten times a day to another. To obtain specific information, the practitioner might ask, "How many times a day (or a week, or a month) does it occur?" Although the practitioner avoids suggesting answers with his questions, occasionally it may be necessary to pursue frequency with leading questions, for example, "Does it occur more often than five times a day?"

The practitioner determines the usual manner of onset for the illness episodes. Any change in onset is specifically mentioned. In the case of many episodes, the longest, shortest, and average durations of the episodes are noted. If there have been only several episodes, the length of each is identified.

In prolonged illnesses, the patterns of remission and exacerbation are described according to their duration and frequency. The practitioner needs to be watchful for environmental or other clues that might be precipitating factors for the illness events.

In recording, there are several suggested methods that can be used in assisting readers to easily identify temporal relationships. The practitioner describes the initial event first and then the subsequent events. The chronological story may be indexed in the lefthand column of the history sheet, using the reference base *prior to admission* (PTA). For example, the index might be listed as follows: "6 years PTA," "3 years PTA," "6 months PTA," "1 day PTA," and so on, with the corresponding narrative alongside and below the temporal index heading.

A method of demonstrating the progression of illness is accomplished by the use of a diagram illustrating the disease process (Fig. 3-2). A diagram is especially helpful in the case of multisymptomatic illnesses.

As the chronological story evolves, the other areas of symptom investigation are integrated into the text of the narrative. Whenever appropriate, the sign's or symptom's location, quality, quantity, setting, associated phenomena, and alleviating and aggravating factors are described, especially whenever there is a change in any of them.

Location. The exact site of the sign or symptom is determined. Subjective events, such as pain, pose some problem. Having a client point to the exact point of pain and trace its radiation with his finger assists in location. In recording location, one uses body hemispheres and landmarks.

Quality. Quality refers to the unique properties of the complaint. Signs, such as discharge, are described according to their color, texture, composition, appearance, and odor. Sound and temperature may be descriptive attributes of other phenomena.

Subjective events, such as pain, challenge the creativity of the practitioner. The quality of pain is frequently characterized as dull, aching, sharp, nagging, throbbing, stabbing, or squeezing.

Whenever appropriate, the client's descriptions are used with quotation marks.

Quantity. Quantity refers to the size, extent, number, or amount, for example, of the pain, rash, discharge, or lesion. With objective signs, the practitioner can use commonly understood measures, such as centimeters, cups, or tablespoons. In describing subjective events, pain, for example, one should note that evaluations such as "a little" or "a lot" have different meanings among persons. The quality of such phenomena can be more accurately understood by describing the client's response to the symptom. For example, does he have to stop and sit or does he continue on with what he is doing?

Setting. Whenever something occurs, the client is somewhere and is either with someone or alone. Physically or psychologically the setting may have an effect on the client, and knowledge of this information may provide the practitioner with clues of the cause of the problem and implications for treatment.

Associated phenomena. Associated phenomena are those symptoms that occur with the chief complaint. They may be related to the chief complaint or may be a part of a totally different syndrome. Often the client will spontaneously identify these events. In addition, the practitioner may ask if there is anything else

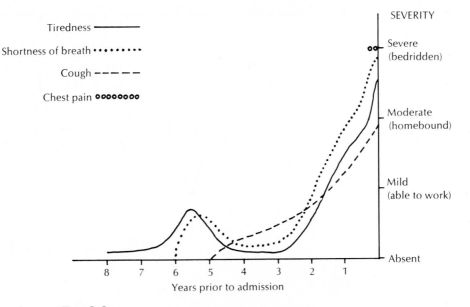

Fig. 3-2
Use of a graph to illustrate symptomatic progress of an illness.

occurring with the chief complaint or ask about the presence or absence of certain specific events. A complete review of the implicated problem system or systems is indicated. Positive responses are recorded with a complete description of all reported symptoms. Negative responses are recorded in the negative information section.

Alleviating or aggravating factors. When an illness occurs, a person often accommodates to it or treats himself. He may decrease activity, eat more or less, wait, or actively medicate and treat himself. The practitioner should nonpunitively probe into the client's actions in response to the problem and into the effect of these actions. If there has been professional intervention, the nature, source, and effect of each intervention are recorded. The client, through treatment or through accommodation, may have discovered something that alleviates the symptom. The client is asked what makes his problem better. The nature of the client's solution may provide valuable therapeutic data and may reflect the nature of his adaptation to illness.

The client is asked about that which makes the chief complaint worse. Usually clients have noticed aggravating factors but may need assistance in recalling them. The practitioner may ask about the effect of movement, positioning, or eating, for example. Again, valuable therapeutic data may be obtained.

Negative information. In analyzing a problem, one may find negative information as significant as positive information in determining the diagnosis.

Each system implicated in the PI section is thoroughly reviewed. All the client's positive replies are recorded in the text of the chronological story. All the negative information is recorded in this separate category of the PI section.

Relevant family history. The client is queried about any problem similar to the chief complaint in his blood relatives. Positive replies are recorded, identifying specifically the relative and his problem. A negative reply is recorded generally, for example, "None of the client's blood relatives has diabetes."

Disability assessment. The practitioner determines the extent to which the symptoms identified in the PI section have affected the client's total life. Not only are the physiological effects determined, but also the sociological, psychological, and financial impacts of the problem.

Past history

The purpose of the past history (PH) section of the health history is to identify all major past health problems of the client.

The following indicates the information to be obtained and recorded in the PH section of the health history:

A. Past illnesses
  1. Childhood illnesses
  2. Injuries
  3. Hospitalizations
  4. Operations
  5. Other major illnesses
B. Allergies
  1. Environmental
  2. Ingestion
  3. Drug
  4. Other
C. Immunizations
D. Habits
  1. Alcohol
  2. Tobacco
  3. Drugs
  4. Coffee, tea
E. Medications taken regularly
  1. By practitioner prescription
  2. By self-prescription

The recording of childhood illnesses is probably more relevant to and more easily obtained for a child's history than for an adult's history. However, all adults should be asked minimally if they have had rheumatic fever. Whenever there is a positive reply, the age of the client at occurrence, the fact or absence of a medical diagnosis, and the sequelae of the disease are determined.

The client is asked to recall accidents and disabling injuries, regardless of whether he was hospitalized for them or was treated on an outpatient basis. The precipitating event, the extent of injury, the fact or absence of medical care, the names of the practitioner and institution, and the sequelae are determined and recorded. The practitioner investigates for patterns of injuries or for the presence of consistent environmental hazards.

Descriptions of hospitalizations include all the times the client was admitted to an inpatient unit. Dates of stay, the primary practitioner, the name and address of the hospital, the admitting complaint, the discharge diagnosis, and the follow-up care and sequelae should all be recorded.

Obstetrical hospitalizations are recorded in the review of systems portion of the health history under the review of the female genital system.

Operations are recorded together, under this specific category. The history should include as complete a description of the nature of the repair or removal as is possible. However, clients are generally and unnecessarily unaware of the nature of their operations. Past records may need to be consulted for accurate and complete information.

Clients may have had major, acute illnesses or chronic illnesses that have not required hospitalization.

The course of treatment, the person making the diagnosis, and the follow-up care and sequelae are noted.

Information under the categories of hospitalizations, operations, and other major illnesses may, in some cases, be redundant. Information is not recorded more than once, but the presence of a past problem is stated, and the reader is referred to the section where the original notation was made.

The practitioner specifically asks about allergies to food, environmental factors, animals, and drugs. (The practitioner should particularly ask about past administrations and reactions are noted in the record.) If the client has an allergy, specific information is obtained about the causative factor, the reaction, the diagnosis of causative factor, the therapy, and the sequelae. Caution must be exercised in assessing drug allergies. A drug reaction may not always be an allergic response; it may be an interaction with a concurrently administered drug, a misdose, or a side effect.

Habits that may have relevance to the health of an individual are excessive alcohol, coffee, or tea ingestion; smoking; and the addictive use of legal or illegal mood-altering substances. In the case of habits, the number of cigarettes, ounces, tablets, and so on, per day are noted along with the duration of the habit.

If therapy is to be logically planned by informed practitioners, it is critical that all medications that are currently being used by the client are known and recorded. Clients usually admit to vague patterns, such as "a white pill once a day for water," but forget to tell the practitioner about the aspirin or antacid they take several times a day unelss they are specifically asked about nonprescription items. Here, the health practitioner has the opportunity to educate clients about the names, doses, and uses of their medications and about the necessity of knowing such information.

Family history

The purpose of the family history (FH) section is to learn about the general health of the client's blood relatives, spouse, and children and to identify any illnesses of environmental, genetic, or familial nature that might have implications for the client's current or future health problems and needs or to their solution or resolution.

The health status of the client's family is significant for several reasons. First, the health status of the client affects and is affected by health conditions in other family members. Communicable diseases are an example. Second, heredity and constitutional factors are associated with the causation of many diseases. A strong family history of certain problems might be important clues in assessment and diagnosis.

The practitioner inquires about the health of the client's consanguineous family members, including maternal and paternal grandparents, parents, siblings, aunts, uncles, spouse, and children. For certain situations, information regarding roommates, sexual partners, and significant others might be relevant to a family history. Information is obtained about the current health status, presence of disease, and current age or age at death of each family member. If a member is deceased, the cause of death is recorded.

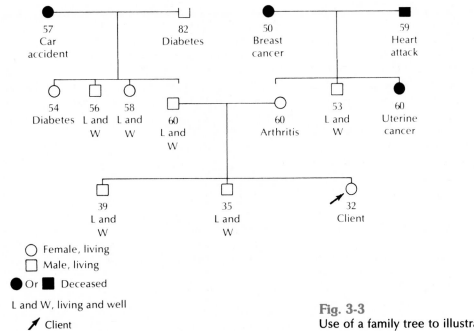

Fig. 3-3
Use of a family tree to illustrate family health.

If the nature of the client's established or possible illnesses have known or suspected familial tendencies, the client is again questioned about similar problems of family members.

Inquiries about the presence of the following diseases are made because of their genetic, familial, or environmental tendencies: alcoholism, allergies, epilepsy, diabetes, hematological disorders (such as hemophilia, sickle cell anemia, thalassemia, hemolytic jaundice, and severe anemia), Huntington's chorea, cancer, hypertension, arteriosclerosis, gout, obesity, coronary artery disease, tuberculosis, and kidney disease. Often printed history forms list these diseases, and the interviewer can check if the client or a family member has the diagnosis. The interviewer may inquire about additional diseases because of the client's family history, occupation, socioeconomic status, ethnic origins, or environment.

The information in the FH section may be outlined in the record or put in the form of a family tree chart. Fig. 3-3 is an example of such a chart. This type of chart is especially useful in situations where genetically transmitted diseases are present or suspected or if the understanding of family composition is an important factor in management.

Review of systems

The review of systems (ROS) portion of the history includes a collection of data about the past and present health of each of the client's systems. This review of the client's physical, sociological, and psychological health status may identify problems not uncovered previously in the history and provides an opportunity to indicate client strengths and liabilities.

Generally, the ROS portion of the history is organized from cephalad to caudad, from physical to psychosocial. Clients are instructed that they will be asked a number of questions. Both beginning and experienced interviewers normally need a checklist or written reminder of the questions usually asked each client.

Physical systems

In the review of physical systems section, the practitioner asks about symptoms or asks a specific question and then pauses, allowing the client to think and respond. If the client responds positively, the examiner analyzes the symptoms according to the characteristics of symptoms discussed in the PI section of the history. The practitioner asks questions quickly enough to be efficient, yet slowly enough to allow the client time to think. Questions generally emphasize the presence of past or current common anatomical or functional problems of the system and the health functioning and maintenance of the system.

Obviously, the signs and symptoms need to be creatively translated into questions and terms that can be understood by the client. For example, questions concerning a symptom such as intermittent claudication would need to be presented in lay, descriptive terms.

The presence or absence of all signs or symptoms regarding which inquiry has been made is stated in the record. The general term *negative* for a total system is meaningless; the reader, if he is not the recorder, does not know which questions were asked and consequently does not know the context of *negative;* if the reader is also the recorder, he probably will not, after time, remember which specific questions were asked. An exception might exist in a health care system where the review of physical systems section is routinized and where *negative* indicates an inquiry into and a negative response to predetermined, universally known, and always-reviewed items of exploration.

In the PI section the practitioner has already reviewed the problem system thoroughly. The practitioner can, under that system in the review of physical systems section, advise the reader to refer to the PI section for information about that system.

Systems and body regions for review and exploration of health status, functional and anatomical problems, and health maintenance in the review of physical systems section are as follows:

General

Usual state of health
Episodes of chills
Episodes of weakness or malaise
Fatigue
Fever
Recent and significant gain or loss of weight (if present, amount, time interval, and possible causes are recorded)
Sweats
Usual, maximum, and minimum weight

Skin

Usual state of health	Masses
Previously diagnosed and treated disease	Odors
	Petechiae
Color changes	Pruritus
Dryness	Temperature changes
Ecchymoses	Texture changes
Lesions	Care habits

Hair

Usual state of health	Use of dyes
Alopecia or hair loss	
Excessive growth or change in distribution	
Texture changes	

Nails

Usual state of health
Changes in appearance
Texture changes

Head and face

Usual state of health
Dizziness
History of trauma
Injuries
Pain

Syncope
Unusual or frequent
  headache

Eyes

Usual state of health
Visual acuity, without and with corrective lenses, if applicable
Cataracts
Changes in visual fields or vision
Diplopia
Excessive tearing
Glaucoma
Date of last ophthalmologic examination
Visual disturbances, such as rainbows around lights, flashing
  lights, or blind spots
Infections
Pain
Pattern of eye examinations
Photophobia
Pruritus
Redness
Unusual discharge or sensations

Ears

Usual state of health
Use of prosthetic devices
Discharge
Hearing ability
Infections
Presence of excessive environmental noise

Tinnitus, buzzing, ringing
Otalgia
Vertigo (subjective or objective)
Care habits, especially ear
  cleaning

Nose and sinuses

Usual state of health
Olfactory ability
Discharge (seasonal associations)
Epistaxis
Frequency of colds
Obstruction

Pain in infraorbital or sinus areas
Postnasal drip
Sinus infection
Sneezing (frequent or prolonged)

Mouth and throat

Usual state of health
Use of prosthetic devices
Abscesses
Bleeding or swelling of
  gums
Change in taste
Dysphagia
Dryness
Excessive salivation

Hoarseness
Lesions
Odors
Pain
Sore throats
Voice changes
Pattern of dental care
Pattern of dental hygiene

Neck and nodes

Usual state of health
Masses
Node enlargement
Pain with movement or palpation

Swelling
Tenderness

Breasts

Usual state of health
Dimples
Discharge
Masses
Pain

Tenderness
Self-examination pattern

Respiratory and cardiovascular systems

Usual state of health
Past diagnosis of respiratory or cardiovascular system disease
Cough
Cyanosis
Dyspnea (if present, amount of exertion precipitating it is
  recorded)
Edema
Hemoptysis
High blood pressure
Orthopnea (number of pillows needed to sleep comfortably
  is recorded)
Pain (exact location and radiation and effect of respiration
  are recorded)
Palpitations
Sputum
Stridor
Wheezing
Paroxysmal nocturnal dyspnea
Date of last roentgenogram or electrocardiogram

Gastrointestinal system

Usual state of health
Appetite
Bowel habits
Previously diagnosed problems
Abdominal pain
Ascites
Change in stool color
Constipation
Diarrhea
Dyschezia
Dysphagia
Flatulence
Food idiosyncrasies

Hematemesis
Hemorrhoids
Hernia
Indigestion
Infections
Jaundice
Nausea
Pyrosis
Rectal bleeding
Rectal discomfort
Recent changes in habits
Thirst
Vomiting
Previous roentgenograms

Urinary system

Usual state of health
Past diagnosed problems
Usual patterns of urination
Anuria
Change in stream

Dysuria
Enuresis
Flank pain
Frequency
Hematuria

Urinary system—cont'd

Hesitancy of stream	Retention
Incontinence	Stress incontinence
Nocturia	Suprapubic pain
Oliguria	Urgency
Polyuria	Urine color change
Pyuria	Urine odor change

Genital system

Male

Usual state of health	Pain
Lesions	Prostate problems
Impotence	Swelling
Masses	

Female

Usual state of health	Obstetrical history (for
Diagnosed problems	each pregnancy)
Lesions	Prenatal course
Pruritus	Complications of preg-
Vaginal discharge	nancy
Frequency of Pap	Duration of pregnancy
smear	Description of labor
Menstrual history	Date of delivery
Age at menarche	Type of delivery (vagi-
Frequency of menses	nal, cesarean sec-
Duration of flow	tion)
Amount of flow	Condition, sex, and
Date of last menstrual	weight of baby
period (LMP)	Postpartum course
Dysmenorrhea	Place of prenatal care
Menorrhagia	and hospitaliza-
Metorrhagia	tion
Polymenorrhea	
Amenorrhea	
Dyspareunia	

Both sexes

Ability to perform and en-	Infertility
joy satisfactory sexual in-	Sterility
tercourse	Venereal disease

Extremities and musculoskeletal system

Usual state of health	Muscles
Past diagnosis of disease	Cramping
Extremities	Pain
Coldness	Weakness
Deformities	Bones and joints
Discoloration	Stiffness
Edema	Swelling
Intermittent claudication	Redness
Pain	Heat
Thrombophlebitis	Limitation of move-
	ment
	Fractures
	Back pain

Central nervous system

Usual state of health	Motor
Past diagnosis of disease	Ataxia
Anxiety	Imbalance
General behavior change	Paralysis
Loss of consciousness	Paresis
Mood change	Tic
Nervousness	Tremor
Seizures	Spasm
Speech	Sensory
Aphasia	Pain
Dysarthria	Paresthesia (hyperesthe-
Cognitive ability	sia, anesthesia)
Changes in memory	
Disorientation	
Hallucinations	

Endocrine system

History of physical growth and development
Adult changes in size of head, hands, or feet
Diagnosis of diabetes or thyroid disease
Presence of secondary sex characteristics
Dryness of skin or hair
Exophthalmos
Goiter
Hair distribution
Hormone therapy
Hypoglycemia
Intolerance of heat or cold
Polydipsia
Polyuria
Polyphagia
Postural hypotension
Weakness

Hematopoietic system

Past diagnosis of disease	Blood type
Anemia	Bruising
Bleeding tendencies	Exposure to radiation
Blood transfusion	Lymphadenopathy

Sociological system

The practitioner cannot effectively diagnose a disorder or treat a client by knowing the client's physical status only. The client is a unique and whole person. For therapy to be effective, the problem must be assessed and treated within the context of that person. The practitioner should, in some organized way, gather information about the sociological status of the client, as well as his psychological, developmental, and nutritional status.

The following is a suggested organization of sociological data:

A. Relationships with family and significant others
1. Client's position in the family
2. Persons with whom client lives
3. Persons with whom client relates
4. Recent family crisis or changes

B. Environment
  1. Home
  2. Community
  3. Work
  4. Recent changes in environment
C. Occupational history
  1. Jobs held
  2. Satisfaction with present and past employment
  3. Current place of employment
D. Economic status and resources
  1. Source of income
  2. Perception of adequacy or inadequacy of income
  3. Effect of illness on economic status
E. Educational level
  1. Highest degree or grade attained
  2. Judgment of intellect relative to age
F. Daily profile
  1. Rest-activity patterns
  2. Social activities
  3. Special weekend activities
  4. Recent changes in daily activities
G. Patterns of health care
  1. Private and public primary care agencies
  2. Dental care
  3. Preventive care
  4. Emergency care

This outline is recommended for gathering the sociological data of the majority of adult clients; obviously, adaptations will need to be made for some individuals. Many clients may be unaccustomed to extensive questioning about nonphysical matters during the taking of a health history. The practitioner may need to explain the use of such data by stating to the client, for example, "To treat you most effectively, it is important that I know something about you as a person."

First, the practitioner asks about the client's role or roles in the family and household. A member may have a societally assigned role, relating to birth, for example, that of son, father, or grandfather, as well as a circumstantially defined role, for example, that of provider, "black sheep," child, and so on. Both should be identified.

Next, the practitioner inquires about the people with whom the client lives and relates on a regular basis. Information can be used to hypothesize, for example, the effect on the family of a long illness of the provider. Also, the practitioner could identify strengths in the presence of strong family or friend relationships. The client should also be asked about the closeness and compatibility of the relationships. Sometimes unsatisfactory social relationships produce stress, which can be a factor in the exacerbation or causation of illness.

It has been epidemiologically demonstrated that there is a higher than expected incidence or morbidity in those who have undergone recent important life crises or changes. Each client should be asked if any recent event has had a significant impact on his life. Resultant positive data might provide clues of causation or implications for prevention of illness.

Physical and psychological environments can have a profound effect on the health status and potential of an individual. The practitioner asks about the client's satisfaction with the appearance and general comfort of his house, his community, and his work situation. The practitioner might ask if the client considers his environment healthy or unhealthy. The pursuit of "why" in the case of negative responses will provide the practitioner some insight into the client's value system, possible information regarding significant health hazards, clues to the cause of the present illness, and a validation of the negative response. The practitioner again asks about recent change or loss. Positive responses are recorded.

Occupational history information can be used to identify past environmental hazards, to determine the fit between personal ability and productivity, and to plan rehabilitation. The practitioner asks about jobs held, satisfaction with those jobs, and the place of current employment.

The practitioner does not, in many cases, need to know the exact annual income; however, he should know the source of income and the client's assessment of its adequacy. Clients whose resources are too insufficient to enable them to follow therapy must be identified early, and appropriate referral for financial assistance made. In the case of probable prolonged illness, financial reserves are discussed and recorded. If the client is covered by any health insurance, the type of insurance, the name of the insurer, and the policy number are recorded.

The educational level of the client is determined. The highest degree or grade completed is recorded. The practitioner may also wish to make a judgment regarding intellectual ability relative to age. Interviewing up to this point in the history has provided the opportunity for extensive observation of the client's understanding, response, and judgment.

Knowledge of the client's daily pattern helps the practitioner know the client as a person, with habits that encourage or impede health. The practitioner asks the client to describe a typical 24-hour day and to indicate weekend differences. Work, activity, sleep, rest, and recreational pursuits are specifically identified in the recording.

Part of the client's past social interaction has been with the health care system, and past responses may be predictive of future patterns. The client is asked about the health agencies that he has used in the past for acute, preventive, and maintenance health care. It can be determined whether the client is a health facility "shopper" or whether care has had continuity.

Psychological system

The following is an outline of the information obtained and recorded in the psychological assessment of the client:

A. Cognitive abilities
1. Comprehension
2. Learning patterns
3. Memory
B. Responses to illness and health
1. Reaction to illness
2. Coping patterns
3. Value of health
C. Response to care
1. Perceptions of the caregivers
2. Compliance
D. Cultural implications for care
1. Patterns of therapy
2. Patterns of illness response

In the assessment of cognitive abilities, the practitioner determines the comprehension ability of the client. Usually this assessment is accomplished more indirectly than directly. Up to this point in the history-taking process, the client has demonstrated his ability to respond to some rather complex questions. The recording is the judgment summary of the practitioner regarding the client's general comprehension ability.

Since education should be an essential component of all therapy, it is useful to determine the client's health-learning patterns. Some clients need personal instructions; others learn best through reading or group discussion. Knowledge of the client's preference can enable efficient use of provider effort and also involve the client in decision making concerning the process of his therapy.

A discussion of the client's behavior in past illnesses and in health will probably be predictive of future responses. The practitioner asks: "What does health mean to you, and what do you do to keep yourself healthy?" "How do you feel, and what do you do when you become slightly ill? When you become very ill?" "Who do you go to for help if you are ill?" Most clients will be able to answer these questions easily. A summary of the client's responses is recorded concisely. Information can alert the practitioner about strengths, weaknesses, and possible problems in therapy.

Skill may be required in learning the client's real responses to care, since he is often placed in a position of subjugation by the health care system. The practitioner might ask the client how comfortable he feels in asking questions of his health care providers and if he has considered himself a partner in care with them. Answers may be recorded verbatim or summarized.

The practitioner asks about the client's amount of compliance to past courses of therapy. If compliance has been minimal, reasons should be determined for noncompliance. Problems resulting from lack of understanding and financial constraints are more easily solved than problems relating to distrust, indifference, or denial.

If the client is of a cultural group different from that of the practitioner and the majority of the care providers, it would be useful to ask the client what he expects of care and therapy, what general things are done in his culture for persons with needs similar to his. If the chief complaint is of an illness, the practitioner asks about the feelings and responses of the client and his significant others to the fact of the illness. Responses may guide the care provider into more efficient and fewer unacceptable routes of intervention.

Developmental data

A detailed description of the developmental assessment is presented in Chapter 4, "Developmental Assessment."

The recording of this data minimally includes a summary of the client's development to date and a statement of current developmental functioning.

Nutritional data

A detailed description of nutritional assessment is presented in Chapter 5, "Nutritional Assessment."

The recording of data minimally includes a description of an average day's food intake; an assessment of adequacy, inadequacy, or excess of the components of the Basic Four food groups; and the presence of any past nutritional problems.

COMPUTER-ASSISTED HISTORIES

Computer science is becoming an important and permanent component of health care technology, and the computer can be used to assist in obtaining the client health history. Studies have demonstrated that the use of the computer in history taking can save practitioner time; can yield a reliable, comprehensive, and readable printout; and is acceptable to clients. In personnel-deficient situations, where time allocated to history taking has been inadequate, the computer-assisted history can be superior to verbal histories.

Computer systems for history taking can be either practitioner-interactive or client-interactive. The client-interactive systems are more commonly used because they are more likely to save practitioner time. A number of client-interactive, computerized, history-taking systems are available. Wakefield and Yarnell (1975) describe a number of both computer-assisted and other self-administered histories that would be very helpful to those considering the use of client self-administered, data collection techniques.

Self-administered histories involve the client's either completing a paper-and-pencil questionnaire or interacting with a computer. In the paper-and-pencil questionnaire situation, the client's responses are computerized in a variety of ways and the practitioner receives a printout of responses. In the client-interactive systems, the client responds to inquiries from a computer terminal. Clients have been generally favorable to computer-assisted interviews, and printouts using such systems have been complete, accurate, and legible.

In any client self-administered system, practitioner time is needed to review the history of the client, but usually this review requires only a relatively small amount of time. The amount of time spent by the client in the history-taking process is not shortened by the computer-assisted methods, however. Client age, number of client's problems, and time required by the client to complete the instructional portion of the computer program are positively correlated with overall time needed to give a computer history, and the number of client's years of formal education is negatively correlated with overall time.

The computer-assisted history is more appropriate to the ambulatory client than to the hospitalized client. The ambulatory client can be scheduled for a computer interview, or he can complete a form for computerization with the printout to be available to the practitioner for an appointment in several days. For hospitalized clients, information is generally immediately needed, and client access to terminals becomes problematical. Also, often the hospitalized client is too ill to complete a questionnaire or to use a computer terminal.

Practitioner-based computer systems for history taking involve either the practitioner's direct interaction with a computer, which is programed for questions relating to the history and into which answers are placed, or the practitioner's completion of a form that is computer-processed at a later time. The computer-interactive systems require a terminal for each practitioner, a situation that may not be cost-effective in ambulatory care situations. The use of the questionnaire for computerization has been used more extensively. The advantage of this latter method is that a legible printout is produced, an improvement over most handwritten documents.

The computer-assisted history can be as effective as the verbal history and may be more effective because remembering items for review is not a problem. Any question that can be asked verbally can be programed

into a computer system, and computer technology allows for additional branching questions if certain significant responses are given. Before additional assessment and therapy it is imperative that any client self-administered history be discussed, reviewed, and verified by the practitioner to determine the validity of significant responses: the client may have misunderstood instructions or there may have been mechanical errors reflected in the information.

As computers become more prevalent in health care systems, especially microcomputers, the use of computer-assisted histories is likely to increase. However, there will always exist situations in which the computer history is not feasible and a verbal history is necessary. Therefore, skill in history taking is, and will continue to be, an important ability of the health care practitioner.

WRITTERN RECORD OF THE HEALTH HISTORY

The written record is the permanent, legal, and working documentation of what was seen, heard, and felt during the examination. It will serve as the baseline by which subsequent changes will be evaluated and therapy advised. It is very often used by a reader who does not have access to the recorder and is consequently subject to interpretation.

It is important that the recorded history be as objective, clear, complete, and concise as possible. The history should be free of recorder bias. The history is not the place for the recorder to bias the reader with opinions of diagnoses. Other portions of a client's record allow for the recorder to elaborate on hypotheses and plans.

In addition, the client's responses should be integrated in an accurate but objective way. This can be accomplished in one of two ways: (1) by paraphrasing the client, using, for example, statements such as "States he had the same symptoms 4 years ago" or "Denies chest pain," or (2) by quoting the client directly, for example, "The pain was so severe, I fell back into the chair I had just gotten up from."

Because most health histories are read over time by multiple health care providers, the clarity of the presentation is very important. A clear presentation is often difficult for the beginning historian, but self, colleague, and instructor feedback about written histories will assist in identifying strengths and deficits in this area. Specific attention to chronology and the quality and quantity of symptoms is needed for most beginners.

The record should be a complete history of the practitioner-client encounter.

The record should be specific enough for the reader to clearly determine what was asked and examined

EXAMPLE OF A RECORDED HEALTH HISTORY: Ill client—cont'd

Back
Denies pain, stiffness, limitation of movement, or disk disease.

Central nervous system
Reports loss of consciousness (1973) following blow to head; duration approximately 30 minutes. Denies clumsiness of movement, weakness, paralysis, tremor, neuralgia, or paresthesia. States he is a "nervous" person but denies hx of nervous breakdown. Hx of drug and alcohol abuse. States he will periodically (every 2 to 3 weeks) have spontaneous jerky movement of legs during rest. There are 4 to 5 movements in each episode. This has never occurred while legs were bearing weight. Denies disorientation or memory disorders. Denies seizures or epilepsy. "Passes out" frequently after heavy alcohol ingestion and sleeps for 5 to 6 hours. Wakes with headache and nausea.

Hematopoietic system
Denies bleeding, bruising, blood transfusion, or exposure to x-rays or toxic agents.

Endocrine system
Denies diabetes, thyroid disease, or intolerance to heat or cold. Growth has been within normal range.

REVIEW OF SOCIOLOGICAL SYSTEM

Family relationships
Has been separated from wife for 6 to 7 months and is in the process of being divorced. States his marital problems do not interfere with seeing his children. Plans to move to his mother's home when discharged from hospital. States relationships with his family are good.

Occupational history
Offset printer since 1981. Presently unemployed. Was advised not to work for 6 months when tuberculosis was diagnosed and has not been "able to get back to work." States he liked that occupation but expresses no urgency to return to work.

Economic status
On disability income, because of tuberculosis and need to rest. States he does not have trouble making ends meet on present income.

Daily profile
Lives alone in a room. States he spends time during the day at home or with friends, drinking. Has no special hobbies or activities to occupy time. Has habit of heavy daily drinking. States "I just hang around all day." Does do some spur-of-the-moment traveling. Weekdays are no different than weekends. States he dropped out of college because of disinterest. Meal patterns are erratic; sleeps 8 to 10 hours every day, usually 1 AM until 9 to 11 AM.

Educational level
States he is "smart enough." Dropped out of college after 2 years because of disinterest. States he has no aspiration except to "get by in life."

Patterns of health care
Has maintained relationship with same physician for the episodic care for the last 10 years. Does return for periodic examinations and follow-up when symptoms "scare him."

Environmental data
Birthplace—New York, N.Y. No travel outside of USA; no armed forces duty.
Home—Plans to move to his mother's home. Will share the 5-bedroom residence with his mother and 2 siblings. Neighborhood is residential; describes it as "beautiful."

REVIEW OF PSYCHOLOGICAL SYSTEM

Cognitive abilities
Oriented to present events. Has fairly adequate vocabulary. Has a fair to poor memory. Cannot recall details of some important events. No history of psychiatric treatment.

Response to illness
States he "quit" drinking when he entered the hospital and plans to abstain in the future. Verbalizes that his health problems are his own fault and that he will die soon if he does not resolve them. States illness does not bother him except when "it gets out of control." Definition of health entails being able to play baseball again.

Response to care

States he has sometimes not followed medical advice, because of fear or because drugs or alcohol did not allow him to think "straight." "People have been nice to me." States all care has been "OK."

Cultural implications

Inactive Presbyterian at present but is concerned about conflict with religious beliefs and life-style. Fourth-generation American.

DEVELOPMENTAL DATA

Adult male who has had problems with interpersonal relationships in his marriage. Has demonstrated drug and alcohol abuse since entering adulthood. Does not express concern regarding his inability to work; has abandoned his college attendance. Immediate plans for the future involve moving in with his mother and trying to stop drinking. Speaks of his children as playmates; expresses few fathering needs or activities.

NUTRITIONAL DATA

States he does not eat when drinking heavily and must build his tolerance to food by taking liquids such as soup or juices after drinking. States he does eat 3 complete meals daily when not drinking. Includes foods from the four basic food groups.

EXAMPLE OF A RECORDED HEALTH HISTORY: Well client

Client: Mary Rose Doe
Address: 1056 N. East St.
St. Louis, Mo. 63047
Telephone: 278-9274
Contact: Mrs. Elsa Smith (mother)
Address: 3496 Oak St.
St. Louis, Mo. 63047
Telephone: 926-8711
Birthdate: Feb. 6, 1955   **Sex:** Female   **Race:** Black
Religion: Methodist (active)   **Marital status:** Married
Social Security number: 396-47-8911
Usual occupation: Grade school teacher
Present occupation: Same—Greenwich School
Birthplace: St. Louis, Mo.
Source of referral: Self
Usual source of health care: St. Louis Health Maintenance Organization
4693 C. Division St.
St. Louis, Mo. 63044
Source and reliability of information: Client; cooperative, apparently reliable
Date of interview: Dec. 12, 1985.

REASON FOR VISIT

Annual physical examination; last exam, 1/84.

PRESENT HEALTH STATUS

Usual health

This is the third St. Louis Health Maintenance Organization (HMO) visit for this 30-year-old black, married, female school teacher who has been in good health for all of her life. Client has been hospitalized twice for the purposes of normal childbirth only. Has no major chronic diseases.

Summary

Client is presently well and requests a physical examination for health maintenance and screening purposes. Is concerned about a strong family history of hypertension and believes that monitoring of her blood pressure status is important.

Also requests a Pap smear and evaluation for continuance of oral contraceptives. Has been taking Ortho-Novum 1+50 since the birth of her last child in 1979. Client enrolled in the health plan a year ago.

PAST HISTORY

Childhood illnesses

Had rubella, chickenpox—not diagnosed by a physician. Has not had rheumatic fever.

Schneiderman, H.: The review of systems: an important part of a comprehensive examination, Postgrad. Med. **71:**151, 1982.

Scully, C., and Boyle, P.: Reliability of a self-administered questionnaire for screening for medical problems in dentistry, Community Dent. Oral Epidemiol. **11:**105, 1983.

Skarfors, E., Waern, U., and Lidell, C.: Findings at a reexamination of a self-administered questionnaire after two and a half years in a sample of sixty-year-old men, Scand. J. Soc. Med. **8:**137, 1980.

Small, I.F., editor: Introduction to the clinical history, Flushing, N.Y., 1971, Medical Examination Publishing Co.

Stout, F., and Doering, P.: The problematic drug history, Dent. Clin. North Am. **27:**387, 1983.

Taking the occupational history, Ann. Intern. Med. **99:**641, 1983.

Truitt, C.A., Longe, R.L., and Taylor, A.T.: The evaluation of a medication history method, Drug Intell. Clin. Pharm. **16:**592, 1982.

Tumulty, P.A.: The effective clinician, Philadelphia, 1973, W.B. Saunders Co.

Wakefield, J.S., and Yarnell, S.R.: The history data base, ed. 3, Seattle, 1975, Medical Computer Services Assoc.

CHAPTER 4

DEVELOPMENTAL ASSESSMENT

In performing the health assessment of a client, there is naturally much emphasis placed on the physical aspects of that assessment. The beginning practitioner is often preoccupied with assimilating new skills, handling new tools and techniques, and remembering lists of questions and components of the history and physical examination. From the onset of the learning process, however, it is important to emphasize a focus on the whole personhood of each client and to gain familiarity with a holistic frame of reference in regard to clients. This involves taking into account the life developmental process of that individual, the series of stages of maturity by which the individual progresses toward a higher level of functioning. This necessitates taking time to discuss and discover the client's world—his interaction and growth within himself, with significant others, and with society at large.

Discussing developmental stages, phases, and crises with clients can provide both practitioner and client with a sharper and deeper perspective of the client's life situation and its relationship to health or illness. An openness to discussing the life tasks of individuals can help them appreciate the appropriateness and normalcy of their feelings and behaviors, or it may assist those who seem blocked in their ability to accomplish their tasks.

It may also help clients to review their past, to compare it to the present, to look at progressive stages and intervals, and to plan for the future, as is appropriate and necessary. Perhaps most importantly, it may serve to help a person appreciate both his similarities to others and his own unique individuality and to gain assurance in his efforts to be most fully and healthily himself.

That growth and development are continuous throughout the life cycle is a premise basic to this approach. To perform a developmental assessment, one must give some thought to what constitutes "growth" and "development." There are numerous components to this broad, diversified, universal, and yet infinitely unique process. These include the physical, emotional, psychological, social, and educational facets of growth. Human development in these and other areas ranges from changes that are slow, subtle, and often elusive to those that occur with almost incredible rapidity. Whatever the rate of changes, one perceives and understands them more fully in the perspective that comes with the passage of time. Gessell, Ilg, and Ames (1956) define growth as "the patterning process whereby the mutual fitness of organism and environment is brought to progressive realization" (p. 25). Growth combines integration and differentiation in all of its aspects—physical, emotional, and social. Change is a central concept; life has the remarkable property of changing with time while maintaining a core of individuality. The problem or challenge of development is "to bring opposites into effectual con-

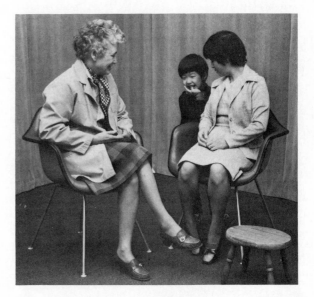

trol and counterpoise . . .in such a manner that the individual achieves integration, choice and direction'' (Gesell and others, 1956, p. 19).

During each phase or stage of human development certain aspects are ascendant or salient, yet the phases are not totally distinct or mutually exclusive. For example, "Childhood does not end nor adulthood begin around adolescence. Rather, the adult is anticipated in the child and the child persists in the adult'' (Katchdourian, p. 51). Stages of development may be defined in different ways. Some are defined by physical changes, others by internal psychological events, still others by external behavior, activities, or life situations.

Erikson suggests eight developmental stages of the ego and identifies for each stage a central task and a threat to the accomplishment of that task. (These will be integrated into the discussion of the various developmental stages.) These central tasks are developmental "crises," although not in the sense of an acute emergency situation, which that word often describes, but rather "as a term designating a necessary turning point, a crucial moment, when development must move one way or another, marshaling resources of growth, recovery, and further differentiation'' (Erikson, 1968, p. 16). It is "a period of increased vulnerability and heightened potential'' (Erikson, 1975, p. 5). He describes a life "cycle" as the "tendency of individual life to 'round itself out' as a coherent experience and to form a link in the chain of generations from which it receives and to which it contributes both strength and fateful discord'' (1975, p. 5).

There is a cyclic aspect to the various developmental stages. For example, young children tend to grow in spurts, then level off for a period, and adolescents tend to have cycles of untoward activity and then inner reflection. Adults also may experience periods of outward and inward involvement. Gesell, Ilg, and Ames suggest that "growth gains are consolidated during recurring periods of relative equilibrium. There is a tendency for stages of increased equilibrium to be followed by stages of lessened equilibrium when the organism makes new inner or outer thrusts into the inner or outer unknown'' (1956, p. 20).

The developmental aspects of infancy and childhood have received much attention and study for several decades, and there is an abundance of literature on these phases, although much still remains to be learned and understood. Of more recent vintage are the studies and theories advanced on adolescence and old age. And latest to surface in the literature on human development is material on that age span between youth and old age, namely, middle adulthood. Similarly, there are numerous tools and tests devised to assess early childhood stages, but few to assess school age children and adults. Several of the

infancy and early childhood assessment tools will be described; with adolescents and adults much developmental assessment is accomplished simply by talking with the client in an accepting, unrushed manner. (Two tools that assist with adult assessment are briefly described.) Nonthreatening questions about thoughts and feelings, work, family, and other activities and an attitude of active listening will encourage clients to share significant discussion about themselves. The practitioner should not expect to learn everything about a client's developmental accomplishments in one or even in several interviews. It is a personal story that takes time and trust to be told, Furthermore, developmental assessment for a client of any age is a continuous, ongoing process. Life is more like a moving picture than a still photograph; it is changing and dynamic and should be regularly reassessed.

The approach used in this chapter will be to organize developmental assessment around seven major life stages: infancy, early childhood, childhood, adolescence, young adulthood, middle adulthood, and late adulthood. Activities characteristic of each stage, including the developmental tasks, will be described. The length of the chronological divisions will increase with age: that is, for infants, monthly changes are described; for adolescents, annual changes; and for adults, decades.

A notation on the clinician's impression of a client's developmental tasks and accomplishments can be placed in the health history after the psychological system review. See examples on pp. 53 and 57.

CONCEPTUAL FRAMEWORK OF DEVELOPMENTAL ASSESSMENT
Pediatrics

The assessment of a child's development is carried out formally or informally by the practitioner during each examination. The opportunity to observe the development of many children enhances the ability to define the parameters of normal development, and the experienced examiner often responds to subtle behavioral cues with an intuitive hunch that all is not well with the child. However, it is usually difficult to verify this initial impression and make a determination of the presence or absence of a developmental deficit while examining a child in a busy clinical setting. The practitioner may need to plan additional time to focus attention on the assessment of the child's development or may need to seek the assistance of experts in child development.

The information obtained from the developmental assessment has many uses. It will aid the practitioner in providing assistance to the parents when they have questions about their child's behavior. Most parents will be interested in learning that their child is developing normally, and with anticipatory guidance they can gain a greater appreciation of ways to support the normal development of their child. The developmental assessment also provides information that can be useful at a future time. For instance, the child who has been developing in a normal fashion and then demonstrates a developmental lag presents a different problem than the child who has been consistently slower in development. Finally, the developmental assessment is helpful in screening for some of the more obvious deficits in development that deserve further investigation.

It is most important to keep in mind that the developmental assessment is not a test of the child's intelligence and does not allow the practitioner to make a diagnosis. It does allow the practitioner to collect data that indicate whether the development of the individual child is within the normal range.

Although there are many theories of development that can provide a framework for observing and assessing the development of children, the discussion in this chapter is limited. However, it is reasonable to expect that each practitioner with an interest in children will be challenged to increase understanding of the behavior presented by children of different ages.

The discussion in this section includes a conceptual framework for organizing the developmental assessment; approaches to the developmental assessment of the child, which can be incorporated into the plan for the health history and examination; and a brief discussion of selected screening tests that can be helpful to the practitioner.

A systematic appraisal of the child's development can be organized in different ways. Although each behavior of the child is part of an indivisible whole, it is clinically useful to separate behaviors into several categories whether the assessment is carried out as a part of the health examination or as a more formal procedure. Different categories of behavior are used, but many of the screening tests commonly focus on three categories: fine and gross motor development, language and communication, and personal-social behavior. These categories are especially useful in the assessment of the infant and preschool child, when observable changes occur most rapidly. When the development of the older child is being assessed, it is important to include questions about the child's adjustment to school and the grade level achieved and about his relationships with peers, siblings, and significant adults.

The stages of motor development have been documented and are well known, as is the relationship of motor skills to neuromotor organization. The practitioner will find information about the expected norms for achieving specific motor skills in most standard text-books of pediatrics or child development. What is not usually discussed in regard to developing motor abilities is the way the child uses these skills. Is the child active and using his skills in a variety of ways? Or is the child quiet, showing little apparent interest or pleasure in walking, running, and climbing? Information as to the amount of activity may lead to questions about the environment. Does it offer too much stimulation or too little? Differences in the use of skills may also be related to organic problems, which are sometimes demonstrated by the hyperactive, impulse-ridden child.

The normal age range for the sequential development of language and communication skills is also well documented, as well as the relationship of speech development to intellectual functioning. The assessment of the child's language and communication skills should provide information about the size of the child's vocabulary, his understanding of language, his clarity of articulation, and his use of phrases and sentences. The speech of the young child is easily disturbed when there are physical problems or problems with the people in the environment. Speech disturbances may be transitory, may indicate an impairment of the hearing or speech apparatus, or may indicate the presence of a mental disability. Although a delay in speech development may be a temporary problem, it is a concern that deserves further investigation even when the child is very young.

The appraisal of the personal-social behavior of the child provides information about the child's developing awareness of himself as a person, his ability to interact with people, and his adaptive behaviors. These abilities can also be described as the intellectual, emotional, and social skills of the child. Erik Erikson's "conceptual itinerary" of the psychosocial stages of life provides a plan, or a guided overview, of the changes and adaptive behaviors of the child in each of the sequential stages of childhood.

Approaches to assessment

The practitioner with limited time would be well served to find ways to incorporate aspects of the developmental assessment into the routine health examination of every child. A good deal of information can be gained by including questions about the child's development in the history. Also, since it is traditional to include observations of the child's behavior as part of the general inspection of the physical examination, it is relatively easy to pay special attention to particular aspects of behavior to obtain data about the child's level of functioning. However, it is also well to keep in mind that the behavior demonstrated may not be typical because of the stress from the unfamiliar environment or the particular problems of the illness that the child is experiencing.

Because there are limited opportunities to observe the child's behavior in the clinical setting, the history becomes the major tool for obtaining information about the child's development. First, the history allows the practitioner to obtain data about the factors that will increase the chances of the child's being at risk for problems that may interfere with his development. Una Haynes outlines many of the factors that contribute to the "at risk" status of the child. This information can be elicited from the past history of the child in the prenatal, natal, and postnatal period of life; from the family history; from the sociological assessment; from the developmental data; and from the history of illnesses and injuries. The history that reveals problems such as prematurity, precipitate delivery, or hyperbilirubinemia in the first 48 hours of life will alert the practitioner that the child is at greater risk than most children for developmental problems. However, this information should not bias the practitioner's perception of the child's development but should encourage a sense of "benign suspicion," a term used by Sally Provence (1968a) to describe the attitude of the examiner.

The pediatric history as outlined in Chapter 24 includes a developmental history that provides information about the age at which the child achieved certain developmental milestones. This information can be used to determine whether the early development was within average or normal limits. The history of the present health or present illness should include a description of the child's current level of functioning. The practitioner can review the achievements expected of the child at a specific chronological age as outlined in many texts on child development. Table 4-1 provides such an outline. Questions about these expected achievements will provide information about the child's current level of development; this information can then be included in the description of the child's present health.

Provence (1968a) mentions two questions that are helpful for the examiner to keep in mind when making judgments about the development of a child: (1) What has the child achieved in the various sectors of development that one can observe, describe, or measure? (2) How does the child make use of the skills and functions available to him? The first question requires the practitioner to find out about the developmental progress of the infant or child from helplessness at birth to his current level of development. The second question requires the practitioner to find out about the adaptation the child is making to his life. The second question is usually more difficult to answer, because it is not based on standardized developmental schedules. However, information about the child's adaptation can be obtained by asking the parent to describe

the child. This description can be broadened by asking whether the child is quiet or active, happy or sad, and mischievous or very good.

Ronald Illingworth (1975) stresses that purely objective tests result in obtaining information about scorable items in the area of sensorimotor skills and that it is of great importance to also determine the child's alertness, responsiveness, and interest in surroundings, which cannot be scored. Arnold Gessell (1947) calls these latter behaviors "insurance factors." If the child demonstrates these behaviors but has delays in some of the sensorimotor behaviors, an opinion should be reserved and the child followed over a longer period of time before judgment is made about the developmental skills of the child.

If there are questions or concerns about a child's development that are identified as the result of the routine appraisal, it would be well to set aside time so that a complete developmental assessment could be done that would include a careful review of the history of the developmental milestones and an appraisal of the child's current level of function. It would be appropriate to use one of the more structured screening tests.

DEVELOPMENTAL SCREENING TESTS

There are several screening tests that the practitioner may find useful in assessing the development of an infant or young child. Most of them require some training for validity of the test to be ensured.

The clinical assessment of gestational age helps the practitioner to determine that the newborn's gestational age is accurate and to anticipate problems that are related to the infant's maturity or immaturity. Several tools designed for use during the first few days of life assess the physical and neuromuscular maturity of the infant. Included in each of the two major categories are selected items that can be scored and the total score obtained allows the practitioner to make a determination of gestational age. One such tool was designed by Dubowitz (see Appendix) and coworkers (1970). A chart to estimate gestational age was developed by Brazie and Lubchenco and can be found in *Current Pediatric Diagnosis and Treatment* (Kempe, Silver, and O'Brien, 1978). Skill in administering these examinations requires practice with the supervision of an experienced clinician.

The Neonatal Behavioral Assessment Scale (see Appendix) developed by Dr. T. Berry Brazelton and associates is designed to assess the infant's interactive behavior during the neonatal period. "It is an attempt to score the infant's available responses to his environment, and so, indirectly his effect on the environment" (Brazelton, 1973, p. 4). The test includes twenty-seven behavioral items and repeated assessments are suggested rather than just one assessment. There are findings that suggest that this tool can be useful in predicting developmental outcomes. It can be used to discriminate between the abnormal baby and the normal baby. It is also very useful in helping parents understand their infant's behavior when parents are included in the testing process. Training in the proper administration of the test is required.*

There are few tools designed to assess infant temperament beyond the first month of life. Therefore, the tool developed by William B. Carey and Sean C. McDevitt is useful. They developed the Carey Infant Temperament Questionnaire for detecting the temperament of infants between 4 and 8 months of age. The questionnaire consists of ninety-five questions relating to behaviors seen during feeding, sleep, elimination, and other activities, and the parent is asked to respond according to a scale from "almost never" to "almost always." Determination of the infant's temperament or behavior is important in understanding how he interacts with his environment. The identification of the infant's temperament profile makes it possible to individualize the help offered to parents in handling and caring for their infant. The questionnaire is available from Dr. Carey.†

The Denver Developmental Screening Test (DDST) developed by W.K. Frankenburg and J.B. Dodds is a tool for the detection of developmental delays during infancy and the preschool years up to 6 years of age (see Appendix). It is not an IQ test but the results help in the estimation of the child's current developmental level. It is a valuable tool in determining the child's developmental needs and provides a basis for planning anticipatory guidance. Items were selected from twelve developmental and preschool intelligence tests on the basis of (1) ease of administration and interpretation and (2) a relatively short time from the point at which a few children could perform an item to the point at which most children could perform the item. The items are organized to give an overall developmental profile with emphasis on gross motor, language, fine motor-adaptive, and personal-social skills. Both professionals and paraprofessionals can learn to administer the DDST with training. Self-instructional units are available so that each individual can learn to use a standardized method of test administration. An instructional unit is also available with a manual, workbook, and film for class instruction, and a proficiency evaluation. Requests for information about the availability of materials for training should be addressed to LADOCA.*

The Denver Articulation Screening Examination (see Appendix) was developed by Amelia F. Drumwright, a speech pathologist, with the purpose of devising a screening test of articulation skill that would "1.) reliably detect disorders in preschool children aged 2½ to 6 years and 2.) be useful and acceptable to speech pathologists, yet readily understandable to other child workers (doctors, nurses, teachers and subprofessionals)" (Drumwright and others, 1973). The examination requires the child to repeat twenty-two words that represent thirty speech sounds. The examiner evaluates sound production and makes an overall judgment about the intelligibility of the child's speech. The norms are presented for children between the ages of 2½ and 6 years. The manuals, test materials, and information about training should be requested from LADOCA.

DEVELOPMENTAL STAGES
Infancy

During the brief period of infancy, from birth to 18 months, the infant develops from a dependent, helpless newborn into a person who walks, talks, and relates to different people in terms of their importance in his life. He begins interacting with his environment from the moment of birth. A rudimentary ego identity, sense of self, evolves as he gradually learns to see himself as separate from his environment and gains feelings of faith and optimism as the core problem "trust vs mistrust" (Erikson, 1968) is initially resolved. He develops intellectual and motor skills that enable him to move from almost total helplessness at birth to being an aggressive explorer at 18 months of age.

The velocity of growth during the first few months and years of life is greater than at any other time but proceeds at a decelerating rate. The newborn infant, on the average, weighs 7 to 7½ pounds at birth and will lose up to 10% of that weight during the first few days of life. The birth weight is usually regained by the tenth day and the infant will then continue to gain steadily. He will double his birth weight during the first 4 months and then triple it by 1 year. During the second year the average weight gain is 6 to 7 pounds. The average length of the newborn is 20 inches, which will increase by 50% during the first year but will not double until 4 years of age.

Marked changes occur in the body contour during infancy. The head grows at a fairly rapid rate during

---

*A list of trained examiners who can provide training can be obtained by writing to the principal investigator, Dr. T. Berry Brazelton. There are also training films available for use with the published manual. These can be obtained by writing to Educational Development Corporations, 8 Mifflin Place, Cambridge, Mass. 02138.
†William B. Carey, M.D., 319 W. Front St., Media, Pa. 19063.

*LADOCA Project and Publishing Co., East 51st Ave. and Lincoln St., Denver, Colo. 80216.

Table 4-1
Child development from 1 month to 5 years—cont'd

6 MONTHS

Motor
1. Supine: lifts head spontaneously.
2. Bounces on feet when held standing.
3. Sits briefly (tripod fashion).
4. Rolls front to back (6-7 months).
5. Grasps foot and plays with toes.
6. Grasps cube with palm.

Language
7. Vocalizes at mirror image.
8. Makes four or more different sounds.
9. Localizes source of sound (bell, voice).
10. Vague, formless babble (especially with family members).

Personal-social-adaptive
11. Holds one cube in each hand.
12. Puts cube into mouth.
13. Resecures dropped cube.
14. Transfers cube from hand to hand.
15. Conscious of strange sights and persons.
16. Consistent regard of object or person (6-7 months).
17. Uses raking movement to secure raisin or pellet.
18. Resists having toy taken away from him.
19. Stretches out arms to be taken up (6-8 months).

8 MONTHS

Motor
1. Sits alone (6-8 months).
2. Early stepping movements.
3. Tries to crawl.
4. Stands few seconds, holding on to object.
5. Leans forward to get an object.

Language
6. Two-syllable babble, such as: a-la, ba-ba, oo-goo, a-ma, mama, dada (8-10 months).
7. Listens to conversation (8-10 months).
8. "Shouts" for attention (8-10 months).

Personal-social-adaptive
9. Works to get toy out of reach.
10. Scoops pellet.
11. Rings bell purposely (8-10 months).
12. Drinks from cup.
13. Plays peek-a-boo.
14. Looks for dropped object.
15. Bites and chews toys.
16. Pats mirror image.
17. Bangs spoon on table.
18. Manipulates paper or string.
19. Secures ring by pulling on the string.
20. Feeds self crackers.

10 MONTHS

Motor
1. Gets self into sitting position.
2. Sits steadily (long time).
3. Pulls self to standing position (on bed railing).
4. Crawls on hands and knees.
5. Walks when held or around furniture.
6. Turns around when left on floor.

Language
7. Imitates speech sounds.
8. Shakes head for "no."
9. Waves "bye-bye."
10. Responds to name.
11. Vocalizes in varied jargon-patterns (10-12 months).

Personal-social-adaptive
12. Plays "pat-a-cake."
13. Picks up pellet with finger and thumb.
14. Bangs toys together.
15. Extends toy to a person.
16. Holds own bottle.
17. Removes cube from cup.
18. Drops one cube to get another.
19. Uses handle to lift cup.
20. Initially shy with strangers.

1 YEAR

Motor
1. Walks with one hand held.
2. Stands alone (or with support).
3. Secures small object with good pincer grasp.
4. Pivots in sitting position.
5. Grasps two cubes in one hand.

Language
6. Uses "mama" or "dada" with specific meaning.
7. "Talks" to toys and people, using fairly long verbal patterns.
8. Has vocabulary of two words besides "mama" and "dada."
9. Babbles to self when alone.
10. Obeys simple requests, such as: "Give me the cup."
11. Reacts to music.

Personal-social-adaptive
12. Cooperates with dressing.
13. Plays with cup, spoon, saucer.
14. Points with index finger.
15. Pokes finger (into stethoscope) to explore.
16. Releases toy into your hand.
17. Tries to take cube out of box.
18. Unwraps a cube.
19. Holds cup to drink.
20. Holds crayon.
21. Tries to imitate scribble.
22. Imitates beating two cubes together.
23. Gives affection.

15 MONTHS

Motor
1. Stands alone.
2. Creeps upstairs.
3. Kneels on floor or chair.
4. Gets off floor and walks alone with good balance.
5. Bends over to pick up toy without holding on to furniture.

Language
6. May speak four to six words (15-18 months).
7. Uses jargon.
8. Indicates wants by vocalizing.
9. Knows own name.
10. Enjoys rhymes or jingles.

Table 4-1

Child development from 1 month to 5 years—cont'd

Personal-social-adaptive

11. Tilts cup to drink.
12. Uses spoon but spills.
13. Builds tower of two cubes.
14. Drops cubes into cup.
15. Helps turn page in book, pats picture.
16. Shows or offers toy.
17. Helps pull off clothes.
18. Puts pellet into bottle without demonstration.
19. Opens lid of box.
20. Likes to push wheeled toys.

18 MONTHS

Motor

1. Runs (stiffly).
2. Walks upstairs—one hand held.
3. Walks backwards.
4. Climbs into chair.
5. Hurls ball.

Language

6. May say six to ten words (18-21 months).
7. Points to at least one body part.
8. Can say "hello" and "thank you."
9. Carries out two directions (one at a time), for instance: "Get ball from table."—"Give ball to mother."
10. Identifies two objects by pointing (or picking up), such as: cup, spoon, dog, car, chair.

Personal-social-adaptive

11. Turns pages.
12. Builds tower of three to four cubes.
13. Puts 10 cubes into cup.
14. Carries or hugs a doll.
15. Takes off shoes and socks.
16. Pulls string toy.
17. Scribbles spontaneously.
18. Dumps raisin from bottle after demonstration.
19. Uses spoon with little spilling.

21 MONTHS

Motor

1. Runs well.
2. Walks downstairs—one hand held.
3. Walks upstairs alone or holding on to rail.
4. Kicks large ball (when demonstrated).

Language

5. May speak fifteen to twenty words (21-24 months).
6. May combine two to three words.
7. Asks for food, drink.
8. Echoes two or more words.
9. Takes three directions (one at a time), for instance: "Take ball from table."—"Give ball to Mommy."—"Put ball on floor."
10. Points to three or more body parts.

Personal-social-adaptive

11. Builds tower of five to six cubes.
12. Folds paper once when shown.
13. Helps with simple household tasks (21-24 months).

14. Removes some clothing purposefully (besides hat or socks).
15. Pulls person to show something.

2 YEARS

Motor

1. Runs without falling.
2. Walks up and down stairs.
3. Kicks large ball (without demonstration).
4. Throws ball overhand.
5. Claps hands.
6. Opens door.
7. Turns pages in book, singly.

Language

8. Says simple phrases.
9. Says at least one sentence or phrase of four or more syllables.
10. Can repeat four to five syllables.
11. May reproduce about five to six consonant sounds. (Typically: m-p-b-h-w).
12. Points to four parts of body on command.
13. Asks for things at table by name.
14. Refers to self by name.
15. May use personal pronouns, such as: I-me-you (2-2½ years).

Personal-social-adaptive

16. Builds five- to seven-cube tower.
17. May cut with scissors.
18. Spontaneously dumps raisin from bottle (without demonstration).
19. Throws ball into box.
20. Imitates drawing vertical line from demonstration.
21. Parallel play predominant.

2½ YEARS

Motor

1. Jumps in place with both feet.
2. Tries standing on one foot (may not be successful).
3. Holds crayon by fingers.
4. Imitates walking on tiptoe.

Language

5. Refers to self by pronoun (rather than name).
6. Names common objects when asked (key, penny, shoe, box, book).
7. Repeats two digits (one of three trials).
8. Answers simple questions, such as: "What is this?"—"What does the kitty say?"

Personal-social-adaptive

9. Builds tower of eight cubes.
10. Pushes toy with good steering.
11. Helps put things away.
12. Can carry breakable objects.
13. Puts on clothing.
14. Washes and dries hands.
15. Eats with fork.
16. Imitates drawing a horizontal line from demonstration.
17. May imitate drawing a circle from demonstration.

Continued.

Table 4-1
Child development from 1 month to 5 years—cont'd

---

3 YEARS

Motor
1. Stands on one foot for at least 1 second.
2. Jumps from bottom stair.
3. Alternates feet going upstairs.
4. Pours from a pitcher.
5. Can undo two buttons.
6. Pedals a tricycle.

Language
7. Repeats six syllables, for instance: "I have a little dog."
8. Names three or more objects in a picture.
9. Gives sex. ("Are you a boy or a girl?")
10. Gives full name.
11. Repeats three digits (one of three trials).
12. Knows a few rhymes.
13. Gives appropriate answers to: "What: swims-flies-shoots-boils-bites-melts?"
14. Uses plurals.
15. Knows at least one color.
16. Can reply to questions in at least three word sentences.
17. May have vocabulary of 750 to 1,000 words (3-3½ years).

Personal-social-adaptive
18. Understands taking turns.
19. Copies a circle (from model, without demonstration).
20. Builds three-block pyramid (⛫).
21. Dresses with supervision.
22. Puts 10 pellets into bottle in 30 seconds.
23. Separates easily from mother.
24. Feeds self well.
25. Plays interactive games, such as "tag."

4 YEARS

Motor
1. Stands on one foot for at least 5 seconds (two of three trials).
2. Hops at least twice on one foot.
3. Can walk heel-to-toe for four or more steps (with heel 1 inch or less in front of toe).
4. Can button coat or dress; may lace shoes.

Language
5. Repeats ten-word sentences without errors.
6. Counts three objects, pointing correctly.
7. Repeats three to four digits (4-5 years).
8. Comprehends: "What do you do if: you are hungry, sleepy, cold?"
9. Spontaneous sentences, four to five words long.
10. Likes to ask questions.

11. Understands prepositions, such as: on-under-behind, etc. ("Put the block *on* the table.")
12. Can point to three out of four colors (red, blue, green, yellow).
13. Speech is now an effective communication tool.

Personal-social-adaptive
14. Copies cross (+) without demonstration.
15. Imitates oblique cross (×).
16. Draws a man with four parts.
17. Cooperates with other children in play.
18. Dresses and undresses self (mostly without supervision).
19. Brushes teeth, washes face.
20. Compares lines: "Which is longer?"
21. Folds paper two to three times.
22. Can select heavier from lighter object.
23. Cares for self at toilet.

5 YEARS

Motor
1. Balances on one foot for 8 to 10 seconds.
2. Skips, using feet alternately.
3. May be able to tie a knot.
4. Catches bounced ball with hands (not arms) in two of three trials.

Language
5. Knows age ("How old are you?")
6. Performs three tasks (with one command), for instance: "Put pen on table—close door—bring me the ball."
7. Knows four colors.
8. Defines use for: fork-horse-key-pencil, etc.
9. Identifies by name: nickel-dime-penny.
10. Asks meaning of words.
11. Asks many "why" questions.
12. Relatively few speech errors remain—90% of consonant sounds are made correctly.
13. Counts number of fingers correctly.
14. Counts by rote to 10.
15. Comments on pictures (descriptions and interpretations).

Personal-social-adaptive
16. Copies a square.
17. Copies oblique cross (×) without demonstration.
18. May print a few letters (5-5½ years).
19. Draws man with at least six identifiable parts.
20. Builds a six-block pyramid from demonstration.
21. Transports things in a wagon.
22. Plays with coloring set, construction toys, puzzles.
23. Participates well in group play.

baby? The infant begins to smile in response to stimuli in the environment and to produce vocal sounds. Most responses are generalized and frequently involve movements of the whole body. The infant during this period has social responses but does not discriminate and any person who can satisfy his needs will be accepted.

By 3 months of age the baby becomes more discriminating. He begins to differentiate mother from others and produces special types of smiles and crying for her, which is the beginning of attachment behavior and the development of awareness of the self as separate from her. Between ages 3 and 6 months he begins to repeat actions that are interesting as well as prolong those that occur accidentally, for instance, repeatedly hitting at toys suspended in the crib to produce movement. He begins to imitate facial movements and sounds. He will look for a displaced object but will not conduct a true search. The infantile reflexes are replaced by purposeful movements, especially those seen in the development of eye-hand coordination. He begins to reach for and grasp objects with a raking motion. The tonic neck reflex and Moro reflex disappear during the fifth or sixth month. At 3 months the infant can, while in the prone position, raise head and chest from the surface with arms extended; at 4 months he can hold his head steadily while being supported in the sitting position; and at 6 months he will begin to sit without support.

The period between 6 and 12 months of life is dominated by the social modality of "taking and holding on" as described by Erikson. It is also described by Bowlby (1969) as being a period of active attachment behavior. The infant at 8 to 9 months of age has a beginning concept of object permanence and becomes fearful that the mother (object) will disappear. He actively initiates contact with her and seeks to maintain that contact. There is true searching for a vanished object, although he may expect to find it in several inappropriate places. His behavior becomes more complex and aggressive. He coordinates earlier repetitive actions into behaviors with a purposeful aim. He now explores objects more fully by rubbing, banging, and chewing them and rapidly discovers correct procedures for manipulating them. Motor development is dramatic as coordination increases. He develops the pincer grasp using the thumb and forefinger, learns to stand, and begins to walk holding on to furniture. He does more vocalizing and begins using pseudowords at about 10 to 12 months of age.

Between 12 and 18 months the infant becomes a toddler. He assumes an upright position and previously acquired motor skills are improved and expanded. Attachment behavior continues to be intense and he

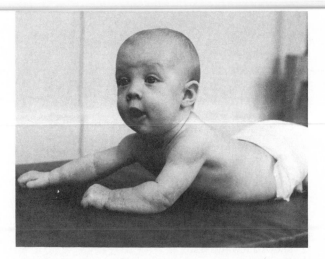

He can raise his chest off the table at 3 months of age.

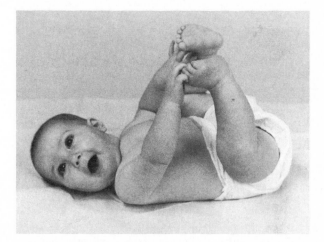

Learning is focused on body actions the first 7 to 9 months of age.

needs his mother close by to explore new places or to cope with threatening situations. Strangers will be treated with caution. However, he thoroughly enjoys his new abilities and is enthusiastically persistent and uninhibited in his attempts to manipulate things in his environment. He continues repetitive play with objects and enjoys putting things in and taking them out of a box as the experimentation with objects and object permanence continues. During the last months of this period cognitive development is such that the infant begins to replace the earlier sensorimotor mental images that are nonverbal and have a highly personal meaning with mental symbols that are the beginning of language and he acquires approximately 20 words besides "mama" and "dada."

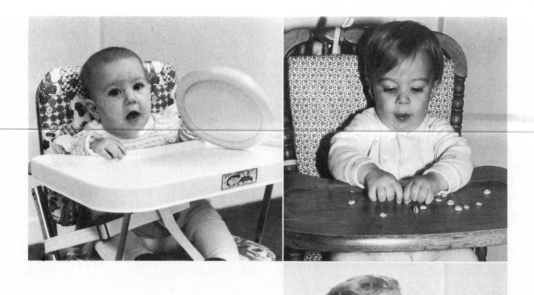

The development of competency is rapid during the first years of life.

Early childhood

The infant moves into the early childhood years well equipped to continue learning about himself and his world. His ability to see himself as separate from his environment, his sense of trust and hope, and his developing intellectual and motor skills allow "autonomy" to blossom. Ego growth is rapid during the second and third years of life as the child continues his exploration and learning about the objects in his environment and gains increasing mastery of his impulses and body functions. He gains a sense of autonomy, a feeling of independence as a separate person.

The ages between 3 and 6 are marked by social, emotional, and intellectual development. The child is developing a sense of himself as a social person in relation to other people. He is also learning about the physical world. As the child identifies with the parents he loves, he is motivated to be what they want him to be as well as to be like them. A conscience, or super-

ego, develops as he begins to internalize the standards of his society as interpreted by his parents. He also becomes involved in the romance with the parent of the opposite sex and learns and accepts a sex role identity. The child's thinking remains egocentric throughout this period. He cannot take the other person's point of view and does not seek to clarify or validate his own point of view. The child learns to use symbols in representational thought and begins to think about objects, people, and actions that are not present.

This period of development is not defined by chronological age because there is overlapping with the infant years and the school years. The core problems described by Erikson are "autonomy vs shame" during the toddler years from 1 to 3 and "initiative vs guilt" during the preschool years between 3 and 6. Cognitive development during this entire period from about 18 months to 7 years is described as "preoper-

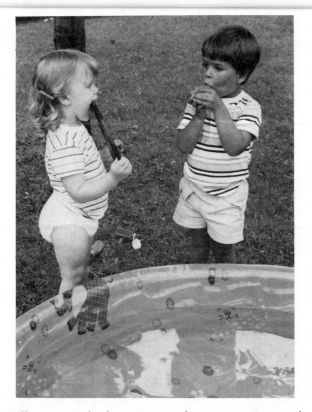

Differences in body contour and posture at 1 year of age and 3 years of age.

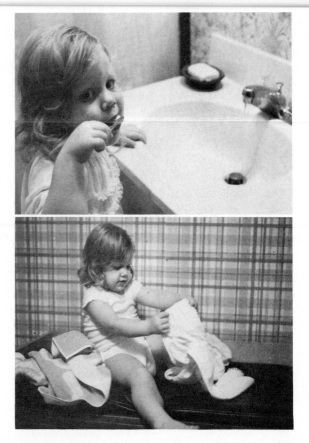

The 3½-year-old takes more responsibility for daily care.

ational" by Piaget and it is during these years that the child begins to acquire mental symbols and develop representational thought.

Growth continues at a decelerating rate. At 2 years the child will have added about 75% of his birth length to his height and at 4 years he will have doubled his birth length. Weight increments continue at a decelerating rate between 2 and 4 years of age, followed by a very gradual acceleration between 4 and 6 years. As the rate of growth in height and weight becomes slower, it also becomes less consistent month by month.

The changes in the child's physical appearance are dramatic. The toddler, as he begins to walk, looks top-heavy with his short legs and his potbelly. Fat pads obliterate the arch of the foot and most young children appear to be flat-footed until 3 or 4 years of age. There is also a tendency for the legs to bow inward and for lordosis to be apparent. The posture and body proportions change. The chest becomes larger in proportion to the head and the abdomen after 2 years of age, the extremities continue to grow faster than the trunk, and the jaw and lower face grow more rapidly than the cranium. The subcutaneous fat decresases rapidly in thickness during the second year and continues to decrease at a slower rate until 5 or 6 years of age, while

muscle tissue continues to grow at a decelerating rate. Because of these changes the child becomes less chubby, the potbelly gradually becomes flatter, and the face loses its babyish look. By the time the child reaches the age of 5 or 6 appearance will be more like that of the older child than that of an infant or young toddler.

Other changes that occur include the improvement in visual acuity. The infant and young child are far-sighted and visual acuity at 2 years of age is estimated to be 20/40, compared to 20/20 between 4 and 5 years of age. The brain will reach 75% of its adult weight by 3 years and approximately 90% by 7 years. The skin changes after the first year and becomes tougher with less water content. The eruption of the primary teeth continues and the child will have the full complement of 20 primary teeth early during the third year when the second molars erupt.

During the second and third years of life, when neuromuscular coordination and intellectual development make it possible for him to actively explore and experiment, the toddler strives to establish a sense of autonomy. He is motivated to assert himself and is uninhibited in the pursuit of his own goals. He has no limiting controls within himself and forges ahead. However, his wish to assert himself can bring him into conflict with his parents when he is confronted with the restrictions that are necessary to help him adapt to society's standards and control his primitive impulses. This is frustrating to him and tantrums are common. It can also be fear-provoking because he needs and wants his parent's love and approval. Despite his omnipotent behavior he is very dependent and wants to please. Therefore, he needs an environment that allows him to make free choices within limits that protect him from making choices that result in disappointing or disastrous consequences. Because he is not always certain of where his impulses will take him, he needs the reassurance that there are limits that protect him. The child gradually accepts limitations as he learns that he is safer and more comfortable when he pays attention to his mother instead of proceeding according to his own wishes. Attachment behaviors continue and, although he becomes increasingly able to play alone for longer

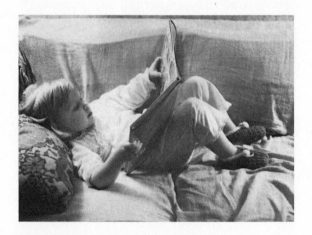

She has learned that she can lie on the couch to read a book like her mother does (3½ years).

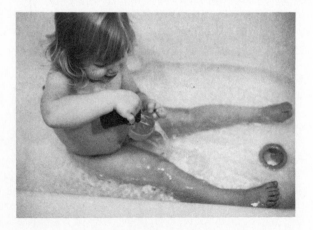

The 3½-year-old enjoys creative water play.

periods of time, he will periodically seek his mother or go to her if threatened in any way. The young child who is faced with a new situation will venture forward with much more assurance if his mother is present. He also needs to turn to her for comfort when things get too difficult. The child during these years is sensitive to changes in the environment because his thinking is organized in a global way. His perceptions are such that, if there is one alteration, the "whole" is changed and becomes strange to him. Therefore, a consistent routine for daily activities is helpful to him. He can anticipate what will happen, learn the behaviors that are expected of him, and gain a feeling of controlling the situation and performing well. Rituals also become important at this age and reach a peak around age 2½. This is most evident at bedtime when the child is dealing with separation. If everything is done the same way each night, he is reassured that his world will not change while he sleeps.

Play during these toddler years begins with exploration and discovery but, as the child gains ability to form mental images, his play becomes imaginative and imitative. He incorporates pieces of reality by imitating. He may imitate an animal or his mother's action. The toddler appears to enjoy the company of other children but does not play with them—he plays beside them. He often treats them as if they were objects and feels free to poke, bite, or push them because he has no inner sense that this is hurtful. His egocentrism is such that if he feels no pain it must be all right. His pleasure in learning about things by touching, feeling, and manipulating is also seen in his early attempts to feed himself, brush his teeth, or drink from a cup. He is naturally messy. However, he is inclined to imitate and copy the behavior of his parents and by 3 years of age will become fairly competent.

Between 3 and 6 years of age the young child becomes more socially responsive and able to give love and affection. The development of initiative is characterized by the wish "to become," a wish to find out what kind of person he can and will be. During the earlier years he achieved a sense of himself as a separate person, a person with some power to influence his environment and control his own impulses and his body. These accomplishments make it possible for him to approach his new tasks with wonderful feelings of confidence and with lots of energy. The social modality is "to make" in the sense of "being on the make" (Erikson, 1963, p. 90). The child becomes intrusive in his desire to attack new situations (and bodies). Erikson says the child at this age intrudes into everyone's space with his locomotion and into everyone's ears with his aggressive talking. The child is noisy, active, and on the move, and thrusts himself into each situation as if driven by his curiosity and imagination. His love and admiration for his parents intensify and his identification with them increases. Sexual identification was begun at an earlier age when the child learned that he was a boy or a girl but during these preschool years it is heightened. It becomes evident as the child begins to model himself to be like the parent of the same sex and becomes acutely aware of sexual differences. His interest in the parent of the opposite sex becomes romantic, which results in conflict as he learns that he cannot displace the parent of the same sex whom he also loves. His feelings of intense love and the wish to be rid of one parent can cause anxiety and fear because the child believes that his wishes are as real as the actual deed. His task is to inhibit his sexual feelings and learn his sexual role and his role in the family. This process allows him to internalize the parents' standards and ideals and gradually develop a sense of moral responsibility. An infantile conscience develops, which makes it possible for him to resist temptation even though his parents are not present. He begins to feel guilt for misbehavior and at approximately 5 years of age he will even feel guilt for wishing to misbehave. This early conscience will be modified throughout the years of childhood as his intellectual abilities increase and his ability to identify reasons for moral action becomes more mature. Play during the preschool years becomes more social and imaginative. The social play of children at this age is complex as they learn to interact with each other while developing concepts, imagination, neuromuscular coordination, and language. Erikson describes this as the play age when the child is offered a microreality in which he uses toys to work out problems and anticipate future roles (Erikson, 1977, p. 99). Through imaginative and creative play the child tries out the roles of different people and also alleviates some of the guilt that occurs as the result of his developing conscience. In play he can be what he wants to be and gain mastery of his fears and alleviate guilt. He can feel strong and adequate instead of little and vulnerable. He can build the biggest castle or paint a beautiful picture. Through play he incorporates the behaviors of his role models, especially his parents, into his own standards of behavior, which helps him understand that he cannot replace his parent but can someday grow up and be a parent himself.

The young child's thinking during these years between 2 and 7 is limited by his egocentrism. He can see only one point of view—his own. He cannot make comparisons mentally so the logic of his own point of view cannot be challenged and he believes that everyone perceives things the same way that he does. He feels no need to justify his own conclusions and takes little notice of how other people think. When communicating with other people, he makes little attempt to relate to what the other person is saying or thinking and, if the listener is not familiar with the incident that he is talking about, his account will make no sense.

Cognitive development is reflected in the child's development of language. Early in the second year of life the child acquires personal, nonverbal mental images of objects and events. His first words and gestures are also invested with unique personal meanings. His vocabulary increases rapidly during these years, which signals the appearance of thought with internal language and signs that allow him to think about objects and people not present and to anticipate future events. However, language does not immediately take the place of action thinking and the young child cannot think through a series of actions. He must actually perform them. His thinking is also characterized by "centering," which means that only one attribute of an object or event stands out in the child's perception. For instance, he can sort objects by color or by form but not by both.

Middle childhood

During the middle years of childhood, from 6 to 10 years, the child moves from the close ties to his family and home to the larger world of peers, his school, and his neighborhood. The family romance is less intense and he is able to go out into the world. It is during this period of latency that the child is free from his earlier concentration on his sexuality and his strong basic drives. He can now direct his energy toward learning the skills and competencies of the mind and body that lead to practical achievements and accomplishments in his culture. There is tremendous intellectual growth during this lull before the storm of adolescence and the child is introduced to learning experiences that help him master the fundamental technology of his culture.

Physical growth and development

Growth during the middle years of childhood is relatively slow and smooth. The characteristic body type has emerged during the preschool years and is confirmed during the middle years; the short child remains short and the tall child remains tall. The increments in weight are less regular than seen in the young infant and child and may remain stationary for weeks at a time. The approximate annual increase in weight is about 5 to 7 pounds. The average annual increase in height is approximately 2 to 3 inches each year. Boys on the average are taller and heavier than girls until the adolescent growth spurt, which occurs earlier in girls. Although the growth spurt will be discussed in relation to the child from 10 to 14 years of age, it is important to recognize that some elementary school age children will already have begun the growth spurt as early as age 8 or 9.

The physical changes that occur make school age children more agile and graceful. They become slimmer, with longer legs and a lower center of gravity than the younger child. They are stronger and better coordinated and are able to fit into the adult physical environment more easily. There is only a slight increase in the size of the cranium because nearly 90% of the growth of the brain is accomplished by age 7. The lower parts of the face continue to grow, giving the child a more mature appearance and making room for the larger teeth to erupt. The first permanent teeth to erupt at 6 to 6½ years of age are usually the mandibular central incisors. The eruption of the large permanent teeth contributes to the so-called ugly duckling appearance of the school age child.

The eyeball continues to grow until 10 or 12 years of age. Visual acuity is usually 20/20 between 4 and 5 years of age, but depth perception is not very accurate until 6 to 7 years of age. Hearing is well established at a much earlier age. Lymphoid tissue increases steadily until puberty and then decreases. This accounts for the abundance of lymphoid tissues such as adenoids and tonsils. The skeleton continues to ossify, with cartilage being replaced by bone. The child has acquired the basic neuromuscular mechanisms by age 6 or 7 and will spend the school years in refining his skills, resulting in an increase in motor skill and coordination.

Thus, the school age child engages in repetition practice in all areas of neuromuscular activities from the fine motor skills of writing to the large motor skills used in baseball, bike riding, and swimming, depending on individual interests.

Psychosocial and cognitive development

By 6 years of age the child's personality has become structured. Through mastery of the earlier developmental crisis he has achieved a concept of self as separate from his environment, acquired a sense of trust, developed autonomy with some power over his own impulses and environment, incorporated standards of his culture as interpreted by his parents, and sublimated the desire "to make" people. According to psychoanalytical theory he has an ego, id, superego, and ego ideal and can deal with the next core problem described by Erikson—industry vs inferiority.

During this period Erikson says the child becomes a worker. He is required to develop intellectual skills, physical skills, and social skills that contribute to his adequacy. The child is sent to school and play is transformed into work, games into competition and cooperation, and the freedom of imagination into the duty to perform (Erikson, 1977, pp. 103-104). The child's attainments in interpersonal and social development are important. The child is now able to see a higher organization of behavior in which he can and does participate. He wants to operate in socially accepted ways

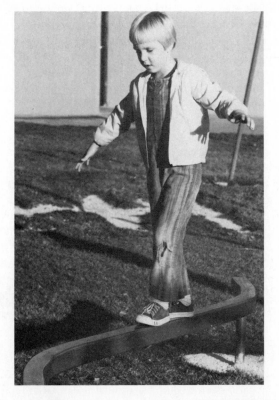

The 6-year-old has good neuromuscular coordination.

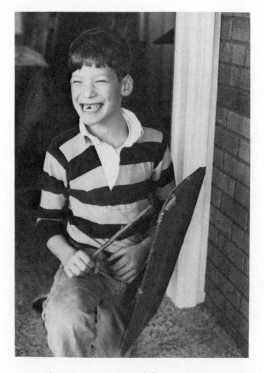

Play is creative and fun at 7 years.

of thinking and behaving. He can take another person's point of view and compare it with his own. He can compare what he hears and sees with what he knows and make judgments about their reality. Also, he is able to reason and can act according to rules, which allows him to benefit from school experiences and to participate in organized play.

As the child moves into the larger world of school and peers, he will continue to need his parents. Demands for conformity are placed on him by people outside the family, such as teachers, scout leaders, and peers. He will continue to need his parents' support and the approval of his teachers and other important adults, but he also needs to find his place in a group of peers. He is ready to be involved in the private world of children where adults are not always welcome. This becomes more apparent toward the end of latency when the child withdraws more into the privacy of his peer group, which is an important socializing agent. Feelings of group solidarity and belongingness are promoted by secret languages and codes as well as a common culture. Together children explore ideas and values as well as their environment.

The cognitive development of the school age child according to Piaget is characterized by the ability to begin to do mentally what he would have had to do with real action at an earlier age. "Piaget illustrated this by presenting 5-, 6-, and 7-year-old children with six sticks in a row and asking them to take the same number from a pile on the table. The younger children solved the problem by placing the sticks beneath the sample and matching the sticks one by one. The older children merely picked up six sticks and held them in their hands. The older children had counted the sticks mentally" (Elkind, 1974, p. 23). The school age child also sees the multiple characteristics of objects rather than centering on only one aspect. For instance, in one study Piaget placed twenty white and seven brown wooden beads in a box and asked individual 5-, 6-, and 7-year-old children if there were more white beads or more wooden beads. The young children could only respond that there were more white beads than brown beads. The older children could determine that there were more wooden beads than white beads because all of the beads were wooden (Elkind, 1974, p. 28). The older children were able to see the whole without losing sight of the uniqueness of the individual parts.

Piaget also found that it is during these years that the child masters the concept of conservation. The child begins to differentiate between the appearances of things and how they really are. Piaget's classic test is to give the child two jars of equal size containing equal amounts of liquid. The contents of one jar are then poured into two smaller containers of equal size and the child is asked whether the amount of liquid poured into the two smaller jars is still the same as that remaining in the other container. The younger children cannot comprehend that the liquid has been conserved when placed in smaller containers. The older children can because they can now make mental comparisons rather than actually manipulating objects, can see the whole as well as the parts, and have mastered the concept of conservation. They are ready for the cognitive task of mastering classes, relationships, and quantities.

However, this new ability to reason and to carry out mental operations in solving problems is limited in a very important respect. They can reason about concrete things but not about verbal propositions. They cannot differentiate between their own assumptions and the facts. In other words, they treat their own hypotheses as if they were facts and reject facts that do not agree with that position. Elkind has defined this as

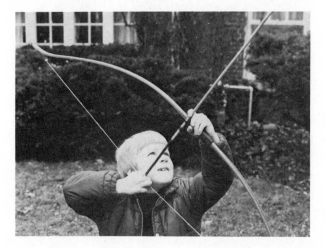

The 8-year-old concentrates on achieving a skill.

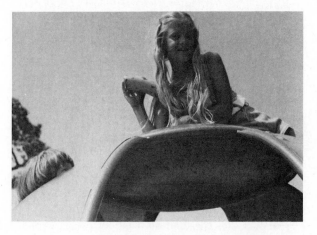

The 10-year-old enjoys her physical skills.

"cognitive conceit" (1974, p. 80). For instance, when the child learns that parents are not always right, there are two prevalent assumptions. One of these is that the adults are not too bright and the other is that the child knows more than the adult. Elkind points out that this behavior is often demonstrated in a spirit of fun or teasing as though the children are aware that they are using a convenient fiction.

"Cognitive conceit" is also useful in understanding the moral behavior of latency age children. Children of this age have internalized rules and know what is right and wrong. However, they continue throughout latency to break the rules they see as being made by adults. The child takes the rules as a challenge to his intellectual superiority and attempts to break them without being caught. School age children continue to operate with this kind of external conscience until the end of childhood when they start to formulate their own rules that will internally regulate their behavior.

Children experience success during this stage of industry as they participate in the many productive activities. They experience a sense of accomplishment that leads to the feelings of adequacy and worth vs the feelings of inferiority that come with repeated failure. School age children's great desire to win at games and willingness to work to achieve a variety of skills demonstate their need to be adequate in their own eyes as well as in the eyes of others.

Preadolescence and adolescence
Preadolescence

The precise parameters of age and developmental levels begin to blend and overlap with the late childhood years. From that point on, a range of years, rather than a precise number, describes each developmental level. Some consider the "late childhood" and "early teen" years as a separate and important category known as "preadolescence." It may be helpful to think in terms of this group as youngsters from ages 9 to 12 in the fifth to eighth grades with tasks, characteristics, and behaviors that differentiate them from children and also from adolescents. Youngsters in this group are at an in-between age; they are no longer cuddly children, nor are they quite yet into the dramatic changes that mark the adolescent's world. It might be said that the tasks of preadolescence have to do with preparation for those adolescent changes that lie only a few years ahead. It is a continuation of the change in primary affiliation with the adult society and the codes of parents to an affiliation with those of their peers. Some of the patterns of the child's personality begin to loosen up and alter in some disorganization preparatory to further growth.

Preadolescents characteristically have great physical restlessness. Running is more natural than walking. Sitting still, even through a meal, may seem nearly impossible. Signs of earlier childhood problems, such as nervous habits or antics or bed-wetting, may reappear temporarily before they are discarded. Muscular strength, skill, and agility are very important. In their quiet moments, which may be rather rare, preadolescents may have imaginative daydreams or may sit and stare blankly into space with apparently little on their minds. Although they may well have fears, worries, or concerns, they are not very interested in talking about them; but they may instead symbolically protect themselves from these problems by possessing toy guns, knives, or flashlights.

These years are often very trying times for parents as the parent-child bonds seem to be loosening and breaking. Although preadolescents do love and feel loyalty toward their parents, they may quite frequently treat them with surprising suspicion, distrust, and irritability. They are easily offended and respond to seemingly minor incidents with the ready accusation that adults do not understand them and, furthermore, treat them wrongly. At the same time, they are seemingly unaware of the effect of any of their own inconsiderateness or the feelings of others and are more or less surprised when it is pointed out to them that their behavior has caused some hurt. Other adults in the neighborhood may receive more admiration than the parents receive. Parental recommendations regarding use of language and matters of appearance and cleanliness are often met with a response of indignation and frequent conflict. They are increasingly sensitive about having a parent see their bodies and about public display of affection.

At this stage, boys and girls have little to do with each other socially, although girls may move through this phase more quickly than boys. Clique and gang formation is a prominent characteristic as they estab-

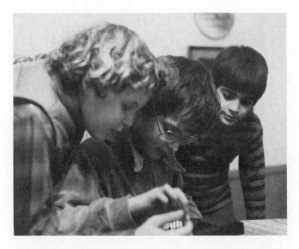

Preadolescence—establishing peer relationships.

lish strong identification with their peer groups. Often their pals and their peer codes do not meet with parental approval, which serves to make them all the more desirable to the preadolescent.

These changes of preadolescence are not easy for the parents, but neither are they easy for the preadolescent. There are often conflicting and painful choices, but the preadolescent must experience these to move on in the establishment of an individual identity.

Adolescence

The terms *adolescence* and *adult* are both derived from the Latin word *adolescere* meaning "to grow up." Both stages of life are, indeed, times of growth; however, the outward manifestations of growth during adolescence are the most dramatic. The age boundaries of adolescence are variable, although generally the teenage years (13 to 19) are used.

Adolescence is eminently a period of rapid and intense physical growth accompanied by profound changes that affect the entire organism. A physiological revolution occurs within and great concern develops over what the adolescent appears to be in the eyes of others compared with what he feels himself to be. According to Erikson (1963, 1968) the task of adolescence is the development of "ego identity" and the danger of the stage is "role confusion." The social world broadens in adolescence and the individual develops a growing sensitivity to the perceived judgments of others; one looks at oneself in comparison to others.

The word *conflict* is often associated with the words teenager and adolescent, and it is truly a stage of conflict and turmoil, as well as one of high growth potential in the physical, sexual, and social areas. The adolescent must learn to cope with increasingly intense impulses, now vested in a maturing genital apparatus, an altering body formation, and a powerful muscle sys-

tem. There is an increased muscular energy and strength, and spurts of physical growth.

Breast development is often the earliest visible sign of puberty in girls, beginning normally between the ages of 8 and 13 and ending between 13 and 18. Girls' pubic hair appears at about age 11, axillary hair about a year later, and the adult pattern of hair distribution is established by about age 14. Most girls begin to menstruate at age 12 to 13, but may normally start as early as 9 or as late as 18; the early cycles tend to be irregular and are often anovulatory.

In boys, testicular enlargement is usually the first pubescent change, starting between 10 and 13 and ending between 13 and 17. The voice begins to deepen at 13 to 14. The growth of pubic hair occurs between ages 12 and 16; the growth of the beard and chest hair is usually somewhat later, around age 16. The first ejaculation usually occurs at 11 to 13 years, but the sperm are immature.

The ages of 10 to 12 mark a spurt in height in girls, and by 14 to 15 their height growth is nearly complete. Boys of 12 to 13 have their rapid growth spurt. For some, this is preceded at about age 11 by a "stocky" or "chubby" period, which begins to decline as the spurt in height begins. By age 16, their height growth is nearly complete.

By the fourteenth year, the body of a girl is more often that of a young woman than that of a child, and for boys that year may mark a transition from boyhood to young manhood.

The behavioral traits of the adolescent years can also be described. The patterns of behavior during adolescence tend to fluctuate between outer- and inner-directedness as though the learnings of one phase need to be tested or reflected upon in the next. The adolescent needs periods for readjustment between the changing organism and the expanding environment. Growth is not a uniform, steady process but may show elements of "grown-up" helpfulness or childish lapses. It is an emotional period; the emotions should be considered symptoms of many forces—fears, struggles, and creative construction. Emotional growth requires creative struggle.

Gesell, Ilg, and Ames (1956) studied the behavioral traits of 10- to 16-year-olds. Their observations are summarized here, although the reader should be cautioned against expecting any set of behaviors during any given year. The sequence and flow of experiences are more important than the exact year during which they occur.

The 10-year-old may be casual and easygoing. He gets along well with parents, siblings (unless they are 1 to 3 years younger than he), and friends. Although the attention span is rather short, there is a zest for learning. There is a delight in physical activity and a sense of

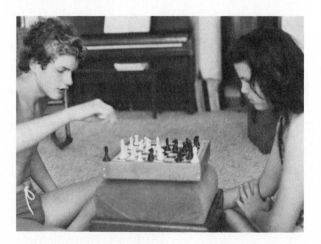

Adolescence—competition and creative conflict.

Major physical changes of adolescence

Female	Male
Breast development	Testicular enlargement
Growth of axillary and pubic hair	Deepening of voice
Onset of menses	Perceptible growth of thyroid cartilage
	Growth of facial, chest, and pubic hair

Both sexes
Spurts of growth in height
Facial and body contours change
Complexion may change with appearance of acne
Increased food intake
Increased muscular strength

Developmental tasks of adolescence

1. Continue to expand the sense of individual identity
2. Cope with increasingly intense impulses—physical, emotional, and sexual
3. Cope with fluctuations between inner- and outer-directedness
4. Develop a changing sense of one's body and new capabilities
5. Begin to develop self-reliance with decision making
6. Develop peer relationships
7. Continue formal learning experiences

fairness and sportsmanship. The 10-year-old may have explosive bursts of anger and may strike out violently, but these episodes tend to be brief and grudges are not harbored. In the area of conscience, he tends to be more aware of what is wrong than of what is right. He tends to be liberal in judgment. The shoulder shrug is a characteristic movement. "It is a golden age of developmental equipoise" (Gesell and others, 1956, p. 37).

The 11-year-old may be sensitive and self-assertive, curious and talkative. He likes to be in motion, loves to argue, and may attempt to mimic and also to criticize parents. The emotional life has variable moods and peaks of intensity, which reflect the relative immaturity of the new emotional developments. In school he is an enthusiastic learner and shows increased concentration. Among friends, he may tend to stir up relationships, moving from hostilities to reconciliations. He senses increased self-reliance and claims the right to make some decisions on his own.

The 12-year-old may be more balanced, more rea-

sonable, and discrete. He relies less on forthright challenges to realize selfhood and tries to win the approval of others. A group of 12-year-olds is a high-spirited one and it has a pervasive role in shaping the attitudes of its members. He is beginning to insist that he is a child no longer. He shows some increased ability to do independent work, though preference for the group is evident. Emotional behavior is coming under increased control, there are signs of insight into self and others, and there is a blend of tolerance, humor, and enthusiasm.

The 13-year-old may be more withdrawn and inner-directed. This is a reflective period—one that may be marked by spells of silence and musing. This new teenager may indulge in numerous private worries in phases of self-absorption. This is an indication of developing inner awareness, a time of releasing and reviewing inner feelings, tensions, and attitudes. Rage tends to be expressed more in words than in physical action as in the past. The 13-year-old is very sensitive to criticism and is more keenly aware of the emotional state of others. Siblings who are 2 to 5 years younger may be a source of great irritation and the parents may be found faulty, especially in problem areas the teenager is trying to resolve.

The 14-year-old may be more expansive and less withdrawn. He seems to enjoy a sense of self-assurance and is anxious to be popular with peers. It is the age of interminable phone conversations, particularly for girls. There is a growing ability to consider two sides of an issue and a development in the use of language. Certain interests acquired may become lifelong ones.

The 15-year-old may be enigmatic and complex, yet desires to be understood by himself and others. He may appear apathetic, while he is acutally preoccupied with inner-feeling states. He may appear resistant, irritable, and suspicious and may nurture feelings of revenge and violence. It is an age of increasing self-perception, a rising spirit of independence, and a loyalty to groups outside the home. Relationships in the home may deteriorate. The adolescent wants to "cut loose"; he is bored by the familiar and eager for new experiences.

The 16-year-old may be often accorded more status and seen as a "pre-adult." He may have achieved some of that sought-after sense of independence, is more self-possessed, and is beginning to think more about the future in terms of a career and family.

These processes and fluctuations continue to some degree for several years in the direction of greater maturation. The task of finding an acceptable work role career, one that is personally and potentially economically adequate, assumes a more central position during the later high school and college years. Sheehy (1974) describes the ages of 18 to 20 as a time of "pulling up roots." College, military service, and short-term trips all provide ways of leaving the family base; peers become substitues for family for periods of time, although rebounds to the family occur from time to time. "The tasks of this passage are to locate ourselves in a peer group role, a sex role, and anticipated occupation, an ideology or world view. As a result, we gather the impetus to leave home physically and the identity to begin leaving home emotionally" (Sheehy, 1974, p. 39). She notes that a stormy progression through this phase probably facilitates the normal progression of the adult life cycle.

Friedenberg notes the difficulty of adolescent passage in our Western society and emphasizes the importance of conflict to the individual and to society:

This process (of establishing a clear and stable self-identification) may be frustrated and emptied of meaning in a society which, like our own, is hostile to clarity and vividness. Our culture impedes the clear definition of any faithful self-image. . . . We do not break images . . . we blur and soften them. The resulting pliability gives life in our society its familiar plastic texture. It also makes adolescence more difficult, more dangerous and more troublesome to the adolescent and to society itself. And it makes adolescence rarer. Fewer youngsters really dare to go through with it; they merely undergo puberty and simulate maturity (p. 17). . . .

The promise of maturity must be fulfilled by those who are strong enough to grow into it at their own rate as full bargaining members. Must there be conflict between the adolescent and society? The point is that adolescence is conflict—protracted conflict—between the individual and society (p. 32). . . .

Adolescent conflict is the instrument by which an individual learns the complex, subtle and precious difference between himself and his environment . . . and leads, as a high synthesis to the youth's own adulthood and to critical participation in society as an adult (Friedenberg, 1959, p. 34).

Young adulthood

During the decade of ages 20 to 30, the major task is to achieve relative independence from parental figures and a sense of emotional, social, and economic responsibility for one's own life. Stevenson (1977) suggests the following developmental tasks:
1. Advancing self-development and the enactment of appropriate roles and positions in society
2. Initiating the development of a personal style of life
3. Adjusting to a heterosexual marital relationship or to another companionship style
4. Developing parenting behaviors for biological offspring, or in the broader framework of social parenting
5. Integrating personal values with career development and socioeconomic constraints

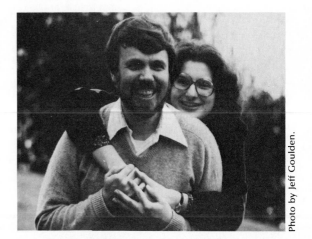

Young adults—choosing a life-style.

Photo by Jeff Goulden.

Erikson (1963), focusing more narrowly on marriage, describes the task of young adulthood as the development of affiliation or intimacy expressed as mutuality with a loved partner of the opposite sex with whom one is willing and able to regulate the cycles of work, procreation, and recreation. This involves the capacity to commit oneself "to concrete affiliations and partnerships and to develop the ethical strength to abide by such commitments, even though they may call for significant sacrifices and compromises" (p. 263). The danger of this stage is isolation or an avoidance of those persons and settings that promote and provide intimacy. A young adult whose identity work is not well underway may settle for sets of stereotyped interpersonal relationships that lead to a deep sense of isolation. This false "intimacy" bypasses the accomplishment of improved understanding of one's own inner resources and those of others.

Young adults may move out of the parental home or establish a more equal role with their parents if they stay in it. They begin to establish a style of single living, a marriage relationship, or another companionship style and adapt to the changes and compromises in expectations that their choice requires. Parenting tasks may be initiated by bearing children, adopting, becoming a foster parent, or reaching out in other ways, such as coaching children's teams or participating in child development–oriented organizations. It should also be noted that with divorce and remarriage, a frequent occurrence in American society, stepparenting and single parenting are fairly common situations. As children develop, parenting roles also develop in a reciprocal manner.

The young adult also chooses an area of study, a career, or a vocation and may begin to consider how one's belief about self and mankind affect that choice. Usually leisure time activities are selected and some young adults include participation in local community and organizational activities in addition to career and family development. Sheehy suggests that the focus of 20s shifts from the interior struggles of late adolescence ("Who am I?" "What is truth?") to a preoccupation with working out external situations ("Where do I go?" "How can I get there?" "How do I put my dreams into effect?"). The tasks revolve around erecting the test structure around the chosen life-style. Becoming caught up in the expectations of others is a pervasive theme, and the impulse to do what one should struggles with the impulses to be experimental and to explore alternative options.

Maturational crises of the 20s occur around these central themes: (1) attempts to increase independence from parents and parental dominance; (2) the choice of a post–secondary education course—school, a job, or the military; and (3) moving into the job or career world and establishing skills.

Middle adulthood

The middle years of adulthood may be thought of as an intermediate stage of life when growth is strongest in the areas of social and emotional development. By this time, individuals have generally chosen a life-style, a family or single pattern of living, and an occupation and are involved in implementing those choices. The span of time considered to cover the middle years is variable; some consider ages 40 to 65 and others, ages

30 to 70 as "middle age." However the boundaries are marked, it is probably the longest stage of an individual's life. The boundaries of this stage of life must be considered tentative and flexible. In this text the framework of 30 to 70 years of age, as described by Stevenson (1977), is used. Stevenson uses the term middlescence to describe this age span and further subdivides it into two categories: (1) the core middle years, or middlescence. I, ages 30 to 50, and (2) the new middle years, or middlescence II, ages 50 to 70. The developmental tasks that she assigns to those subcategories of the middle years are presented in the boxed material below.

During the ages between 30 and 50, major goals and activities are in the areas of self-development, assistance to both the younger and older generations, and organizational endeavors. Individuals feel a need to come to terms with their own and with society's value orientations, and with the similarities and discrepancies therein. One's own value orientation may undergo a major change or numerous minor changes during these years when patterns are beginning to seem quite set but may not seem comfortably so. Individuals move into various roles and stations in a variety of settings: in the family, at work, in religious organizations, and in community and civic affairs. In Western society, much of the implementation of the goals of major institutions, including business, industry, government, education, religion, and charitable agencies,

---

Developmental tasks

**Developmental tasks of middlescence I,
the core of the middle years (30–50)**

1. Developing socioeconomic consolidation
2. Evaluating one's occupation or career in light of a personal value system
3. Helping younger persons (eg., biological offspring) to become integrated human beings
4. Enhancing or redeveloping intimacy with spouse or most significant other
5. Developing a few deep friendships
6. Helping aging persons (eg., parents or in-laws) progress through the later years of life
7. Assuming responsible positions in occupational, social, and civic activities, organizations, and communities
8. Maintaining and improving the home or other forms of property
9. Using leisure time in satisfying and creative ways
10. Adjusting to biological or personal system changes that occur

**Developmental tasks of middlescence II,
the new middle years (50–70)**

1. Maintaining flexible views in occupational, civic, political, religious, and social positions
2. Keeping current on relevant scientific, political, and cultural changes
3. Developing mutually supportive (interdependent) relationships with grown offspring and other members of the younger generation
4. Reevaluating and enhancing the relationship with spouse or most significant other or adjusting to their loss
5. Helping aged parents or other relatives progress through the last stage of life
6. Deriving satisfaction from increased availability of leisure time
7. Preparing for retirement and planning another career when feasible
8. Adapting self and behavior to signals of accelerated aging processes

From Stevenson, J.S.: Issues and crises during middlescence, New York, 1977, Appleton-Century-Crofts.

is performed by the middle-aged population. Work is a major activity and motivating force. For some the work itself is rewarding and gratifying; for others, the only rewards are the paycheck and the fringe benefits.

Much time during these years goes into promoting the growth of significant others, including one's children, parents, spouse, and friends. Erikson's seventh stage of life, generativity vs stagnation, addresses this issue of producing either another generation or something that may be passed on to the next generation. For some this means parenthood, for others this means generativity through creative acts of expression of altruism. Failure to advance to this stage or develop this task can result, according to Erikson, in a stagnation of self or narcissistic self-indulgence. It should be noted that much of the economic effort and gain of the employed middle-aged population goes toward the support of the younger and older generations. It is important that, while providing these various forms of support and assistance, the middle-aged avoid a need to completely control these other age groups.

As leisure time increases in the society, the activities that fill that larger portion are worthy of thoughtful consideration. People may choose to develop skills and

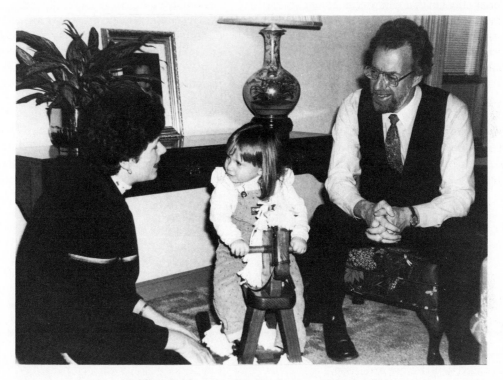

Middle adulthood—the development of a family.

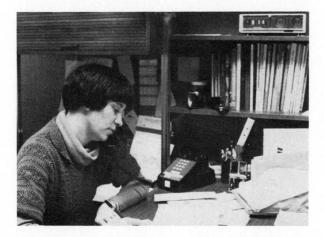

Middle adulthood—the development of a career.

talents that will serve them well in the present and in the future event of retirement. Part of self-knowledge and self-acceptance is an acknowledgment of the changes at the physical, emotional, and intellectual levels that accompany the aging process. The physical alterations may be the most difficult to accept in a culture where the signs of youthfulness are most highly acclaimed. It is most helpful to find some balance between accepting the inevitable changes in appearance while striving to maintain a high level of health with positive approaches toward exercise, diet, and the socioemotional environment. The changes of added years can also be appreciated in terms of emotional and intellectual benefits that can accrue.

During the decades of the 30s and 40s there are several maturational crises that do occur and various situational crises that can occur. Maturational crises are developmental transitions; they are stresses that occur periodically in the life cycle. Situational crises are events that occur with less frequency and predictability, and for only certain individuals. Some of the predictable maturational crises in the core middle years occur in the early 30s and again in the early to mid-40s and have to do with the direction one's life seems to be taking. "Why am I doing this and not something else?" "Why am I with this person and not someone else?" "Why this career or talent or role and not another?" "Have I defined myself too narrowly?" are some of the common questions. Much soul-searching about priorities occurs and may lead to changes in residence, job, career, or spouse or to a reevaluation and acceptance of things as they are. Individuals may approach the 30s realizing that they have expended both time and energy in doing the things their family and society indicated they "should" do. They may begin to feel too restricted by the career and personal choices made earlier and to realize that other aspects of themselves are struggling to surface and find expression. New choices and alternatives, as well as the old ones, are reconsidered and commitments may be altered or deepened. This may involve an uprooting of the life that seemed to be so well grounded and striking out after a new vision. A job or career change may be sought, single people may renew the search for a partner, married people may feel discontent leading to a serious review of the marriage and perhaps to separation or divorce. Childless couples reconsider having children, while those who have spent a number of years raising young children may move toward involvement outside the home.

Once these struggles are decided in some way, the following few years may be characterized by a more settled situation during which people put down roots, invest in property, and work earnestly on climbing some particular career or social ladder. Much time and energy are involved in work and child rearing; satisfaction with a marriage may change.

For many individuals, the mid-30s mark a significant milestone. An awareness of life being at its halfway mark emerges. Time's passage may be felt as never before. There may be a diminishing acceptance of stereotyped roles and acknowledgment that few answers are absolute. Sheehy (1974) refers to the years of 35 to 45 as the "Deadline Decade," a time of reevaluating choices, purposes, and the expenditure of resources. It is a period of uncertainty and opportunity, a chance to restructure a narrower, earlier identity. Individuals may stumble on new aspects of themselves if they give themselves the permission to do so.

Davitz and Davitz (1976) have focused on the decade of 40 to 50 and found some similarities as well as a number of differences in the way men and women handle those years. There seems to be a generally increased awareness of one's own mortality as age-group acquaintances begin to develop illnesses and to die, often as a result of a heart attack. People in their 40s become aware, perhaps for the first time, that younger people view them as being in an older age group. Identity questions surface again, as they do with some frequency throughout the adult years, and individuals wonder: "What have I done?" "What have I become?" "Am I doing what is most fulfilling, rewarding, and satisfying for me?" "Who am I now?" Occasionally, they wonder what things might be like if they could begin again, but there is also the realization that although one might still make changes, one cannot go back to the beginning.

Parenting may be difficult, especially if the children are adolescents and working out identity problems of their own. Some parenting behaviors may be resented, although the parents may believe they are merely trying to prevent a repeat of their own mistakes. Parents may be attempting to relive their own lives through their maturing children and this is often understandably met with resentment from offspring who are seeking to lead their own lives. Concerns about aging parents also become more prominent.

During the early 40s, men may be enjoying success and promotions at work or may harbor a concern that this is the last chance to make it. Some experience tension from a fear of being passed by and are very sensitive to any indications that peers or superiors are losing confidence. While much energy goes into work or much frustration is experienced there, a sense of boredom with marriage and family life may emerge. Fears regarding sexual drive and loss of potency and masculinity may be experienced. Frustrations may be acted out at home, which tends to be the safest setting, producing more strain on the marriage and family relationship. Extramarital affairs are not uncommon. The emotions are fluctuating, moving from anger to affection and warmth and reflecting some of the internal conflicts about identity at work and at home. These conflicts occur in a context of responsibilities from which the person usually feels he or she cannot escape.

During the mid-40s, the attitude toward work may change from one of total involvement to one of lesser interest with a growing interest in developing a sport or hobby. The meaningfulness of activities is a frequent theme, as daily routines at work and home are rethought and belief in religion, politics, and relationships are reevaluated. This situation offers potential for psychological growth and a reintegration and stabilization of identity. Toward the second half of the 40s, some of the conflicts may be resolved. The stress on the marriage may promote a change in the relationship with a greater acceptance of interdependency or it may lead to a divorce and, possibly, to remarriage. Greater sexual maturity can provide an enhanced capacity to give and receive pleasure. Work may become more acceptable and viewed more in terms of its responsibilities than in terms of power. During these years aspects of the personality and talents that have been latent may begin to emerge. Physical changes are moderate; weight may increase and recovery time after exertion may be longer.

In our Western society, a woman approaches the age of 40 with a complex mixture of feelings: a sense of greater self-assurance and poise may be counterbalanced with a sense of apprehension. A woman of 40 is frequently thought of a middle-aged, settled, and mature. This set of role expectations may frustrate her, especially if she does not see herself conforming to that model. Involvement in a career may be a source of strength for a woman, as work brings its own rewards and sense of personal accomplishment and her identity is not entirely tied up with her family. It may also be a source of strain as demands from both work and family may be very high. Women in the work world who may already have experienced some discrimination can find promotions increasingly rare and even resented by a husband who has not been similarly recognized. A woman who has devoted years to home and family may be eager to get into the outside world of school, business, or involvement in community activities.

Weight may become an eminent concern: a battle against weight gain may also be a battle against aging, the loss of physical attractiveness, and all that that implies in our culture. Difficulties in this area may well depend on the amount of self-esteem that has been previously derived from physical attractiveness. Gray hair is yet another manifestation of a physical change accompanying aging and may be a source of distress.

A woman confronted with her own concerns about aging might find these reinforced by her husband's behavior if he appears to be dissatisfied with the marriage. If divorce results, new friends and a new life-style must be developed. If the marital storms are weathered, a closer bond may be forged. Expectations of each spouse for the other may become more based in the facts than the fantasies of the relationship, and mutual dependence is accepted, as well as the individual strengths and differences.

Single persons may experience a change in their relationships with married couples; aloneness may become a more prominent theme, despite the positive aspects of independence. The previous choice of career over marriage may be reconsidered, particularly if the parents have died.

Menopause, which normally occurs during the 40s or early 50s, involves both physical and psychological changes. The hormonal imbalance may result in episodes of emotional instability, rapid mood shifts, nervousness, irritability, insomnia, and fatigue. Some depression may be involved, but many women react with equanimity. The reaction to menopause may depend on how other developmental crises have been handled. Menopause may be followed by a heightened sexual drive and enjoyment of sex as concerns about pregnancy are diminished.

During the "new" middle years, generally ages 50 to 70, individuals have an opportunity to define and integrate the emotional and intellectual growth that has occurred during the earlier adulthood years. It may be a time of changes within the outside of the family resulting in the time and energy to develop new areas of interest. In the work world, many have attained much or most of what they can, although for a few, advancement is still possible. In certain arenas, such as in legislative, business, governmental, religious, and community service areas, these years may be the prime years of activity. Many of the highest positions in these areas are occupied by people in the new middle years. Within the family setting, spouses may be back to the couple stage, or fast approaching it, and need to readjust to the contracted nuclear family or to life alone if a spouse should die. Grandparenting is a new role often acquired during this stage. Parents need to reassess their relationships with their children and move from the adult-child type of interactions to adult-adult interactions with their offspring who have reached adulthood. Men may become more aware of, less fearful of, and more accepting of their tendencies to provide care and nurturance, while women may accept and develop more fully their assertiveness through an interest in business, politics, or other organizations and activities outside the home. The aging parents of 50- to 70-year olds often require assistance emotionally,

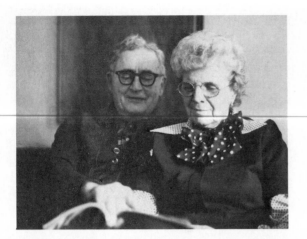

Middle adulthood—the preparation for retirement.

physically, and/or financially. It continues to be important to help both the older and younger generations continue their own development and not to stifle either with overwhelming controls.

People in this age group, as in any age group, are confronted with rapid changes in technology and in the social environment. However, they often prefer to advise some caution and restraint in the type and rate of change. Life experiences have, hopefully, brought some sense of wisdom and judgment to the middle-aged; and although some younger people may view them as overly cautious and nonprogressive, the balance between the two views is important. At the same time, openness and flexibility continue to be important characteristics to health and well-being. Those who stay current with new ideas and trends will have a more positive approach to life and less need of maintaining a defensive posture and will probably communicate more effectively with younger individuals.

Preparation for retirement is a very important task, perhaps especially for people who have been employed outside the home, but also for those who have maintained the housework. Both must readjust to more shared time. Preparation through adult education or development of new or latent skills can pave the way for a refocusing of talent. In a way, preparation for retirement is lifelong, in that a person brings to retirement all that he has become throughout the years. Specific planning for retirement should not be delayed until retirement is imminent.

Late adulthood

As is the case with other stages of adulthood, the parameters of later adulthood and old age are not easy to define. Almost everyone is acquainted with someone who seems "old" at 40 and with someone else who seems "young" at 65. Some gerontologists have

attempted to deal with this situation by setting apart the years from 60 to 75 as early old age and the years from 75 on as later old age.

Later adulthood has become a subject of increasing interest to more people over the past several years. Factors influencing this increased interest include the longer life span and the decline in death rates in Western society, leading to increased numbers of the elderly in the population. However, changes in the social and family structure of this society, along with attitudes toward aging and the aged, have created many problems for these ever-larger numbers of old people. Institutional forms of care have been developed but have often proved unsatisfactory; major pieces of legislation have been passed on behalf of the elderly, but often this has not eased the passage of time and the financial, social, and emotional problems that develop. The emphasis on youth and their culture, behavior, and attitudes is accompanied by a negative attitude toward those on the other end of the age spectrum. It is often said that in this culture, all wish to live long but no one wishes to grow old. This is in marked contrast to other cultures, where old age is respected and even revered.

Later adulthood is similar to all other developmental stages in that certain adaptations are necessary and certain developmental tasks need to be achieved. Yet these developmental tasks are different from earlier ones in that these are the final ones in life.

Among the most significant developmental and adjustive tasks in later adulthood are:
1. Maintaining or developing activities that enhance self-image, contribute to a sense of worth in society, and help to retain functional capacity
2. Developing new roles as in-laws and/or grandparents
3. Adapting to numerous losses—economically, socially, emotionally (such as job, friends, spouse)
4. Adapting to physical changes
5. Performing a life review
6. Preparing for one's own death

As both demands from work and family and living arrangements change somewhat with the onset of retirement, time to do other things becomes more available. It is very important that preparation be made for the use of time far in advance of the retirement years. Failure to do so can make the change in time utilization and availability come as a shock and the hours may seem empty, heavy, or endless. If, on the other hand, preparation has been made, time can be used to advantage in the development of new careers, hobbies, sporting skills, or community activities. This should enhance both self-worth and functional capacity. Educational opportunities for adults of all ages are increasing. For the older adult, continuing education can provide an opportunity to learn again simply for the pleasure of learning or to enable them to develop another set of skills or an avocation. It is important to both physical and mental well-being that individuals continue to be involved in and contributing to society. If one or both spouses of an elderly couple have been employed, they must also learn to adjust to having more time together and to intermeshing their lives effectively.

New roles emerge for older adults as their children marry and have children of their own. Acceptance of their children's spouses into the family network is very instrumental in the ongoing interaction of the family. Interaction with grandchildren can be a very pleasant aspect of aging if it does not become too time consuming or burdensome. Grandparents need to be able to enjoy their grandchildren without having to be overly responsible for them. Another family role that may continue or may begin in early later adulthood is the caretaking of elderly parents who may be ill or at least more dependent. Individuals need to reevaluate personal identity in light of these new roles in life.

It is abundantly evident that numerous losses do accompany the later years of life. Retirement and its consequences must be dealt with. The loss of a job after many years of employment may be one of the greatest developmental and situational crises in the life of an individual. As stated earlier, it is very important to plan far in advance for postretirement activities that enhance self-respect. The loss of a job often includes the loss of the social relationships that were a part of that setting. It may also mean the loss of opportunities for certain kinds of recognition and achievement.

Couples or individuals must learn to adapt their lifestyle to a retirement income. As retirement incomes become relatively smaller in an inflationary era, this lowered income becomes more of a loss. Homes, entertainment styles, and lifelong travel plans may have to be given up or diminished in scope to meet the costs of necessities for food, housing, and health care.

Other losses may include the deaths of friends, a spouse, or other family members. These losses are among the most difficult aspects of later adulthood. Coping with bereavement for one with whom one has shared life experiences, memories, and plans leaves a great personal void: it is important to experience the profound emotions that accompany the loss and then to go on living one's own life and fostering the development of new relationships.

Adaptation to physical changes may also be viewed as a series of losses. Physical strength and vigor do tend to decline gradually over the years. In the 60s and 70s this change is often accompanied by diminishing

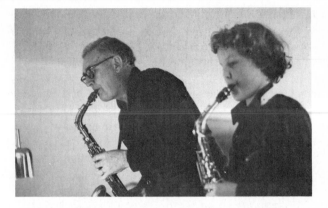

Later adulthood—grandparenting.

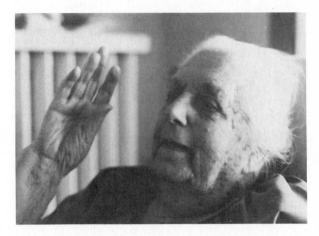

Later adulthood—the life review.

sensory acuity of the eyes, ears, and taste. The emergence of one or several chronic illnesses may also impinge on strength, self-image, and independent status. The older population does become more dependent on the health care system for more frequent intermittent care and, for a small percentage of them, for full institutional care in various types of nursing homes. The majority of the elderly do continue to live at home and to receive some care from family or significant others; however, their more independent status is decreased. Major tasks are to accept physical changes and their limitations and to conserve strength and resources as necessary.

The process of performing a life review is an important developmental task of later adulthood. Most older persons do spend some time reflecting on their accomplishments and failures, satisfactions, and disappointments in an effort to integrate and evaluate the diverse elements of a life lived so that a reasonably positive view of their life's worth can be reached. Failure to accomplish this task may lead to serious psychological problems. The life review process is far more than useless reminiscence. It allows for some gratification and also for the revision in understanding and clarification of experiences that may have been poorly understood or accepted at the time of their occurrence. It is an inventory that helps put past successes and failures into some perspective. It is often important for the older person to share some of this material with others, particularly with the younger generation. This can be mutually beneficial because it gives the older person a sense of usefulness and some credit for their age and wisdom and can provide the younger person with a sense of history. Today's older Americans have lived through more changes than any other single group in human history. This life developmental task is well described by Erikson (1963) as the eighth cycle of man: ego integrity vs despair. "It is the acceptance of one's one and only life cycle as something that had to be and that, by necessity, permitted of no substitutions" (p. 268).

Preparation for one's own death, views on death, and the possibility of an afterlife may very likely evolve from the life review process. For many, if not all, it is important to consider the issue of their own death and to prepare for it in terms of finishing one's business or setting one's affairs in order. This takes many forms: finalizing a will, achieving some goal, resolving some or many interpersonal relationships, and saying one's farewells to significant family members and friends. If the dying process is prolonged in the presence of some chronic illness, the individual will go through several phases of dealing with their eventual death. Both popular and professional literature are making available knowledge and information about the process of dying as the final phase of life. To die in a way as close as possible to what the individual desires may be thought of as life's final developmental task.

Although there are few tools to assess life changes and their effects on adults, two that have been developed are the Recent Life Changes Questionnaire and the Life Experiences Survey. Both of these are an attempt to assess life stresses and to indicate a possible relationship between life stresses and susceptibility to physical and psychological problems or illnesses.

The Recent Life Changes Questionnaire (Rahe, 1975) is a self-administered questionnaire containing a list of events that subjects respond to by checking those events that they have experienced in the previous 6 months to 1 year (Table 4-2). To determine the scores for these events the researchers had a large group of subjects rate each of the items, with "marriage" assigned to an arbitrary value, with regard to the amount of social readjustment each event required. Mean values for each items were taken to represent the average amount of social readjustment required. The values, called Life Change Units, were added to yield a life stress score. Studies using this tool have shown correlations between high recent life change scores and the development of health problems. This tool does combine a life stress score based on both desirable and undesirable events and it may be important to take these differences into account in the assessment of an individual's life change and its impact on health. It is also important to consider an individual client's own assessment of both the intensity of the life changes and his assessment of the strength of his coping abilities.

The Life Experiences Survey (Sarason, Johnson, and Siegel, 1978) is a self-report tool that allows respondents to indicate events they have experienced over the past year (Table 4-3). It includes events that occur fairly frequently and allows respondents to weigh the desirability or undesirability of events. Ratings are on a seven-point scale from extremely negative (-3) to extremely positive ($+3$). A positive change score is obtained by adding those events rated as positive, the negative change score is obtained by adding the negatively rated events, and a total change score is obtained by adding those two values. Studies by Sarason and others (1978) suggest that there is a relationship between negative life change as measured by the Life Experiences Survey and problems of a psychological nature. Although the cause-effect relationship is often unclear between life changes and health status and the effect of life changes or stresses differs from person to person depending on their unique characteristics, including the degree of perceived control over events and the degree of psychosocial assets, yet these tools may be useful ones to the clinician in obtaining some assessment of the active and recent change factors, some of which may be considered developmental tasks, and their importance in a client's life.

Table 4-2

Recent life changes questionnaire

Scoring weight	

HEALTH

Within the time periods listed, have you experienced:

53   1. An illness or injury which:
        (a) Kept you in bed a week or more, or took you to the hospital?
        (b) Was less serious than described above?

15   2. A major change in eating habits?

16   3. A major change in sleeping habits?

19   4. A change in your usual type and/or amount of recreation?

    *5. Major dental work?

WORK

Within the time periods listed, have you:

36   6. Changed to a new type of work?

20   7. Changed your work hours or conditions?

29   8. Had a change in your responsibilities at work:
        (a) More responsibilities?
        (b) Less responsibilities?
        (c) Promotion?
        (d) Demotion?
        (e) Transfer?

23   9. Experienced troubles at work:
        (a) With your boss?
        (b) With co-workers?
        (c) With persons under your supervision?
        (d) Other work troubles?

39   10. Experienced a major business readjustment?

45   11. Retired?

47   12. Experienced being:
        (a) Fired from work?
        (b) Laid off from work?

    *13. Taken courses by mail or studied at home to help you in your work?

HOME AND FAMILY

Within the time periods listed, have you experienced:

20   14. A change in residence:
        (a) A move within the same town or city?
        (b) A move to a different town, city or state?

15   15. A change in family "get-togethers"?

44   16. A major change in the health or behavior of a family member (illness, accidents, drug or disciplinary problems, etc.)?

25   17. Major change in your living conditions (home improvements or a decline in your home or neighborhood)?

100   18. The death of a spouse?

63   19. The death of a:
        (a) Child?
        (b) Brother or sister?
        (c) Parent?
        (d) Other close family member?

37   20. The death of a close friend?

    *21. A change in the marital status of your parents:
        (a) Divorce?
        (b) Remarriage?

    (NOTE: Questions 22-32 concern marriage. For persons never married go to Item 33.)

50   22. Marriage?

35   23. A change in arguments with your spouse?

29   24. In-law problems?

    25. A separation from spouse:
[45]   (a) Due to work?
65   (b) Due to marital problems?

From Rahe, R.H.: Epidemiological studies of life change and illness, Int. J. Psychiatry Med. 6(1-2):133-146, 1975. © Baywood Publishing Co., Inc.
*New questions.

[ ] Scaling weight derived from an earlier (military) scaling study.

Continued.

Currently, drug-induced malnutrition is another cause of concern. Subacute deficiencies of nutrients as a result of drug interference in the bioavailability of the nutrient to the cell are sometimes encountered in clients receiving prolonged drug therapy.

In consideration of these factors, it would appear very desirable to make every health professional aware of the existing and potential nutritional problems in their communities and institutions. Every individual in the United States has a right to receive adequate health care, and an integral part of health care is nutritional care.

Nutritional care is a problem-solving process involving assessment before implementation of the care plan and during the period that the plan is carried out. So that nutritional care may be provided to each individual, as many health professionals as possible should be trained to evaluate the nutritional status of individuals or populations. This assessment is one of the techniques necessary to the implementation of the preventive aspects of health care.

Nutritional status may be defined as the state of health enjoyed as a result of nutrition. The World Health Organization has defined health as a state of "complete physical, mental and social well-being and not merely the absence of disease or infirmity."

Nutritional assessment aids in (1) identifying malnutrition in an individual or in a population, of current nutritionally high-risk groups in the community, and of factors related to the cause of malnutrition; (2) providing information on resources available in planning efforts to overcome malnutrition; and (3) evaluating the efficacy of the nutritional care provided to the individual or the efficacy of the nutritional programs implemented in the community.

DEVELOPMENT AND NATURE OF MALNUTRITION

Malnutrition results from faulty or imperfect nutrition. At its fundamental level, it represents an inadequate supply of nutrients to the cell. A series of factors may be responsible for cellular malnutrition. Psychosocial, economic, and political factors and personal likes and dislikes of foods may contribute to inadequate intake of food or nutrients, resulting in *primary malnutrition.* On the other hand, factors such as inadequate digestion, improper absorption, faulty utilization, and increased requirement or excretion of nutrients may lead to decreased bioavailability of the nutrient to the cell, causing *secondary malnutrition.* Fig. 5-1 should be helpful in determining factors related to the bioavailability of nutrients.

Although both primary and secondary malnutrition ultimately result in similar manifestations, the cause

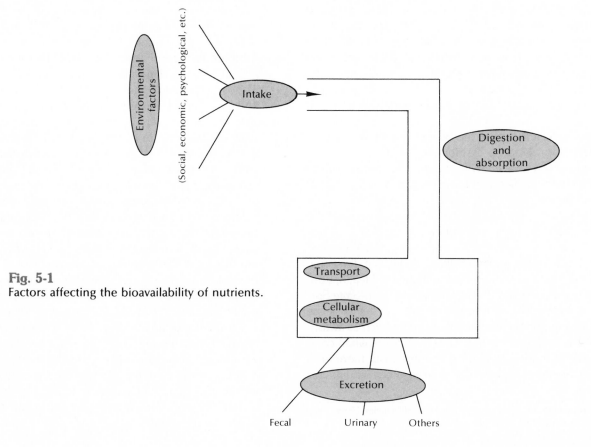

Fig. 5-1
Factors affecting the bioavailability of nutrients.

needs to be identified to treat the condition. For instance, the vitamin A deficiency resulting from a lack of intake could be overcome by administering this nutrient through foods or supplements. However, the secondary deficiency of this vitamin observed in severe protein deficiency can be alleviated only by instituting protein therapy. Malnutrition may be *acute*, that is, the result of temporary adverse conditions that can be rapidly overcome, leaving no long-standing effects. Malnutrition may also be *chronic*, that is, the result of adverse conditions continued without relief over a period of time. Chronic malnutrition may lead to irreparable losses, such as blindness and growth retardation, and occasionally may even lead to death.

Fig. 5-2 describes the steps in the development of a nutrient deficiency. As to how fast and to what degree the deficiency of a nutrient would proceed is determined by the level of dietary intake and by the previous nutritional status, reflecting the extent of body stores and the body's ability to adapt to lower levels of the nutrient intake. Irrespective of the rate of progression, the general pattern in which the disease develops is similar to the one shown.

In the gradual development of a nutrient deficiency, tissue reserves are first mobilized in an effort to maintain the necessary supply of the nutrient to the cells. This is reflected in a reduced concentration of the nutrient in the blood or tissues and in decreased urinary excretion of the nutrient. As the deficiency progresses, the tissue reserves are depleted, resulting in an inadequate supply of the nutrient to the cell. This leads to biochemical lesions such as changes in enzymes, coenzymes, and metabolites, the levels of which would be altered in the blood and in the tissues. Further progression of the deficiency is manifested in the anatomical lesions and clinical symptoms detectable in a thorough physical examination by an alert practitioner. Clinical manifestations of vitamin deficiencies such as beriberi, pellagra, and scurvy are easily recognized.

In summary, it is possible to identify the development of a nutrient deficiency at the intake level, at the blood and tissue level, and during a physical examination. This is the principle on which the major methods of nutritional assessment, namely food intake studies, biochemical parameters, anthropometric measurements, and clinical examinations, are based.

PROCEDURES FOR ASSESSMENT

Whether the assessment is of a single individual or of a group of people in a population, the procedures are basically the same. However, when individual cases are considered, a more thorough nutritional assessment can be made, including an accurate nutritional history and sophisticated laboratory studies. When population groups are assessed, general methods, simple and fast, perhaps with less accuracy and precision,

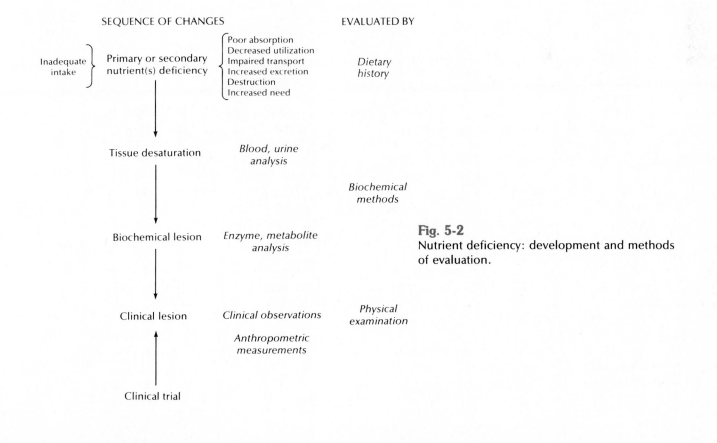

Fig. 5-2
Nutrient deficiency: development and methods of evaluation.

may have to be resorted to because of limitations of time, personnel, and facilities.

The nutritional profile of a community can be determined from various sources, such as food balance sheets, vital statistics, and agricultural data. Although food balance sheets provide information on the per capita availability of food and nutrients to the population, they do not consider individual food consumption and the variation in intakes as a result of age, sex, socioeconomic condition, personal preference, or other factors affecting the food intake. Likewise, vital statistics may be helpful in the identification of morbidity and mortality but may not be reliable in tracing the mortality and morbidity to the nutritional status.

Four major methods are important in the assessment of nutritional status:

1. Dietary surveys
2. Clinical appraisal
3. Anthropometry
4. Biochemical appraisal

In all these methods, data obtained from various techniques have to be evaluated in relation to "norms" or standard guidelines. Uses and limitations of individual guidelines are discussed under each method. However, one point worth stressing is that the norms used here are statistical norms obtained from a sample of the "healthy" population. Whether these are identical with the biological norms compatible with good health is a matter of debate.

Dietary surveys

Dietary surveys, or food intake studies, deal with collecting information on the dietary practices of people, including intakes of specific foods or nutrients over a known period of time. Populations subsisting on marginal intakes may not show physical signs of deficiency, or lesions. For these "subclinical" states, food intake studies have advantages because biochemical methods are extensive in comparison. In addition, this method serves as a check on the validity of the biochemical and clinical observations and vice versa.

Dietary surveys, if carried out appropriately, provide information on (1) the food or nutrient intake of the individual or population group, (2) the nutritional practices of the individual or population group, (3) ration allowances in emergency situations, (4) menu preparation and food procurement, and (5) the nutritional quality of foods available and of those foods actually consumed.

In communities, dietary surveys also help in identifying resources that can be used in programs for improving the nutritional status of the population. Information gathered is also applied when plans are developed for modifying existing economic, agricultural, and food management policies and programs.

A word about ethnic foods would be in place here. Many people partially, if not fully, still adhere to food habits developed in the country of origin. A knowledge of ethnic/cultural food is essential in analyzing the diets and in nutrition education.

It must be remembered that dietary surveys yield information of the situation during a limited time, whereas much of the clinical and biochemical evidence reflects the long-term nutrition of the individual. A recently improved diet would not immediately relieve the biochemical and clinical lesions; thus, a discrepancy between dietary and other findings can be expected and explained.

Dietary surveys are carried out in a number of ways. Each has merits and limitations. The method of choice depends on several factors, such as the size of the sample; background of the individual or population group surveyed; availability of personnel; and provisions for data collection, analysis, and interpretation.

Two types of food intake studies are mainly in vogue: the family or group method and the individual food intake method.

Family or group method. The family or group method is useful in obtaining information on the intake of a homogenous population, such as persons in the same institution or in a family sharing a common kitchen. Common methods of gathering information include the food record method and the food list method. In both methods, full cooperation from the individual in charge of the food service is essential. One of the drawbacks is in the need for estimating the food wastage occurring during the period of the study. About 10% of the energy value of the diet has been estimated as this loss, although it varies from study to study.

Food record method. The food record or inventory method consists of keeping a record of all the foods in the kitchen at the beginning of the survey, of all foods obtained during the period of the survey (2 to 4 weeks), and of all the foods remaining at the end of the survey. Food waste occurring during the study and foods eaten away from home also are recorded. From these lists, amounts of foods consumed over the period are determined.

Food list method. In the food list method, an estimate of the quantities of foods used during a given period of time is obtained through an interview with the person responsible for the food service.

Individual food intake method. Individual food intake studies generally consider both qualitative and quantitative aspects. Three approaches have usually been in practice. These include the food intake record, the 24-hour recall method, and the dietary history method.

Food intake record. Food intake at each of the meals is recorded concurrently over a known period of time by means of weights, household measures, or estimates of quantities of specific foods. How many days this survey should last and which of the weekdays is to be included are debatable points. In view of the fact that the day-to-day diet varies in the United States, a 1-day intake is not representative of the usual intake. It is desirable to include more than 1 day. The longer the duration, the better the reliability; however, since subjects tend to lose interest in keeping records after a while, it is advantageous to limit the record keeping to short periods.

A 3-day food intake record appears to be quite satisfactory, both in terms of the subject's cooperation and in terms of obtaining reliable information. Since a person's eating pattern tends to change during the weekend, inclusion of a weekend day may be advocated. Some researchers have found that inclusion of a weekend day along with 3 weekdays provides a satisfactory record.

Weighed-food records are a modified version of the food intake method and involve weighing all the foods consumed by the subject. The subject may be trained to weigh the foods accurately, or an investigator may be assigned to do this. This version is expensive and is mainly used in metabolic research studies.

In general, the food intake record has the disadvantage of making the subject conscious of his eating pattern, and this consciousness might make him modify his intake. When the subject is asked to estimate his intake, discrepancies related to the concept of serving size might also occur.

Twenty-four hour recall method. The 24-hour recall method is very practical and useful in nutrition clinics. Intake of specific foods is recalled in terms of either estimates or quantities determined by means of weights or household measures. In view of the importance of enteral and parenteral feeding, particularly in the hospitals but becoming more common at home for certain patients, the intake through these routes also should be considered. From the memory point of view, the best recall period appears to be the immediate past 24 hours. A trained interviewer, generally a dietitian, usually carries out this method. To improve the reliability of the informant's memory, cross-check methods have been devised. The same questions are asked in different ways at different times in the interview. However, this procedure is time consuming and expensive and may be used only when the interviewer's time is not a limiting factor.

The accuracy of this method will vary. Women appear to be more accurate than men, and younger people more than elderly people, in giving data. Intake determined by the 24-hour method tends to be higher than that reported in a 7-day record. The day-to-day variation in meal pattern and in food intake makes the 24-hour recall method not entirely representative of the individual's usual intake. Validity of the data obtained from the recall method has also been questioned. However, for all practical purposes, this method seems to provide sufficient information. It has been shown that for group comparisons, 24-hour recall records on a larger number of people provide better criteria than long-term studies on a limited population.

Dietary history method. The dietary history method yields qualitative information on long-standing food habits. This information is useful in interpreting the biochemical and clinical findings because the latter are indicative of long-standing food habits. The individual is asked to report his current or past intake in terms of frequency of occurrence of food items, changes in meal pattern, methods of food preparation, food likes and dislikes, shopping practices, and any other pertinent information. The history not only reflects the individual's food behavior but also is informative in terms of identifying the cause of nutritional problems. The dietary history also is a check for the validity of the intake reported in the 24-hour recall method. Dietary histories in conjunction with a 24-hour recall enhance the accuracy of the information. Nutrient intake calculated from food records is generally lower than that calculated from diet histories.

Tactics for eliciting data. Since individuals' food habits are of a very intimate nature, much of the success in eliciting suitable information on food habits depends on the interview. All the tactics described for an effective interview would be helpful here, also. Rapport between the interviewer and the informant is of utmost importance. A positive environment enhances the interaction between the interviewer and the interviewee. On an individual basis, a 30- to 45-minute interview using a suitable questionnaire or nutrition history form will yield useful information. Highly trained personnel can obtain very reliable information if the proper interview techniques are used (Table 5-1).

To facilitate communication, the interviewer may use various sizes of glasses, spoons, bowls, and food models to help the subject estimate food quanitities more accurately. Repetition may be necessary to cross-check information. Data on meal patterns over weekends and holidays help in deciding the days to be included for the food intake study. Observation of food intake, if possible, would further help cross-check the information given by the individual. This is possible only if one visits the home or institution.

Eliciting an accurate diet history and food intake is an art. Food habits are so personal to people that they may not be telling the truth for a variety of reasons, for example, embarrassment or apprehension. The interviewee oftentimes likes to tell the interviewer what the

Table 5-1
Data collected and implications from diet history

Host factor	Information sought	Implication
Demographic	Age; sex	Determine nutrient needs
Food intake	Actual foods consumed; frequency of foods; food likes and dislikes; vitamin and other supplements—dosage	Judge dietary pattern and adequacy; cross-check information; help plan diets and counsel (megavitamin therapy)
Type of feeding	Oral; enteral; parenteral	Supplement intake data
Appetite	Taste and smell perception; loss or gain of appetite; anorexia	Help plan diet; aid in identifying nutrient deficiencies or disease conditions
Physical activity	Occupation; length and types of exercise; duration of sleep	Determine caloric needs (of particular importance in obesity)
Food avoidances	Allergies and intolerances; reasons for avoiding foods	Help plan diet; identify conditions needing intervention (of particular importance for children)
Dental-oral health	Teeth and gum health; fitting dentures; salivation; swallowing	Help plan diet; identify conditions needing intervention (of particular importance for elderly)
Gastrointestinal	Heartburn; bloating; gas; distention; diarrhea; constipation; gastrointestinal fistula	Help plan diet; identify conditions needing intervention
Medications	Antacids and laxatives; other medications—frequency of usage, dosage	Help plan diet; drug-nutrient interaction (of particular importance in hospitalized patients and elderly)
Home life-style	Who shops; who cooks; type of cooking and storage facilities; number in household	Aid in family counseling in relation to life-style at home; referral if needed
Economic condition	Source of income and food dollars	Help plan diet, particularly in relation to economic priorities; educate to wise use of food dollars
Ethnicity	Ethnic, cultural, religious background; if migrants, which generation	Determine food habits; help plan diets in accordance with their choice

Table 5-2
Basic Four food guide (1956)

Food group	Essentials of an adequate diet
Milk and milk products	Children, 3 to 4 cups Adults, 2 or more cups
Fruits and vegetables	
Green and yellow vegetables	4 servings
Citrus fruits or raw cabbage	1 serving
Potatoes, other vegetables, and fruits	1 serving
Meat, poultry, fish, and eggs	2 or more servings
Bread, flour, and cereal (enriched or whole grain)	4 or more servings

interviewer would like to know rather than the truth. This might lead to a tendency to overestimate or underestimate the serving sizes. The combined problems of reliability and accuracy make it apparent that the quality of data obtained is determined by the skill, personality, and sensitivity of the interviewer and the honesty of the client.

A diet history may be brief or detailed. A detailed diet history not only helps in assessing the nutritional status but also is useful in identifying factors that affect food behavior and cause malnutrition. This, in turn, is helpful in nutrition planning. For this reason, a diet history could also include information on the client's medical and social background in addition to the data on food intake and habits.

Analysis and evaluation of data. Food intake data are evaluated in terms of either the foods in the diets or the nutrients, or both. Tools used for analysis and evaluation include the Basic Four food guide, food consumption tables, and chemical analysis.

Basic Four food guide. The Basic Four food guide, though not perfect, serves as a practical tool for rapid analysis and evaluation of diets. The guide was recommended by the U.S. Department of Agriculture (USDA), based on the essentials of an adequate diet. Table 5-2 describes the Basic Four food guide. The intake of the recommended number of servings of

Table 5-3
Mean heights and weights and recommended energy intake

Age and sex group	Weight		Height		Energy		
					Needs		
	kg	lb	cm	in	MJ	kcal	Range in kcal
INFANTS							
0.0-0.5 yr	6	13	60	24	kg × 0.48	kg × 115	95-145
0.5-1.0 yr	9	20	71	28	kg × 0.44	kg × 105	80-135
CHILDREN							
1-3 yr	13	29	90	35	5.5	1,300	900-1,800
4-6 yr	20	44	112	44	7.1	1,700	1,300-2,300
7-10 yr	28	62	132	52	10.1	2,400	1,650-3,300
MALES							
11-14 yr	45	99	157	62	11.3	2,700	2,000-3,700
15-18 yr	66	145	176	69	11.8	2,800	2,100-3,900
19-22 yr	70	154	177	70	12.2	2,900	2,500-3,300
23-50 yr	70	154	178	70	11.3	2,700	2,300-3,100
51-75 yr	70	154	178	70	10.1	2,400	2,000-2,800
76+ yr	70	154	178	70	8.6	2,050	1,650-2,450
FEMALES							
11-14 yr	46	101	157	62	9.2	2,200	1,500-3,000
15-18 yr	55	120	163	64	8.8	2,100	1,200-3,000
19-22 yr	55	120	163	64	8.8	2,100	1,700-2,500
23-50 yr	55	120	163	64	8.4	2,000	1,600-2,400
51-75 yr	55	120	163	64	7.6	1,800	1,400-2,200
76+ yr	55	120	163	64	6.7	1,600	1,200-2,000
Pregnancy						+300	
Lactation						+500	

From Recommended Dietary Allowances, revised 1980, Food and Nutrition Board, National Academy of Sciences–National Research Council, Washington, D.C. The data in this table have been assembled from the observed median heights and weights of children, together with desirable weights for adults for mean heights of men (70 in) and women (64 in) between the ages of 18 and 34 years as surveyed in the U.S. population (DHEW/NCHS data).

Energy allowances for the young adults are for men and women doing light work. The allowances for the two older age groups represent mean energy needs over these age spans, allowing for a 2 percent decrease in basal (resting) metabolic rate per decade and a reduction in activity of 200 kcal per day for men and women between 51 and 75 years; 500 kcal for men over 75 years; and 400 kcal for women over 75. The customary range of daily energy output is shown for adults in the range column and is based on a variation in energy needs of ±400 kcal at any one age, emphasizing the wide range of energy intakes appropriate for any group of people.

Energy allowances for children through age 18 are based on median energy intakes of children of these ages followed in longitudinal growth studies. Ranges are the 10th and 90th percentiles of energy intake, to indicate range of energy consumption among children of these ages.

determined amounts from each of the food groups is assumed to provide an optimum diet. The 24-hour intake is divided into foods of the four groups: milk, meat, fruits and vegetables, and cereals and cereal products. The servings in each group are compared to the recommended ones for judging the dietary adequacy. A discussion of the uses and limitations of the Basic Four food guide may be found in any textbook on nutrition.

Currently, ethnic foods and vegetarian diets are becoming popular. It is advisable to be knowledgeable about the nutritive value of these foods and diets. The ingredients that go into the combination dishes are important. Once the foods are identified, Basic Four

analysis follows the same principle. In a vegetarian diet, meat substitutes (nuts, legumes, and lentils) will take the place of meat foods.

Food composition tables. It is possible to calculate the amount of nutrients provided by a diet from food composition tables if the food is described in the table. The standard food composition table is the *Agriculture Handbook No. 456* (Adams). Data compiled from various laboratories sometimes consider the variety of foods, the method of preparation, and other factors that affect the nutritive value of foods.

With the influx of convenience foods in the market, it is rather hard to analyze diets with these tables because so many of the foods are not listed. Some-

Table 5-5
Estimated safe and adequate daily dietary intakes of additional selected vitamins and minerals

Age group	Vitamins			Trace elements*						Electrolytes		
	Vitamin K (µg)	Biotin (µg)	Pantothenic acid (mg)	Copper (mg)	Manganese (mg)	Fluoride (mg)	Chromium (mg)	Selenium (mg)	Molybdenum (mg)	Sodium (mg)	Potassium (mg)	Chloride (mg)
INFANTS												
0.0-0.5 yr	12	35	2	0.5-0.7	0.5-0.7	0.1-0.5	0.01-0.04	0.01-0.04	0.03-0.06	115-350	350-925	275-700
0.5-1.0 yr	10-20	50	3	0.7-1.0	0.7-1.0	0.2-1.0	0.02-0.06	0.02-0.06	0.04-0.08	250-750	425-1,275	400-1,200
CHILDREN AND ADOLESCENTS												
1-3 yr	15-30	65	3	1.0-1.5	1.0-1.5	0.5-1.5	0.02-0.08	0.02-0.08	0.05-0.1	325-975	550-1,650	500-1,500
4-6 yr	20-40	85	3-4	1.5-2.0	1.5-2.0	1.0-2.5	0.03-0.12	0.03-0.12	0.06-0.15	450-1,350	775-2,325	700-2,100
7-10 yr	30-60	120	4-5	2.0-2.5	2.0-3.0	1.5-2.5	0.05-0.2	0.05-0.2	0.1-0.3	600-1,800	1,000-3,000	925-2,775
11 + yr	50-100	100-200	4-7	2.0-3.0	2.5-5.0	1.5-2.5	0.05-0.2	0.05-0.2	0.15-0.5	900-2,700	1,525-4,575	1,400-4,200
ADULTS	70-140	100-200	4-7	2.0-3.0	2.5-5.0	1.5-4.0	0.05-0.2	0.05-0.2	0.15-0.5	1,100-3,300	1,875-5,625	1,700-5,100

From Recommended Dietary Allowances, Revised 1980. Food and Nutrition Board, National Academy of Sciences–National Research Council. Because there is less information on which to base allowances, these figures are not given in the main table of the RDAs and are provided here in the form of ranges of recommended intakes.
*Since the toxic levels for many trace elements may be only several times usual intakes, the upper levels for the trace elements given in this table should not be habitually exceeded.

on clinical appraisal. The auxiliary health worker would then alert the physician to the presence or absence of clinical symptoms.

Clinical appraisal is the least sensitive technique among the methods used in the nutritional assessment. Some reasons for this are as follows:

1. Subjectivity of the examiner or examiner bias is involved in the judgment. Different evaluators differ regarding the identification and degree of malnutrition of the same lesion. The more nonspecific a lesion is, the more differing are the opinions. An example of this is seen in the examiner variability observed in the recordings of three examiners in an area included in the recent Ten-State Nutrition Survey (Table 5-8). Another example is that of the examiner who judges the leanness of a male subject's body in relation to his own and that of the female subject's in relation to the contour of his wife. Therefore, standardization of examiners' parameters must be carried out often. Color slides would be very useful in the identification and standardization of signs of deficiency.

2. Because of the nature of the development of nutrient deficiencies, clinical assessment may or may not correlate well with the food intake data or with the biochemical parameters.

3. The nonspecific nature of clinical lesions encountered may complicate the diagnosis. The same lesion could be traced to a deficiency of one or more nutrients. The lesion could also be a result of some other reason, such as allergy or trauma.

In spite of its drawbacks, clinical appraisal does have a definite role in the total assessment procedure:

1. It provides information to supplement that obtained in anthropometric, dietary, and biochemical methods.

2. As seen in Fig. 5-2, anatomical lesions do not appear until the deficiency is far advanced. The presence of clinical symptoms in some individuals of a community would indicate the possibility of a subclinical deficiency in others. This identification could lead to correction at earlier stages.

3. Clinical assessment may reveal a host of other diseases not diagnosed earlier that merit diagnosis and treatment.

4. A physical examination may detect nutritional deficiency not detected by dietary or biochemical methods.

Table 5-9 summarizes certain of the symptoms associated with specific nutrient deficiencies in human beings. Some of the observations made on specific tissues that are useful in the assessment procedure are briefly discussed here. One should note, however, that

Table 5-6
Suggested guide to interpretation of nutrient intake data

	Deficient	Low	Acceptable	High
Protein (g/kg)	<0.5	0.5-0.9	1.0-1.4	>1.5
Iron (mg/day)	<6.0	6-8	9-11	>12
Calcium (g/day)	<0.3	0.30-0.39	0.4-0.7	>0.8
Vitamin A (IU/day)	<2,000	2,000-3,499	3,500-4,999	>5,000
Ascorbic acid (mg/day)	<10	10-29	30-49	>50
Thiamine (mg/100 kcal)	<0.2	0.20-0.29	0.3-0.4	>0.5
Riboflavin (mg/day)	<0.7	0.7-1.1	1.2-1.4	>1.5
Niacin (mg/day)	<5	5-9	10-14	>15

From Manual for nutrition surveys, ed. 2, Washington, D.C., 1963, Interdepartmental Committee on Nutrition for National Defense.

Table 5-7
Dietary standards used by the U.S. Public Health Service in evaluating dietary intake in the National Nutritional Survey, 1970

Age	Energy (kcal/kg)	Protein (g/kg)	Calcium (mg)	Iron (mg)	Thiamine (mg/kcal)	Riboflavin (mg/kcal)	Vitamin A (IU)	Ascorbic acid (mg)
6-7 yr	82	1.3	450	10	0.4/1,000	0.55/1,000	2,500	30
10-12 yr								
Male	68	1.2	650	10	0.4/1,000	0.55/1,000	2,500	30
Female	64	1.2	650	18	0.4/1,000	0.55/1,000	2,500	30
17-19 yr								
Male	44	1.1	550	18	0.4/1,000	0.55/1,000	3,500	30
Female	35	1.1	550	18	0.4/1,000	0.55/1,000	3,500	30
Adults								
Male	38	1.0	400	10	0.4/1,000	0.55/1,000	3,500	30
Female	38	1.0		18	0.4/1,000	0.55/1,000		
Pregnant	+200	+20	800	18	0.4/1,000	0.55/1,000	3,500	30
Lactating	+1,000	+25	900	18	0.4/1,000	0.55/1,000	4,500	30

From Guthrie, H.A.: Introductory nutrition, ed. 4, St. Louis, 1979, The C.V. Mosby Co.

although prolonged and severe deficiencies of nutrients are manifested in anatomical lesions, not all the changes observed can be traced to nutritional origin.

Sometimes complaints from patients who have deficiencies of specific nutrients aid in diagnosing the symptoms faster. Examples of these complaints are general weakness, chronic fatigue, loss of appetite, loss of weight, bleeding gums, and soreness of the eyes and mouth.

Eyes. Dryness of the cornea and conjunctiva and corneal opacity (xerophthalmia) are usually associated with vitamin A deficiency. Infiltration of the cornea by blood vessels is associated with vitamin B_2, or riboflavin, deficiency.

Skin. Some of the dermatitides are associated with certain vitamin deficiencies. In niacin deficiency, dermatitis of skin exposed to sunlight is observed. In vitamin A deficiency, xerosis or roughness of skin caused by the hardness of papillae at the base of the hair follicle is seen. Nasolabial dermatitis is often considered a pyridoxine deficiency. Essential fatty acid deficiency

Table 5-8
Percentage of adult clinical findings by three examiners in a selected area of the Ten-State Nutrition Survey

	Examiners		
	1	2	3
Number of examinations	1,123	1,127	589
Filiform papillary atrophy	4.1	1.1	11.2
Follicular hyperkeratosis	4.0	0.6	6.8
Swollen red gums	2.8	3.7	4.1
Angular lesions	0.4	0.4	1.2
Glossitis	0.6	0.4	0.5
Goiter	3.6	6.6	3.6

From Laboratory tests for assessment of nutritional status, Sauberlich, H.E., Dowdy, R.P., and Skala, J.H., CRC Crit. Rev. Clin. Lab. Sci. **4**:215, 1973. © CRC Press, Inc. 1973. Used by permission of CRC Press, Inc.

Table 5-9

Clinical syndromes associated with deficiencies of specific nutrients

Calories: Underweight, underheight, weight loss, lethargy, anemia, edema, marasmus

Protein: As above, fatty liver, kwashiorkor

Fat: Dermatoses in infants (essential fatty acid deficiency), deficiencies of the fat-soluble vitamins A, D, E, and K

Vitamin A: Growth failure, follicular hyperkeratosis, night blindness, xerophthalmia, keratomalacia, impairment of vestibular balance, impaired immunity

Vitamin D: Rickets, tetany, osteomalacia

Vitamin E: Unknown, macrocytic anemia

Vitamin K: Decreased plasma prothrombin activity with prolonged coagulation time and hemorrhages

Thiamin: Anorexia, beriberi, polyneuropathy, toxic amblyopia, heart disease, the ophthalmoplegia of Wernicke's syndrome

Riboflavin: Photophobia, corneal vascularization, angular stomatitis, glossitis, dermatitis

Niacin: Pellagra, dermatitis, glossitis, diarrhea, mental confusion and deterioration, encephalopathy

Pantothenic acid: Nutritional melalgia (burning feet syndrome)

Folic acid: Glossitis, achrestic anemia, megaloblastic anemia of infancy, megaloblastic anemia of pregnancy, nutritional macrocytic anemia, sprue

Pyridoxine: Anemia, convulsions (infants), polyneuropathy, seborrheic eczema

Vitamin B_{12}: Glossitis, macrocytic anemia, peripheral neuropathy, combined system disease (posterolateral column degeneration), mental changes and deterioration

Biotin: Seborrheic dermatitis

Choline, inositol, and carnitine: Unknown

Ascorbic acid: Scurvy, scorbutic gums, subperiosteal hemorrhages, petechial hemorrhages, anemia, impaired wound healing

Iron: Anemia, achlorhydria, glossitis

Iodine: Simple goiter

Fluorine: Dental caries

Calcium: Osteomalacia, a role in the production of senile osteoporosis has been suggested but not proven

Magnesium: Neuromuscular irritability, tetany

Potassium: Alkalosis, muscle weakness and paralysis, cardiac disturbances

Salt (NaCl): Anorexia, nausea, vomiting, lassitude, asthenia, muscle cramps, circulatory collapse

Water: Thirst, dehydration, oliguria, mental changes progressing to coma

Adapted from Goodheart, R.S., and Wohl, M.G.: Manual of clinical nutrition, Philadelphia, 1964, Lea & Febiger.

Table 5-10

Metropolitan height and weight tables (1983)*

Men					Women				
Height		Small frame	Medium frame	Large frame	Height		Small frame	Medium frame	Large frame
Feet	Inches				Feet	Inches			
5	2	128-134	131-141	138-150	4	10	102-111	109-121	118-131
5	3	130-136	133-143	140-153	4	11	103-113	111-123	120-134
5	4	132-138	135-145	142-156	5	0	104-115	113-126	122-137
5	5	134-140	137-148	144-160	5	1	106-118	115-129	125-140
5	6	136-142	139-151	146-164	5	2	108-121	118-132	128-143
5	7	138-145	142-154	149-168	5	3	111-124	121-135	131-147
5	8	140-148	145-157	152-172	5	4	114-127	124-138	134-151
5	9	142-151	148-160	155-176	5	5	117-130	127-141	137-155
5	10	144-154	151-163	158-180	5	6	120-133	130-144	140-159
5	11	146-157	154-166	161-184	5	7	123-136	133-147	143-163
6	0	149-160	157-170	164-188	5	8	126-139	136-150	146-167
6	1	152-164	160-174	168-192	5	9	129-142	139-153	149-170
6	2	155-168	164-178	172-197	5	10	132-145	142-156	152-173
6	3	158-172	167-182	176-202	5	11	135-148	145-159	155-176
6	4	162-176	171-187	181-207	6	0	138-151	148-162	158-179

Source of basic data *1979 Build Study*, Society of Actuaries and Association of Life Insurance Medical Directors of America. Courtesy of the Metropolitan Life Insurance Company, 1983.

*Weights for adults age 25 to 59 years based on lowest mortality. Weight in pounds according to frame size in indoor clothing (5 pounds for men and 3 pounds for women) wearing shoes with 1-inch heels.

results in eczematic skin, particularly in infants. Ascorbic acid defiency resulting in capillary fragility is the cause of perifollicular petechiae.

Oral cavity. Riboflavin deficiency is considered to be the cause of cheilosis or angular stomatitis, that is, cracks and fissures in the lips, particularly at the corners of the mouth. Often this is followed by redness, swelling, and ulceration of the lips. Riboflavin deficiency sometimes causes the tongue to have a magenta hue, which could also be caused by folic acid or vitamin B_2 deficiencies. A scarlet, raw appearance of the tongue with a loss of papillae is a sign of niacin deficiency. Bleeding gums are associated with ascorbic acid deficiency, and mottled teeth are associated with excessive intake of fluoride. Dental caries may be a result of fluoride deficiency or faulty nutritional practices after tooth eruption.

Hair. Lack of luster, depigmentation, and decreased hair diameter are often the outcomes of protein deficiency.

Glands. Enlargement of the thyroid gland, goiter, is a manifestation of a lack of iodine availability to the thyroid cells.

Anthropometry

Anthropometry deals with the measurements of a part or whole of the body. Because nutrition is one of the determinants of growth and development, it is not surprising that over the decades researchers have attempted to establish this criterion as a measure of nutritional adequacy. Anthropometry is of particular interest in the nutritional assessment during the growing years. However, the nonspecificity of this method should be kept in mind in light of present findings that the ultimate growth and development of an individual is the result of a complex web of factors, such as genetic tendencies, maternal and childhood nutrition, infections and diseases influencing the growth process from the time of conception to maturity, and environmental factors.

The most commonly used parameters in anthropometry are height; weight; skinfold thicknesses; and the circumferences of the arm, chest, and head.

Height and weight

Data collection. Exact height and weight data depend on the accuracy of instruments used, as well as on correct techniques. Weighing machines are convenient. Regular checking and recalibration of the scales may be necessary. Lever balances are more reliable than spring balances. In practice, however, many modifications to accuracy need to be made, depending on the situation. Ideally, the nude weight of the individual should be considered, but this is often impractical. An indirect and practical method of determining the nude weight is to recommend that similar amounts of clothing be worn by the individual each time he is weighed. The deduction of this weight from the total weight would yield an estimate of the nude weight.

Standing height should be measured on a standard scale. The individual should stand erect, and a sliding headpiece may be helpful in judging accuracy. With infants, recumbent length is considered. Here again, innovative methods are often employed when measuring is carried out in developing countries.

Norms. Efforts to correlate height and weight in relation to age and sex with nutritional status have been met with limited success, mainly because of the norms used for comparison. If the standards for height and weight consider body builds without defining the builds—small, medium, or large frame—as was done in the 1959 Build and Blood Pressure Study by the Society of Actuaries, a great deal of subjectivity enters the evaluatory mechanism. On the other hand, if stature is not considered, too high a degree of homogeneity may be assumed, which would also contribute to errors in assessment. The lateral bony chest measurement by roentgenographic determination may be used as a stature reference, but the procedure is expensive and may not be practical in population studies.

The most commonly used standard height and weight tables for age 25 and over were first published in 1960 (Table 5-10). These were derived from the Build and Blood Pressure Study and give ideal or desirable weights in relation to heights for different statures (frames). The ranges of weight given in the tables are those that were associated with lowest mortality. It should be remembered that these tables are based on people who buy insurance and may not be a representative example of the population.

Smoothed average weights for adult men and women by age and height are given in Table 5-11. Published by the National Center for Health Statistics, U.S. Public Health Service, these data on height, weight, and selected body dimensions were collected in 1960 to 1962 and were based on a nationwide probability sample. They are, therefore, more representative of the adult civilian, noninstitutionalized population in the United States than are data from the Build and Blood Pressure Study, which represents an insured population.

Height and weight standards used for children are the Harvard growth charts and the Iowa growth charts, which mainly reflect the growth rate of middle-class white children. The more recent standards by Falkner (Table 5-12) include the 5th, 50th, and 95th percentile heights and weights for white North American children from birth to 18 years. Falkner suggests that children

Table 5-11
Smoothed average weights for men and women (by age and height: United States 1960-1962)*

Height (in inches)	Weight (in pounds)						
	18-24 years	25-34 years	35-44 years	45-54 years	55-64 years	65-74 years	75-79 years
MEN							
62	137	141	149	148	148	144	133
63	140	145	152	152	151	148	138
64	144	150	156	156	155	151	143
65	147	154	160	160	158	154	148
66	151	159	164	164	162	158	154
67	154	163	168	168	166	161	159
68	158	168	171	173	169	165	164
69	161	172	175	177	173	168	169
70	165	177	179	181	176	171	174
71	168	181	182	185	180	175	179
72	172	186	186	189	184	178	184
73	175	190	190	193	187	182	189
74	179	194	194	197	191	185	194
WOMEN							
57	116	112	131	129	138	132	125
58	118	116	134	132	141	135	129
59	120	120	136	136	144	138	132
60	122	124	138	140	149	142	136
61	125	128	140	143	150	145	139
62	127	132	143	147	152	149	143
63	129	136	145	150	155	152	146
64	131	140	147	154	158	156	150
65	134	144	149	158	161	159	153
66	136	148	152	161	164	163	157
67	138	152	154	165	167	166	160
68	140	156	156	168	170	170	164

From Obesity and health: a source book for professional health personnel, U.S. Department of Health, Education, and Welfare, U.S. Public Health Service. Adapted from National Center for Health Statistics: Weight by height and age of adults, United States, 1960-1962, *Vital Health Statistics.* PHS Pub. No. 1000—Series 11, No. 14, May 1966.
*Estimated values from regression equations of weights for specified age groups. NOTE: See Appendix B for 1983 data and method of determining frame size.

Table 5-12
Height and weight of children 4 to 18 years of age

Ages (years)	Height (inches)			Weight (pounds)		
	5th P*	50th P	95th P	5th P	50th P	95th P
BOYS						
4	38.3	40.8	43.3	30.0	36.1	42.2
5	40.3	43.4	46.4	33.0	40.3	47.6
6	42.8	45.9	49.0	36.0	44.7	53.4
7	44.8	48.1	51.4	40.3	50.9	61.5
8	46.9	50.5	54.1	44.4	57.4	70.4
9	48.8	52.8	56.8	48.0	64.4	80.4
10	50.6	54.9	59.2	51.4	71.4	91.4
11	51.9	56.4	60.9	53.3	78.9	102.5
12	53.5	58.6	63.7	60.0	86.0	113.5
13	55.2	61.3	67.4	65.3	98.6	131.9
14	57.5	64.1	70.7	75.5	111.8	148.1
15	61.0	66.9	72.8	88.0	124.3	160.6
16	63.8	68.9	74.0	97.8	133.8	169.8
17	65.2	69.8	74.4	106.5	139.8	174.0
18	65.9	70.2	74.5	110.3	144.8	179.3
GIRLS						
4	38.1	40.7	43.3	28.8	36.1	43.4
5	40.6	43.4	46.2	32.2	40.9	49.6
6	42.8	45.9	49.0	35.5	45.7	55.9
7	44.5	47.8	51.1	38.3	51.0	63.7
8	46.4	50.0	53.6	42.0	57.2	72.4
9	48.2	52.2	56.2	45.1	63.6	82.1
10	49.9	54.5	59.1	48.2	71.0	95.0
11	51.9	57.0	62.1	55.4	82.0	108.6
12	54.1	59.5	64.9	63.9	94.4	124.9
13	57.1	62.2	66.8	72.8	105.5	138.2
14	58.5	63.1	67.7	83.0	113.0	144.0
15	59.5	63.8	68.1	89.5	120.0	150.5
16	59.8	64.1	68.4	95.1	123.0	150.1
17	60.1	64.2	68.3	97.9	125.8	153.7
18	60.1	64.4	68.7	96.0	126.2	156.4

From Falkner, F.: Some physical growth standards for white North American children, Pediatrics **29**:448, 1962.
*P, percentile.

falling outside the 5th and 95th range may have to be further assessed for nutritional imbalances.

Many factors, such as secular trends and healthier mothers with better nutrition giving birth to larger babies, have contributed to significant increases in average heights and weights of the present generation. In view of this, height and weight norms developed a decade or more ago would tend to become obsolete.

Again, growth charts developed for a specific population may or may not be applicable for another population. However, unavailability of reliable standards have often made these charts useful for practical purposes in nutritional surveys.

Skinfold thickness

The rising incidence of obesity has necessitated the screening of obese individuals from those that are of above-average weight. Obesity is the excessive accumulation of fat in the adipose tissue as a result of caloric surplus in the system. Therefore, efforts are directed toward evolving methods to measure body fat. Fatness can be determined from such variables as body density, lean body mass, and soft tissue roentgenograms; but the most inexpensive and simple, and therefore practical, method of assessing body fat is to measure the skinfold thickness. Skinfold measurements are indicative of subcutaneous fat and of the caloric status. However, this variable appears to be more useful in

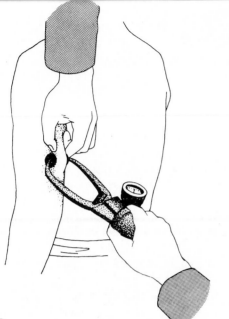

Fig. 5-3
Measuring triceps skinfold with calipers. (From Guthrie, H.A.: Introductory nutrition, ed. 3, St. Louis, 1975, The C.V. Mosby Co.)

Table 5-13
Percentiles for midarm circumference for whites of the Ten-State Nutrition Survey, 1968 to 1970

Age group	Age midpoint (years)	Triceps skinfold percentiles (mm)				
		5th	15th	50th	85th	95th
MALES						
0.0-0.4	0.3	4	5	8	12	15
0.5-1.4	1	5	7	9	13	15
1.5-2.4	2	5	7	10	13	14
2.5-3.4	3	6	7	9	12	14
3.5-4.4	4	5	6	9	12	14
4.5-5.4	5	5	6	8	12	16
5.5-6.4	6	5	6	8	11	15
6.5-7.4	7	4	6	8	11	14
7.5-8.4	8	5	6	8	12	17
8.5-9.4	9	5	6	9	14	19
9.5-10.4	10	5	6	10	16	22
10.5-11.4	11	6	7	10	17	25
11.5-12.4	12	5	7	11	19	26
12.5-13.4	13	5	6	10	18	25
13.5-14.4	14	5	6	10	17	22
14.5-15.4	15	4	6	9	19	26
15.5-16.4	16	4	5	9	20	27
16.5-17.4	17	4	5	8	14	20
17.5-24.4	21	4	5	10	18	25
24.5-34.4	30	4	6	11	21	28
34.5-44.4	40	4	6	12	22	28
FEMALES						
0.0-0.4	0.3	4	5	8	12	13
0.5-1.4	1	6	7	9	12	15
1.5-2.4	2	6	7	10	13	15
2.5-3.4	3	6	7	10	12	14
3.5-4.4	4	5	7	10	12	14
4.5-5.4	5	6	7	10	13	16
5.5-6.4	6	6	7	10	12	15
6.5-7.4	7	6	7	10	13	17
7.5-8.4	8	6	7	10	15	19
8.5-9.4	9	6	7	11	17	24
9.5-10.4	10	6	8	12	19	24
10.5-11.4	11	7	8	12	20	29
11.5-12.4	12	6	9	13	20	25
12.5-13.4	13	7	9	14	23	30
13.5-14.4	14	8	10	15	22	28
14.5-15.4	15	8	11	16	24	30
15.5-16.4	16	8	10	15	23	27
16.5-17.4	17	9	12	16	26	31
17.5-24.4	21	9	12	17	25	31
24.5-34.4	30	9	12	19	29	36
34.5-44.4	40	10	14	22	32	39

From Frisancho, A.: Triceps skinfold and upper arm muscle size norms for assessment of nutritional status, Am. J. Clin. Nutr. **27**:1052, 1974.

assessing normal and moderately fat people rather than really obese people.

Data collection. Calibrated calipers are used in measuring skinfold thickness. Lange's calipers and Herpenden's calipers are examples. The calipers allow most of the assessors to obtain reasonably reliable numerical values, provided the interpersonnel and intrapersonnel variabilities in measurement are overcome. Standardization with the instrument and with the assessor are needed. The skinfold is pinched up to the point where the sides are parallel. Care should be taken not to touch the muscle or the bone. The thickness is then measured by means of standard calipers, using constant pressure. Selection of the site for measurement is critical, since not all the sites are practical or reliable as indicators of fatness. The lower thoracic site appears to be ideal but impractical. The most commonly selected sites are the deltoid triceps, the subscapular region, and the upper abdomen. Measurement of triceps skinfold (TSF) with Herpenden's calipers is shown in Fig. 5-3. According to some researchers, a single skinfold measurement of the triceps is useful in diagnosing obesity.

Norms. Normal values for this variable are presented in Table 5-13. These norms are derived for the American white population and are more applicable to this specific group. If used for other groups, discretion is indicated. However, these norms are invariably used for all groups because of the unavailability of any other standard.

Measurement of circumferences

Head. With the present concern, although controversial, over the relationship between nutrition and mental development, the need for methods to assess brain growth is being recognized. Measurement of head circumference is being used as a tool for this purpose.

This parameter is of importance in infancy because it is an indicator of brain development, most of which is complete in the first year of life. Head circumference is more satisfactory if taken with the infant lying on his back. The measuring tape is passed around the head. The largest circumference is measured by placing the tape anteriorly over the lower forehead just above the supraorbital ridges and by passing it posteriorly over the most prominent part of the occiput. Values ranging from 31 cm to 37 cm at birth have been considered normal. Lower values should be a matter of concern.

Arm. Midarm circumference (MAC) measurement is a useful criterion for the musculature and therefore in determining the extent of protein calorie malnutrition. A soft tape measure calibrated in centimeters is placed around the arm, usually the left arm at its midpoint. The tape should be firmly wrapped around without compressing the underlying muscle. Table 5-14 gives the standard values for this variable. For further discussion refer to Jellife (1966).

Midarm muscle. Midarm muscle circumference (MAMC) has been a more useful criterion to assess the somatic protein—muscle mass—status of an individual. This is of particular importance in assessing the protein calorie status of hospitalized patients because the muscle mass is reflective not only of the protein calorie status of the individual but also of the general exercise and increased usage of certain muscle groups (Jellife, 1966).

MAMC can be calculated from the formula:

$$C_2 = C_1 - \pi S$$

where C_2 = MAMC in cm
 C_1 = MAC in cm
 S = TSF in cm
 π = 3.143

C_1 and S can be measured as already discussed and C_2 calculated. Table 5-15 gives the standards for adults for midarm muscle circumference measurement.

Invariably, anthropometrists have attempted to construct formulas based on various anthropometric measurements to provide an index of nutritional status. In some cases they have proved useful in the nutritional diagnosis; however, in others they have been less satisfactory. Therefore, height and weight are still the choice criteria in community assessment. Depending on the resources and enthusiasm of the assessor, other criteria could be included.

Biochemical appraisal

The biochemical method—or laboratory assessment, as it is sometimes called—measures levels of nutrients; their metabolites; and enzymes associated with or even compounds clearly related to the nutrient under consideration in blood, other body fluids, urine, or tissues such as liver and bone. Because tissue biopsies are hazardous and difficult techniques are involved, tissues are rarely used for analysis; rather, blood or urine is used.

Biochemical assessment is more objective than clinical and dietary methods. In addition, this method detects marginal or subclinical deficiencies before overt clinical lesions appear. It can also indicate metabolic alterations caused by a deficiency of the detected nutrient. Generally, two types of tests are used: (1) measurement of the circulating nutrient in blood or urine and (2) a functional test to evaluate biochemical functions that are dependent on an adequate supply of nutrients. Whereas the former aids in detecting the presence of the problem in earlier stages, the latter indicates the severity.

Specimen collection, handling, and storage are of critical importance, as is the standardization of various laboratory methods to overcome the interpersonnel and interlaboratory variabilities. A detailed discussion of this can be found in the manual by the ICNND. Recent changes in the quantity and quality of the diet may result in variations in blood and urine composition. The composition of nutrients in blood and urine has also been noted to vary during the day. Therefore, blood samples are usually collected for analysis from a fasting subject.

Parameters. Although nutritional status cannot be completely asessed by the biochemical method, different parameters may be used to assess the status of specific nutrients. The parameter to be chosen for a specific nutrient depends on the physiological significance of the test and also on the facilities and resources available, including the cost. Some test methods are still in the experimental stages. Some are used only in research or in individual assessments. However, the parameter should be sensitive enough to assess the status of the particular nutrient. Table 5-16 describes some of the parameters used to assess the status of certain specific nutrients.

Table 5-14

Percentiles for upper arm circumference for whites of the Ten-State Nutrition Survey, 1968 to 1970

Age group	Age midpoint (years)	No.	Arm circumference percentiles (mm)				
			5th	15th	50th	85th	95th
MALES							
0.0-0.4	0.3	41	113	120	134	147	153
0.5-1.4	1	140	128	137	152	168	175
1.5-2.4	2	177	141	147	157	170	180
2.5-3.4	3	210	144	150	161	175	182
3.5-4.4	4	208	143	150	165	180	190
4.5-5.4	5	262	146	155	169	185	199
5.5-6.4	6	264	151	159	172	188	198
6.5-7.4	7	309	154	162	176	194	212
7.5-8.4	8	301	161	168	185	205	233
8.5-9.4	9	287	165	174	190	217	262
9.5-10.4	10	315	170	180	200	228	255
10.5-11.4	11	294	177	186	208	240	276
11.5-12.4	12	294	184	194	216	253	291
12.5-13.4	13	266	186	198	230	270	297
13.5-14.4	14	207	198	211	243	279	321
14.5-15.4	15	179	202	220	253	302	320
15.5-16.4	16	166	217	232	262	300	335
16.5-17.4	17	142	230	238	275	306	326
17.5-24.4	21	545	250	264	292	330	354
24.5-34.4	30	679	260	280	310	344	366
34.5-44.4	40	616	259	280	312	345	371
FEMALES							
0.0-0.4	0.3	46	107	118	127	145	150
0.5-1.4	1	172	125	134	146	162	170
1.5-2.4	2	172	136	143	155	171	180
2.5-3.4	3	163	137	145	157	169	176
3.5-4.4	4	215	145	150	162	176	184
4.5-5.4	5	233	149	155	169	185	195
5.5-6.4	6	259	148	158	170	187	202
6.5-7.4	7	273	153	162	178	199	216
7.5-8.4	8	270	158	166	183	207	231
8.5-9.4	9	284	166	175	192	222	255
9.5-10.4	10	276	170	181	203	236	263
10.5-11.4	11	268	173	186	210	251	280
11.5-12.4	12	267	185	196	220	256	275
12.5-13.4	13	229	186	204	230	270	294
13.5-14.4	14	184	201	214	240	284	306
14.5-15.4	15	197	205	216	245	281	310
15.5-16.4	16	187	211	224	249	286	322
16.5-17.4	17	142	207	224	250	291	328
17.5-24.4	21	836	215	233	260	297	329
24.5-34.4	30	1153	230	243	275	324	361
34.5-44.4	40	933	232	250	286	340	374

From Frisancho, A.: Triceps skinfold and upper arm muscle size norms for assessment of nutritional status, Am. J. Clin. Nutr. **27**:1052, 1974.

Table 5-15

Percentiles for midarm circumference for whites of the Ten-State Nutrition Survey, 1968 to 1970

Age group	Age midpoint (years)	Midarm circumference percentiles (mm)				
		5th	15th	50th	85th	95th
MALES						
0.0-0.4	0.3	81	94	106	125	133
0.5-1.4	1	100	108	123	137	146
1.5-2.4	2	111	117	127	138	146
2.5-3.4	3	114	121	132	145	152
3.5-4.4	4	118	124	135	151	157
4.5-5.4	5	121	130	141	156	166
5.5-6.4	6	127	134	146	159	167
6.5-7.4	7	130	137	151	164	173
7.5-8.4	8	138	144	158	174	185
8.5-9.4	9	138	143	161	182	200
9.5-10.4	10	142	152	168	186	202
10.5-11.4	11	150	158	174	194	211
11.5-12.4	12	153	163	181	207	221
12.5-13.4	13	159	169	195	224	242
13.5-14.4	14	167	182	211	234	265
14.5-15.4	15	173	185	220	252	271
15.5-16.4	16	186	205	229	260	281
16.5-17.4	17	206	217	245	271	290
17.5-24.4	21	217	232	258	286	305
24.5-34.4	30	220	241	270	295	315
34.5-44.4	40	222	239	270	300	318
FEMALES						
0.0-0.4	0.3	86	92	104	115	126
0.5-1.4	1	97	102	117	128	135
1.5-2.4	2	105	112	125	140	146
2.5-3.4	3	108	116	128	138	143
3.5-4.4	4	114	120	132	146	152
4.5-5.4	5	119	124	138	151	160
5.5-6.4	6	121	129	140	155	165
6.5-7.4	7	123	132	146	162	175
7.5-8.4	8	129	138	151	168	186
8.5-9.4	9	136	143	157	176	193
9.5-10.4	10	139	147	163	182	196
10.5-11.4	11	140	152	171	195	209
11.5-12.4	12	150	161	179	200	212
12.5-13.4	13	155	165	185	206	225
13.5-14.4	14	166	175	193	221	234
14.5-15.4	15	163	173	195	220	232
15.5-16.4	16	171	178	200	227	260
16.5-17.4	17	171	177	196	223	241
17.5-24.4	21	170	183	205	229	253
24.5-34.4	30	177	189	213	245	272
34.5-44.4	40	180	192	216	250	279

From Frisancho, A.:Triceps skinfold and upper arm muscle size norms for assessment of nutritional status, Am. J. Clin. Nutr. **27**:1052, 1974.

Table 5-16

Assessment of nutritional status

Nutrient	Blood	Urine*	Others
Protein	Protein (P)†	Total nitrogen	
	Albumin (P)	Urea	
	Albumin (S)†	Creatinine	Creatine-height index
	Transferrin (S)	Hydroxyproline	
	RBP (S)‡		
	Amino acids (P)		Nitrogen balance
	Lymphocyte counts		
Iron	Hemoglobin		Complete blood count (CBC);
	Hematocrit		size and color of cells
	Transferrin (S)		
	Iron (S)		
Vitamin A	Vitamin A (P)		
	Carotene (P)		
Vitamin C	Vitamin C (S)	Vitamin C	Vitamin C load test
	Vitamin C (WBC)†		
Thiamin	Transketolase (E)	Thiamin	
Riboflavin	Glutathione reductase (E)	Riboflavin	
Niacin		N-methyl nicotinamide	
Vitamin B_6	GOT (E)§	Xanthurenic acid	Tryptophan load test
	GPT (E)§	Pyridoxine	
Folic acid	Folic acid (S)	FIGLU (formiminoglutamic acid)	
Vitamin B_{12}	Vitamin B_{12} (S)		CBC; size and color of cells
Iodine		Iodine	

*Urinary values are often considered per unit weight of creatinine excreted.
†P, Plasma; S, serum; WBC, white blood cell; E, erythrocyte.
‡Retinol binding protein
§Glutamic-oxaloacetic transaminase; glutamic-pyruvic transaminase.

Table 5-17

Criteria for evaluating some frequently used biochemical measures of nutritional status
(levels indicative of a deficiency state)

	Adult males	Children 2-5 years	Children 6-12 years
Blood data			
Hemoglobin (g/dl)	<12	<10	<10
Hematocrit (% packed cell volume)	<37	<30	<30
Serum albumin (g/dl)	<2.8	*	*
Serum ascorbic acid (mg/dl)	<0.1	<0.1	<0.1
Plasma vitamin A (μg/dl)	<10	<10	<10
Serum iron (μg/dl)	<60	<40	<50
Transferrin saturation (%)	<20	<20	<20
Serum folacin (mg/ml)	<2	<2	<2
Serum vitamin B_{12}	<100	<100	<100
Plasma vitamin E (mg/dl)	<0.2	<0.2	<0.2
Urinary data			
Thiamine (μg/g creatinine)	<27	<85	<70
Riboflavin (μg/g creatinine)	<27	<100	<85
Tryptophan load (100 mg/kg) (mg xanthurenic acid/24 hr)	>75	>75	>75

From Guthrie, H.A.: Introductory nutrition, ed. 4, St. Louis, 1979, The C.V. Mosby Co. Modified from Christakis, G., editor: Nutritional assessment in health programs, Am. J. Public Health **63**(suppl.):1, 1973.
*No values available.

Biochemical parameters have also been used to identify and screen certain diseases. For instance, elevated levels of serum cholesterol and triglycerides have been implicated in heart disease. Efforts are being continued to evolve more sensitive parameters and newer and more accurate techniques. Hair biopsy sample analysis for certain trace minerals and protein status is being considered. Urinary hydroxyproline as an index for detecting protein-calorie malnutrition is another more recent parameter being used. However, the need for large numbers of parameters is being questioned. Whether fewer variables could be used for screening population groups is also being debated. Much more experimentation and study are necessary before a decision can be made.

Methods. The biochemical methods used vary in cost, reliability, and the degree of technical expertise. They are also constantly being revised and improved. Analytical techniques for evaluating constituents of blood have been adopted for use with very small samples. These microtechniques have enabled the determination of fifteen to twenty biochemical constituents in as small a sample as 1 ml of blood. Microtechniques have not only added to the convenience of the individual being tested but have also facilitated the usage of more biochemical parameters in the nutritional assessment. The selection of a test and method and the interpretation of results depend on resources available and on the preference of the researcher.

Norms. Norms for biochemical parameters that are frequently used have been developed by the Interdepartmental Committee on Nutrition for National Defense (ICNND). These standards refer to the adult man only. Therefore, in the National Nutrition Survey, standards referring to all age groups are derived on the basis of research findings and the ICNND standards (Table 5-17).

The norms used are often criticized. The arbitrarily chosen cutoff points, indicative of some degree of risk (deficient, marginal, and acceptable), are a matter of controversy. This is not surprising in view of the fact that the specificity of laboratory evaluation of nutrients and the physiological significance of the tests used are still not conclusive.

Interpretation. Biochemical data indicate the deviation from the norm but not always the cause of the deviation. Further difficulty in interpretation is encountered when the body's homeostatic mechanisms, which could cause a nutrient deficiency, are considered. Only when the body's homeostatic mechanisms fail do deficiencies in specific nutrients become apparent.

Currently, immune response of the host is also being considered in assessing nutritional status. Cell-mediated immunity (CMI), as judged by a failure to develop cutaneous hypersensitivity to various allergens, is depressed in protein-calorie malnutrition. Lymphocyte counts are also reduced in this condition.

Conclusion

More positive correlation between biochemical parameters and dietary intake data have been found in nutrition surveys than between laboratory and clinical findings. This is not surprising in consideration of the nonspecific nature of clinical lesions and the development of biochemical variations before physical abnormalities are apparent.

This does not mean that the clinical method is not of importance or that one method of assessment is better than the other. The data from all the methods should be collected, integrated, and then interpreted to be assured of a reasonable degree of diagnostic accuracy and sensitivity.

Nutritional assessment is an expensive procedure. Presently, the need for large numbers of variables is being questioned. Christakis states that all the variables discussed before do not always have to be considered every time. The screening procedures could be determined by the levels of approach. In some cases, such as a well baby clinic, a minimum level of assessment inclusive of simple indices such as height, weight, hemoglobin level, and food habits may be sufficient. In some situations, an "in-depth" approach may be necessary. For a detailed discussion see Christakis.

Efforts are being made to reduce the number of tests necessary to identify nutritionally vulnerable individuals and groups without reducing the diagnostic potential. Statistical analysis (factor analysis) of the data collected on more than 25 variables in the Ten-State Survey indicated that perhaps as few as 8 to 10 of these parameters would provide as much information as that provided by all the variables together. For example in children, consumption of as few as two nutrients, calories and iron, seem to reflect that of all the nutrients. With this, time, effort, and money may be efficiently and effectively used.

An example of a simple data-gathering form for nutritional assessment follows.

Sample data-gathering form for nutritional assessment

GENERAL INFORMATION

Name: _____ Date of interview: _____

Address: _____ Interviewer: _____

Age: _____ Sex: _____ Marital status: _____

Occupation (type): _____

Educational attainment: _____

Primary diagnosis (if hospitalized) (include medical history): _____

_____

_____

Chronic conditions, if any (diabetes, PVK, etc.): _____

_____

Living arrangements: ☐ Family ☐ Alone ☐ Institution ☐ Other (specify): _____

Number in the household: _____

Ethnic background: _____

Religion (food restrictions, if any): _____

Economic conditions

   Amount of money spent on food: _____

   Participation in food programs: ☐ WIC ☐ Food stamps ☐ Other (specify): _____

Physical activity (specify type, duration, and frequency)

   Sleep _____ hours/day

   Feeding problems (if any) (chewing, swallowing, dependent feeding, others [specify]) _____

_____

   Food allergies or intolerances: _____

   Food preferences: _____

   Vitamin-mineral supplement (specify type and amount): _____

_____

24-HOUR FOOD INTAKE

(can be completed by the interviewer or interviewee)

Meal	Time	Foods consumed (specify type, additions, ingredients, etc.)
Breakfast		
Snack(s)		
Lunch		
Snack(s)		
Dinner		
Snack(s)		

Sample data-gathering form for nutritional assessment—cont'd

ANTHROPOMETRIC MEASUREMENTS

Height (cm) _____
Weight (kg) _____
Tricep skinfold (TSF) (mm) _____
Midarm circumference (MAC) (cm) _____
Midarm muscle circumference (MAMC) (cm) _____

LABORATORY DATA OF IMPORTANCE

(depends on the nutrients in which you are interested)
Hemoglobin _____ g/ml
Hematocrit _____ %
Serum albumin _____ g/dl
Serum transfusion _____ g/dl
You can transfer these data from medical chart.

AFTER COLLECTION OF DATA

1. Assess the adequacy of diet using
   a. Basic-Four food guide
   b. RDA (after calculating the nutrient intake using food composition table):
      Caloric intake: _____ kcal
      Protein intake: _____ g
      Other nutrients according to the nature of assessment.
2. Compare the anthropometric measurements to standards:
   Weight for height (% standard)
   MAC: Percentile rank
   MAMC: Percentile rank
3. Compare the laboratory values to appropriate norms:
   From the data gathered, identify the nutritional need(s) of the subject.
   To cross-check information, gather data on frequency of foods consumed. This list can be concise or detailed depending on the nature of assessment.

Food	Amount	Frequency of consumption		
		Daily	Weekly	Monthly
Milk group				
Meat group				
Fruit and vegetable group				
Bread and cereal group				
Other				

BIBLIOGRAPHY

Adams, C.F.: Nutritive value of American foods in common units, Agriculture Handbook No. 456, Washington, D.C., 1976, Agriculture Research Service, U.S. Department of Agriculture.

Arroyave, G.: Biochemical evaluation of nutritional status of man, Fed. Proc. **20**:39, 1960.

Beal, V.A.: The nutritional history in longitudinal research, Am. J. Diet Assoc. **51**:426, 1967.

Bollet, A.J., and Owens, S.: Evaluation and nutritional status of selected hospitalized patients, Am. J. Clin. Nutr. **26**:931, 1973.

Butterworth, G., and Blackburn, G.: Hospital malnutrition, Nutr. Today **10**:8, 1975.

Christakis, G.M., editor: Nutritional assessment in health programs, Am. J. Pub. Health **63**(suppl.):1, 1973.

Food and Nutrition Board: Recommended dietary allowances, Revised 1980, Washington, D.C., 1980, National Academy of Sciences–National Research Council.

Frisancho, A.: Triceps skinfold and upper arm muscle size norms for assessment of nutritional status, Am. J. Clin. Nutr. **27**:1052, 1974.

Garn, S.M.: The applicability of North American growth standards in developing countries, Grad. Med. Assoc. J. **93**:914, 1965.

Grant, A.: Nutritional assessment guidelines. Available from A. Grant, Box 25057, Northgate Station, Seattle, Wash. 98125.

Gueney, M.J., and Jellife, D.B.: Arm anthropometry in nutritional assessment: monogram for rapid calculation of muscle circumference and cross sectional muscle and fat areas, Am. J. Clin. Nutr. **26**:912, 1973.

Guthrie, H.A., and Guthrie, G.M.: Factor analysis of nutritional status data from Ten-State Survey, Am. J. Clin. Nutr. **29**:1238, 1976.

Guthrie, H.A., Owens, G.M., and Guthrie, G.M.: Factor analysis of measures of nutritional status of preschool children, Am. J. Clin. Nutr. **26**:497, 1973.

Hillman, R.W.: Concordance among clinical signs suggestive of malnutrition, Am. J. Clin. Nutr. **20**:1118, 1967.

Hollingsworth, D.: Dietary determination of nutritional status, Fed. Proc. **20**:50, 1960.

Howells, G.R., Wharlon, B.A., and McCance, R.A.: Value of hydroxyproline indices in malnutrition, Lancet **1**:1082, 1967.

Interdepartmental Committee on Nutrition for National Defense (ICNND): Manual for nutrition surveys, Bethesda, Md., 1963, ICNND.

Jelliffe, D.B.: The assessment of the nutritional status of the community, WHO Monogr. Ser. **53**:3, 1966.

Kelsey, J.L.: A compendium of nutritional status studies and dietary evaluation studies conducted in the United States, 1957-1967, Part II, J. Nutr. **99**(suppl. 1):123, 1969.

Klevay, L.M.: Hair as a biopsy material: assessment of zinc nutriture, Am. J. Clin. Nutr. **23**:284, 1970.

Krehl, W.A., and Hodges, R.E.: The interpretation of nutrition survey data, Am. J. Clin. Nutr. **17**:191, 1965.

Leevy, C.M., and others: Incidence and significance of hypovitaminemia in a randomly selected municipal hospital population, Am. J. Clin. Nutr. **19**:259, 1965.

Medical assessment of nutritional status: report of the Joint FAO/WHO Expert Committee, WHO Techn. Rep. Ser. 258, 1963.

Pearson, W.N.: Biochemical appraisal of the vitamin nutritional status in man, JAMA **180**:49, 1962.

Pekkarinen, M.: Methodology in the collection of food consumption data, World Rev. Nutr. Diet **12**:145, 1970.

Plough, I.C., and Bidforth, E.B.: Relations of clinical and dietary findings in nutritional surveys, Public Health Rep. **75**:699, 1960.

Selzer, C.C., Goldman, R.F., and Mayer, J.: The triceps skinfold as a predictive measure of body density and body fat in obese adolescent girls, Pediatrics **36**:212, 1965.

Standard, K.L., Lovell, H.G., and Garrow, J.S.: The validity of certain physical signs as indices of generalized malnutrition in young children, J. Trop. Pediatr. **11**:100, 1966.

Suaberlich, H.E., Dowdy, R.P., and Skala, J.H.: Laboratory tests for the assessment of nutritional status, CRC Crit. Rev. Clin. Lab. Sci. September, 1973, p. 215.

U.S. Department of Helath, Education, and Welfare: Ten-state nutritional survey, 1968-1970, vols. 1-5, Atlanta, Ga., Health Services and Mental Health Administration.

Wilson, C.S., and others: A review of methods used in nutrition surveys conducted by the Interdepartmental Committee on Nutrition for National Defense (ICNND), Am. J. Clin. Nutr. **15**:29, 1965.

CHAPTER 6

ASSESSMENT OF SLEEP-WAKEFULNESS PATTERNS

CLINICAL IMPLICATIONS OF HUMAN CIRCADIAN RHYTHMS

Normal human beings are characterized as organisms that adapt bodily functions in such a way as to have a different physiochemical and psychological makeup for each hour of the day. Yet each of these changes is carefully regulated for the given hour. And the variations of one day closely resemble those of each other day. This ability to maintain a relative internal constancy has been termed *homeostasis* or, more precisely, *homeokinesis*. Thus, healthy individuals represent the integration of a myriad of cyclical alterations of psychophysiological functions.

Biological rhythms have been described for all levels of biological functions. The external stimuli that are most likely to affect the human are those whose periods most closely correspond to endogenous rhythms.

Considerable evidence has supported the possibility of endogenous timekeeping. Circadian rhythms persist even when an organism is isolated from time cues (free-running cycles). Humans who have been placed in a chamber where the levels of light, temperature, food, and sounds are kept constant have circadian rhythms that more directly reflect the behavior of the human clock(s). The most prevalent rhythms, when freed from the effects of the environment, are periods of 23 to 25 hours called circadian. *Circadian rhythms* are defined as those functions with a period of 20 to 28 hours. However, there is a wide range of biological rhythms with periods of less than a second to more than a year (Table 6-1). *Ultradian rhythms* are those periods less than 24 hours. Ultradian rhythms in the human being include the electrical activity of the brain as recorded by electroencephalogram (EEG), heartbeat, and breathing. *Infradian rhythms* are characterized by periods longer than 28 hours, an example of which is the menstrual period. The suprachiasmatic nuclei of the hypothalamus have been demonstrated to be the anatomical structures that are necessary to the control of many circadian rhythms, including the sleep-wakefulness cycle. However, it is known that circadian rhythms are controlled by more than one oscillator. Two key properties must be demonstrated for a biological structure to be considered a biological clock. First, the structure must count the passage of time independently of any periodic input from the environment and, second, the structure times of the events in the body. It is known that relatively few chemical compounds interfere with circadian rhythms. One class of chemicals that is known to reset the timing of circadian clocks is methylxanthines. Caffeine is the most common substance in this family of chemicals.

Table 6-1

Types of biological rhythms

Rhythm	Time period	Example
Ultradian	< 24 hours	Electrical activity of brain (EEG) Heartbeat Respiratory rate Sleep cycles
Circadian	20-28 hours	Most human rhythms Vital signs Serum electrolyte values Urine electrolyte values Hormones of the pituitary gland
Infradian	> 28 hours	Menstrual cycle Sexual hormones

Since the cyclical nature of human function has been defined, a good deal of experimentation has been focused on determining whether one or more factors in the environment are the cause of the rhythms. Further work has been devoted to locating receptors in humans that sense these external factors and are responsible for the establishment of the rhythms.

Human beings adapt to environmental cues of an immediate nature, as well as to external sequences or cycles of regularly changing conditions. Examples of regular external periodicities that are thought to be incorporated into organisms' adaptive behavior are the tides, the light-dark cycle, the lunar cycle, and the seasons. This adaptive process involves the establishment of an endogenous rhythm that approximately corresponds to the environmental stimulus. These rhythms are known as the biological clocks that allow the organisms to adjust to the changes occurring outside. Once the internal rhythm is established, the environmental cue that caused the change becomes a synchronizing stimulus and is called a *Zeitgeber* (Ger. *Zeit*, time; and *Geber*, giver).

It has been shown that cells may be influenced directly by gravity and electrostatic magnetic fields. The nervous system seems important to the control of rhythms in higher organisms, particularly as related to photoperiodicity. At least one researcher has hypothesized different levels of rhythm organizations: neural, endocrine, and cellular. In this system, the neural system is thought to be entrained by dominant synchronizers and cellular elements by weaker synchronizers. In human beings, it is necessary to include a fourth level, psychosocial organization, which may serve to modify rhythmical trends.

In the human, social cues are considered to be important *Zeitgeber's.* An experiment comparing groups of subjects isolated from time cues exhibited free-running periods different from each other. When a subject was moved from one group to another, a progressive phase shift occurred to resynchronize with the new group.

The influence most frequently observed in plants and animals is the day-night, or light-dark, cycle. Such circadian (L. *circa,* about; and *dies,* day) rhythms have been identified for all cells and functions of the human body from enzyme levels to complex neural events. Because most human rhythms are 23 to 25 hours in length, they are termed circadian. However, although most human functions are entrained by a period approximating 24 hours, the peaks (high-function point) and troughs (low-function point) of daily rhythms for various functions can occur at different times; and although these functional records show phase relationships to each other, it is not known if all the rhythms for the various functions are entrained by *Zeitgeber* stimuli or by other rhythms internal to the person.

It has been hypothesized that functions such as the sleep-wakefulness cycle are weakly entrained, whereas functions such as urinary output, body temperature, adrenocortical secretion, enzyme production, and cellular division are more strongly incorporated. Data to support this hypothesis are those from experiments wherein subjects are placed in lightproof and soundproof enclosures for weeks to months. As many stimuli as possible are removed, and this is termed the free-running condition, which means that cyclical events occur in the absence of their respective *Zeitgeber.* The sleep-wakefulness cycle becomes desynchronized to 30 to 33 hours. The more deeply entrained cycles, the vegetative functions, retain a 25-hour cycle. Thus, many endogenous cycles may be in new phase relationships.

Table 6-2

Time of maximum amplitude of physiological rhythms in a person whose sleep cycle is 11 PM to 7 AM

	Peak of cycle*
Vital signs	
Temperature (rectal)	4-6 PM
Heart rate	4 PM
Respiratory rate	2-3 PM
Blood pressure	7-10 PM
Cardiac output	Midnight
Venous pressure	Midnight
Oxygen consumption	Midnight
Physical vigor	3-4 PM
Optical reaction time	3 AM
Grip strength	2-8 PM
Blood	
Sodium	4-5 PM
Calcium	9-10 PM
17-Hydroxycorticosteroid	7-8 AM
Hematocrit	9-10 PM
Polymorphonuclear cells	12-1 PM
Lymphocytes and monocytes	11-3 AM
Urine	
Sodium	12-1 PM
Potassium	12-1 PM
Calcium	3-4 PM
Magnesium	1 AM
Dopamine	3 PM
Catecholamines	5-7 PM
Vanillylmandelic acid	5-7 AM
17-Hydroxycorticosteroid	9-10 AM
Rate of excretion	8-9 AM
Mitosis-epidermal	11-12 PM
Body weight	6-7 PM

*The valley or low period for these values occurs approximately 12 hours later.

The 24-hour temperature rhythm was defined soon after the development of the clinical thermometer in the eighteenth century. However, a refined experimental approach to the study of biological rhythms in human physiology had its origin in the 1920s when it was shown that rhythms occur even in metabolism. Table 6-2 reflects some of the data useful to the health care professional in this still relatively unknown field.

The measures of physiological function that have been used as diagnostic indicators have been shown to exhibit a circadian rhythm. The human body has been shown to have a diurnal rhythm of peaks and troughs for nearly every laboratory value and physiological measurement.

The variation from high (peak) to low (trough) for some values may be minor, as little as 10% of plasma potassium concentration, but the changes over a 24-hour period may be markedly variable as in the case of plasma cortisol, which is quite low before sleep and reaches a daily peak just before awakening. It is now considered good practice to take into account the time of day at which the plasma cortisol was obtained.

It has been shown that the sensitivity to many pharmacological agents, such as morphine and ethanol, to bacteria, and to carcinogens varies over the 24-hour period. Thus, the time the client takes a given medication may influence the effectiveness of the drug.*

Some cycles appear to be significantly related to one another; for instance, the pulse rate and respiratory rate in the normal adult demonstrate a 4:1 ratio, and any long-term deviation from this ratio may be the diagnostic feature of abnormal function.

Nocturnal diuresis has been given as an example of a phase change (180 degrees) in a biological rhythm; the change in time for this function was recognized as abnormal and given diagnostic significance long before circadian rhythms were well defined.

Periodic mood changes are described in both normal mental states and in emotional illnesses. Dramatic changes in affect occur in manic-depressive illness. One group has reported that some hormonal functions may free run whereas other rhythms adhere to the 24-hour cycle and has correlated depression with the times when hormonal functions are out of phase.

ALTERATIONS IN ENVIRONMENTAL TIME

The human being, like most other species on earth, evolved in a regular 24-hour light-dark cycle. Yet many changes have occurred in human life-style that have an effect on circadian rhythmicity. The invention of the light bulb caused an interference with light-dark cycles.

*The body is more sensitive to toxic effects of some drugs at specific times of the day.

Persons who have experienced unconventional sleep-wake schedules, such as persons working evening and night shifts and persons traveling across time zones, may have disruption of circadian rhythms. That is, the rhythm of such individuals may be out of phase with persons sleeping in the nighttime hours and with the majority of persons in that time zone.

The hospital environment may disrupt the circadian rhythms of patients subjected to relatively constant levels of noise, light, and activity around the clock, such as occurs in intensive care units.

A good deal of work has been devoted to determining whether interference with circadian rhythms results in disorders in the affected individual. Two particularly fruitful areas for this study have been work situations requiring a change in the sleep-wakefulness pattern and rapid travel across time zones.

Industrial shift workers demonstrate changes in accuracy and accident proneness. Workers who change shifts give an indication of some imbalance in rhythms.

Some 16% of workers in the United States and about 60 million persons worldwide are known to rotate between day and night shifts or to be assigned permanently to evening or night work.

The major health disruptions associated with shift work are disruptions of sleep and digestive disorders. It is not feasible for shift workers to sleep at the normal phase of the circadian cycle. Sleep may occur at the phase of maximum arousal of the endogenous rhythm. Other persons in their lives may be awake and making noise as the shift worker tries to sleep. Food may be available only at times of days when the hormones and enzymes of the gastrointestinal tract are at low ebb. Many persons (as high as 80%) who rotate shifts report sleep disruption, including insomnia and sleepiness at work. Disruptions of the circadian cycle have been associated with emotional disturbance and impaired coordination. Temperature changes over the 24-hour period are reduced in amplitude. The work schedules of health professionals, particularly house officers and nurses, are often disruptive of circadian synchrony.

Travel

Translongitudinal passage or long-distance travel across time zones results in a derangement of rhythms so that several days are required to adapt to local time. A 5-hour flight westward results in a readjustment period of 2 days for the sleep-wakefulness cycle, 5 days for body temperature, and 8 days for cortisol secretion.

Travel by airplane has produced rapid shifts in environmental light-dark cycles. At one time travel in an easterly or westerly direction was sufficiently slow that the time zones below the Arctic Circle (500 to 1000

6. Avoidance of caffeine (Explanation: Caffeine is known to modify circadian rhythms.)
7. Avoidance of smoking (Explanation: Both nicotine and the resultant increased carbon monoxide blood levels may cause arousal.)

It is recommended that persons with insomnia not stay in bed tossing and turning but get up and find an absorbing and satisfying activity until they feel tired again.

Disorders of excessive somnolence

Hypersomnia. *Hypersomnia* is the term used to describe the condition wherein an individual has a tendency to sleep for excessive periods. In some clients the sleep period may be extended to 16 to 18 hours a day. The episodes of hypersomnia may be acute or chronic. The EEG sleep patterning is normal. Victims of hypersomnia are found to have higher pulse and respiratory rates than normal individuals during both sleep and wakefulness.

Perihypersomnia is a condition that is described as an increased need for sleep (18 to 20 hours a day) that lasts for only a few days, following which the client is fine.

Hypersomnia has been correlated with uremia, increased intracranial pressure, and diabetic acidosis. The hypothyroid client may report longer hours spent in sleep and sleepiness when awake.

In some cases hypersomnia may be a conversion symptom. The severely anxious client may be escaping discomfort in sleep. The hysterical personality and the depressed individual are predisposed to conversion symptoms. This mechanism should be looked for particularly when the need to sleep occurs repeatedly in conjunction with potentially troublesome experiences, such as "Whenever my mother-in-law comes for a visit."

Narcolepsy. Narcolepsy ("sleep attacks") is the term used to describe the excessive daytime drowsiness or uncontrolled onset of sleep. Although the pathophysiology of narcolepsy is not clearly understood, it is safe to say that the condition is a disorder in the sleep regulatory mechanism. The episode of sleep occurs when the client is engaged in what are considered to be wake-time activities. Some 10% of diagnosed narcoleptics have described situations of falling asleep while driving and causing accidents. Others have fallen asleep in such unusual activities as standing at attention while in the military service or while eating. It is particularly important to be alert to the evidence that will establish the diagnosis so that treatment may be instituted, since the untreated narcoleptic is dangerous to himself and to others. The annual incidence is thought to be at least 0.07% in the United States.

The episodes of involuntary sleep may begin just before puberty, that is, at approximately 12 years of age in girls and 14 years of age in boys. The range of age for the first attack may occur any time between 10 and 40, however. The familial involvement should be explored, since family members show an incidence of narcolepsy twenty times that of the general population.

Clinical records indicate that affected individuals may have the condition for as long as 15 years before it is diagnosed. This is particularly reprehensible, since the attacks can be eliminated by amphetamines or methylphenidate (Ritalin) hydrochloride.

Because most normal people feel sleepy from time to time during the day, particularly at quiet times, such as during a dull lecture or television broadcast, a careful history is necessary to differentiate this dozing phenomenon from narcolepsy.

Automatism is sometimes reported by the narcoleptic victim's relatives. He appears to be awake but may act irrationally. The client does not remember the episode.

Diagnosed narcoleptics are observed to sleep fewer hours than their normal counterparts, and the sleep they do obtain is interrupted and restless. They fall asleep remarkably quickly, sometimes within 15 seconds after lying down, and complain of difficulty in waking up.

Narcolepsy has been described as a tetrad of four symptoms: sleep attacks, cataplexy, hypnagogic hallucinations, and sleep paralysis. The final two symptoms occur in the transition period between sleep and wakefulness and are only indicative of narcolepsy when accompanied by the preceding symptoms.

Sleep attacks. The uncontrolled sleep in the early stages of the disorder occurs infrequently and under conditions that are described by normal people as sleep inducing. The episodes increase in number and occur in increasingly bizarre circumstances. Eventually the episodes occur 3 to 5 times a day, lasting 5 to 15 minutes. Some of these victims fall asleep without warning, whereas others feel sleepy for minutes or hours before succumbing to sleep.

Cataplexy. Approximately 4 to 5 years after the disorder is initiated, cataplexy may be experienced by the client. Cataplexy is abrupt weakness or paralysis of voluntary muscles and is seen predominantly in the muscles of the arms, legs, and face. There are many gradations of the loss of voluntary skeletal contraction. The episode may be experienced as only a fleeting weakness or as the inability to move quickly. On the other hand, all the skeletal muscles may be paralyzed. The intraocular muscles are a frequent exception. The client may still be capable of perceiving his external environment. He may describe the attacks as "My knees buckled," "My jaws sagged," "I couldn't speak," "The muscles of my neck were twitching," or "I couldn't walk."

The cataplectic attack may last from a half second to 10 minutes, and the client may experience them only once or twice a year or as often as 100 times a day. The attacks appear to be triggered by strong emotion, loud noise, a startle reaction, or sudden fright. Hearty laughter has frequently been implicated as a stimulus to the episodes.

Hypnagogic hallucinations. These attacks may be described as dream episodes. They are generally disturbing or frightening dreams that occur as the client is falling asleep. The client describes the dream as very real—"As if I were right there"—and the feeling as one of being awake. This can occur in the normal individual.

Sleep paralysis. The phenomenon of sleep paralysis is a skeletal muscle paralysis of varying degrees that occurs when the client awakes or is falling asleep. The client describes the arousal as one of waking and being aware of external conditions but unable to move or speak. If undisturbed, the client recovers gradually. However, if he is stimulated, as by touching, paralysis ameliorates quickly. It must be borne in mind that sleep paralysis may occur in as many as 2% to 3% of the normal population.

Relation to REM sleep. Although narcolepsy has been linked to epilepsy in the past because of similar EEG patterning, it is not the same; nor can narcolepsy be logically attributed to depression or schizophrenia. More acceptable in the light of research findings is that narcolepsy is related to REM sleep. REM activity can be recorded during sleep attacks. The victim has a REM period at the beginning of his long sleep period. Some individuals with cataplexy experience REM sleep before recovery. Both hypnagogic hallucinations and sleep paralysis in normal individuals have been associated with REM activity.

Treatment of narcolepsy includes good sleep hygiene and the use of stimulants such as dextroamphetamine, methylphenidate, and pemoline. Cataplectic attacks are treated with imipramine, clomipramine, or protriptyline (antidepressants). Support groups have been sponsored by the American Narcolepsy Association.

Secondary sleep disorders

Secondary sleep disorders are those sleep disturbances that occur in individuals who have clinical disorders. Those clinical entities most often accompanied by sleep disorders are alterations in thyroid hormone secretion, chronic renal insufficiency, depression, schizophrenia, alcoholism, and anorexia nervosa.

Alterations in thyroid hormone secretion. Individuals with both hyposecretion and hypersecretion of the thyroid have derangements of stage 3 and 4 sleep. Individuals with hyperthyroid conditions have decreased stages 3 and 4 sleep time, whereas persons with hypothyroid conditions show increases. Sleep patterns return to normal with adequate treatment to bring the client into the euthyroid range.

Chronic renal insufficiency. The client who undergoes dialysis treatments for chronic renal insufficiency has been observed to have sleep disturbances that occur with greatest frequency just before dialysis and are improved after the dialysis. Investigation has shown that sleep disturbances correlate with the uremic condition.

Depression. Depression is both a mental illness and a symptom. Depression is seen in the grieving process over significant loss or when things otherwise go badly. The depressed client has prolonged latency in achieving sleep, more rapid transition from stage to stage, more frequent awakening, less slow-wave sleep, less total sleep time, and more REM activity.

Depression as a mental illness is that which is incurred without significant loss. A subgroup of depressives is made up of those individuals who alternate between periods of depression and mania. The classical clinical description of the sleep pattern in depression is that of early morning awakening. Stage 4 sleep decreases in both manic and depressive clients. During the manic phase the client is observed to have decreased total sleep time and decreased REM activity. Depressed periods are associated with normal sleep time.

Schizophrenia. Some investigators have reported anorexia and a reduction in REM sleep in the early phases of schizophrenia. Stages 3 and 4 sleep are also significantly reduced in the schizophrenic. Greater eye movement has been reported in hallucinating schizophrenics than in nonhallucinating individuals.

Alcoholism. Studies have shown that the subject who has drunk 6 ounces of 95% alcohol before sleep shows REM deprivation during his sleep period, whereas the person who drinks small amounts of alcohol may not show changes in the sleep pattern. The client who drinks three to four drinks a day may feel tremulous in the morning and "need" a drink to calm down. Because alcohol is a CNS depressant, it may help the client get to sleep; but because it is a short-acting drug, it does not affect sleep maintenance. Furthermore, it may diminish REM sleep in the early hours of the sleep period and therefore contribute to a rebound increase of REM activity in the latter hours of sleep. Withdrawal studies of chronic alcoholics showed that sleep periods were made up almost entirely of REM sleep. These alcoholics frequently awakened from REM to experience hallucinations.

Both slow-wave and REM sleep appear to be

decreased in acute alcoholic psychosis. Initially, slow-wave activity appears to increase, whereas REM sleep is suppressed. As the condition progresses both may disappear. As mentioned above, REM rebound has been employed as an explanation for the hallucinations that occur on withdrawal of alcohol. The rebound of slow-wave sleep has been cited as the harbinger of recovery from the psychosis.

Anorexia nervosa. The individual experiencing anorexia nervosa has a protein-calorie deficiency that is accompanied by a patterned sleep disturbance. There is a reduction of the deeper sleep stages, 3 and 4, as well as of REM sleep. Although stage 1 sleep is increased, there is a reduction in total sleep time (boxed material below).

Parasomnias (disorders of arousal)

Parasomnia is the term used for those patterns of waking behavior that appear during sleep. Some of those most common behaviors are night terrors, somnambulism (sleepwalking), sleep talking, bruxism (teeth grinding), nocturnal erection, and enuresis (bedwetting).

Night terrors and dream anxiety attacks (nightmares). Night terrors occur during slow-wave sleep (stages 3 and 4). Children who experience night terrors generally do not display daytime anxiety, whereas adults are likely to have anxiety symptoms.

Night terror–sleep terror. The individual with night or sleep terror has repeated episodes of abrupt awakening with symptoms of anxiety that last about 1 to 10 minutes. The episodes generally occur between 30 and 200 minutes after onset of sleep during sleep stages 3 and 4. Anxiety symptoms include tachycardia, rapid breathing, dilated pupils, sweating, and piloerection, indicating sympathetic arousal. Efforts to comfort the victim of night terrors are generally unsuccessful.

Dream anxiety attacks. Dream anxiety attacks are the most common and are considered to be milder than night terrors. They occur in the middle of sleep or later. Autonomic anxiety signs may or may not accompany these episodes. Mental confusion frequently occurs, particularly if the sleeper is awakened suddenly.

Somnambulism. Sleepwalking is common (1% to 6%) in children between the ages of 5 and 12 years. It occurs more often in children than in adults. Furthermore, boys are affected more frequently than girls. Sleepwalking has familial relationships; it is more common among family members than among the general population. Both sleepwalking and night terrors occur during stages 3 and 4 of sleep, usually between 30 and 200 minutes after onset of sleep. The sleepwalker may not awaken during the episode if he is active less than 3 to 4 minutes but will show an awakening pattern if he stays up longer. During ambulation the sleeper functions at a low level of awareness and critical skill.

The essential feature of sleepwalking is repeated episodes of a sequence of complex behaviors, including leaving the bed and walking. The walking periods may last from a few minutes to half an hour. The sleepwalker does not appear to be conscious and is amnesic for the episode. The face of the sleepwalker is expressionless, and efforts to communicate with the somnambulist produce little response. Although the sleepwalker appears able to see and does walk around objects in his path, coordination is poor and stumbling and falling are hazards, particularly in going down stairs. Some sleepwalkers have walked through windows.

It is important to teach the family to protect the sleepwalker from injury by installing safety rails or guards, locks on windows, and having the somnambulist's bedroom on the ground floor.

Sleep talking. Articulation during sleep appears to be a frequent occurrence. Talking during sleep generally occurs during NREM sleep and during body movement.

Sleep disorders

Conditions associated with excessive daytime sleepiness	Conditions associated with chronic insomnia
Sleep apnea	Pain
Narcolepsy	Sleep apnea
Stimulant dependency	Restless legs syndrome
Shift change ⎤ Circadian	Nocturnal myoclonus
Change of ⎬ rhythm	Alpha sleep
time zone ⎦ disruption	Depression—nonpsychotic, i.e., loss of a loved one
Resulting from:	Exercise just before sleep
Hypothyroidism	Caffeine
Brain tumor	Coffee > 4 cups
	Tea
	Colas
	Resulting from:
	Aging
	Hyperthyroidism
	Anorexia nervosa
	Psychoses:
	Depression
	Manic-depressive illness
	Schizophrenia
	Change of ⎤ Circadian
	time zone ⎬ rhythm
	Shift change ⎦ disruption
	Pain
	Environmental discomfort
	Noise
	Cold
	Drug dependency and drug withdrawal
	Steroid administration
	Alcoholism

Nocturnal erections. Nocturnal erections occur during REM sleep and are said to occur at a frequency of approximately 80% in young men. Although there is considerable variation in the frequency of penile erection in men in their 70s, with some individuals showing a marked decrement in REM sleep erection, many of these older men maintain the young adult frequency to age 80. The penile circumference during REM sleep erection is markedly decreased as frequency wanes. Frequently, the client who is impotent in the awake state can achieve an erection during sleep. However, the erection abates soon after awakening.

Although clients may report that the sleep they obtain following sexual intercourse is more relaxed and restful, no significant changes in EEG patterning have been noted.

Bruxism. The grinding of the teeth during the sleep period, called bruxism, may occur in as many as 15% of the population. Evidence of the practice may be seen in damaged teeth or supporting structures. EEG studies demonstrate that bruxism generally is seen during stage 2 sleep.

Enuresis. The problem of enuresis has long been considered a genitourinary problem, although a pathological condition of this system is seldom found. Primary enuresis is bed-wetting during sleep. It persists from birth to at least the age of 6. Secondary enuresis refers to bed-wetting during sleep by an individual who has physiological control of micturition. This is primarily a disorder of childhood that is identified in 5% to 15% of all preadolescent children, and it may have a familial pattern. However, enuresis has been observed to exist in some sample adult groups at a rate of 1% to 2%.

Enuresis occurs more frequently in boys than in girls. Researchers have demonstrated more frequent bladder contractions and greater heart rate during the entire sleep period of those individuals affected, although the act of urination occurs in stage 2. The episode of bed-wetting occurs during slow-wave sleep. Children with enuresis are generally described as deep sleepers, that is, difficult to rouse from sleep. Whereas primary enuresis may be the result of a pathophysiological defect, secondary enuresis may be reflected to psychological factors.

In assessing the enuretic child, one should explore the affective state surrounding this condition with both the child and his parents. Although data from sleep laboratories demonstrate that 90% of enuretic children are asleep when bed-wetting occurs, in most cases studied the parents believed that the child had control over the occurrence. The parents punished the child, producing shame, embarrassment, guilt, or anxiety. To investigate how the episodes have been dealt with, the following questions might be used.

To the parents: "How have you felt about your child's wetting the bed?" If this question is nonproductive, more specific information might be gained by asking, "Do you feel he (she) could prevent the bed-wetting?" or "Do you punish him (her) when he (she) wets the bed?"

To the child: "How do you feel when you wake up after wetting the bed?"

Sleep apnea. Sleep apnea is a periodic cessation of breathing that occurs during sleep. A cessation of diaphragmatic movement may occur. This is called diaphragmatic apnea. Obstructive apnea is obstruction as a result of the relaxation of muscles of the nasopharynx, hypopharynx, and pharynx, which also occurs during sleep. Enlarged adenoids or tonsils predispose to this disorder. The bed partner may describe breathing of the affected individual as labored with long periods of apnea or as heavy snoring. The period of apnea leads to progressive hypercapnia, hypoxemia, increased pulmonary arterial pressures, sinus bradycardia, and other arrhythmias. This is known as upper-airway sleep apnea. A mixed form of apnea is both central and upper airway. Sleep apnea is thought to play a role in sudden infant death syndrome (SIDS). Serious arrhythmias are associated with sleep apnea.

Sleep apnea is a frequent cause of insomnia and excessive daytime sleepiness. Several important types of sleep apnea have been described:

1. *Obstructive, upper airway or occlusive:* The victim of obstructive sleep apnea is typically a middle-aged plethoric man with a history of hypertension who complains of daytime sleepiness. He may also have personality changes including irritability, impotence, morning headache, and lack of coordination and slurred speech on arising. It has also been demonstrated that alcoholics have a higher incidence of sleep apnea than nondrinking persons.

   Diagnosis is made in the sleep laboratory by demonstrating that there is no nasal or oral airflow despite persistent respiratory effort. The periods of sleep apnea may make up 50% to 60% of total sleep. The client is hypoxic and hypercarbic and may have cardiac arrhythmia. Tracheostomy reverses the symptoms.

2. *Central sleep apnea:* The client with central sleep apnea has an absence of respiratory effort and the lack of nasal and oral airflow. Persons with sleep apnea have responded to treatment with imipramine, clomipramine, and theophylline.

   Sleep apnea is often seen as a mixture of obstructive and central sleep apnea.

3. *Pickwickian syndrome:* Pickwickian syndrome is a clinical diagnosis for the client who is markedly obese with the attendant restriction of respira-

tion. The client has a history of hypertension. The sleep symptoms are similar to obstructive apnea. Treatment for pickwickian syndrome focuses on weight loss and proper pulmonary toilet.

Sleep apnea in children resembles obstructive apnea in adults. The affected children fall asleep during the day. Parents describe loud snoring, and the children may have enuresis, morning headaches, and irritability.

Sleep-provoked disorders: sleep patterns in chronic illness

The sleep-provoked disorders include symptoms and signs of chronic clinical diseases that are elicited during sleep (Table 6-6).

Pain. Clients who experience chronic pain may complain of "tossing and turning all night." These clients awaken frequently and stay awake for long periods of time. What has been shown through observation of individuals with angina pectoris is that they tend to underestimate their actual number of movements. Clients with angina experience pain during REM sleep. On awakening they may or may not report an upsetting dream. A direct cause-and-effect relationship has not been established.

Duodenal ulcer. Clients with duodenal ulcer often awaken in the night and complain of epigastric pain, which is relieved by food or antacid. It has been shown that these incidents are correlated with an increased secretion of gastric hydrochloric acid (three to twenty times greater than normal), particularly related to REM sleep; normal subjects studied did not demonstrate this increase in secretion.

Cardiovascular symptoms. The pain of myocardial ischemia frequently accompanies REM sleep. Observations of patients with myocardial infarctions have shown that premature ventricular contractions (PVCs) are increased during or immediately following REM sleep. The horizontal position generally assumed during sleep results in an increased plasma volume as gravity effects on the fluid compartments are obviated. The increased cardiac input may lead to left ventricular failure, resulting in pulmonary edema and dyspnea. Because many of the manifestations of heart disease do occur during the sleep period, many clients express a fear of going to sleep. This fear of falling asleep is particularly true of the client with angina pectoris or cardiac arrhythmia.

Respiratory alterations. Clients with emphysema have increased carbon dioxide tension and decreased oxygen saturation during sleep.

Children with asthma have been shown to have a decreased amount of stage 4 sleep as compared to normal children. In children asthmatic attacks originate in the late part of the sleep period, when the child is not in stage 4 sleep. In adults they may occur in any sleep stage. There is a decrease in total sleep time and frequent awakenings.

Asthmatics frequently have bronchial spasm during REM sleep periods.

Metabolic disorders. Individuals with diabetes mellitus have been shown to have variable levels of blood glucose during the sleep period. Thus, diabetic individuals who are being regulated for the first time or who are out of control may need special surveillance during sleep.

Rheumatoid arthritis. Early morning stiffness is a frequent symptom of the victim of rheumatoid arthritis. Short periods of disuse lead to stiffness.

Migraine headaches. Individuals with migraine headaches and with cluster headaches who suffered severe headache on awakening were monitored by EEG, which showed that the headache began during REM sleep.

ASSESSMENT OF SLEEP HABITS

The sleep-wake cycle is an obvious function of temporal organization. If the client cannot sleep at night or falls asleep during the daytime, it is likely that help will be sought to correct these subjective symptoms. Sleep disruptions may be debilitating and interfere with daytime activities.

Table 6-6
Clinical observations associated with stages of sleep

Stage of sleep	Associated clinical condition
NREM sleep	
Stage 1	Myoclonic jerks
	Bruxism
Stage 2	Bruxism
	Enuresis most likely to occur
Stage 3	Night terrors
	Sleepwalking
	Sleep talking
	Hypothyroidism—metabolic rate most depressed
All stages	Enuresis
	Bronchial asthma—except stage 4 in childhood
REM sleep	Nocturnal erection or emission
	Migraine headaches
	Gastric acid secretion increased
	Duodenal ulcer—incidence of epigastric pain
	Coronary atherosclerosis
	ECG changes
	Anginal attacks
	Bronchial asthma in children

The simplest and probably most accurate way, outside a sleep laboratory, to evaluate sleep-wake disorders is to have the client record the times of going to sleep and awakening for sleep periods, including naps, for a month. In most cases the health care provider sees the client for the first time in an ambulatory setting and must interview the client to obtain the information that will help to define the characteristics of the disorder and the 24-hour sleep-wakefulness pattern. Additional information may be obtained from the bed partner of the client.

In most cases it is more productive to allow the client to describe his sleep habits in his own words. An open-ended question may provide the stimulus to the client to give all the information pertinent to assessment. Examples of such questions are as follows:

"How have you been sleeping?"
"Can you tell me about your sleeping habits?"
"Are you getting enough rest?"
"Tell me about your sleep problem."

An adequate history includes a general sleep history, a psychological history, and a drug history. The description obtained of the sleep problem should include the 24-hour pattern of sleep and wakefulness.

There are times when the practitioner will have to ask more specific questions to understand the client's sleep habits. The suggested questions (see p. 132) may serve as a guide for this assessment. Only those questions need be used that will elicit the information not given by the more general query.

A technique that might more clearly define the sleep-activity cycle of the client is to provide him with a graph form on which to record his hours of sleep. He should be encouraged to keep a record over a long enough period that the pattern is well demonstrated on the graph.

He might be taught to color code his various activities to give the examiner, as well as himself, a clearer picture of his circadian rhythm. Even a simple written daily record of the sleep-activity cycle may prove helpful. At any rate, a diary of several days' sleep-activity cycles will allow the examiner a broader data base from which to advise the client.

The medication the client has been taking must be assessed. Cases of insomnia resulting from drug interaction have been recorded, and many drugs currently prescribed for induction of sleep may change the EEG activity pattern. Some of these changes are summarized in Table 6-7. The drugs listed in this table should be given particular attention in assessing the client's sleep pattern.

Table 6-7
Effects of pharmaceutical agents on the sleep cycle

Decrease time		Increase time		Allow normal time	
Drug	Dosage	Drug	Dosage	Drug	Dosage
REM sleep					
Placidyl	500 mg	Reserpine	1-2 mg	Chloral hydrate	0.5 g
Doriden	500 mg	LSD	30 µg		1.0 g
Seconal	100 mg				1.5 g
Phenobarbital	200 mg				
Nembutal	100 mg			Dalmane	15-30 mg
Quaalude	300 mg			Quaalude	150 mg
Benadryl	50 mg			Librium	50-100 mg
Scopolamine	0.006 mg/kg			Valium	5-10 mg
Morphine					
Heroin					
Alcohol	1 g/kg				
Tofranil	50 mg				
Elavil	50-75 mg				
Miltown	1,200 mg				
Amphetamine	15 mg				
Stage 4 sleep					
Doriden	500 mg	Antidepressants in the			
Nembutal	100 mg	presence of depression			
Valium	10 mg				
Librium	50 mg				
Reserpine	0.14 mg/kg				
Chloral hydrate	1.5 g				

Aspects of sleep pattern	Questions to elicit sleep pattern
Time retired Initial insomnia	"What time do you usually go to bed?" "Do you fall asleep right away?" "How long does it take you to fall asleep?" "How often do you have trouble falling asleep? Does it occur every night? Every other night? Just the weekend? Every Monday?" "How do you feel before you fall asleep?"
Maintenance insomnia	"Do you wake up in the night? How often does this occur?" What wakes you up once you have fallen asleep? Is there something that helps you get back to sleep?"
Arousal-terminal insomnia	"What time do you wake up? How often do you get up this early? What wakes you up at this early hour?" "What do you do once you wake up?"
Quality of sleep (affective response)	"How do you feel when you get up?" "Do you feel rested after a night's sleep?"
Naps	"Do you nap during the day?"
Dreams, night terrors	"Do you dream at night?" "Are your dreams ever frightening?" "Do your dreams ever wake you?" "How do you feel when you wake up from a bad dream?"
Bruxism	"Has anyone ever told you that you grind your teeth in your sleep?"
Somnambulism	"Has anyone ever told you that you walk in your sleep?" "Have you ever awakened in some place different than the one in which you went to sleep?" "Have you ever awakened to find furniture or other objects moved around in your home?"
Daytime activity work pattern	"What kind of work do you do?"
Shift change	"What hours do you work?"
Recreation, exercise	"What kind of activity is involved in your work?" "What do you do for fun?" "Are you engaged in any exercise?"
Home responsibilities	"Do you work at home? What kind of work do you do at home?"
Sleep environment	
Bedding (mattress, pillows, blankets)	"Do you need any special bedding to help you sleep?" "How many pillows do you use?"
Light	"Do you sleep with the lights off?" "Does having a light on at night bother you?"
Noise	"Do you have to have it very quiet to sleep?" "Do noises keep you awake at night? Wake you up?"
Ventilation	"Do you open the window at night?"
Temperature	"Do you need the bedroom to be cold [warm] to sleep well?"

Aspects of sleep pattern	Questions to elicit sleep pattern
Special activities associated with sleep	
Bath, massage	"What do you do just before going to bed?"
Food	"Do you eat before you go to bed?" "Do you like to have a snack before bed?"
Drink (warm milk, water)	"Do you like a drink before going to bed?" "What do you prefer as your bedtime beverage?"
Medication	"Do you take any medicine to help you sleep?" "Are you taking anything to keep you awake in the daytime?" "Are you taking any medicine at all?"
Personal beliefs about sleep	"How much sleep do you think you should have to stay healthy?" "What will happen if you don't get enough sleep?"
Internal stimuli	"How does the way you sleep affect your family?"
Psychiatric disorders (anxiety, depression, schizophrenia)	"How have your spirits been?" "Have you had a lot of worries lately?"
Alteration as a result of physical condition (stimulus, electrolyte imbalance)	"How have you been sleeping?"

BIBLIOGRAPHY

Aschoff, J.: Circadian systems in man and their implications, Hosp. Pract. **11**:51, 1976.

Aschoff, J., and others; Reentrainment of circadian rhythms after phase-shifts of the zeitgeber, Chronobiologica **2**:22, 1975.

Baker, R.M., and others: Lots of things you should know (and probably were never taught) about sleep, Patient Care **4**:24, 1970.

Bale, P., and White, M.: The effects of smoking on the health and sleep of sports women, Br. J. Sports Med. **16**(3):149, 1982.

Brown, C.C., and others: Sleep disorders: help for the patient who can't sleep, Patient Care **4**:24, 1970.

Brown, F.A.: The "clocks" timing biological rhythms, Am. Sci. **60**:756, 1972.

Bünning, E.: The physiological clock, London, 1973, The English Universities Press, Ltd.

Conroy, R.T., and Mills, J.N.: Human circadian rhythms, London, 1970, J. & A. Churchill.

Dement, W.C.: Some must watch while some must sleep, San Francisco, 1976, San Francisco Book Co., Inc.

Folk, G.E.: Biological rhythms. In Folk, G.E., editor: Textbook of environmental physiology, Philadelphia, 1974, Lea & Febiger.

Frankel, B., Patten, B., and Gillin, C.: Restless legs syndrome, JAMA **230**(9):1302, 1974.

Freemon, F.R.: Sleep research: a critical review, Springfield, Ill., 1972, Charles C Thomas, Publisher.

Ganten, D., and Pfaff, D., editors: Sleep: clinical and experimental aspects, New York, 1982, Springer-Verlag New York, Inc.

Guilleminault, C., Tilkin, A., and Dement, W.C.: The sleep apnea syndromes, Ann. Rev. Med. **27**:465, 1976.

Guilleminault, C., and Dement, W., editors: Sleep apnea syndromes, New York, 1978, Alan R. Liss, Inc.

Hartmann, E.L.: The functions of sleep, New Haven, 1973, Yale University Press.

Hudgel, D.: Diagnosis and therapy of sleep apnea, J. Fam. Pract. **12**(6):1001, 1981.

Kales, A., editor: Sleep physiology and pathology, Philadelphia, 1969, J.B. Lippincott Co.

Kales, A., and Kales, J.: Sleep disorders, N. Engl. J. Med. **290**:487, 1974.

Kales, A., Soldatos, C., and Kales, J.: Taking a sleep history, Am. Fam. Physician **22**(2):101, 1980.

Kales, A., and others: Sleep and dreams: recent research on clinical aspects, Ann. Intern. Med. **68**:1078, 1968.

Kales, J.D.: Aging and sleep. In Goldmann, R., and Rockstein, M., editors: Physiology and pathology of human aging, New York, 1975, Academic Press, Inc.

Kales, J.D., and others: Resource for managing sleep disorders, JAMA **241**:2413, 1979.

Kiester, E., Jr.: I keep falling asleep: what's wrong with me? Today's Health **54**:40, 1976.

Kleitman, N.: Sleep and wakefulness, Chicago, 1963, University of Chicago Press.

Kupfer, D., and Reynolds, C., III: Sleep disorders, Hosp. Pract. **18**(2):101, 1983.

Luce, G.C.: Biological rhythms in psychiatry and medicine, U.S. Department of Health, Education, and Welfare, National Institute of Mental Health, Public Health Service Publ. No. 2088, 1970, U.S. Government Printing Office.

Mendelson, W.: Sleep and its disorders, New York, 1977, Plenum Publishing Corp.

Miles, L.E., and Dement, W.C.: Sleep and aging, Sleep **3**(2):119, 1980.

Moore-Ede, M., Sulzman, F., and Fuller, C.: The clocks that time us, Cambridge, Mass. 1982, Harvard University Press.

Orem, J., and Bames, C., editors: Physiology in sleep, New York, 1980, Academic Press, Inc.

Orr, W., Altshuler, K., and Stahl, M.: Managing sleep complaints, Chicago, 1982, Year Book Medical Publishers, Inc.

Rechtschaffen, A., and Kales, A.: A manual of standardized terminology, techniques and scoring for sleep stages in human subjects, National Institute of Health Publ. No. 204, Washington, D.C., 1968, U.S. Government Printing Office.

Soldatos, C.R., Kales, A., and Kales, J.D.: Management of insomnia, Ann. Rev. Med. **30**:301, 1979.

Sollberger, A.: Biological rhythm research, New York, 1965, Elsevier Publishing Co.

Usdin, G., editor: Sleep research and clinical practice, New York, 1973, Brunner/Mazel, Inc.

Webb, W.: Sleep: an experimental approach, New York, 1968, Macmillan, Inc.

Webb, W., editor: Biological rhythms, sleep and performance, New York, 1982, John Wiley & Sons, Inc.

Wever, R.: Internal phase-angle differences in human circadian rhythms: causes for changes and problems of determinations, Int. J. Chronobiol. **1**:371, 1973.

Williams, R.L., and Karacan, I.: Sleep disorders: diagnosis and treatment, New York, 1975, John Wiley & Sons, Inc.

Williams, R.L., Karacan, I., and Hursch, C.J.: Electroencephalography (EEG) of human sleep: clinical applications, New York, 1974, John Wiley & Sons, Inc.

Zarcone, V.: Narcolepsy, N. Engl. J. Med **288**:1156, 1973.

Recent studies have shown the glass thermometer to be subject to inaccuracy. Furthermore, in most subjects the oral thermometer must be left in place for 8 minutes for women and 9 minutes for men to obtain full registration of the instrument at room temperatures of 65° to 75° F (18.3° to 23.9° C). Thus, the readings obtained for shorter registration periods must be considered to be approximations of the actual temperature of the client.

Other disadvantages in the use of the glass thermometer are frequent breakage and danger to the client through the use of rigid glass rod. Several instances of perforation of the rectal wall have occurred through inappropriate placement of a glass thermometer.

The examiner may also build in error through improper reading of the thermometer. The eyes must be at a 90 degree angle to the meniscus of the mercury to avoid parallax error.

Electronic thermometry. The electronic thermometer has been in use over the past decade. The advantages to be realized with the fully charged, correctly calibrated instrument are speed and accuracy of measurement. The probes used in these thermometers are unbreakable, thus obviating damage from broken glass and mercury ingestion, which are hazards with the traditional clinical thermometer.

The electronic thermometers are claimed to provide increased accuracy over glass thermometers by providing correct readings within 0.2° F. Thirty seconds is required for registration without lip closure. Less examiner time is required in the use of these thermometers.

Oral, rectal, and axillary temperature assessment

Differences in temperatures recorded from the mouth, rectum, or axilla have been shown to reflect the length of time the thermometer is allowed to register rather than actual variation in temperature from one site to another.

Oral temperature. The oral temperature registration is the most convenient method for the client. This site for temperature determination is the one used unless the client is an infant, unconscious, confused, or has shown erratic behavior.

A 5- to 15-minute wait is recommended before temperature assessment if the client has ingested hot or iced liquids, to allow the temperature to stabilize. Small temperature increases will occur if the client has smoked in the 2 minutes preceding the temperature assessment. The oral thermometer may take as long as 8 to 9 minutes to reach maximum registration. Other assessment procedures may be done at this time.

Rectal temperature. The rectal site for temperature registration is preferable for the confused or comatose client, the individual who is unable to close his mouth, the client who is receiving oxygen or the client who may bite the thermometer for other reasons.

The rectal temperature is routinely ordered as the general mode of temperature registration in some agencies.

The thermometer placed in the rectum will register adequately within a 2-minute time span in adults and within 3 minutes in premature infants.

Axillary temperature. Eleven minutes has been shown to be the maximum length of time necessary for the full registration of axillary temperature. This method has been shown to be safe and accurate for infants and small children.

Correlation of pulse and temperature

It should be noted that marked increases in temperature are accompanied by increments in pulse and respiratory rates because oxygen requirements are known to increase 7% for every 1° F (10% for every 1° C) rise in temperature. Since reducing cellular temperatures results in a decreased rate of cell metabolism, oxygen consumption is lessened in hypothermia; therefore, pulse and respiratory rates also decline.

Fever

Fever, or pyrexia, is the elevation of body temperature above normal limits as compared with a given individual's basal data. Fever may be a valid diagnosis when the temperature is found to be 98.6° F (37° C) for a specific client if his normal temperature ranges about 97° F (36.1° C).

Not all causes of fever are related to disease. Exercise may cause a temporary elevation of temperature, which subsides when the activity is stopped.

It has been suggested that a temperature above 97° F in a client who has been lying in bed (whose metabolism is basal) indicates the presence of disease. The association of an elevated temperature with disease is called a fever.

Fever is caused by those conditions that contribute to heat production, that prevent heat loss, or that affect the heat-regulating centers of the CNS.

Fevers are described according to the chronological pattern of occurrence and amplitude. Frequently, the recognition of the pattern may help to establish the diagnosis. The following paragraphs present descriptions of fever.

A *continuous* or *sustained fever* is one in which there is a persistent elevation of temperature without a return to normal values for that individual. This pattern is typical of typhoid or typhus fever.

An *intermittent fever* is one in which there are major diurnal variations, so that there is a daily elevation of temperature with a drop to subnormal or normal values in the same 24-hour period. When there is a marked difference between the peaks and the troughs of the temperature, the fever is called *hectic* or *septic*. This type of fever is seen in pyrogenic infection.

Remittent fever is characterized by a temperature elevation that does not return to normal level but shows marked spikes of even further increased temperature on the febrile baseline. This appears in sustained or continuous fever, in which there are only slight variations from the elevated set point.

Relapsing fever is one in which febrile periods alternate with periods of normal temperature. This pattern of fever is seen in malaria, relapsing fever, and the Pel-Ebstein fever of Hodgkin's disease.

Fever may also be described by the rate pattern of dissolution. *Lysis* is the gradual disappearance of fever, whereas *crisis* is the rapid (less than 36 hours) decrease of temperature to normal.

Stages or chronology of fever. The development of the febrile condition and its abatement have been described in three stages, called cold, hot, and defervescence.

The period of a developing increase in core temperature is characterized by heat conservation reactions. The affected individual has diminished cutaneous circulation, and the skin looks blanched and feels cold. Heat production is attested to by shivering and piloerection ("goose pimples"). Chills and rigor are the extremes of shivering that produce rapid increases in temperature.

The hot stage is the period after the fever has peaked (regulated at the new set point). During this stage blood flow to the periphery is increased. The affected individuals' body radiates excess heat, feels hot, and is flushed.

The stage of defervescence is the period of fever abatement and is characterized by heat loss mechanisms; particularly prominent is vasodilation and sweating. Diaphoresis is diffuse perspiration, which may accompany fever abatement.

Respiratory pattern

The assessment of the respiratory pattern is discussed in Chapter 15, "Assessment of the Respiratory System."

Pulsation

The assessment of central pulses discussed in Chapter 16, "Cardiovascular Assessment: the Heart and Neck Vessels," should be read before this section.

Assessment of the peripheral arterial pulse has been a part of the health professional's routine procedure throughout recorded medical history. The peripheral arterial pulse is a pressure wave transmitted from the left ventricle to the root of the aorta to the peripheral vessels.

Examination of the peripheral (radial) arterial pulsation gives less information concerning left ventricular ejection or aortic valvular function than does the assessment of the more central (carotid) arteries because the normal arterial pulse expands normal peripheral arteries only slightly. The information obtained is a necessary part of the data base, however, because the nature of the peripheral pulse gives an indication of cardiac function and of perfusion of the peripheral tissues. These peripheral pulsations are evaluated in terms of rate, amplitude (indicating volume), rhythm, and symmetry regularity. They may also be auscultated for the presence of bruits.

Arterial pulses are most accurately examined while the client is reclining with the trunk of the body elevated about 15 to 30 degrees.

Parameters of arterial pulsation

Visual and palpable pulsations result from diameter changes incurred through vessel filling and through straightening of the vessel. These pulsations are referred to as arterial pulse waves.

Pressure changes in the wall of the artery are felt through the overlying skin and subcutaneous tissue. The arterial pressure pulse wave is sensed through the pressure receptors in the pads of the examiner's fingers, which are superimposed on the vessel wall, as in pressure of paired arterial pulses exerted against the wall. The pulse is best palpated over arteries that are close to the surface of the body and that lie over a bony surface. The arteries that are palpated during the health examination include the superficial temporal, carotid, brachial, ulnar, radial, femoral, popliteal, dorsal pedal (dorsalis pedis), and posterior tibial.

Rate. As defined by the American Heart Association, the heart rate is normal when it is between 50 and 100 beats per minute.

The pulse rate is counted for 1 full minute to evaluate rate, rhythm, and volume accurately. Some authorities recommend counting for 15 to 30 seconds for those pulses that are normal on palpation and to

Table 7-5

Chronological variations in pulse rate

Age	Pulse rate (beats/min)
Birth	70-170
Neonate	120-140
1 year	80-140
2 years	80-130
3 years	80-120
4 years	70-115
Adult	60-100
Conditioned athlete	≅50

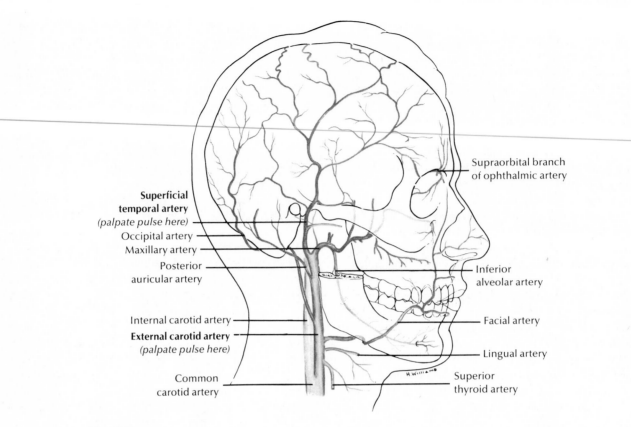

Fig. 7-5
Arteries of the head and neck. (Modified from Francis, C.C., and Martin, A.H.: Introduction to human anatomy, ed. 7, St. Louis, 1975, The C.V. Mosby Co.)

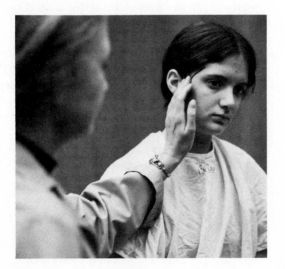

Fig. 7-6
Palpation of the superficial temporal artery.

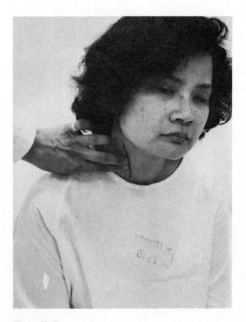

Fig. 7-7
Palpation of the carotid artery.

extend the period of evaluation only when irregularities are detected.

A diurnal rhythm is noted for pulse rate. The lowest rate is seen in the early morning hours, and the most rapid rates are observed in the late afternoon and evening.

Chronologically the pulse rate decreases from infancy through the middle years; there is a tendency for it to increase in the older client (Table 7-5).

A sex difference is noted in that women have demonstrated a rate 5 to 10 beats per minute faster than men.

Volume. Pulse volume is estimated from the feel of the vessel as blood flows through it with each heartbeat. Bounding is the descriptive term used to describe the full pulse that is difficult to depress with the fingertips. The normal pulse is easily palpable and does not fade in and out and is not easily obliterated. Weak, feeble, and thready are descriptive words for the pulse of a vessel that has low volume. The artery in this case is readily compressed. The absent pulse is not palpable.

Amplitude. The strength of the left ventricular contraction is reflected in the amplitude of the pulsation. This may be recorded as follows:

3+ Bounding, hyperkinetic
2+ Normal
1+ Weak, thready, hypokinetic
0 Absent

Elasticity of the arterial wall

Elasticity of the arterial wall is reflected by the expansibility or deformability of the artery as it is palpated by the examiner's fingers. The normal artery is soft and pliable, whereas the sclerotic vessel may be more resistant to occlusion, even hard and cordlike. The artery may feel beaded and tortuous to touch in the individual with arteriosclerosis.

Palpation of arterial pulses—pulse points

Superficial temporal pulse. The superficial temporal artery is accessible to palpation anterior to the tragus of the ear and upward to the temple and is frequently used in the clinical evaluation of pulsation (Figs. 7-5 and 7-6).

Carotid pulse. Examination of the carotid and jugular pulse is described in Chapter 16. Fig. 7-7 shows one method of palpation of the carotid artery.

The carotid pulse is easily accessible and is frequently the pulse evaluated in emergency situations.

The easiest method of locating the carotid is by placing the fingers lightly over the trachea and allowing them to slide into the trough between the trachea and the sternocleidomastoid muscle. The carotid will be felt immediately below the examining fingers. The pulse is palpated in the lower half of the artery to avoid pressure on the carotid sinus. Care should be taken to avoid undue pressure on the carotids to avoid stimulation of the baroreceptors of the carotid sinus and a resultant slowing of the heart and a decrease in blood pressure. All symmetrical pulses except the carotid may be measured simultaneously. The carotid pulses should not be measured simultaneously. Excessive biarterial pressure may dangerously occlude the blood supply to the brain.

Radial pulse. The radial pulse is the one most frequently used as an initial indication of the rate and rhythm of pulsation, the pattern of pulsation, and the shape (consistency) of the arterial wall. This pulse is easily accessible to the examiner, and its evaluation causes little inconvenience to the client. Other pulses easily evaluated in the upper extremity are the ulnar and brachial pulses (Fig. 7-8).

The radial pulse is readily assessed by placing the pads of the examiner's second and third (or first, second, and third) fingers on the palmar surface of the relaxed and slightly flexed wrist medial to the radial styloid process (Fig. 7-9). Occasionally the arteries run a deeper and more lateral course. Both radial pulses should be felt simultaneously for an assessment of symmetry. The fingers should exert sufficient pressure to occlude the artery during diastole, yet allow the vessel to return to normal contour during systole.

Ulnar pulse. The ulnar artery may be compressed against the ulna on the palmar surface of the wrist. It is not used as frequently as the radial artery in evaluation.

Brachial pulse. Brachial pulse assessment by auscultation is a part of the blood pressure evaluation. The pulse is palpated as it passes through the upper half of the cubital fossa at the midline (anterior surface of the elbow joint) because halfway through the fossa it bifurcates into the radial and ulnar arteries. The brachial artery is palpated medial to the biceps tendon. The brachial artery may be used to determine the arterial waveform, as can the carotid artery. The waveform of more peripheral arteries may be distorted and therefore provide less valuable data.

Femoral pulse. The pads of the examiner's fingers explore the groin in the area just inferior to the midpoint of the inguinal ligament. This is also approximately midway between the anterior superior iliac spine and the symphysis pubis (Figs. 7-10 and 7-11).

Popliteal pulse. Since the popliteal artery is situated relatively deeply in the soft tissues behind the knee, the knee should be flexed for examination of the pulsation in this artery. The pulse may be readily examined with

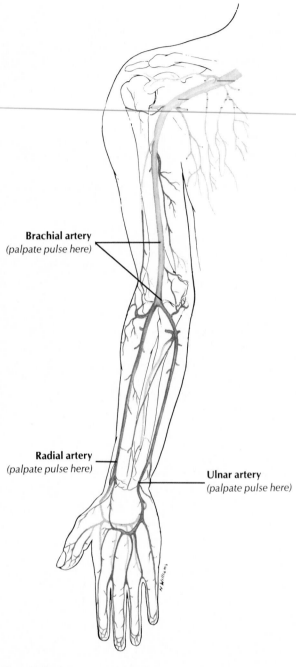

Brachial artery
(palpate pulse here)

Radial artery
(palpate pulse here)

Ulnar artery
(palpate pulse here)

Fig. 7-8
Arteries of the upper extremity. (Adapted from Francis, C.C., and Martin, A.H.: Introduction to human anatomy, ed. 7, St. Louis, 1975, The C.V. Mosby Co.)

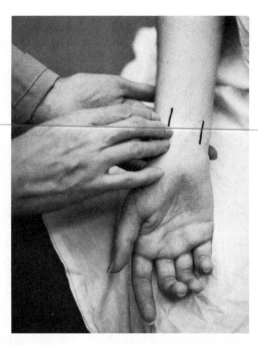

Fig. 7-9
Palpation of the radial pulse. The site for palpation of the ulnar artery is also marked.

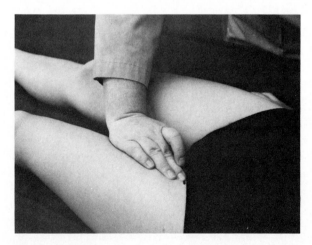

Fig. 7-10
Palpation of femoral pulse.

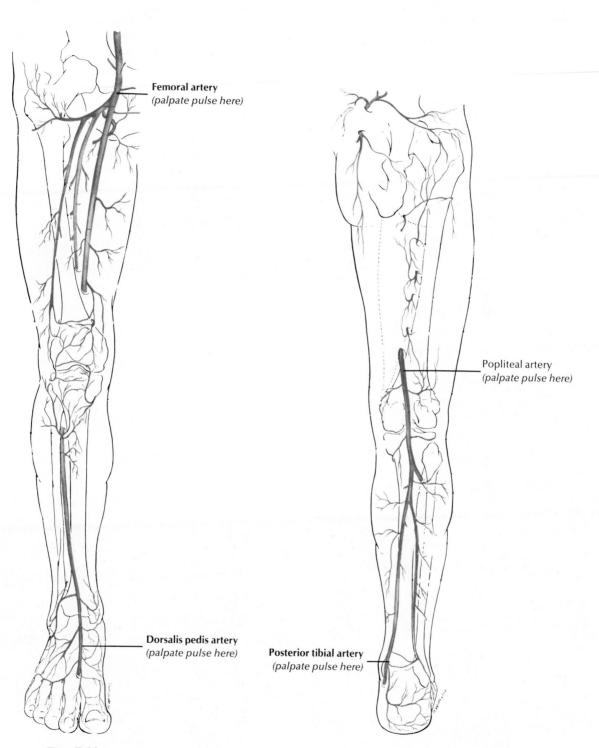

Femoral artery
(palpate pulse here)

Popliteal artery
(palpate pulse here)

Dorsalis pedis artery
(palpate pulse here)

Posterior tibial artery
(palpate pulse here)

Fig. 7-11
Arteries of the lower extremity. (Adapted from Francis, C.C., and Martin, A.H.: Introduction to human anatomy, ed. 7, St. Louis, 1975, The C.V. Mosby Co.)

the client in either the dorsal recumbent (Fig. 7-12) or prone position (Fig. 7-13). The fingertips are pressed deeply into the popliteal fossa.

Dorsal pedal pulse. The pads of the examining fingers examine the dorsum of the foot. The foot should be dorsiflexed to obviate traction on the artery, preferably to 90 degrees (Fig. 7-14).

When the dorsal pedal pulse is congenitally absent, pulsation may sometimes be discerned in the lateral tarsal artery, located in the proximal dorsum of the foot, or in the peroneal artery, anterior to the lateral malleolus.

Although only one pedal pulse can occasionally be palpated, this need not necessarily indicate arterial insufficiency; it may be a result of clinically insignificant congenital variation in the arteries to the foot.

One or both dorsal pedal pulses have been noted to be absent in 12% of children and in 17% of adults. Whereas whites seldom show an absence of the posterior tibial pulse, a 9% incidence of absence has been found in black adults.

Posterior tibial pulse. The pads of the examining fingers palpate posterior or inferior to the tibial medial malleolus while the client's foot is dorsiflexed, preferably to 90 degrees (Fig. 7-15).

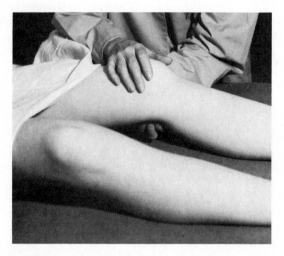

Fig. 7-12
Palpation of the popliteal pulse with client in the dorsal recumbent position.

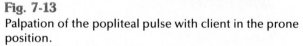

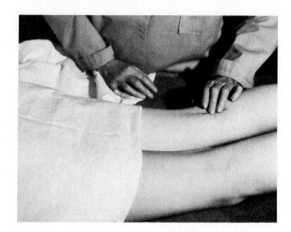

Fig. 7-13
Palpation of the popliteal pulse with client in the prone position.

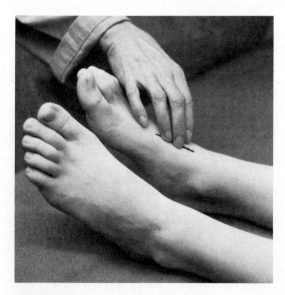

Fig. 7-14
Palpation of the dorsal pedal pulse.

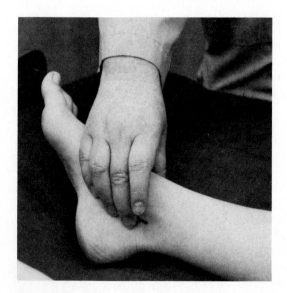

Fig. 7-15
Palpation of posterior tibial pulse.

The examination of the pulses of an extremity begins with the most distal pulse point. Normal pulses in the dorsal pedal and posterior tibial arteries indicate that there is no disruption of flow to the extremity, whereas a weak or absent pulse is expected to be found distal to an obstruction. However, the observation of an indication that an individual has a disease known to produce a peripheral vascular change, such as circulatory impairment or diabetes, dictates the examination of all the superficial pulse points. A thorough assessment includes assessment of all pulse points.

Irregularities in pulsation (Fig. 7-16)

Tachycardia. Rates persistently over 100 beats per minute (tachycardia) suggest some abnormality (Table 7-6). However, hyperkinetic heart action can be the result of exercise, anger, anxiety, or fear in the normal client. Heart rates are increased during fever, anemia, hypoxia, and low volume states (shock).

Bradycardia. A slow heart rate less than 50 beats per minute is known as bradycardia (Table 7-7). These slow rates may indicate stimulation of the parasympathetic system or failure in the electrical conduction system of the heart. Bradycardia may be iatrogenically produced through overdoses of digitalis.

The well-trained athlete may have cardiac rates less than 50 beats per minute.

Irregular rhythm—pulse deficit. Cardiac arrhythmias, that is, atrial fibrillation, atrial flutter with block, and second degree heart block resulting in dropped beats, irregular sinus depolarization, and premature complexes result in an irregular rhythm of the pulse.

Pulse deficit means that the number of pressure waves palpable at the peripheral pulse point is less than the actual number of muscular contractions of the heart. Pressure waves initiated by weak, premature ventricular contractions may not be transmitted to the periphery. Simultaneous measurement at the precordium and peripheral pulse point reveals this deficit.

Bigeminal pulse. A pulse that alternates in amplitude from beat to beat may be produced by a small, premature ventricular beat after a strong beat, resulting from normal electrical cardiac conduction. The strong pulse occurs after a long diastolic filling phase following the premature beat. The pulse is irregular. This condition is called bigeminal pulse and can be identified by simultaneously palpating the radial pulse and listening at the precordium.

Pulsus alternans. Pulsus alternans is a pulse that alternates between strong and weak beats while the rhythm is regular. When the variation is marked, the alternation from weak to strong beats is palpable. However, it may be necessary to use the sphygmomanometer and stethoscope to determine minor changes. The examiner will hear the alternation of loud and soft sounds in pulsus alternans. (See assessment of pulsus alternans in the section on blood pressure in this chapter).

Pulsus paradoxus. Arterial pressure is known to fluctuate physiologically with the respiratory cycle, falling with inspiration and rising with expiration. This variation is detectable at normal respiratory amplitude but is more marked during forced respiratory volumes. Two mechanisms appear to explain this effect. First, the changes in pleural pressure during respiration appear to affect the arteries and veins as they enter or leave the thoracic cage, altering the gradients whereby blood enters or leaves the thorax. Second, the relationship between the ventricles of the heart is such that distention of one results in alteration of the filling characteristics (distensibility or compliance) of the other. Reduction in pleural pressure during inspiration increases the return of systemic venous blood to the right ventricle. The increase in right ventricular filling pressure results in a shift of the interventricular septum leftward, thus reducing the amount of blood that is accepted by the left ventricle. The resultant decrease in left ventricular end diastolic pressure decreases the stroke work of the subsequent left ventricular systole. Thus, although there is an increase in right ventricular output, left ventricular output is decreased. In conditions characterized by distention of the venous system, for example, right ventricular failure as a result of severe obstructive lung disease or pericardial tamponade, a greater fall in pleural pressure and, thus, arterial pressure occurs. This is called pulsus paradoxus.

The variation in arterial pressure may be objectively measured only through the use of a stethoscope and sphygmomanometer. Following detection of systolic pressure, the first noted Korotkoff sound, the pressure is allowed to decrease very slowly until sounds can be heard throughout the respiratory cycle. The decrease in arterial pressure during inspiration in the normal individual may be 10 ± 5 mm Hg. A difference greater than 15 mm Hg is indicative of pulsus paradoxus.

Palpitations. In the resting state the normal individual is unaware of the beating of his heart. *Palpitation* is the term used to record a description given by the client of his perception of the feeling of his heartbeat (Table 7-8). Such expression as "pounding," "thudding," "fluttering," "flopping," and "skipping" are common descriptive terms used by clients to describe this phenomenon. Palpitation is more common just before falling asleep or during sleep.

Physiological palpitations may be experienced by the normal individual following strenuous exercise or when he is aroused emotionally or sexually. In this

NORMAL PULSE

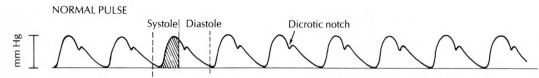

Systole| Diastole   Dicrotic notch

mm Hg

Graphic recording of pulse pressure as obtained from electrical transducer. The normal pulse is easily palpable but may be obliterated by pressure. The wave of a single pulsation rises in systole, reaches a summit, and descends more slowly in diastole. The secondary rise in pressure, noted in diastole, is associated with closure of the aortic valve. The point at which the increase in pressure changes the downward slope is known as the dicrotic notch. This may not be palpable. The difference in pressure from the endpoint of diastole to the summit is the amplitude. Normal amplitude (30-40 mm Hg) is recorded as 2 +. A pulse of greater amplitude is called strong, and one of lesser amplitude is weak or faint.

SMALL, WEAK PULSE

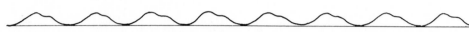

A weak pulse may be difficult to feel, and the vessel may be obliterated easily by the fingers. The pulse may "fade out" (be impalpable). This pulse is recorded as 1 +. The pulsation is slower to rise, has a sustained summit, and falls more slowly than the normal. A pulse that is weak and variable in amplitude is called thready.

LARGE, BOUNDING PULSE

The large, bounding (also called hyperkinetic or strong) pulse is readily palpable. It does not "fade out" and is not easily obliterated by the examining fingers. This pulse is recorded as 3 +.

WATER-HAMMER PULSE

The water-hammer pulse (also known as collapsing) has a greater amplitude than the normal pulse, a rapid rise to a narrow summit, and a sudden descent.

PULSUS ALTERNANS

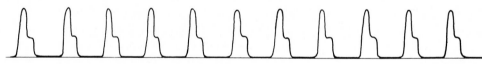

Pulsus alternans is characterized by alternation of a pulsation of small amplitude with the pulsation of large amplitude while the rhythm is normal.

Fig. 7-16
Table of pulses.

POSSIBLE CAUSE

Partial arterial occlusion
Myocardial infarction
Myocarditis
Pericardial effusion shock
Stenosis of valves: aortic,
   mitral, pulmonic, tricuspid

Hypovolemia
Physical obstruction to
   left ventricular output,
   e.g., aortic stenosis

Exercise
Anxiety
Fever
Hyperthyroidism
Aortic rigidity or
   atherosclerosis

Patent ductus arteriosus
Aortic regurgitation

Left ventricular failure
More significant if pulse
   slow

	POSSIBLE CAUSE
BIGEMINAL PULSE	Disorder of rhythm

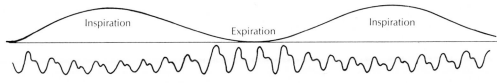

Bigeminal pulsations result from a normal pulsation followed by a premature contraction. The amplitude of the pulsation of the premature contraction is less than that of the normal pulsation.

PULSUS PARADOXUS

Pulsus paradoxus is characterized by an exaggerated decrease (>10 mm Hg) in the amplitude of pulsation during inspiration and increased amplitude during expiration. (See text for measurement with sphygmomanometer.)

Premature cardiac contraction

Tracheobronchial obstruction
Bronchial asthma
Emphysema
Pericardial effusion
Constrictive pericarditis

PULSUS BISFERIENS

Pulsus bisferiens is best detected by palpation of the carotid artery. This pulsation is characterized by two main peaks. The first is termed percussion wave and the second, tidal wave. Although the mechanism is not clear, the first peak is believed to be the pulse pressure and the second, reverberation from the periphery.

Aortic stenosis combined
with aortic insufficiency

IRREGULAR PULSE RHYTHM

Pulse deficit means that the number of pressure waves palpable at the peripheral vessel is less than the cardiac contractions.

Cardiac arrhythmia
Atrial fibrillation
Atrial flutter with block
Second-degree heart block
Irregular sinus depolarization
Premature complexes
Weak, premature ventric-
ular contractions

Fig. 7-16, cont'd
Table of pulses.

Table 7-6
Characteristics of common forms of tachycardia

Type	Rhythm, amplitude	Most common ventricular rate (beats/min)	Onset	Termination	Effect of carotid sinus massage
Sinus tachycardia	Regular; constant ampli-tude	Usually 170	Gradual	Gradual	Gradual slowing and return to previous state
Paroxysmal atrial tachycardia (PAT)	Regular; constant ampli-tude	170	Abrupt	Abrupt	Sudden slowing of heart rate or no change
Paroxysmal atrial flutter	Flutter, regular; uniform amplitude	170	Abrupt		Sudden diminution of rate or temporarily irregular rhythm
Ventricular tachycardia	Irregular; variable ampli-tude	140	Sudden		No effect

Table 7-7

Characteristics of common forms of bradycardia

Type	Rhythm, amplitude	Most common ventricular rate (beats/min)	Effect of exercise
Sinus bradycardia	Regular; constant amplitude	40	Rate increases appropriately through varying degrees of exercise
Incomplete heart block	Constant amplitude	40	May double or become irregular in response to exercise
Complete heart block		40	Increases only slightly in response to exercise

Table 7-8

Guide to causes of palpitations

Possible cause	Signs and symptoms
Menopausal symptom	Associated with heat "flashes" or perspiration
Drugs known to produce a hyperkinetic heart	History of ingestion of monoamine oxidase inhibitors, thyroid replacement or stimulatory drugs, adrenergic drugs, alcohol, tea, coffee
Hemorrhage, hypoglycemia, pheochromocytoma	Sudden occurrence of palpitation not related to exercise or emotional arousal
Hypervolemia	Blood pressure is elevated
Psychopathology	Clinical examination reveals no evidence of hyperkinetic heart or irregularity of rate
Postural hypotension	Palpitations occur when individual stands
Anemia, fever, atrial fibrillation, thyrotoxicosis, exposure to environmental heat	Clinical examination reveals hyperkinetic heart
Extra systoles	Irregular "skips"

case the cardiac contraction is of greater rate and amplitude. Several pathophysiological states are also associated with a hyperkinetic heart (anemia, fever, hypoglycemia, and thyrotoxicosis). Irregularities in cardiac rhythm have also been associated with palpitations, particularly extra systoles and ectopic tachycardia. The chief complaint of palpitations is frequently correlated with psychopathology.

A common feature of the anxiety state, palpitations may be related to the increased adrenergic activity that is present in this arousal state. This relationship creates some problem for the examiner; since the presence of palpitations frequently creates anxiety, careful questions will be necessary to minimize this effect.

Arterial insufficiency

Assessment of the arterial pulsation is particularly important in those individuals suspected or diagnosed as having diseases known to compromise the arterial circulation. Some of these pathophysiological conditions are diabetes, atherosclerosis, Buerger's disease, Raynaud's disease, and arterial aneurysm.

Signs and symptoms of arterial insufficiency include intermittent claudication, increased pallor on elevation of the extremity, a prolonged venous filling time following elevation of the extremity, flush incurred by gravitational effect if the extremity is below the level of the heart, and tissue death (gangrene). Symptoms may also include easy fatigability. Ischemic pain may be incurred by simple resistance exercises. Intermittent claudication is the transient ischemic pain encountered by the client in his arms when he is working with them or in his legs when he is walking.

The impaired flow of arterial insufficiency may be adequate to serve the metabolic activities of the muscle at rest but does not maintain the circulation necessary to the increased metabolic rates of exercise. The pain is theorized to be the result of the buildup of metabolic acids that stimulate the sensory nerves. It is described as cramping or "tightness" and sometimes likened to being in a vise. Many clients, however, do not recognize the discomfort as pain but describe aching, cramping, burning, tiredness, numbness, or weakness of the calf muscles.

Intermittent claudication in the arms may be confused with the pain of angina pectoris. The examiner must carefully define the fact that the pain occurred with work and disappeared with rest. Subclavian arterial insufficiency may result in dizziness and faintness.

In both arterial insufficiency and venous stasis, calf pain is experienced that is relieved during sleep (see comparison in boxed material on p. 159).

Physical examination of the client thought to have arterial insufficiency includes auscultation of the arteries, palpation of the pulses, and observations of cuta-

Differentiation of arterial insufficiency from venous stasis

	Client's response	
	Arterial insufficiency (intermittent claudication)	**Venous stasis**
Interview		
When does the pain occur?	Walking	Standing
What makes the pain worse?	Cold	
What helps to get rid of the pain?	Standing	Elevation
	Stopping to rest	
Do you notice swelling in your feet or legs?	No	Yes
Inspection of involved extremity		
Pulses	Decreased amplitude or absent	
Skin	Cool to touch	Brownish pigmentation
	Pallor, rubor on elevation	
	Shiny	
	Hair loss	
	Nails thickened, ridged	
If ulcer present	Irregular edges	Shallow exudate covering
	Pale, boggy, granulation tissue	
	Eschar covering	Located on side of ankle
	Gangrene possible	No gangrene
	Located on toes or sites of trauma	

neous color; examination should be done before and after exercise.

Absence of pulsation in the femoral artery and at least one peripheral vessel is a criterion for the diagnosis of arterial insufficiency.

Arterial insufficiency in the arm, although generally thought to be less frequent than that of the leg, may frequently be demonstrated through changes in murmurs, pulses, and skin color after exercise.

Importance of exercise testing in determining arterial insufficiency of the extremities. Exercise testing of the poorly perfused limb is based on the inability of the occluded vessel to increase blood flow to meet the increased demands for oxygen. Bruits that were present only in systole continue into diastole, since there is a relatively decreased diastolic pressure distal to the obstruction, which promotes forward flow (Fig. 7-17). (See also Fig. 16-31.)

In clients with intermittent claudication the pulses diminish in amplitude following exercise. Cutaneous ischemia may be apparent.

The amount of the exercise needed to produce these vascular changes is usually not more than that which is part of daily living. Flexion-extension exercises of the arms and legs (deep knee bends) or walking may produce these changes.

Homans' sign. Thrombosis of the deep veins of the calf muscles may be detected by forced dorsiflexion of

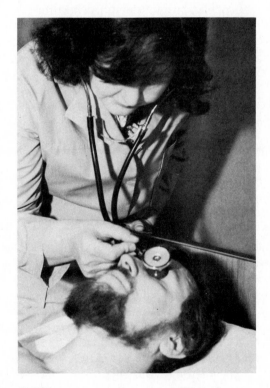

Fig. 7-17
Listening for an ocular bruit. The bell of the stethoscope is applied to form a right seal around the orbit. (From Burnside, J.W.: Physical diagnosis: an introduction to clinical medicine, ed. 16, Baltimore, 1981, Williams & Wilkins.)

the foot. This maneuver compresses the veins and causes pain. The complaint of pain by the client when this maneuver is performed indicates Homans' sign. It is important to remember that deep venous thrombosis may be silent, that is, not give rise to pain.

Auscultation for arterial murmurs

All accessible arteries should be ausculated in the client suspected of arteriovascular disease. Murmurs are not present over major arteries in the normal adult, and only faint ones are heard in the normal child.

Arterial murmurs (bruits) may result from hyperdynamic cardiac states or from irregularity of arterial walls.

The bell of the stethoscope is used to detect bruits over major vessels. The instrument is lightly held to avoid occluding the underlying vessel. Should the examiner detect a murmur, the limb is exercised if no contraindication exists, and the auscultation is repeated. The auscultation of a systolic murmur that extends into diastole in the postexercise state connotes some degree of arterial obstruction.

Sphygmomanometer detection of arterial flow

Failure to palpate pedal pulsation may indicate the use of the sphygmomanometer for detection of arterial flow. The pneumatic cuff is inflated to a pressure between the systolic and diastolic blood pressure. Oscillation of the needle (aneroid) or mercury column (mercury) in synchrony with the ventricular contraction is indicative of blood flow to the extremity. A disadvantage of this method is that it does not indicate the adequacy of the flow volume.

Blood pressure

Arterial blood pressure is the force exerted by the blood against the wall of the artery as the heart contracts and relaxes. *Systolic arterial blood pressure* is the force exerted against the wall of the artery when the ventricles are contracted, and *diastolic arterial blood pressure* is the force when the heart is in the filling or relaxed phase. *Pulse pressure* is the difference between the *systolic* and *diastolic* blood pressures.

The blood pressure is determined by the cardiac output and peripheral resistance. Thus, the blood pressure reflects the volume of fluid in the cardiovascular system and elasticity of the arterial walls.

The screening examination is especially important to the recognition of the client who has a disorder in blood pressure, particularly hypertension (persistently elevated blood pressure). Because hypertension may be present without symptoms, it is known as the silent disease. The client who does not feel ill does not usually come to a clinic or hospital for health care. Thus, this examination may be instrumental in getting the hypertensive client into the therapeutic milieu in time to prevent some of the sequelae of hypertension.

A measure of the functions of the cardiovascular system may be accomplished through the assessment of peripheral arterial blood pressure. The peripheral blood pressure is the force exerted against the walls of the vessels and the force responsible for the flow of blood through the arteries, capillaries, and veins. The pressure is the result of the interaction of cardiac output and peripheral resistance and is dependent on the velocity of the arterial blood, the intravascular volume, and the elasticity of the arterial walls.

Stephen Hales made the first recorded direct measurement of blood pressure in 1733 when he cannulated the artery of a horse, allowing the blood to rise in a glass tube. He was also able to demonstrate the changes in blood pressure that occur in systole and diastole as he watched the blood rise and fall in the tube with each heartbeat. Almost a century later (1828), Poiseuille attached a mercury-filled tube to a cannulated artery. Since mercury is 13.6 times heavier than blood or water, the column in the tube was much shorter. Several instruments for the indirect method of blood pressure measurement were devised in the late 1800s.

The systemic arterial blood pressure may be assessed either by direct or indirect methods. The direct method requires cannulation of the artery but is the trusted method of measurement. Routine, direct arterial blood pressures are not measured, because of the potential sequelae, though the risks are small. Indirect blood pressure measurement can be made without opening the artery. The valid methods of indirect measurement are those that are closest in values to those made from direct techniques. Direct blood pressure standards are used to calibrate indirect pressure instruments.

Indirect measurement

Indirect methods of blood pressure measurement involve the following three physiological facts: (1) the arterial wall may be occluded by direct pressure, resulting in the obliteration of the pulse distal to the compression; (2) oscillations that vary directly with the amount of pressure being applied may be measured from the compressed artery; and (3) the normal extremity blanches (pales) when its arterial blood supply is occluded by pressure, and there is flushing or return of color when the pressure is removed.

The most commonly used method of indirect assessment of blood pressure is the auscultatory technique. For the procedure a sphygmomanometer and a stethoscope are used.

The two types of sphygmomanometers commonly used in the assessment of arterial blood pressure are

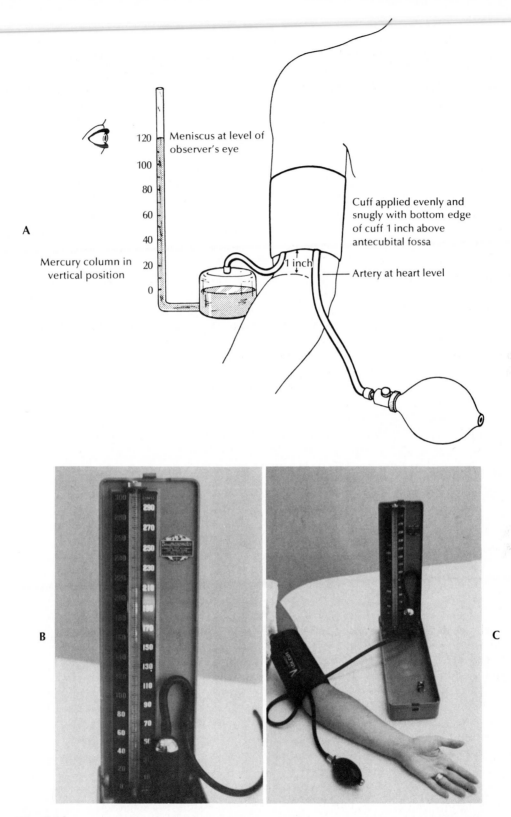

120 — Meniscus at level of observer's eye

Cuff applied evenly and snugly with bottom edge of cuff 1 inch above antecubital fossa

Mercury column in vertical position

1 inch

Artery at heart level

Fig. 7-18
A, Mercury gravity manometer (diagrammatic). **B,** Mercury manometer. **C,** Mercury sphygmomanometer applied to client. (**A** from Burch, G.E., and DePasquale, N.P.: Primer of clinical measurement of blood pressure, St. Louis, 1962, The C.V. Mosby Co. **B** and **C** reproduced with permission from *Blood pressure measurement: a handbook for instructors,* © 1979, Chicago Heart Association.)

the mercury gravity and the aneroid instruments. Each instrument includes a pressure manometer, an inflatable rubber bladder encased in a cloth cuff, and a rubber hand bulb with a pressure control valve.

The air distensible bladder encased in the cloth cuff is used to occlude an artery. The cuff is long enough to encircle the extremity and be fastened securely in place. The covering cuff must be made of elastic material so pressure is applied evenly to the limb.

The mercury gravity manometer (Fig. 7-18) is made up of a straight glass tube connected to a reservoir of mercury. The reservoir in turn is connected to the pressure bulb, so that pressure created on the bulb causes the mercury to rise in the tube. Because the weight of mercury is dependent on gravity, a given amount of pressure will always support a column of mercury of the same height, given the tube is straight and of uniform diameter. The mercury manometer does not need further calibration after the initial setting.

The aneroid sphygmomanometer (Fig. 7-19) is made up of a metal bellows connected to the compression cuff. Changes in pressure within the apparatus cause the bellows to expand and collapse. The movement of the bellows rotates a gear that moves a pointer across the calibrated dial. The aneroid sphygmomanometer is calibrated against a mercury manometer, since the more complex mechanisms have been shown to need frequent adjustment. This is simply done by using a connecting Y tube between the manometers.

Electronic blood pressure measurement. Electronic cuff manometer consoles are available. They are easier to manipulate, since no stethoscope is required. This type of equipment is especially advantageous for hearing-impaired health professionals and for clients who are hearing impaired and who monitor their own blood pressure.

Some models have error indicators.

The electronic models are more expensive than the aneroid or mercury manometers. The opportunity for error is greater, since the electronic units are less accurate and are battery dependent. Another disadvantage is that calibration may be performed only by the manufacturer.

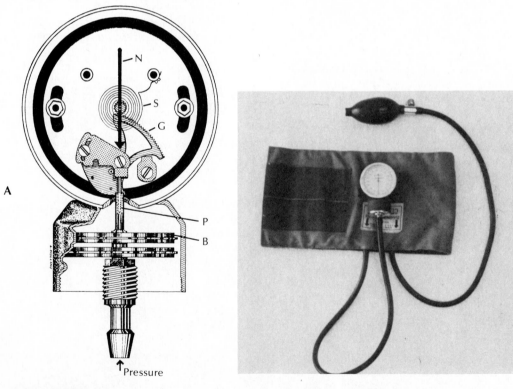

Fig. 7-19

A, Aneroid sphygmomanometer (diagrammatic). Variations within the bellow (B) activate a pin (P), which sets a gear (G) into motion. The gear, in turn, operates the spring (S), which causes the needle (N) to move across the face of a calibrated dial. **B,** Aneroid sphygmomanometer. (**A** from Burch, G.E., and DePasquale, N.P.: Primer of clinical measurement of blood pressure, St. Louis, 1962, The C.V. Mosby Co. **B** reproduced with permission from *Blood pressure measurement: a handbook for instructors,* © 1979, Chicago Heart Association.)

*Taking blood pressure**

1. Assist the client to a comfortable sitting position, with arm slightly flexed, forearm supported at heart level, and palm turned up. Expose the upper arm fully.
2. Palpate the brachial artery. Position the cuff 2.5 cm (1 inch) above the site of brachial artery pulsation (antecubital space). Center the arrows marked on the cuff over the brachial artery.
3. Be sure the cuff is fully deflated. Wrap the cuff evenly and snugly around the upper arm. Be sure the manometer is positioned at eye level.
4. If you do not know the client's normal systolic pressure, palpate the radial artery and inflate the cuff to a pressure 30 mm Hg above the point at which radial pulsation disappears. Deflate the cuff and wait 30 seconds.
5. Place the stethoscope earpieces in the ears and be sure sounds are clear, not muffled.
6. Relocate the brachial artery and place the diaphragm (or the bell) of the stethoscope over it.
7. Close the valve of the pressure bulb clockwise until tight.
8. Inflate the cuff to 30 mm Hg above the client's normal systolic level.
9. Slowly release the valve, allowing the mercury to fall at a rate of 2 to 3 mm Hg per second. Note the point on the manometer at which the first clear sound is heard. Continue to deflate the cuff gradually, noting the point at which a muffled or dampened sound appears. Continue cuff deflation, noting the point on the manometer at which sound disappears.
10. Deflate the cuff rapidly and remove it from the client's arm unless you need to repeat the measurement. If repeating the procedure, wait 30 seconds.

Measurement of blood pressure by palpation. The brachial artery is palpated below the cuff, and the cuff is inflated to 30 mm Hg beyond the point at which the pulse is obliterated. The air pressure in the bladder is released at a rate of 2 to 3 mm Hg per heartbeat, and systolic blood pressure is recorded at the point at which pulsations first become palpable. The diastolic pressure is said to coincide with the cessation of vibrations in the artery. The diastolic value is difficult to obtain. However, in a test situation, more than 79% of the values obtained were within ±4 mm Hg of those obtained by auscultatory procedures.

*Modified from Potter, P.A., and Perry, A.G.: Fundamentals of nursing: concepts, process, and practice, St. Louis, 1985, The C.V. Mosby Co.

Auscultatory method of arterial blood pressure assessment. When the cuff is properly placed on the limb, the arterial blood can flow past the cuff only when arterial pressure exceeds that in the cuff. Partial obstruction of arterial blood flow disturbs the laminar flow pattern, creating turbulence. This turbulence produces sounds called Korotkoff sounds and can be heard over arteries distal to the cuff through a stethoscope (Fig. 7-20).

The bell of the stethoscope is more effective than the diaphragm in transmitting the low-frequency Korotkoff sounds. The bell is applied snugly over the artery; care is taken not to press hard enough to close the artery.

The deflated cuff is applied, without wrinkles, snugly around the upper arm so that the edge of the cuff is 2 to 3 cm above the site at which the bell of the stethoscope is to be placed. The artery is palpated, and the cuff is inflated at a rate of 12 to 20 mm Hg per second to a peak of 30 mm Hg higher than the point at which the pulse was obliterated. The cuff is then deflated at a rate of 2 to 3 mm Hg per heartbeat. The level of the meniscus of the mercury column at which the Korotkoff sounds are changed is noted.

The *systolic blood pressure* is recorded for that point at which the Korotkoff sounds are initially heard. This

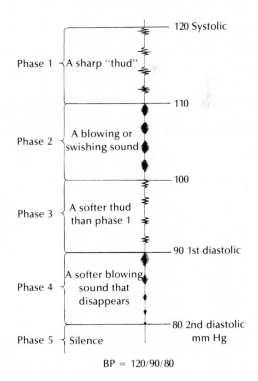

Fig. 7-20
Phases of the Korotkoff sounds. (From Burch, G.E., and DePasquale, N.P.: Primer of clinical measurement of blood pressure, St. Louis, 1962, The C.V. Mosby Co.)

is also the beginning of *phase 1,* which starts with faint, clear, and rhythmic tapping or thumping noises that gradually increase in intensity. At this point the intraluminal pressure is the same as the cuff pressure but not great enough to produce a radial pulse.

Phase 2 is characterized by a murmur or swishing sound heard as the vessel distends with blood, creating eddies and producing vibration of the vessel wall. *Phase 3* is the period during which the sounds are crisper and more intense. In this phase the vessel remains open in systole but obliterated in diastole.

The *muffling* of the Korotkoff sounds is the guidepost for the beginning of *phase 4* and the pressure at this point is believed by many authorities to be the closest to the *diastolic arterial pressure* measured by a direct method. At this point the cuff pressure falls below the intraluminal pressure. It is frequently called the first diastolic pressure. The second diastolic pressure and *phase 5* are said to be present when the Korotkoff sounds are no longer heard. Phase 5 marks the period wherein the vessel remains open during the entire cycle.

If muffling of the Korotkoff sounds is established as indicative of diastolic level, the value will be about 8 mm Hg greater than that obtained by the direct method.

Disappearance of the Korotkoff sounds is a risky criterion for diastolic pressure, since the sounds do not abate in some individuals until a pressure well below the diastolic value is reached.

Thus, three values are recorded: the systolic pressure, the point of muffling of the Korotkoff sounds, and the disappearance of the sounds. An example of the record might be 120/78/54. This method has the approval of the World Health Organization and the American Heart Association.

Korotkoff sounds may be heard all the way to zero on the sphygmomanometer scale. This occurs frequently in normal children and in certain hyperdynamic states such as the aftermath to vigorous exercise, in thyrotoxicosis, or in severe anemia. In this case the pressure at the beginning of phase 4 is noted and recorded, as well as a description of sound heard to 0 mm Hg.

Cuff size. If the cuff is too narrow, the blood pressure reading will be erroneously high. A wide cuff increases the risk of an erroneously low reading.

The sphygmomanometer cuff should be 20% to 25% wider than the diameter of the extremity in which the blood pressure is being taken. Another recommendation is that the bladder width be equal to two fifths the circumference of the limb. A more liberal approximation suggests that the cuff should cover two thirds of the upper arm. Ideally, the bladder should completely encircle the extremity and should be snugly applied. Cuffs may be obtained in several sizes (Table 7-9).

CAUTION: The cuff size is determined by the diameter of the limb, not the age of the client.

The examiner's eye must be at a direct line with the level of the meniscus of the mercury column to avoid parallax error, and the mercury column must be kept in a vertical position.

The cuff should be deflated completely (0 mm Hg) between successive readings. At least a 15-second interval is allowed between readings, with the cuff completely deflated, to avoid spurious readings as a result of venous congestion.

The bladder and the pressure bulbs should be monitored for leaks. Erratic inflation or deflation usually indicates a leak.

Measurement of blood pressure in the leg. The blood pressure in the leg may be measured with the client in either the supine or prone position. The Korotkoff sounds are evaluated over the popliteal artery.

In the popliteal artery, the systolic arterial blood pressure is higher (10 ± 5 mm Hg) than in the brachial artery, whereas the diastolic pressure is generally lower. This difference is magnified in aortic insufficiency and in some hyperdynamic states such as after exercise.

Increasing audibility of the Korotkoff sounds in infants and the flush test. Occasionally the Korotkoff sounds are not heard over the brachial artery in infants. A suggestion for making the sounds audible is to hold the infant's arm upright for 1 to 2 minutes with the cuff in place. The pressure is measured immediately on lowering the arm.

In the event that the Korotkoff sounds cannot be obtained, a flush pressure that approximates the mean blood pressure may be measured in the upper or lower extremity. The procedure for this test is as follows: The properly sized cuff is placed around the infant's wrist or ankle. An elasticized bandage is placed around the extremity distal to the cuff to promote vascular emptying. The bladder pressure of the sphygmomanometer is raised to approximately 150 mm Hg. The bandage is removed, and the cuff pressure is decreased at a rate of 2 to 3 mm Hg per heartbeat until a vascular flush (rubor) is observed. The appearance of the flush is correlated with the sphygmomanometer reading.

Auscultatory gap. Occasionally, as the pneumatic cuff is being deflated, the Korotkoff sounds disappear and then are heard 10 to 15 mm Hg later. This is called auscultatory gap. The examiner records systolic blood pressure at the onset of the first sound. Thus, the auscultatory gap will not be cause for error if the cuff was inflated to 20 mm Hg above the point at which the artery was occluded as determined by palpation.

Table 7-9
Dimensions for appropriate size cuff

	Range of dimensions of bladder (cm)	
	Width	**Length**
Newborn	2.5- 4.0	5.0-10.0
Infant	6.0- 8.0	12.0-13.5
Child	9.0-10.0	17.0-22.5
Adult	12.0-13.0	22.0-23.5
Large adult arm	15.5	30.0
Adult thigh	18.0	36.0

From The National Heart, Lung, and Blood Institute's Task Force on Blood Pressure Control in Children: Report of the Task Force on Blood Pressure Control in Children, Pediatrics Supplement 59 (suppl.5): 797, 1977. Copyright American Academy of Pediatrics 1977.

Normal systolic and diastolic pressure. In adults the systolic blood pressure has a normal range of 95 to 140 mm Hg; 120 mm Hg is cited as average (when measured in the brachial artery). Normal diastolic pressure ranges from 60 to 90 mm Hg; 80 mm Hg is average.

The systolic blood pressure in the neonatal period may range about 60 mm Hg. It has been recommended that a systolic blood pressure less than 55 mm Hg be considered hypotension. Blood pressure gradually increases until adolescence, when an accelerated rise is incurred. Thus, at about 17 or 18 years, blood pressure reaches adult levels.

The proper application of the auscultatory method yields values that are within ±4 to 5 mm Hg of the direct method of measurement.

Normal variations in blood pressure recordings. The blood pressure in a normal individual varies continually with respiration, autonomic state, emotional levels, and biological rhythms. Furthermore, successive readings of indirect measures of blood pressure by the same or different observers may differ by as much as 10 mm Hg.

In the normal individual, the *change from a supine to an erect position* causes a slight decrease in systolic blood pressure (less than 15 mm Hg) and in diastolic pressure (less than 5 mm Hg). Marked drops in pressure (greater than 30 mm Hg) incurred when the individual stands may be indicative of a vasopressor defect or of hypovolemia.

The blood pressure also shows a *24-hour, or circadian, pattern.* Consistent with the other vital signs, the blood pressure has higher values in the afternoon and evening hours and lower values in the late hours of sleep.

Because blood pressure is readily altered by *stressful events,* an effort should be made to relax the client as much as possible before taking the blood pressure.

Food and exercise also affect the blood pressure. It is recommended that the individual should not eat or exercise in the 30 minutes before the determination is made. The extremity should be at heart level for a period of approximately 5 minutes.

Differences in blood pressure indicating disease. The initial examination of blood pressure should include a measurement in both arms and one from the leg. Differences in blood pressure between the two arms may be caused by congenital aortic obstruction (coarctation), by acquired conditions such as aortic dissection, or by obstruction of the arteries of the upper arm.

Constriction or obstruction of the aorta may be suspected when the pressure assessed in the client's arms exceeds that in the legs, particularly when the differences are great.

Coarctation of the aorta must be suspected when the brachial pressure markedly exceeds that of the popliteal artery. This reversal of gradient may also accompany other obstructive lesions of the aorta or obstructive lesions in proximal arteries of the leg.

Assessment of pulsus paradoxus. Arterial blood pressure in normal human beings is known to vary as much as 10 mm Hg during relaxed respiration. The decrease with inspiration may be 10 ± 5 mm Hg, whereas on exhalation proportionate increase is noted. A difference greater than 15 mm Hg is indicative of pulsus paradoxus. These fluctuations may be more accurately assessed by raising the cuff pressure to a level greater than systolic pressure and by allowing the cuff to deflate very slowly while the client breathes normally.

Assessment of pulsus alternans. Pulsus alternans is pulse beat to pulse beat variation in systolic pressure. Although the presence of pulsus alternans may be readily determined from palpation of the pulse, when it is marked, it may be accurately assessed through the use of the sphygmomanometer.

The cuff is inflated to 20 mm Hg above the systolic pressure as determined via palpation. On deflation to phase 1, only alternate beats are heard. Later all beats are audible and palpable. After still further deflation all beats are of equal intensity. The difference between this point and the peak systolic level is often used in determining the degree of pulsus alternans.

Pulse pressure. The pulse pressure is the difference between systolic and diastolic pressure. The normal value is generally 30 to 40 mm Hg. The heart rate may influence the pulse pressure. With a slowly beating heart the period of flow or "runoff" from the aorta to the periphery is lengthened, lowering the diastolic pressure, thus increasing the pulse pressure.

A wide pulse pressure accompanied by bradycardia

frequently indicates increased intracranial pressure, aortic insufficiency, patent ductus arteriosus, and arteriovenous fistula. The pulse pressure is also increased in hyperkinetic states such as hyperthyroidism or after vigorous exercise. Although the stroke volume may be greater, rapid runoff may result in low diastolic recordings.

With increased peripheral resistance, runoff to the peripheral circulation is less; thus, more blood accumulates in the aorta, and both systolic and diastolic blood pressure increase.

A small stroke volume will tend to decrease the pulse pressure.

Hypertension and hypotension

Hypertension. The World Health Organization defines hypertension as a persistent elevation of blood pressure greater than 140/90. The American Heart Association recommends that 160/95 be the defining point for hypertension in the client over 40 years of age. Elevation of either systolic or diastolic blood pressure is an indication for further diagnostic tests.

If the definition of hypertension in the adult is accepted as a diastolic pressure in excess of 90 mm Hg, then about 15% of whites and 30% of blacks in the United States have hypertension. One study estimated that one half of hypertensive persons have not been identified.

The structures most frequently observed to suffer damage as peripheral resistance is increased are the heart, the kidneys, and the brain. Vessel changes are best observed in the retina. Sclerosis, hemorrhage, and exudates typify the alterations seen in hypertension.

The incidence of cerebrovascular accident (CVA) is increased by high pressure in the vessels in the brain.

An exaggerated pulsus paradoxus is observed in pericardial effusion, constrictive pericarditis, severe chronic obstructive pulmonary disease, and hypovolemia.

Increased cardiac work is required to pump the blood against the increased peripheral resistance. Thus, congestive heart failure, left ventricular hypertrophy, or angina pectoris may result from hypertension.

The examiner must bear in mind other signs and symptoms that accompany hypertension. These might include severe headache, blurred vision, and signs of renal disease.

Pulsus alternans may be detected in tachypnea if the respiratory rate is half the heart rate, immediately following ventricular ectopic contractions, in myocardial failure resulting from severe organic heart disease, and in bigeminal rhythm.

Clinical assessment of hypertension in children. Although it is accepted that the routine measurement of blood pressure in all children from newborn through adolescence is imperative to the diagnosis of hypertension, this practice is frequently neglected. The screening examination may yield an incidence of hypertension of approximately 2.3% in children 4 to 15 years of age. Early detection of these hypertensive children may mean that diagnosis and treatment may be initiated in time to prevent the sequelae of the underlying disease process. It has been shown that 90% of adults are subject to essential or idiopathic hypertension, whereas this is true only for 20% of children. The blood pressure is recorded each time the child is seen and is considered with other developmental data.

Hypertension is said to exist in children when either the systolic or diastolic blood pressure is greater than the 95th percentile for age, that is, two standard deviations above the mean. Fig. 7-21 shows the range of blood pressures obtained in children.

The blood pressure as measured by Doppler technique has demonstrated that blood pressure rises rapidly from between 4 days and 6 weeks and then remains reasonably stable until the first year. The 95th percentile for blood pressure between 6 weeks and 6 years is about 115 mm Hg. Note the progressive increase in blood pressure that is incurred from 1 year to age 15.

The observation of a brachial blood pressure of 150 mm Hg or more may be indicative of secondary hypertension resulting from renal or endocrine disease or coarctation of the aorta. Coarctation of the aorta is also suspected when the blood pressure in the arms exceeds that in the legs by 30 mm Hg. The normal difference in the infant is that the brachial blood pressure is 17 ± 10 mm Hg greater than in the legs.

The findings of an elevated blood pressure in the pediatric client alert the examiner to look for indications of hypertensive encephalopathy (hyperactivity, excitablity, and fundal changes).

The National Heart, Lung, and Blood Institute recommended (1984) that nondrug therapies such as diet, exercise, and behavior modification be pursued aggressively in treating the mildest cases of high blood pressure. The recommendations were made in response to research data indicating toxicity and side effects of antihypertensive drugs.

Weight reduction was recommended with the justification that weight loss often results in a substantial decrease in blood pressure even when ideal weight is not achieved. The report advised that high blood cholesterol levels be reduced even though definitive information of the effect on blood pressure is not available. Restriction of dietary sodium to an amount equal to 2 g was also recommended. Alcohol consumption was advised to be less than 4 ounces of hard liquor, 16 ounces wine, or 48 ounces of beer a day.

A regular program of exercise was recommended, as well as behavior modification therapies such as relaxation and biofeedback. The committee said a diastolic pressure less than 85 mm Hg can be considered normal, but a reading of 85 to 89 mm Hg is high-normal and should be watched.

Hypotension. Hypotension has been defined as a persistent blood pressure less than 95/60.

Hypotension in the absence of other signs or symptoms is generally innocent. In fact, lower blood pressures may be considered beneficial because the heart does not have to pump as hard to circulate the blood. The blood pressure must be high enough to assure an adequate blood supply to the kidneys, brain, and other body tissues.

However, sudden changes in blood pressure may produce changes in body function. Sudden drops in normal blood pressure may result in fainting. This is observed in orthostatic hypotension. In this case, the

blood pressure may be normal when the individual is reclining but drops when the individual rises to a sitting or standing position, particularly when the position change is a rapid one. Faintness and dizziness from orthostatic hypotension is common in individuals who have been confined to bed or have diseases of the nervous system.

A drop in blood pressure may also follow severe injury, hemorrhage, and endotoxin-producing infections. In hypovolemic or endotoxic shock, the Korotkoff sounds will be less audible or absent. Since the peripheral blood pressure is an important parameter for determining the method of treatment, ultrasonic direct or invasive techniques of blood pressure assessment may be used. Some other signs of shock might include increased pulse and respiratory rates, dizziness, confusion, blurred vision, diaphoresis, and cold and clammy skin.

Respiratory rate, volume, and rhythm assessment are described in Chapter 15 on assessment of the respiratory system.

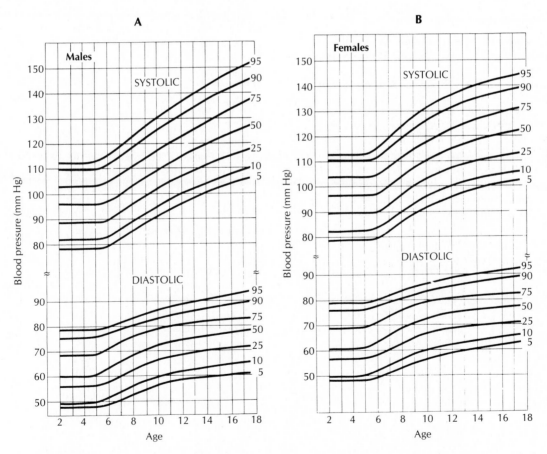

Fig. 7-21
Percentiles of blood pressure measurement (right arm, seated). **A,** Men. **B,** Women. (From the National Heart, Lung, and Blood Institute's Task Force on Blood Pressure Control in Children: Pediatrics **59** (suppl. 5):797, 1977. Copyright American Academy of Pediatrics 1977.)

BIBLIOGRAPHY

Atkins, E., and Bodel, P.: Fever, N. Engl. J. Med. **286:**27, 1972.

Baker, N.C., and others: The effect of type of thermometer and length of time inserted on oral temperature measurements of afebrile subjects, Nurs. Res. **33**(2):109, 1984.

Barnhorst, D.A., and Barner, H.B.: Prevalence of congenitally absent pedal pulses, N. Engl. J. Med. **278:**264, 1969.

Blood pressure measurement: a handbook for instructors, Chicago, 1979, Chicago Heart Association.

deSwiet, M., and others: Blood pressure in infancy. In Harper, P., and Muir, J., editors: Advanced medicine, ed. 15, Bath, England, 1979, Pitman Press.

Draper, G., Dupertuis, C., and Caughey, J., Jr.: Human constitution in clinical medicine, New York, 1944, P.B. Hoeber, Inc.

DuBois, E.F.: Heat loss from the human body, Harvey Lecture, Bull. N.Y. Acad. Med. **15:**143, 1939.

DuBois, E.F.: Fever and the regulation of body temperature, Publ. No. 13, American Lecture Series, Springfield, Ill., 1948, Charles C Thomas, Publisher.

DuBois, E.F.: The many different temperatures of the human body and its parts, West. J. Surg. **59:**476, 1951.

Folk, C.E.: Temperature regulation. In Folk, G.E., editor: Textbook of environmental physiology, Philadelphia, 1974, Lea & Febiger.

Fowler, N.O.: Inspection and palpation of venous and arterial pulses, New York, 1970, American Heart Association.

Garn, S.M.: Types and distribution of hair on man, Ann. N.Y. Acad. Sci. **53:**498, 1951.

Garrison, G.E., Floyd, W.L., and Orgain, E.S.: Exercise and the physical examination of peripheral arterial disease, Ann. Intern Med. **66:**587, 1967.

Geddes, L.A.: The direct and indirect measurement of blood pressure, Chicago, 1970, Year Book Medical Publishers, Inc.

Gold, J.J.: Hirsutism and virilism. In Gold, J.J., editor: Gynecologic endocrinology, New York, 1975, Harper & Row, Publishers.

Gruskin, A.: Clinical evaluation of hypertension in children, Primary Care **1:**233, 1974.

Haddock, N.: Blood pressure monitoring in neonates, MCN **5:**131, 1980.

Hochberg, H.M., and Salomon, H.: Accuracy of an ultrasound blood monitor, Curr. Ther. Res. **13:**129, 1971.

Hurst J.W., editor: The heart, ed. 4, New York, 1974, McGraw-Hill Book Co.

Karvenen, N.J., Telivuo, L.J., and Jarvinen, E.J.: Sphygmomanometer cuff size and accuracy of indirect measurement of blood pressure, Am. J. Cardiol. **13:**688, 1964.

King, G.E.: Errors in clinical measurement of blood pressure in obesity, Clin. Sci. **32:**233, 1967.

King, G.E.: Taking the blood pressure, JAMA **209:**1902, 1969.

Leon, M., and others: Biosynthesis of testosterone by a Stein-Leventhal ovary, Acta Endocrinol. **39:**411, 1962.

Londe, S.: Blood pressure in children as determined under office conditions, Clin. Pediatr. **5:**71, 1966.

Londe, S., and others: Hypertension in apparently normal children, J. Pediatr. **78:**569, 1971.

McCutcheon, E.P., and Rushmer, R.F.: Korotkoff sounds, Circ. Res. **20:**149, 1967.

McGregor, M.: Pulsus paradoxus, N. Engl. J. Med. **301**(9):480, 1979.

Meninger, K.: A psychiatrist's world: the selected papers of Karl Meninger, M.D., New York, 1959, The Viking Press, Inc.

The National Heart, Lung, and Blood Institute's Task Force on Blood Pressure Control in Children: Report of the Task Force on Blood Pressure Control in Children, Pediatrics **59**(suppl. 5):797, 1977.

Nichols, G.A.: Taking adult temperatures: rectal measurements, Am. J. Nurs. **72:**1092, 1972.

Nichols, G.A.: Time analyses of afebrile and febrile temperature readings, Nurs. Res. **21:**463, 1972.

Nichols, G.A., and Kucha, D.H.: Taking adult temperatures: oral measurements, Am. J. Nurs. **72:**1090, 1972.

O'Rourke, M.F.: The arterial pulse in health and disease, Am. Heart J. **82:**687, 1971.

Recommendations for human blood pressure determination by sphygmomanometer, New York, 1967, American Heart Association.

Roaf, R.: Posture, New York, 1977, Academic Press, Inc.

Simpson, J.A., and others: Effect of size of cuff bladder on accuracy of measurement of direct blood pressure, Am. Heart J. **70:**208, 1965.

Sorlie, P., Gordon T., and Kannel, W.B.: Body build and mortality, JAMA **243:**1828, 1980.

Sphygomomanometers: principles and precepts, Copiague, N.Y., 1965, W.A. Baum Co.

Ur, A., and Gordon, M.: Origin of Korotkoff sounds, Am. J. Physiol. **218:**524, 1970.

Williams, R.: Textbook of endocrinology, Philadelphia, 1974, W.B. Saunders Co.

Wu, R.: Behavior and illness, Englewood Cliffs, N.J., 1973, Prentice-Hall, Inc.

CHAPTER 8

ASSESSMENT OF MENTAL STATUS

The major focus of the mental status examination is the identification of the individual's strengths and capabilities for interaction with the environment. Although it is important to detect the weaknesses and maladaptations that hamper daily living, the examiner must assess the individual's resources for environmental and social adjustment. The information to be obtained includes educational development, occupation, economic status, marital status, responsibilities for the family, stresses in living, and goals toward which the client is striving.

The objective of the mental status examination is to assess those thoughts or mental processes that interfere with the individual's ability to reach an optimum level of function. Thus, the examiner is alert to behaviors that may interfere with happiness, life satisfaction, or social adjustment. The examiner further seeks to understand the origin of those behaviors and the development of them to the present time. The developmental history plays an essential role in the mental status examination. The three categories of information assessment include the individual, his experience, and socioeconomic factors. From a *neurological viewpoint* the examiner is assessing *cerebral function.*

The interview is the initial and most important tool in health assessment for obtaining data about the client's behavior and interactions with his environment. Although the client's self-report may not be entirely factual, the client's report and/or those of significant others are often the only data base available to the examiner from which to analyze the client's behavior.

The interview is a richer source of behavioral data than questionnaires or interactive computer methods. The examiner has a good deal more flexibility, such as being able to devote more time to exploring specific areas of importance to the client. In addition, the interviewer has the advantage of being able to observe the client's nonverbal behaviors.

The method of interviewing most frequently observed, that is, eliciting feelings and facts for the history, is a combination of asking questions and waiting while appearing alert and interested as the client provides the answers in his own language. This method allows for an observation of awareness, cognitive function, and affect. The questions asked the client are aimed at obtaining more data about symptoms, family and medical history, the parameters of the client's life situation, and an evaluation of his support systems.

In assessing the mental status of the client, the examiner usually deals with symptoms—the thought processes or behavior and how the client feels about them. Some signs may be available, such as behavior that is disturbing to others. The examiner elicits the evolutionary history of the client's complaints and makes his own observations. Because what the client reports may change with each examination and because the client's words may have different connotations for different examiners, it is difficult to obtain agreement in the terminology of the assessment of behavioral symptoms. The most helpful record is one that describes the *client's behaviors and words accurately and succinctly.*

The choice of words used to describe behavior during the interview should be carefully selected. The interviewer would do well to avoid words that are semantically unacceptable to the client. For instance, the individual may find it acceptable to be termed hypersensitive but not irritable, or meticulous but not compulsive.

The record should be kept as simple and direct as possible; hazy terminology should be avoided. Words such as *anxious, cheerful,* and *suspicious* are loaded words, fraught with individual variation in connotation. They mean different things to different readers. A more meaningful record describes observations of appearance and behaviors of the client in objective, that is, measurable units.

It must be borne in mind that the behaviors elicited in the mental status examination are no more than a sample of the individual's thoughts and feelings.

The appraisal of mental status is a process that may be built into the interview and the physical examination. However, the client who demonstrates dysfunction in affect or thought processes may indicate the need for further exploration.

A full mental status examination is indicated when loss of memory or aphasia is encountered in the client.

The only materials that may be helpful in the examination of mental status are a pencil, paper, and a newspaper.

PHYSICAL APPEARANCE AND BEHAVIOR

The examiner carefully observes the client's physical appearance, manner of dress, facial expression, and body posture as a measure of mental function. In essence, assessment of neural status will be the composite of the way the client looks, acts, and feels (see also Chapter 7 on general assessment). Particular attention is given to posture.

Assessment of motor behavior—movement
Posture, behavior, and reaction time

The posture is important in providing clues to the client's feelings. The client who walks slowly into the room, barely lifting his feet, and who slumps in the chair while avoiding the examiner's glance may be eloquently describing a lack of affect or depression. On the other hand, the person who bounds into the room, energetically shaking the examiner's hand while rapidly glancing around the room may be demonstrating significant overreaction. The tense muscles and furrowed forehead or the furtive, darting eyes, coupled with the wet handshake of the individual with anxiety should alert the examiner to look for further symptoms to corroborate this impression. With each interchange the speed and appropriateness of reaction are evaluated to detect the client's position on the continuum of poverty of movement to hyperactivity.

Coordination

General coordination of movement may be assessed through observation of the gait. To assess the complex acts of coordination, the examiner may give the client simple phrases to write and simple geometric figures to draw. The client is asked to draw more fundamental figures such as a circle, square, or triangle followed by more complex figures such as a house or flower. Persons with Alzheimer's disease are unable to make accurate copies of the figures.

Grooming and apparel

Failure of the client to give attention to personal cleanliness is a clue to underlying emotional problems. Thus, dirty hair or a dirty body, uncombed hair, or unkempt nails in a previously healthily groomed person warrant further exploration. The nails are examined for evidence of nail biting by the client. The female client with carelessly or bizarrely applied cosmetics should also be examined further. (On the other hand, lack of makeup may have no significance, since the client may have an allergy to the chemicals in cosmetics or her makeup may look so natural that it is not detected by the examiner. Deterioration in grooming occurs in depression, schizophrenia, and organic brain disease. One-sided neglect has been observed in association with parietal lesions. What is looked for in the behaviors is a pattern.) The clothing is examined to determine its appropriateness to the occasion (place, time) and the client's position in life. Bright yellow and red have been associated with euphoria, whereas drab olive green and black have been associated with depression. Attention is given to the amount and type of jewelry worn by the client. The sexual impression conveyed by the clothing may also have diagnostic value. The female client who appears dressed in masculine clothing with closely cropped hair may be giving a message of her sexual identity (or may just be exhibiting the unisex nature of dress popular in the 1970s and 1980s).

Interaction and relationship with examiner

An overall assessment of whether the client is cooperative, recalcitrant, friendly, hostile, or ingratiating is made. The examiner is alert to his or her own feelings whether they are consciously understood or arise from reasons not clearly understood. The feelings are recorded whether the feelings are positive, neutral, or negative. Many examples have been reported of examiners feeling fear in the presence of clients who later proved violent. The feeling is not discounted until sufficient data accrue to support ignoring the emotion. In other cases the examiner found a client irritating. This feeling may be provoked in others in the client's environment and cause the client's problems in daily life. Thus, intuitive feelings should be noted.

Speech

The manner of speech may give clues of the status of thought processes. Comprehension of and ability to use the spoken language may be readily assessed during the interview and the assessment procedure. The answers to the examiner's questions and the ability to follow instructions ("Change into this gown," "Please sit on this chair") give valuable data about the client's comprehension and willingness to cooperate.

The nature of responses to the examiner's questions is important. The normal individual answers questions frankly. Failure to answer a question, circumlocution, or other evasive replies should be noted. Criticism given to the examiner by the client and whether the client talks up or down to the examiner may be recorded.

Rapid-fire conversation should be noted, as well as slow and halting delivery. These observations should be mentally positioned on a continuum of poverty of movement to hyperactivity. The client who monopolizes the interview should also be noted. Slow, monotonous speech is characteristic of parkinsonism. The client, just as the professional, chooses the words he feels are best suited to his companion of the moment. Thus, the words chosen by the client usually give a good idea of his general intelligence, educational level, social level, and level of functioning.

Articulation is assessed. This includes fluency, ease of expression, rhythm, hesitancies, stuttering, and repetitiousness. The omission or addition of letters, syllables, and words, or their transposition, and the misuse of words suggest aphasia. In addition, the client may be observed to practice circumlocution or to attempt to express his thoughts nonverbally (pantomime) to avoid revealing that he has forgotten a word. Repetitious, abnormal thought patterns revealed in speech are recorded. These would include neologisms, verbigeration, or echolalia.

Disorders of the structures responsible for speech may be evident during conversation with the client. These include the following:

1. *Dysphonia:* Difficulty or discomfort in making laryngeal speech sounds, such as hoarseness. *Dysphonia puberum* is difficulty in controlling laryngeal speech sounds that occur as the larynx enlarges in puberty.
2. *Dysarthria:* Difficulty in articulating single sounds or phonemes of speech; individual letters *(f, g, r)*; labials—sounds produced with the lips *(b, m, w,* rounded vowels) (cranial nerve [CN] VII); gutterals—sounds produced in the throat (CN X); and linguals—sounds produced with the tongue *(l, t, n)* (CN XII). Dysarthria may be demonstrated by asking the client to repeat a phrase such as "Methodist Episcopal" or by asking him to read a short paragraph containing all of these letters.
3. *Dysprosody:* Difficulty in speech such that inflection, pronunciation, pitch, and rhythm are impaired.

Aphasia. Aphasia is a general term for a dysfunction or loss of ability to express thoughts by speech, writing, symbols, or signs or to interpret sensory input (Table 8-1). These disorders are caused by lesions of the brain (Fig. 8-1). The term *aphasia* excludes those disturbances of expression related to abnormalities of neurons to the muscles of speech, disorders of the anatomical structures that participate in the production of speech and mental deficiency. Aphasia encompasses *agnosia,* the impaired ability to recognize once-familiar objects, and *apraxia,* the impaired ability to carry out purposeful activity related to language. The most common cerebral pathological condition associated with aphasia is vascular disease. Although the cerebral hemispheres share equal responsibility in controlling the two sides of the body in general, language requires the simultaneous input of both and is controlled by one. The hemisphere in which language is controlled is called the dominant hemisphere. It has been shown that 95% of these individuals who are right-handed and have a language deficit have lesions of the left cerebral hemisphere, whereas 70% of left-handed individuals with language impairment also have a lesion of the left cerebral hemisphere.

Aphasia may be evaluated during the initial interview with the client. The ability of the client to comprehend auditory verbal stimuli may be tested against the client's ability to answer questions and carry out instructions. Visual verbal ability is assessed from the client's ability to read and to explain the content he has read (see boxed material on p. 173). Further data may be obtained by asking the client to identify familiar objects or geometric figures.

The client may be able to express himself in some forms of speech when his free-flowing conversational speech is impaired. Some of these are included in Table 8-2.

Agnosia. *Agnosia* is a general term for the dysfunction or loss of ability to interpret sensory stimuli. These disorders have been termed receptive aphasia. Individuals with visual agnosia have the primary reception of the visual image but are unable to associate the previous experience that allows interpretation of what is being viewed. Specific cerebral cortical regions make it possible for the individual to recognize visual, auditory, and tactile stimuli. Testing for tactile interpretation is a part of the sensory examination of the neurological examination.

Apraxia. Comprehension is normal in apraxia. *Ideational apraxia* is the term for dysfunction or loss of ability to formulate the ideational concepts necessary to carry out a skilled motor act. The individual is unable to conceive the idea or retain it. This disability accompanies diffuse cerebral disorders, for example, arteriosclerosis.

Motor apraxia is decline of kinesthetic motor patterns necessary to a motor act. This disability may be related to a lesion of the precentral gyrus.

Ideomotor apraxia is the term that is used to define the situation in which an individual has lost the skills for

Causes of coma	
Toxic and metabolic	**Disorders involving physical damage to the brain**
Exogenous toxins	Tumor
Alcohol	Edema
Drugs	Stroke
Metabolic	Intracerebral hemorrhage
Uremia	Contusion
Hepatic failure	
Hypoxia	
Hypercapnia	
Hypercalcemia	

Orientation

Orientation is assessed from the client's awareness of person, place, and time.

A typical kind of protocol used in obtaining this information is as follows:

Person
"What is your name? Address? Telephone number?"
"Do you know who I am?"
"Do you know what my job is?"

Place
"Tell me where you are. What is the name of this place?"
"Do you know the name of the town you are in?"
"Who brought you here?"

Time
"Do you know what day this is? Month? Year?"

The degree of disorientation is recorded. Descriptions should include enough data to allow the reader to know if the client has no awareness of a particular parameter, limited or dysfunctional awareness, or exact perception.

Time orientation is the one most frequently disordered in clients with mental disease. The feeling that time is passing slowly is characteristic of anxious or depressed clients who tend to underestimate the passage of time. On the other hand, obsessive-compulsive individuals are highly cognizant of the exact time. A disturbance in time orientation is an early finding in organic brain syndrome, as well as toxic or metabolic central nervous system alterations.

A disturbance of place orientation may accompany organic brain syndrome or schizophrenia. An individual may not be oriented as to person in the aftermath of cerebral trauma or seizures or in amnesic fuguelike conditions.

Loss, disappointment, and suffering are associated with withdrawal and isolation in normal persons. They may complain of feelings of depersonalization and deny the reality of what is happening to them. The normal person is able to accept the circumstances causing his pain when the stress abates. The less integrated individual may become progressively more depersonalized or develop amnesia.

The individual with schizophrenia may have behavior characterized by marked withdrawal and isolation, symbolism, and grandiose gesture. In addition, body image may be distorted as to shape and movement, as well as feelings of weight.

Attention span

An appraisal of the individual's attention span is a worthwhile task of the mental status examination. This includes the examiner's description of the client's ability to maintain interest and his ability to concentrate.

The attention span is one of the first functions of the sensorium to suffer disturbance. Allowing the client to talk over a short period of time gives evidence of his stream of consciousness. The continuity of ideas is evaluated. The client's response to questions and directives will provide evidence of his attentiveness to external conditions. When a new idea is introduced in the interview, the normal client processes this alteration and responds appropriately. The client may be given a series of numbers to repeat immediately or two or three sentences that he is asked to memorize and repeat at a later time in the interview, as in memory testing. Sometimes a fictitious name and address are employed.

Attention span may be impaired in normal individuals who are fatigued, anxious, or drugged. In many pathological states attention span is shortened. The client may be easily distractible, confused, or negativistic.

Memory

Memory is a function of general cerebral competence. Impairment of memory occurs in both neurological and psychiatric disorders. Some general questions that may help the examiner establish a disorder in memory are as follows:

"Have you noticed any loss of memory?"
"How well do you remember what you are told? What has happened to you?"
"Do you remember those things that happened years ago best or those that happened today or yesterday?"

Immediate memory (verbalized remembering immediately after presentation). Immediate memory is tested by digit recall. Two sample tests follow:

"Please allow me to test your memory skills. I'd like you to repeat these numbers after me:
7, 4
9, 6, 5, 3
8, 9, 4, 1, 5
3, 8, 7, 4, 1, 6."

"I will say some numbers; you say them backward. For instance, I say *8, 2*; you say *2, 8*:

3, 8

7, 2, 0

5, 9, 2, 7."

The normal individual can generally repeat five to eight digits forward and four to six digits backward.

Recent memory may be impaired in temporal lobe trauma, senile dementia, and Korsakoff's psychosis.

Recent memory (verbalized remembrances after several minutes to an hour). Examples of questions and exercises for assessing recent memory are as follows:

"How long have you been here?"

"Why did you come here?"

"What were you doing before you came here?"

"What time did you get up today?"

"How many meals have you eaten today?"

"What did you eat for breakfast today?"

The client may be given some simple information and asked to reproduce it after a few minutes.

Remote memory (verbalized remembrances after hours, days, or years). The client may also be given three to five unrelated words to remember and repeat back. Examples of questions for assessing remote memory are as follows:

"Where were you born?"

"Tell me the name of the high school you attended."

"What was your mother's maiden name?"

Remote memory is lost in widespread cortical damage such as the late stages of dementia. It may be dysfunctional in schizophrenic illnesses.

In testing for memory the examiner does not ask questions for which he does not have access to answers. Memory loss in organic dementia may involve disorders for immediate and recent events while clients may be able to recall events from childhood with accuracy. Memory disturbances are observed in febrile and toxic conditions, as well as in mania and hysteria. Frontal lobe lesions are often associated with memory loss.

Amnesic conditions are those in which memory is lost for a specific period of time or for certain life situations. In spite of memory loss the individual with amnesia remains aware of his environment. Amnesia is frequently associated with the posttrauma periods and epileptic disorders.

Confabulation is an attempt by the client to "fill in the gaps" with fabricated or made-up answers when he is unable to remember.

Abstraction ability. To assess abstraction ability, the examiner may ask the client to give the meaning of familiar proverbs:

"A bird in the hand is worth two in the bush."

"People in glass houses should not throw stones."

"When the cat's away, the mice will play."

"Don't count your chickens before they hatch."

"A rolling stone gathers no moss."

"A stitch in time saves nine."

Individuals with schizophrenia or organic brain syndrome may give concrete explanations. Inability to provide an adequate explanation may indicate lack of intelligence, brain damage, or organic brain syndrome.

Similarities. The following exercises may be used to assess the client's ability to determine similarities:

"Tell me how the following are like each other: bird and butterfly; dog and goldfish; fish and plankton; window and door; German person and Swiss person; pencil and typewriter."

"Try to finish these comparisons for me: beer is to glass as coffee is to _____; engine is to airplane as pedal is to _____."

The assessment of the ability to define the fine but essential differences between objects or between events is the objective in testing the perception of dissimilarities. Some examples of items that may be used to assess this ability are as follows:

"Tell me how these objects differ: a bush and a tree; a rock and a plant."

Lesions of the left hemisphere may impair the client's ability to recognize similarities and to discriminate objects and events.

Ability to learn (comprehension). The ability to learn includes abilities in perception retention, association (interpretation), and recent memory. These processes are thought of as registration, storage, and retrieval. The client is given an address or a sentence that does not contain familiar associations. The material may be presented in writing or may be spoken. The client is asked to remember the content verbatim:

"Listen to me carefully, I am going to give you an address that I want you to remember. Later on, I will ask you to repeat it for me: Apartment 13, Dover Hill Building."

Or the client might be given a sentence such as the Babcock sentence:

"One thing a nation must have in order to become rich and great is a large and secure stock of wood."

Or the rest may consist of four unrelated words. An approximate 5- to 10-minute interval is allowed before the client is asked to repeat the material.

Computation. The following exercise may be used to assess the client's computational abilities:

"Subtract 7 from 100. Continue on subtracting 7 from the resulting remainder."

The ability to calculate may be impaired in diffuse brain disease and lesions of the angular gyrus. The normal individual is able to complete the computation in 1½ minutes with less than four errors.

Organic brain syndrome may be the reason for slowness in computation or increased numbers of errors. However, computation skills may be impaired in depression or anxiety.

Ability to read. A copy of a current newspaper or popular periodical is generally available and may be used to determine the client's reading skills. The examiner should be certain that the client is wearing corrective lenses if they are needed for reading.

Impairment of the ability to read is called dyslexia.

General knowledge—general information

Health assessment may include an evaluative estimate of what the client has learned in school and an estimate of his awareness of current events. The examiner should *match* his *inquiries* to the *educational, sociocultural,* and *life experiences of the client.* The client might be asked questions about well-known national leaders such as the president, capitals of countries, or names of oceans. The questions of current events should include generally known phenomena. The examiner might base these questions on recent newspaper headlines that dealt with important current issues.

Intellectual level

The examiner has obtained several criteria that are a part of human intellectual capacity: vocabulary, memory, calculation, reading, writing, and general knowledge. There is no need, in a screening assessment, to administer intelligence tests. However, the incorporation of selected items from the Stanford-Binet test may provide enough information to allow the examiner to further assess whether referral is necessary. It has been suggested that test items be selected from the 10-year-old level for initial presentation and then move to progressively more difficult tasks.

The intellectual level of the client may be deduced from his perceptive grasp of the comments and questions directed toward him, his level of general information and vocabulary, his exercise of logic, range and originality of thought, and cultural attainments.

Higher intellectual functions of judgment, analysis, synthesis, and abstraction are impaired in acute brain injury even when specific receptive, expressive, or memory functions are intact. On the other hand, cognitive abilities may remain operant when specific expressive and memory functions are dysfunctional.

Expressive functions are speaking, drawing, writing, and other physical movement, including nonverbal behaviors. All mental activity must be inferred from the expressive functions. Disorders of the expressive functions are known as apraxias.

Judgment

Judgment is a term that encompasses all the cognitive processes that include the processes of evaluation, assessment, and decision making, particularly those in which two or more experiences are related to one another. The individual who is able to evaluate a situation and determine the appropriate reaction(s) is said to have good judgment or reasoning ability. Assessment of judgment is accomplished through evaluation of the client's expressed attitudes to his social, physical, vocational, and domestic status and his plans for the future. Judgment may be inferred to be intact if the client's business affairs are in order and he is meeting social (including family) obligations. The client might also be asked to tell the examiner how he would respond in certain social situations.

Simple tests of reasoning power include an explanation indicating the meaning of abstractions. Judgment has been observed to be impaired in highly charged emotional states, mental retardation, organic brain syndrome, and schizophrenia.

Two examples of questions that may elicit indicators of judgment are as follows:

"What would you do if you were in a theater when fire broke out?"
"What would you do if you found four, stamped, addressed envelopes?"

Thought processes

The thoughts expressed by the client are evaluated in reference to his ability to be logical, coherent, relevant, and goal directed. Thought processes are the subjective ideations, comprehensions, and interpretative experiences of the client. The examiner must rely on what the client expresses verbally and nonverbally in drawing conclusions concerning the client's thought processes. The examiner should consider affect, insight, and the content of communication.

Patterns of thinking are analyzed for appropriateness of sequence, logic, coherence, and relevance. The examiner listens carefully to the thought content and associative processes. The examiner should be able to follow the sequence of ideas expressed by the client. The words, sentences, and ideas should be logical and goal directed.

Disturbances in thought processes are observed in the form of thinking, in the stream of thought, and in the thought content. *A disturbance in the form of thinking* is called *dereistic* and is illogical. The mental activity is incongruent with reality and does not adhere to the laws of logic and experience. The schizophrenic individual expresses thoughts indicative of psychic activity that is not synchronized with reality. The ideation expressed by autistic individuals is thought to be derived from unconscious processes, and the terms *autism* and *dereistic thinking* are considered to be synonymous.

Variation from normal in the rate or nature of associative processes is a *disturbance in the stream of thought* such as perseveration, stereotypy, neologism blocking, magical thinking, intellectualization, and circumstantiality. *Blocking or thought deprivation,* is characterized by a pause in the middle of a thought, phrase, or sentence. The most common cause of interruption of the thought process is unconscious and a result of emotional conflicts of which the client is unaware. The client is aware of the pause and frequently is made anxious because he does not understand why the interruption occurred. The words that follow the pause may be unrelated to the thought that preceded the pause. Blocking is most commonly observed in schizophrenic persons. However, blocking is occasionally seen in normal persons.

Magical thinking. The conviction that certain thoughts or behaviors can protect the individual from dreaded actions or evil or can lead to the fulfillment of wishes is called magical thinking. Magical thinking or behaviors constitute a disturbance in the stream of thought. The magical behaviors may be simple gestures or postures or complex activities. Magical thinking plays a prominent role in many cultures, and therefore, the examiner must understand magical behaviors that are a part of various social classes and cultural groups. Magical thinking is normal in children who do not understand the scientific cause and effect for events in their milieu. The magical behavior is thought to provide a defense against helplessness and anxiety.

Intellectualization. Intellectualization is a process of thinking excessively about the philosophical or theoretical ideas such that the stream of thought is interrupted and emotionally charged impulses are avoided. The adolescent who is obsessed with religion may be using the intellectual absorption in religious ideas as a mechanism for avoiding disturbing sexual impulses. The client who has conducted a scholarly search of the literature regarding a particular sign of disease may be involving himself so thoroughly in the intellectual delineation of the sign that he is able to avoid the feeling of fear engendered by the sign that is in fact indicative of a threat to life. Thus, the defense mechanism of intellectualization may interfere with reality and carried to the extreme may lead to obsessive thought and even paranoia.

Circumstantiality. Interruption in the stream of thought as a result of excessive associations of an idea reaching the conscious level is called circumstantiality. The verbalization of the extraneous ideas and the digression from the thought serve to avoid emotionally charged areas. Circumstantiality is observed in obsessive disorders, in schizophrenia, and in organic brain syndromes.

Perseveration. Perseveration is an interruption in the stream of thought, characterized by repetition of a word or phrase that persists although the client recognizes the repetition and is able to express a desire to say something more appropriate. Perseveration is frequently observed in clients with pathological disorders of the premotor region of the frontal cortex. Perseveration has also been described in schizophrenic persons.

Stereotypy. An interruption in the stream of thought resulting from continual repetition of a behavior (action or speech) or sequence of behaviors is called stereotypy. Stereotyped behavior is seen most frequently in schizophrenic individuals.

Disturbances in thought content. Mental dysfunction or psychiatric symptoms are referred if some relief of symptoms can be anticipated. The symptoms that are most worthy of attention are those that are uselessly repetitive in nature, uncomfortable for the client, and disabling.

The common disorders of emotion and thought processes are defined here. Familiarity with this symptomatology may help the examiner focus questioning and recognize a cluster of symptoms. As with the physical examination, the examiner is looking for a pattern.

delusion A false belief of great magnitude, not influenced by experience, improbable in nature, and not related to the cultural and educational background of the client.

Delusions are subdivided according to their content:

delusion of being controlled A fixed belief that the individual feelings, thoughts, and actions are being imposed by some external force.

bizarre delusion A false belief characterized by incongruous, even ridiculous, content.

grandiose delusion A false belief with content that includes an exaggerated sense of one's importance, power, knowledge, or identity.

delusional jealousy A false belief that one's sexual partner is not faithful.

mood-congruent delusion A belief consistent with either a depressed or manic mood.

mood-incongruent delusion A false idea in which content is not consistent with a depressed or manic mood.

nihilistic delusion A false belief with content that involves the nonexistence of the self or part of the self, others, or the world.

persecutory delusion A false belief with content that has the theme of a person or group being attacked, harassed, cheated, persecuted, or conspired against.

delusion of poverty A false belief that a person will lose his personal possessions.

delusion of reference A false belief that the people in a person's immediate environment have unusual significance, usually negative.

somatic delusion A false belief with a theme that pertains to the function of the body.

• • •

depersonalization Feelings that one is not real or has lost his identity may occur alone. Some individuals describe feeling mechanical.

derealization Feelings that environmental objects or the world around one is unreal; almost always associated with depersonalization.

eidetic imagery Vivid imagery of past event, present in some artists; original experience more intense, however; 50% to 60% of children up to age 12 able to visualize previously perceived object.

hallucination Perception for which no external stimuli can be ascertained. An endogenous experience in an individual whose sensorium is clear. *Simple hallucination:* simple perception, such as seeing light. *Complex hallucination:* more detailed experiences, such as seeing figure of a person. Although any sensory system might be involved, *auditory hallucinations* are reported most commonly. The client may perceive a voice or sound of some type coming from outside his head. The voice may be that of a parent or close object relationship. The messages that the client reports may be condemning or accusatory or by contrast may be complimentary and encouraging. In some cases the voice is described as clear and distinct, whereas for others the voice is faint or inaudible. *Visual hallucinations* have been described as vivid images of persons or animals or conversely as shadowy figures. Visual hallucinations are often associated with organic conditions. *Tactile hallucinations* have been described as the feeling of bugs or worms crawling on the surface of the skin or below the surface of the skin. Tactile hallucinations have been described in organic disease, i.e., alcohol withdrawal.

ideas of reference Falsely interpreting external events as relating to oneself. Normal individuals often voice this symptom, that is, suspecting that a partially overhead conversation refers to oneself. (Ideas of reference are less firmly held than delusions).

illusion Perception based on an actual external stimulus with misinterpretation or distortion of the event.

paranoid ideation Feeling that one is being persecuted or plotted against; feeling that one is controlled or manipulated by others (influence); feeling that one is being communicated with or controlled from the outside (reference).

Hallucinations occur in many mental illnesses and brain disorders. The most frequently reported hallucination is the one of hearing voices, which occurs most often in schizophrenia. Highly organized and detailed hallucinations like "watching television" are recounted most often by individuals with hysteria. Hallucinations or perceptual disturbances are a part of the effect of psychedelic drugs, that is, the tryptamine group, the phenylethylamine group, Ditran, tetrahydrocannabinol (the active principle of *Cannabis),* phencyclidine and lysergic acid diethylamide (LSD).

Emotional status, affect

Affect is defined as the feeling tone or emotion. The examiner is generally able to develop an estimate of the client's prevailing mood and emotional status or affective state from his verbal and nonverbal behavior. Affects may be found to be labile: repeated, rapid, and abrupt shifts.

Affective responses, the feelings associated with ideas, are noted throughout the interview process. The examiner notes appropriateness and degree of affect to a given idea, as well as the range of affect to a variety of situations. A range of affect may be described as broad (normal), restricted (constricted), blunted, or flat.

The depressed individual may have blunted affect. The depressed individual who expresses suicidal feelings needs immediate attention. Flat affect may characterize the schizophrenic individual, and apathy may be observed in persons with organic brain syndrome. Extreme emotional responses may be observed in manic behavior. Bizarre behavior may be seen in the person with schizophrenia.

An interview protocol to help the examiner bring out the feelings of the client when he does not offer spontaneous data might contain the following:

"How do you feel inside?"
"How have your spirits been?"
"Do you feel this way most of the time?"
"Are you in good spirits, happy [unhappy] most of the time?"
"Do you let people know how you feel?" *If no,* "Are you afraid to let people see how you feel?"
"Can you control how you feel?"
"When do you feel the best, in the morning or in the evening?"
"How do you feel life has treated you?"
"Do you enjoy your life?"
"Is life worth living for you?"
"What does the future look like?" *If a negative reply,* "Does everything look hopeless? Do you think you will see tomorrow?"
"What plans have you made for your future?"
"Have you ever considered hurting yourself?" *If yes,* "Did you follow through and actually hurt yourself?"
"Do you think about dying?"

Some adjectives used to describe mood include the following:

appropriate Feelings that correspond to environmental situation

inappropriate Mood does not match culturally normal feeling state that would accompany client's life situation or what he is saying

flat Unresponsive

depressed Sad, feels deserted without help, hopeless, feels a burden to others

anxiety Worried and concerned, fearful, alarmed, apprehensive, tense (perception of danger that may be internal or external)

agitated Feels in turmoil, perturbed, disturbed

elated Lively, joyful, high spirits, more cheerful than usual

manic Excitation, euphoria, irritability possible (accompanied by hyperactivity, rapid speech rate, and other signs of an excited state)

labile Feelings characterized by repeated, rapid, and abrupt shifts

euphoric Exaggerated feeling of well-being

euthymic A mood in the "normal" range

expansive Lack of restraint in expressing one's feelings

irritable Feelings of tension, easily annoyed

The client's mood may be altered in both organic and psychogenic disorders.

Insight

Insight is the client's ability to perceive himself realistically and to understand himself. The evaluation of insight involves the assessment of the client's understanding of and attitude toward the cause and nature of his illness. Simple questions such as "Why did you decide to come here (name of health care facility) at this time?" allow the client to explain in his own words his comprehension of his health status and his realization of physical and mental symptoms.

It is important to elicit the individual's attitude and willingness to accept professional advice and treatment. When an apparent lack of insight is found, the examiner should attempt to determine if a real loss has occurred or whether the client may be attempting to hide his problems. Insight may be lost in the euphoria of mania. Difficulties may be ascribed to external sources in paranoia.

The elicitation of the chief complaint and the data of present illness may provide information about the client's insight to the examiner. Helpful questions with which to conclude the analysis of the chief complaint are as follows:

"Have you noticed any change in yourself or in your outlook on life?"
"Have you noticed any change in your feelings?"

The appraisal of emotional status includes an investigation of the client's life situation and personality (general coping behavior). An interview protocol to elicit this information might be similar to the one that follows.

Queries

Frequently recorded responses

Present (chief) complaint
"Tell me why you are here."

Present illness
"When did you last feel well?"
"What changes have you noted in yourself?"
"When did you first notice the problem?"
"How long did it last?"
"What do you feel is causing the problem?"
"Have you had any other troubling bodily or psychological feelings (symptoms)?"
"How are you sleeping? Eating?"
"Do you feel better in the morning or in the evening?"
"Have you gained or lost any weight?"

Family history
"How old is your father? Is he employed?"
"What does [did] he do for a living?"
"How old is your mother? Is [was] she employed?"
"Did either your father or your mother have any other marriages?"
"How well did they get along?"
"Tell me about their personality [temperament]?"
"How did you feel about your parents?"
"Was your home a comfortable place?"
"Did any of your family have any emotional problems? Ever need to see a doctor because of a nervous problem?"

Affectionate, warm, easygoing, strict, cold, always worried, always in debt, drunk all the time

Childhood and premorbid personality
"What were you like as a child?"
"How did your parents [brothers, sisters] describe you to others?"
"What did your teachers think of you?"
"Did you like to be with people?"
"Tell me how you would describe yourself."

Friendly; happy; nervous; jumpy; shy; self-conscious; delicate; enuresis; nail biting; fears—of the dark, small rooms, open spaces, high places, crowds; depressed; loner; read all the time; hated sports; successful; unsure of self

Medical history
"Have you ever been diagnosed as having a disease?" *If yes,* "Explain this to me."

Psychological history
"Have you ever been in counseling or treatment for an emotional problem?"

Queries	Frequently recorded responses
Recent stress	
"Have you had any recent cause for grief?"	
"Have you been bereaved over the loss of a loved person?"	
"Are all your relatives and friends in good health?"	
"Are there any problems with your job?"	
"Is money a problem for you?"	
"Are there problems in your marriage? Love life?"	
Education	
"Where did you go to school?"	
"What was the highest grade you attended?"	
"How did you feel about school?"	
"How well did you do in school?"	Overachievement, truancy, suspension
Employment	
"What kind of work do you do?"	
"Tell me where you have worked and how long you worked at each job?	Long periods of unemployment, frequent job turnover
"Have you ever served in a military service?"	
"Do you enjoy working?"	
"How do you get along with your boss? People who work for you?"	
Delinquency	
"Have you ever been in trouble with school? The police?"	
Drug history	
"Have you ever been given a prescription for medicine by a doctor?" *If yes,* "Tell me about it."	
"Have you ever used drugs available in the street?" *If yes,* "How much? How long? Are you taking drugs now?"	Grass (marijuana), uppers, downers, hash, tic (phencyclidine [PCP]), horse (heroin)
"Do you drink beer? Wine? Whiskey? How much? How long?" *or* "How much and what are you drinking these days?"	
"Do you drink soda pop? How much?"	
Marital history	
"How old is your wife [husband]?"	
"How long have you been married?"	
"How do you feel about your marriage?"	Hate to go home, often go out with the guys
"How many children do you have?"	
"Were there any other pregnancies?"	
"How do you get along with your children?"	
"What kinds of things do you do as a family?"	
"How many times were you engaged?"	
"Were you ever married before?" *If yes,* "Tell me about it."	

Queries	Frequently recorded responses
"Is your sexual relationship satisfactory to you?" *If no,* "How do you manage?"	Masturbation, homosexuality, extramarital intercourse
"Do you have any extramarital relationships?"	
Social milieu	
"Tell me about your friends."	
Support systems	
"Who would you turn to if you were in trouble?"	
"Do you feel that you need someone to turn to?"	
Insight	
"Do you consider yourself different now than before your problem began?"	
"What do you think about your problem?"	
"Do you think you are sick?" *If yes,* "Do you think you will get over it?"	
"Do you think you need help?"	
"In what way would you change if you had a choice?"	
"Do you think the same way now that you always have?"	
"Do your thoughts come slower [faster] than they used to?"	

Self-drawings made by the client on blank pieces of paper may help the examiner in his examination of body image. ("Draw yourself for me.") The drawing is inspected with special reference to size of image, the facial expression (affect), the activity of the figure, the amount and nature of detail, and the diminution or exaggeration of body parts. Another useful device is that of asking the client to fill in an outline of the human body. ("Draw your insides.") The heart, lungs, and intestines are the structures most frequently added. The placement and size of the organs drawn by the client may provide clues of their meaning to him.

Once a symptom has been identified as a chief complaint (that is, phobia, depression, compulsion, psychosomatic dysfunction), the history relevant to its development is explored. The individual's previous personality (characteristic behavior pattern) is explored in relation to behaviors that led to the exacerbation of the symptom in response to stress. In addition, the potential for resolution of the problem is identified. That is, the individual's personal, social, and environmental resources are determined.

Coping behaviors

In an evaluation of the individual's resources for adjusting to life's experiences, it is valuable to know the coping behaviors he has found helpful in reducing stress, such as contact sports, jogging, meditation, and reading.

Defense mechanisms. Unconscious defense mechanisms include the following:

projection Attribution of one's feelings, attitudes or desires to others, that is, blaming others for one's faults

rationalization Creation of self-satisfying but erroneous reasons for one's behaviors

denial Failure to recognize internal or external reality

displacement Transposition of feelings such as anger from an appropriate to an inappropriate (less threatening) object

The examiner must be aware of thoughts expressed by the client indicating the exercise of these defenses.

Organic brain syndrome

Organic brain syndrome is a diagnostic term used to describe those individuals with signs indicating medical or neurological dysfunction causing an impairment of orientation, memory, or other mental functions (see boxed material at top right). Affective symptoms, delusions, hallucinations, and obsessions may also be present. An acute brain syndrome (delirium) is one of short duration that is usually reversible. A chronic brain syndrome (dementia) is long standing and often progressive in nature; its prognosis is less favorable.

Affective disorders

The client with an affective disorder runs the gamut from depression to exaggerated euphoria or mania. The highs and lows show little correlation with the life situation (see boxed material at bottom right).

During the down mood period the client evidences such symptoms as anorexia, insomnia, sense of worthlessness, sense of being a burden, and thoughts of self-destruction. On the high mood cusp the client may describe flights of ideas or hyperactivity.

Primary affective disorders are those observed in a client who has had no previous psychiatric disorders. *Secondary affective disorders* are those seen in a client who has been previously diagnosed as having psychiatric illness.

A *bipolar affective disorder* is diagnosed when mania is present whether or not depression occurs. Depression occurring in the absence of mania is known as a *unipolar affective disorder*.

The client with an affective disorder often tells the examiner that "something is wrong with my mind."

Paranoid ideations have been reported in clients with affective disorders. These thoughts appear to be augmented ideas of reference related to the feeling of worthlessness.

Organic brain syndrome: characteristic symptoms and signs

Acute delirium	**Dementia**
Impairment of consciousness	May be disoriented
Delusions possible	Attention span impaired
Hallucinations possible	Judgment impaired
May be disoriented	Recent memory impaired
Attention span impaired	Mood swings
Judgment impaired	Irritability
Mood swings	
Recent memory impaired	
Restlessness	
Anxiety	
Fear	

Affective disorders: characteristic symptoms and signs

Mania

	Somatic
Euphoria	
Irritability (sometimes)	Hyperactivity
Flight of ideas—generally comprehensible	Rapid speech rate
Distractibility	Rhyming
Delusions possible (may be of grandeur)	Punning
	Decreased sleep
Passivity—sensation that body is under external control	
Depersonalization	

Depression

	Somatic
Dejection	Pain
Discouragement	Tachycardia
Despondency	Dyspnea
Depression	Gastrointestinal dysfunction
Feeling of being down in the dumps, blue	Anorexia
Irritability	Constipation
Fearfulness	Sleep disorders
Loss of interest in daily activities	Insomnia
Social withdrawal	Hypersomnia
Guilt	Lack of energy
Inability to focus thoughts	Psychomotor retardation
Indecisiveness	Frequent crying
Recurring preoccupation with suicide, death	Impotence (in men)
Thoughts of self-destruction	Restlessness
Hopelessness	Pacing, wringing of hands
Feeling of gloomy future, impending doom	
Loss of interest in sexual activity	
Delusions possible (frequently involving self-deprecation)	

lips, earlobes, or nail beds can be gently pinched to see how quickly the color returns. The color usually returns quickly, but if the delay is prolonged, there may be decreased oxygenation of the blood or decreased blood flow to the skin.

Skin palpation

Palpation of the skin is used to amplify the findings observed on inspection and is usually carried out simultaneously as each body part is examined. Changes in temperature, moisture, texture, and turgor are detected by palpation.

Temperature of the skin is increased when blood flow through the dermis is increased. Localized areas of skin hyperthermia are noted in the presence of a burn or a localized infection. Generalized skin hyperthermia involving all of the integument may occur when there is fever associated with a localized or systemic disease. Temperature of the skin is reduced when there is a decrease in blood flow in the dermis. Generalized skin hypothermia occurs when the client is in shock, whereas localized hypothermia occurs in conditions such as arteriosclerosis.

The moisture found on the skin will vary from one body area to another. It is normal to find the soles of the feet, the palms of the hands, and the intertriginous areas—where two surfaces are close together—containing more moisture than other parts. The amount of moisture found over the entire integument also varies with changes in the environmental temperature, with muscular activity, and with the body temperature. The skin functions in the regulation of body temperature and produces perspiration that evaporates, thus cooling the body when the temperature is increased. The skin is normally drier during the winter months, when environmental temperatures and humidity are decreased, and with the increase in age of the individual. Abnormal dryness of the skin occurs with dehydration; the skin will feel dry even when the temperature is increased. Dryness of the skin is also found in conditions such as myxedema and chronic nephritis.

Texture refers to the fineness or coarseness of the skin, and changes may indicate local irritation or trauma to defined skin areas or may be associated with problems of other systems. The skin becomes soft and smooth in hyperthyroidism and rough and dry in hypothyroidism.

Turgor refers to the elasticity of the skin and is most easily determined by picking up a fold of skin over the abdomen and observing how quickly it returns to its normal shape. There is a loss of turgor associated with dehydration, and the skin demonstrates a laxness and a loss of normal mobility, returning to place slowly. Loss of turgor is also associated with aging; the skin

Table 9-2
Alopecia—hair loss

Type of alopecia	Description
Androgen (in female)	Thinning of scalp hair; male pattern hirsutism on body
Areata	Circumscribed bald areas; sudden onset, usually reversible
Chemical	Hair brittle; breaks off
Cicatricial	Permanent localized loss of hair associated with scarring
Drug or radiation	Loss of hair caused by antineoplastic agents, such as gold, thallium, and arsenic, or by radiation
Male pattern	Regression of anterior hairline, temples, and vertex; hereditary
Mucinosis	Erythematous papules or plaques without hair
Syphilitic	Generalized thinning of hair or baldness; mucous patches without hair

becomes wrinkled and lax. Increased turgor is associated with an increase in tension, which causes the skin to return to place quickly when pinched.

Hair

The hair over the entire body is examined to determine the distribution, quantity, and quality. There is a normal male or female hair pattern that evolves after puberty, and a deviation may be indicative of an endocrine problem. Changes in the quantity of the hair are of importance. Hirsutism, increased hair growth, is found in conditions such as Cushing's syndrome and acromegaly. Decreased hair growth or loss of hair may be associated with hypopituitarism or a pyogenic infection. Types of alopecia, or hair loss, are listed in Table 9-2. The quality of the hair is determined by the color and texture. Changes in color such as graying occur normally with aging, but patchy gray hair may develop following nerve injuries. Changes in texture of hair associated with hypothyroidism include dryness and coarseness, and changes associated with hyperthyroidism include increased silkiness and fineness.

Nails

The assessment of the nails is important to determine not only their condition but also possible evidence of systemic diseases. The nails are examined for shape, normal dorsal curvature, adhesion to the nail bed, regularity of the nail surface, color, and thickness. The skin folds around the nails are examined for any color changes, swelling, increased temperature, and tenderness (Fig. 9-3).

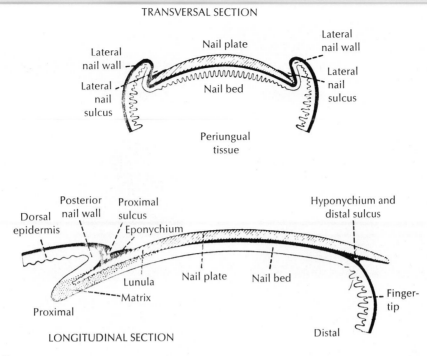

Fig. 9-3
Scheme of nail anatomy in transversal and longitudinal sections. (Diagram based on Achten, 1959. From DeNicola, P., and Morsiani, M.: Nail diseases in internal medicine, Springfield, Ill., 1974, Charles C Thomas, Publisher.)

The nails are keratinized appendages of the epidermis, as are hairs. The nails consist of (1) the nail matrix (root), wherein the nail plate is developed; (2) the nail plate; (3) the nail bed, which is attached to the nail plate; and (4) the periungual tissue, including the eponychium and the perionychium.

The nail matrix is not visible. The lunula, located at the base of the visible nail, has the shape of a half moon. The whiter color of the lunula compared to the more distal nail is caused by the uptake of keratolytic granules and by the lunula's looser connection to the underlying vascularized derma. A bluish hue is observed in the nails of more darkly pigmented subjects. The size of the lunula is variable and may not be visible in older subjects.

The nail plate is a horny, semitransparent structure with a dorsal convexity. The nail bed lies distal to the lunula and is not known to participate in nail formation. The visible nail has a roughly rectangular shape. Normal thickness of the nail is 0.3 to 0.65 mm, being somewhat thicker in men.

The free edge of the nail fold is continuous with the cuticle, which is an extension of the stratum corneum of the dorsum of the finger. The eponychium lies below this and is the anterior extension of the roof of the nail fold on the nail plate. The hyponychium is the portion of the fingertip underlying the free portion of the nail. The perionychium is the epidermis bordering the nail.

Nail growth

The nail plate is formed continuously and uniformly at all points in the matrix. The plate is pushed forward by cells of the germinative layer of the matrix. The fingernail growth rate in the normal adult has been reported variously as 0.1 to 1 mm per day. The rate varies with nutrition, age, and activity level.

Nail growth also has a circadian and seasonal rhythm. It is greater in the morning, lessening progressively in the afternoon and the night. Nail growth is greater in warm seasons than in cold, and accelerated growth has been observed in warm climates. The growth rate slows with aging. The total time required for reaching the free margin of the nail from the lunula is called the migration time and is normally 130 days. The time required for complete renewal of the fingernail (regeneration time) is 170 days, while that of the toenail is 1 to 1½ years.

Nail absence

Anonychia is the complete absence of the nail. This condition is usually congenital.

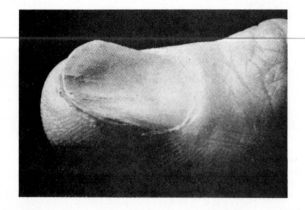

Fig. 9-4
Koilonychia. (From Samman, P.D.: The nails in disease,
London, 1978, William Heinemann Medical Books,
Ltd.)

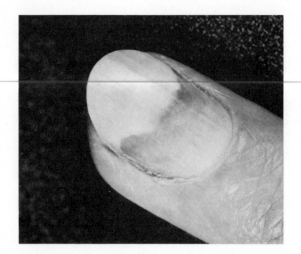

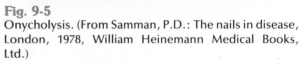

Fig. 9-5
Onycholysis. (From Samman, P.D.: The nails in disease,
London, 1978, William Heinemann Medical Books,
Ltd.)

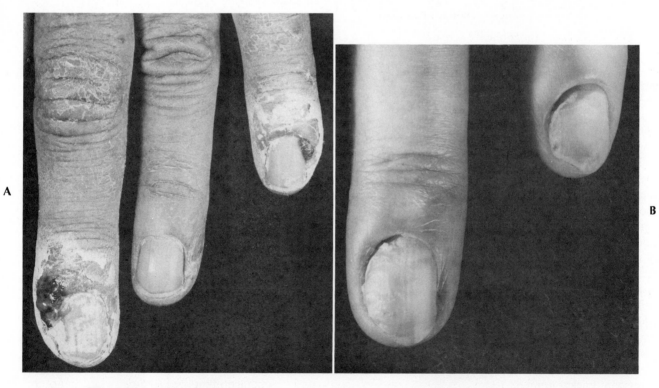

Fig. 9-6
A, Acute paronychia. **B,** Chronic paronychia—early stage. Note loss of cuticle and bolstering
of posterior nail fold. (From Samman, P.D.: The nails in disease, London 1978, William Heinemann Medical Books, Ltd.)

Changes in nail curvature

Platyonychia is flattening of the nails, although color, consistency, and thickness are not altered. This may be hereditary or may be the forerunner of koilonychia.

Koilonychia describes a nail that has the general shape of a spoon. The color is generally white, and the nail is opaque. The concave portion of the nail is particularly fragile. When all the nails are not involved, the cause may be chronic eczema or a tumor of the nail bed. Systemic diseases associated with koilonychia are hypochromic anemias, chronic infections, malnutrition, pellagra, and Raynaud's disease (Fig. 9-4).

Racket nail is a flattened and expanded nail, usually the thumb. It has been considered a sign of secondary syphilis.

Changes in nail adhesion

Onycholysis is separation of the nail from the nail bed, originating at the free edge and progressing proximally. Although the condition may be congenital, it has also been associated with disorders of the thyroid—both hypothyroidism and hyperthyroidism—repeated trauma, peripheral arteriospasm (as in Raynaud's disease), hypochromic anemias, syphilis, eczema, and acrocyanosis (Fig. 9-5).

Onychomadesis is the separation of the nail starting at the roof of the nail and progressing to the free margin. This condition is the result of a lesion of the matrix and the hyponychium. The separation may be the result of peripheral neuritis, amyotrophy, hemiplegias, thrombosis, vascular disease, frostbite, exanthemas (scarlet fever, measles), or hypocalcemia.

Paronychia is an inflammation of the folds of tissue surrounding the nails leading to erythema, with inflammation, swelling, and induration of the nail fold accompanied by pain and tenderness. It is the most common complaint related to the nails. Drops of pus may be extruded from beneath the nail fold ulceration. The ulceration tends to involve surrounding tissues. The lesion generally involves the distal third of the nail, which may be broken or destroyed as necrosis progresses. This condition is common in diabetic persons. *Candida albicans,* staphylococci, and streptococci are most frequently involved. Third-stage syphilis and leprosy may lead to paronychia (Fig. 9-6).

Changes in the nail surface

Beau's lines (Beau's striations, transverse sulci) are striations approximately 1 mm deep and 0.1 to 0.5 mm wide running across the entire nail perpendicular to the longitudinal axis. Beau's lines appear on all fingers. The color is the same as the remainder of the nail. Beau's lines are thought to be caused by an arrest of nail growth at the matrix. If the retardation of growth is repeated, another line may result. Because the nail grows at a rate of approximately 0.1 mm per day and the eponychium is about 3 mm long, it is possible to calculate the point in time at which the hiatus in nail production occurred. Beau's lines have been associated with the acute phase of infectious diseases, malnutrition, and anemia (Fig. 9-7).

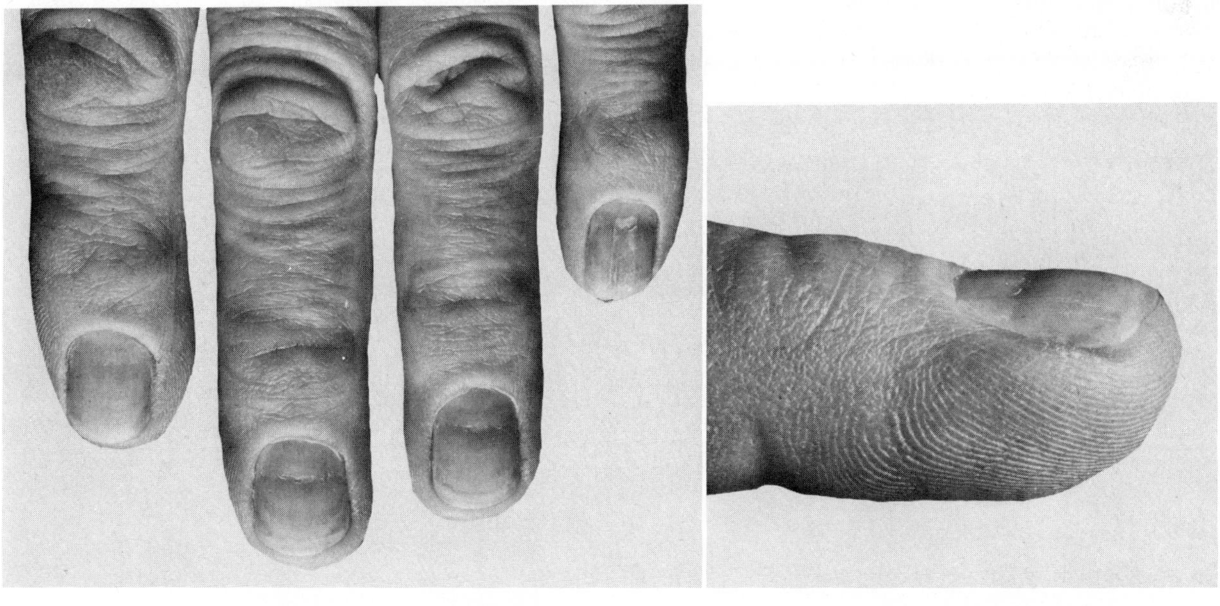

Fig. 9-7
A, Beau's lines. **B,** Beau's lines, side view. (From Samman, P.D.: The nails in disease, London, 1978, William Heinemann Medical Books, Ltd.)

Pitting deformities of the nail may vary from pinpoint to pinhead size and may be linear or irregular in distribution. These depressions have been observed in psoriasis, peripheral vascular disease, diabetes, and infectious diseases such as syphilis and tuberculosis (Fig. 9-8).

Mees' lines are crescent-shaped transverse lines similar in color to the lunula. They have been observed in arsenic poisoning.

Striated nails are characterized by longitudinal ridges running the length of the nail and are associated with increased fragility. Nail striations have been observed in malnutrition, anemia, defective peripheral circulation, chronic infections, and psoriasis. Nail striations are frequently observed in the elderly.

Changes in nail color

Leukonychia is characterized by white striations or 1- to 2-mm dots that progress to the free edge of the nail as growth proceeds. The white areas may result from trauma, infections, vascular disease, psoriasis, and arsenic poisoning.

Leukonychia totalis (white nails) is a condition in which the entire nail plate is white. Although the white nail may be congenital, this type of nail has been associated with hypocalcemia, severe hypochromic anemia, leprosy, hepatic cirrhosis, and arsenic poisoning. Paired narrow white bands parallel to the lunula have been associated with hypoalbuminemia. These white lines affect the nail bed rather than the nail plate.

Melanonychia is the presence of brown color in the nail plate resulting from a melanin redistribution in the melanophore cells. Normal nails in white persons are not pigmented, but the nails are pigmented in black persons from adolescence. An increase in pigment of the nails may be seen in Addison's disease and malaria.

Pigment band is a single black or brown streak in the nail of a white person. The development of such a line may be caused by junctional nevus in the nail matrix. Brown striations are common in black persons (Fig. 9-9).

Bluish nails are observed in cyanosis and venous stasis. Sulfhydric acid poisoning results in the formation of sulfhemoglobin, which creates a blue tinge as it

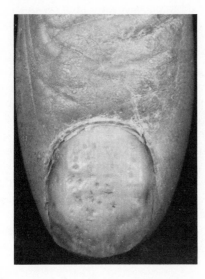

Fig. 9-8
Psoriasis—nail pitting. (From Samman, P.D.: The nails in disease, London, 1978, William Heinemann Medical Books, Ltd.)

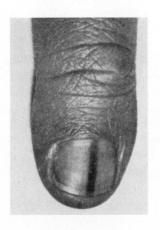

Fig. 9-9
Pigment band probably caused by a junctional nevus. (From Samman, P.D.: The nails in disease, London, 1978, William Heinemann Medical Books, Ltd.)

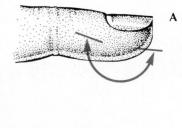
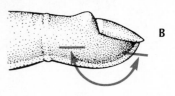
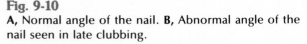

Fig. 9-10
A, Normal angle of the nail. **B,** Abnormal angle of the nail seen in late clubbing.

circulates in the capillary bed beneath the nail. Wilson's disease has been associated with a bluish tint of the lunula. *Pseudomonas aeruginosa* infection is associated with a bluish gray color of the entire nail.

Changes in nail thickness

Thickening or hypertrophy of the nail is generally caused by trauma. The nail of the small toe is often the only one affected; it takes on a clawlike shape. Thickening of the nails has been associated with psoriasis, fungal infection, defective vascular supply, and trauma. Thinning of the nail has been linked to defective peripheral circulation and nutritional anemias.

Brittleness of the nails is a common sign. Systemic diseases associated with brittle nails are nutritional anemias and impaired peripheral circulation. Prolonged exposure to water and alkaline substances has also been associated with brittle nails.

Clubbing of fingers

Clubbing of fingers (drumstick fingers) is associated with a decrease of oxygen supply in general. The resultant changes in the nail have been called *hippocratic* or *watch-glass* nails. The watch-glass nail is longer in the longitudinal axis than in the transverse axis, and the dorsal convexity is increased (Fig. 9-10). The nail is thickened, hard, shiny, and curved at the free end. The matrix atrophies. Early in the process the normal angle of the nail to the nail base (160 degrees) is lost. The nails are flatter and may be at a 180-degree angle to the nail base. In advanced cases the entire nail is pushed away from the base at an angle greater than 180 degrees and feels "spongy." (The student may simulate this spongy feel by grasping the distal phalanx on the lateral aspects of a finger at the level of the nail bed of one hand firmly between thumb and middle finger of the opposite hand. After a second or two the lunula will feel spongy when pressed down by the nail of the index finger of the examining hand.) The distal phalanx becomes enlarged as the condition progresses. Clubbing is associated with respiratory (emphysema, chronic obstructive lung disease, carcinoma of the lung) and cardiovascular diseases and cirrhosis (Fig. 9-11).

Sebaceous glands

The sebaceous glands, which are more numerous over the face and scalp areas, normally become more active during adolescence, resulting in increased oiliness of the skin. A sudden increase in the oil of the skin at other ages would not be normal and may be suggestive of an endocrine problem.

SKIN LESIONS: DESCRIPTION AND CLASSIFICATION

The initial examination of any skin lesion should be carried out at a distance of 3 feet or more to determine the general characteristics of the eruption. This first observation should provide the opportunity to determine the location, distribution, and configuration of the lesions. A closer examination is required next to determine the color, size, shape, texture, firmness, and morphological characteristics of the individual lesions.

It is not possible to discuss the particular manifestations of the many skin problems that the examiner may find in practice. This discussion is limited to a few examples that demonstrate some of the different characteristics of skin lesions that will assist the examiner in describing the problem when consulting a dermatologist or a textbook on dermatology.

The distribution of skin lesions is fairly simple to describe according to the location or body region affected and the symmetry or asymmetry of findings in comparable body parts. The examiner must keep in mind that there are characteristic patterns that provide the major clue in the diagnosis of a specific skin problem. Fig. 9-12 illustrates a few distribution patterns by specific problems.

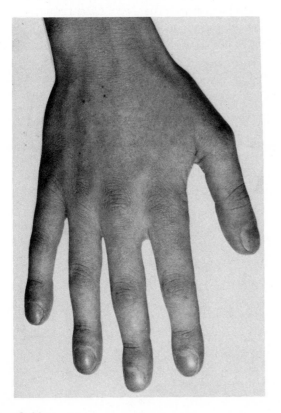

Fig. 9-11
Finger clubbing. (From Samman, P.D.: The nails in disease, London, 1978, William Heinemann Medical Books, Ltd.)

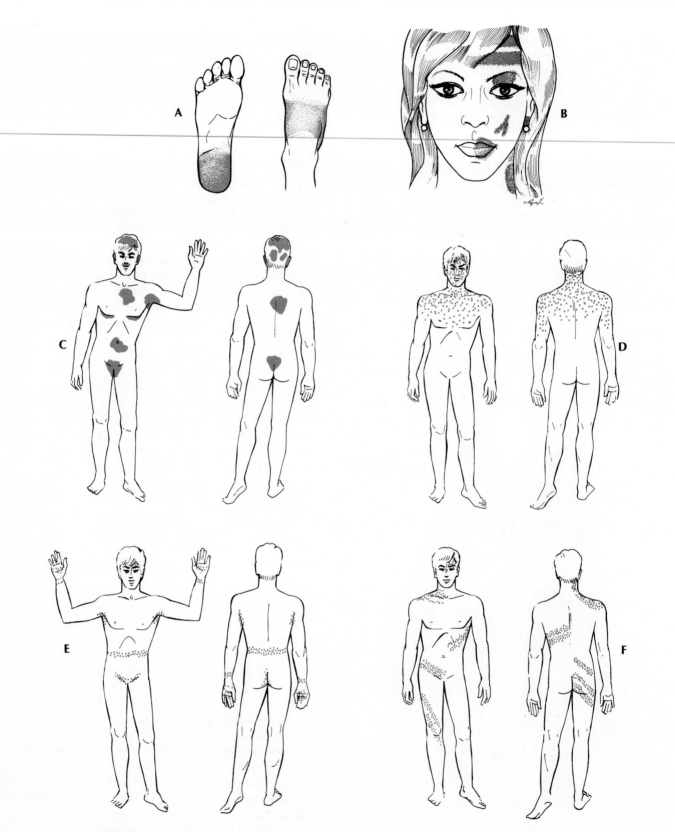

Fig. 9-12
Distribution of lesions in selected problems of the skin. **A,** Contact dermatitis (shoes). **B,** Contact dermatitis (cosmetics, perfumes, earrings). **C,** Seborrheic dermatitis. **D,** Acne. **E,** Scabies. **F,** Herpes zoster.

The configuration of skin lesions is equally important in defining the problem. Configuration refers to the arrangement or position of several lesions in relation to each other. For example, the skin lesions of tinea corporis, ringworm of the body, have an annular configuration that is circular. Some of the terms used to describe the configuration of skin lesions are as follows:

Grouped	Lesions clustered together
Herpetiform or zosteriform	Multiple groups of vesicles erupting unilaterally following the course of cutaneous nerves
Linear	Lesions arranged in a line
Annular	Lesions arranged in a circle, ring-shaped
Polycyclic	Multiple annular arrangements of lesions
Arciform	Lesions arranged in an arc, bow-shaped
Reticular	Lesions meshed in the form of a network
Confluent	Lesions become merged together; not discrete

Fig. 9-13 illustrates some of the different configurations that occur.

The color of the individual lesion should be described. There may be no discoloration, or many colors may be seen, as with ecchymosis when the initial dark-red and dark-blue colors are fading and a yellow color is seen. The lesions may be well defined with the color changes limited to the borders of the lesion and are referred to as "circumscribed," or the borders may be undefined with the color changes spread over a large area and described as "diffuse." Diascopy is used to observe for color changes of a lesion when pressure is applied. A transparent slide is pressed against the skin to express blood from the capillaries and superficial venules. Telangiectases will blanch, whereas petechial or purpuric lesions will not.

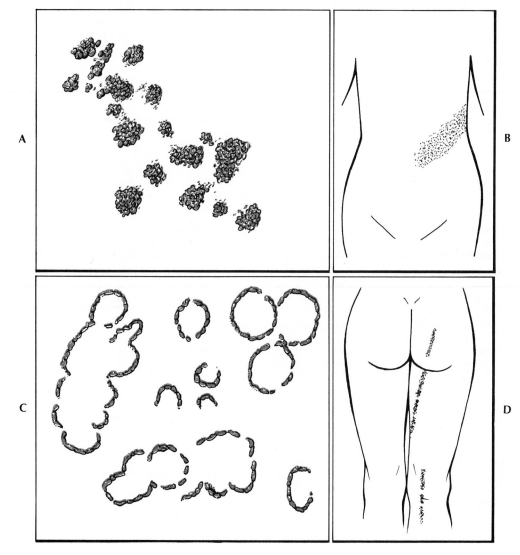

Fig. 9-13
Examples of different configurations of skin lesions. **A,** Grouped. **B,** Zosteriform. **C,** Annular (circular) and arciform (arc). **D,** Linear.

Table 9-6
Common raised lesions—cont'd

Condition	Lesion	Location
FROM INFESTATION		
Pediculosis corporis (body lice)	Wheal; central hemorrhagic spot; linear excoriations; later dry, scaly pigmentation	Trunk; can be generalized
Pediculosis pubis (pubic lice)	Papules; discrete; excoriated; gray-white dots at base of hair—nits; lice may be seen at base of hairs	Genital region; lower abdomen; chest; axillae; eyebrows; eyelashes
	Gray-blue macules	May be present on abdomen; thighs; axillae
Scabies	Vesicles; papules; pruritus	Skin folds

SUMMARY

I. General observation while client is standing, if possible, and with the examiner 3 feet or more away
   A. General skin color
   B. Hair distribution, texture, and quantity over body
   C. Sun-exposed areas (face, ears, back of neck, dorsum of hands and arms) compared with less-exposed areas
   D. Pigmented labile areas (dorsal flexor surfaces of hands and wrists, face around mouth, axillae, areolae, midline of abdomen, and genital area)
   E. Vascular flush areas (from cheek to cheek across bridge of nose, neck, upper chest, flexor surface of extremities, and genital area)
   F. Location and distribution of any rash, birthmarks, scratches, bruising, or swelling

II. Closer observation and palpation of skin while client is sitting or lying down
   A. Nails
      1. Color, contour, and thickness of nails and their adherence to the nail beds
      2. Temperature, color, shape, and tenderness of skin folds around nails
      3. Grooming
   B. Hair of scalp
      1. Quantity
      2. Color
      3. Texture
      4. Grooming
   C. Mucosa of nose and mouth
      1. Color
      2. Moisture
      3. Texture
   D. Each part of the body as examined
      1. Color
      2. Temperature
      3. Moisture
      4. Texture
      5. Turgor
   E. Abnormal changes or lesions of the skin
      1. Color
      2. Configuration and arrangement
      3. Morphological structure of individual lesions
      4. Size of individual abnormality, such as a lesion, birthmark, or bruise (to be measured)
      5. Moisture
      6. Number (count when possible)
      7. Depth and consistency
      8. Temperature
      9. Tenderness

BIBLIOGRAPHY

Binnick, S.A.: Skin diseases: diagnosis and management in clinical practice, Menlo Park, Calif., 1982, Addison-Wesley Publishing Co., Inc.

DeNicola, P., and Morsiani, M.: Nail diseases in internal medicine, Springfield, Ill., 1974, Charles C Thomas, Publishers.

Fitzpatrick, T.G., et al.: Dermatology in general medicine, ed. 2, New York, 1979, McGraw-Hill Book Co.

Lazarus, G.S., and Goldsmith, L.A.: Diagnosis of skin disease, Philadelphia, 1980, F.A. Davis Co.

Rook, A., and Wilkerson, D.S.: Textbook of dermatology, ed. 3, Oxford, Mass., 1979, Blackwell Scientific Publications, Inc.

Samman, P.D.: The nails in disease, London, 1978, William Heinemann Medical Books, Ltd.

Sauer, G.C.: Manual of skin diseases, ed. 4, Philadelphia, 1980, J.B. Lippincott Co.

Stewart, W.D., Danto, J.L., and Maddin, S.: Dermatology: diagnosis and treatment of cutaneous disorders, ed. 4, St. Louis, 1978, The C.V. Mosby Co.

CHAPTER 10

ASSESSMENT OF THE EARS, NOSE, AND THROAT

The examination of the ears, nose, and throat is an important part of every physical examination because it provides the opportunity to inspect directly or indirectly most parts of the upper respiratory system and the first division of the digestive system. The clinical examination of these body orifices can provide information about the client's general health, as well as information about significant local disease. The methods of examination are primarily inspection and palpation.

The client should be seated for the ear, nose, and throat examination with the examiner's head at approximately the same level as that of the client. The necessary equipment includes an otoscope with various sizes of speculums, tongue blades, 4- by 4-inch gauze sponges, rubber gloves or finger cots, and a tuning fork (512 cycles per second [cps]). A good light source such as a gooseneck lamp with a 100- to 150-watt bulb is helpful, but if not available, a penlight can be used. A dental mirror and a nasal speculum may also be helpful.

Discussion is focused on each of the three areas: the ears, the nose and paranasal sinuses, and the mouth and oropharynx. The portion of the chapter on each area includes a brief review of the anatomy and physiology, a description of the methods to be used in the examination, and some of the common findings of which the examiner should be aware when examining the particular area.

EARS
Anatomy and physiology

The ear is a sensory organ that functions both in hearing and in equilibrium. It has three parts: the external ear, the middle ear, and the inner ear. Fig. 10-1 illustrates the structures of the ear.

The external ear has two divisions, the flap called the auricle or pinna and the canal called the external auditory canal or meatus. Stretching across the proximal portion of the canal is the tympanic membrane, which separates the external ear from the middle ear. The auricle is composed of cartilage, closely adherent perichondrium, and skin. The main components of the auricle are the helix, anthelix, crus of helix, lobule, tragus, antitragus, and concha (Fig. 10-2). The mastoid process is not part of the external ear but is a bony prominence found posterior to the lower part of the auricle.

The external auditory canal, which is about 1 inch in length, has a skeleton of cartilage in its outer third and a skeleton of bone in its inner two thirds. It has a slight curve with the outer one third of the canal directed upward and toward the back of the head, whereas the inner two thirds is directed down and forward. The skin of the inner ear is very thin and sensitive.

The tympanic membrane, which covers the proximal end of the auditory canal, is made up of layers of skin, fibrous tissue, and mucous membrane (Fig. 10-3). The membrane is shiny, translucent, and a pearl gray color. The position of the ear drum is oblique with respect to the ear canal. The anteroinferior quadrant is most distant from the examiner, which accounts for the cone of light or the light reflex. The membrane is slightly concave and is pulled inward at its center by one of the ossicles, the malleus, of the middle ear. The short process of the malleus protrudes into the eardrum superiorly, and the handle of the malleus extends downward from the short process to the umbo, the point of maximum concavity. Most of the membrane is taut and is known as the pars tensa. A small part superiorly is less taut and is known as the pars flaccida. The dense fibrose ring surrounding the tympanic mem-

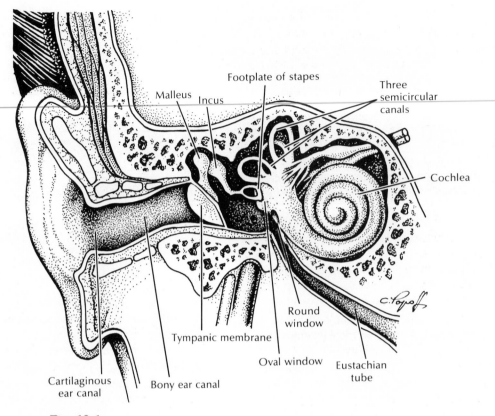

Fig. 10-1
External auditory canal, middle ear, and inner ear.

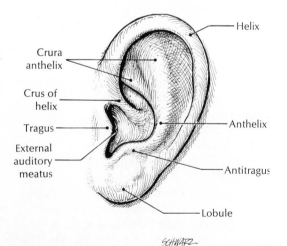

Fig. 10-2
Structures of the external ear.

brane, with the exception of the anterior and posterior malleolar folds superiorly, is the anulus.

The middle ear is a small, air-filled cavity located in the temporal bone. It contains three small bones called the auditory ossicles: the malleus, the incus, and the stapes. The middle ear cavity contains several openings. One is from the external auditory meatus and is covered by the tympanic membrane. There are two openings into the inner ear, the oval window into which the stapes fits and the round window covered by a membrane. Another opening connects the middle ear with the eustachian tube. The middle ear performs three functions: (1) it transmits sound vibrations across the ossicle chain to the inner ear's oval window, (2) it protects the auditory apparatus from intense vibrations, and (3) it equalizes the air pressure on both sides of the dividing tympanic membrane to prevent the tympanic membrane from being ruptured.

The inner ear is made up of two parts, the bony labyrinth and, inside this structure, a membranous labyrinth. The bony labyrinth consists of three parts: the vestibule, the semicircular canals, and the cochlea. The vestibule and the semicircular canals comprise the organs of equilibrium. The cochlea comprises the

Plate 1

Some common dermatoses and cutaneous manifestations of systemic disorders.

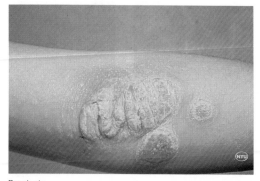

Psoriasis

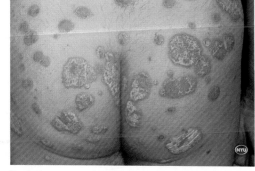

Psoriasis

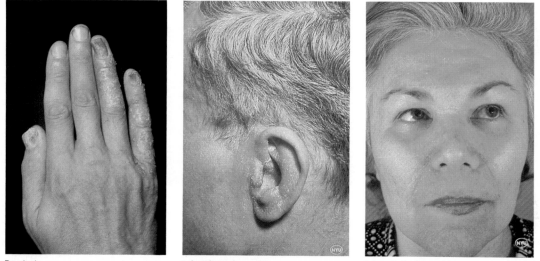

Psoriasis

Seborrheic dermatitis

Seborrheic dermatitis

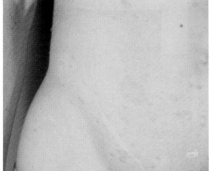

Pityriasis rosea

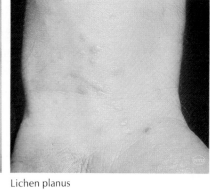

Lichen planus

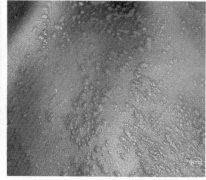

Lichen planus

Continued.

Plate 3
Nose.

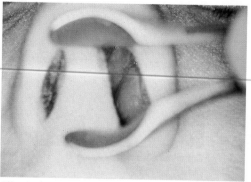

Allergic rhinitis

Plate 4
Mouth.

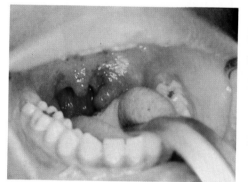

Acute viral pharyngitis

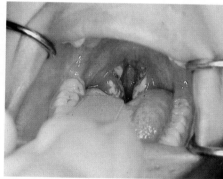

Tonsillitis, pharyngitis

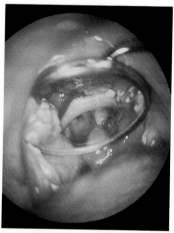

Yeast infection, lingual tonsil, hypopharynx

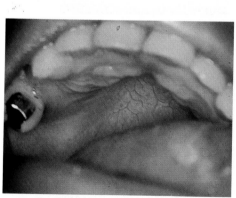

Leukoplakia

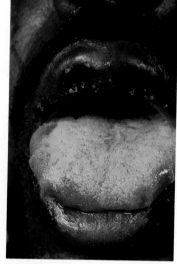

Acute bacterial stomatitis

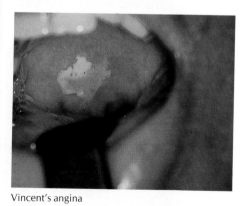

Vincent's angina

Continued.

Plate 4, cont'd
Mouth.

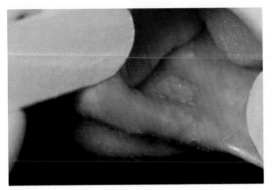

Herpes zoster

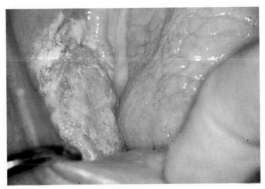

Squamous cell carcinoma

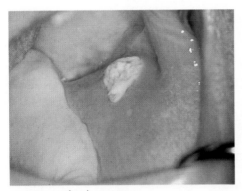

Carcinoma of oral mucosa

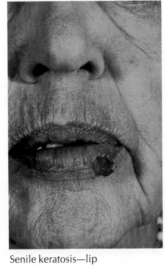

Senile keratosis—lip

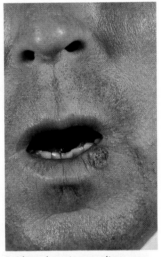

Epidermal carcinoma—lip

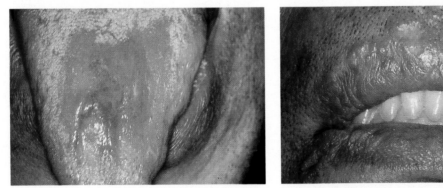

Drug reaction—tongue

Drug reaction—lip

Plate 4. Courtesy Dr. Edward L. Applebaum, Head, Department of Otolaryngology, University of Illinois Medical Center, Chicago, Illinois.

Plate 5

Eyes.

A

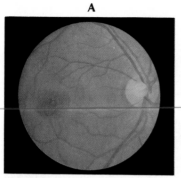

Normal fundus in a young person (right eye). Note the retinal background, optic disc, retinal arterioles and veins, and macular area.

B

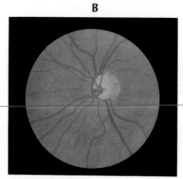

Glaucomatous cupping of the optic disc (left eye). The disc is pale, atrophic. Note the course of vessels at the disc.

C

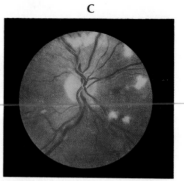

Hypertensive retinopathy with cotton wool exudates and hemorrhage (right eye).

D

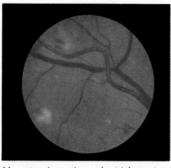

Hypertensive retinopathy (right eye). Note arteriovenous crossing change, hemorrhages, and exudates.

E

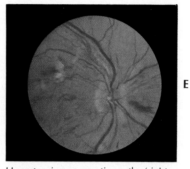

Hypertensive neuroretinopathy (right eye). Note blurred optic disc margins of papilledema.

F

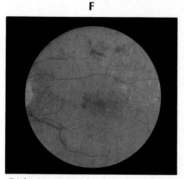

Diabetic retinopathy (left eye). Note hemorrhages and exudates.

G

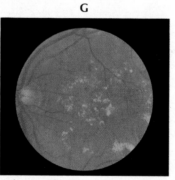

Left eye in old diabetic. Note numerous hard exudates and microaneurysms.

H

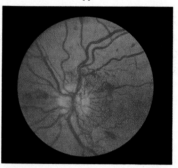

Proliferative diabetic retinopathy (left eye). Note neovascularization near optic disc.

I

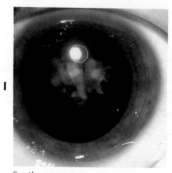

Senile cataract.

J

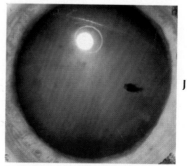

Snowflake cataract of diabetes.

Plate 5. **A** to **H** from Larsen, H.W.: The ocular fundus, Copenhagen, 1976, Munksgaard International Publishers, Ltd. **I** and **J** from Donaldson, D.D.: Atlas of diseases of the eye. The crystalline lens, vol. V, St. Louis, 1976, The C.V. Mosby Co.

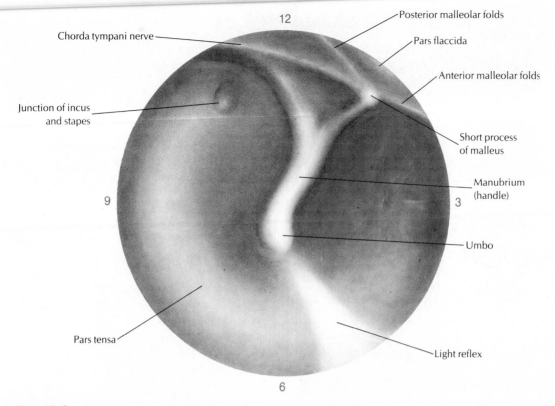

12

Chorda tympani nerve

Posterior malleolar folds

Pars flaccida

Anterior malleolar folds

Junction of incus
and stapes

Short process
of malleus

Manubrium
(handle)

9

3

Umbo

Pars tensa

Light reflex

6

Fig. 10-3
Usual landmarks of right tympanic membrane with "clock" superimposed. (From Whaley,
L.F., and Wong, D.L.: Nursing care of infants and children, ed. 2, St. Louis, 1983, The C.V.
Mosby Co.)

organ of hearing. The cochlea is a coiled structure that contains the organ of Corti, which transmits stimuli to the cochlear branch of the auditory nerve (cranial nerve [CN] VIII).

Hearing occurs when sound waves enter the external auditory canal and strike the tympanic membrane, causing it to vibrate at the same rate as the sound waves striking it. The auricle does not direct or amplify sound and has little apparent usefulness. The vibrations are transmitted through the auditory ossicles of the middle ear to the oval window. From the oval window the vibrations travel via the fluid of the cochlea, winding up at the round window, where they are dissipated. The vibrations of the membrane cause the delicate hair cells of the organ of Corti to beat against the membrane of Corti, acting as a stimuli setting up impulses in the sensory endings of the cochlear branch of the auditory nerve (CN VIII).

Hearing loss

There are several types of hearing loss. However, almost every form may be classified under one of three headings: conductive hearing loss, sensorineural or perceptive hearing loss, or mixed hearing loss.

Conductive hearing loss occurs when there are external or middle ear disorders such as impacted cerumen, perforation of the tympanic membrane, serum or pus in the middle ear, or a fusion of the ossicles. The vibrations are not adequately transmitted to the inner ear through the ear canal, tympanic membrane, middle ear, and ossicular chain; and a partial loss of hearing occurs.

Sensorineural, or perceptive, hearing loss occurs when there is a disorder in the inner ear, the auditory nerve, or the brain. Vibrations are transmitted to the inner ear, but an impairment of the cochlea or auditory nerve attenuates the nervous impulses from the cochlea to the brain.

Mixed hearing loss is a combination of conductive and sensorineural loss in the same ear.

Examination

The examination of the external ear begins with an inspection of both auricles to determine their position, size, and symmetry. Then the lateral and medial surfaces of each auricle and the surrounding tissues are inspected to determine the skin color and the presence of deformities, lesions, or nodules. The auricles and mastoid areas are palpated for evidence of swelling, tenderness, or nodules.

Manipulation of the auricle can also be helpful. Ordinarily there is no discomfort if the client has an otitis media. If pressure on the tragus or gently pulling on the auricle causes pain, the client has an external otitis. Although fairly simple, this part of the examination is frequently neglected.

Examination of the external auditory canal and tympanic membrane requires additional lighting. It is suggested that the examiner become acquainted with the use and maintenance of the electric otoscope. For the otoscope to be effective, the batteries should be changed frequently to ensure optimum efficiency. The focus of light should be directed out of the end of the speculum. Some speculum carriers are movable and can be out of alignment with the bulb carrier. Some older models have a bulb carrier that can be bent, causing the light to be deflected to one side of the speculum.

Before insertion of the speculum in the ear, the opening of the auditory canal should be carefully inspected for redness, swelling, narrowing of canal, a foreign body, or discharge. Any discharge should be described in terms of appearance and odor. A putrid odor is usually indicative of mastoid disease with bone destruction. After this inspection, the speculum can be inserted. The following points should, however, be remembered:

1. Use the largest speculum that can be inserted in the ear without pain.
2. The client's head should be tipped toward the opposite shoulder for easy examination of the canal and tympanic membrane.
3. In adults the ear canal may be straightened by pulling the auricle upward and backward; in young children and infants it may be straightened by pulling the auricle downward (Fig. 10-4).
4. The inner two thirds of the external meatus, which has a bony skeleton, is sensitive to pressure. Insert the speculum gently and not too far to avoid causing pain.
5. The angle at which the speculum is inserted into the meatus must be varied, or only a limited area of the tympanic membrane will be seen.

The auditory canal should be inspected for cerumen, redness, or swelling. The appearance of the normal canal varies in diameter, shape, and growth of hairs. Hair growth is limited to the outer third of the canal, but the hairs may be numerous.

Another aspect of the examination of the auditory canal is the evaluation of cerumen, which is produced by the sebaceous glands and the apocrine sweat glands in the canal. There are apparently racial variations in color, and black or brown cerumen will be noted in the client with darker skin coloring. There is also some difference in the color of fresh cerumen as compared to older, drier cerumen; the former is a lighter, yellow or even pink color, and the latter is a darker, yellowish brown color. A small amount of cerumen will not interfere with the examination; the examiner can look past it and visualize the tympanic membrane. However, if the wax is excessive, it may be necessary to remove it.

Two of the methods that can be used for the removal of wax are curettement and irrigation. *Curettement* is appropriate if the wax is soft or there is a question of perforation of the tympanic membrane. However, it should not be done except by a skilled clinician. The closeness of the blood vessels and nerves to the surface make it easy to cause bleeding and pain. There is also a risk of perforating the tympanic membrane if the client moves or the curette is used with too much vigor. *Irrigation* may be used when the wax is dry and hard but should not be carried out if there is a possibility that the membrane is perforated. Lukewarm water is used for the irrigation, which is done by repeatedly injecting the water from a syringe toward the posterosuperior canal wall. This procedure will cause the client to feel dizzy.

The examination of the tympanic membrane (see Fig. 10-3) requires a careful assessment of the color of the membrane and the identification of landmarks. The membrane is usually a translucent pearl gray color; in disease the color may be yellow, white, or red. Some membranes have white flecks or dense white plaques that are the result of healed inflammatory disease. The landmarks are identified, beginning with the light reflex, which is a triangular cone of reflected light seen in the anteroinferior quadrant of the membrane. A diffuse or spotty light is not normal. At the top point of the light reflex toward the center of the membrane is the umbo, the inferior point of the handle of the malleus. Anterior and superior to the umbo is the long process of the malleus, which appears as a whitish line extending from the umbo to the juncture of the malleolar folds, where the small white projection of the short process of the malleus can be seen. The malleolar folds and the pars flaccida, the relaxed portion of the membrane, are superior and lateral to the short process. Finally, an attempt should be made to follow the anulus around the periphery of the pars tensa. It is in the areas close to the anulus that perforations are frequently noted.

Fluid in the middle ear may sometimes be identified by air bubbles or a fluid level seen through the tympanic membrane.

Bulging of the tympanic membrane may occur when pus forms in the middle ear. The pressure

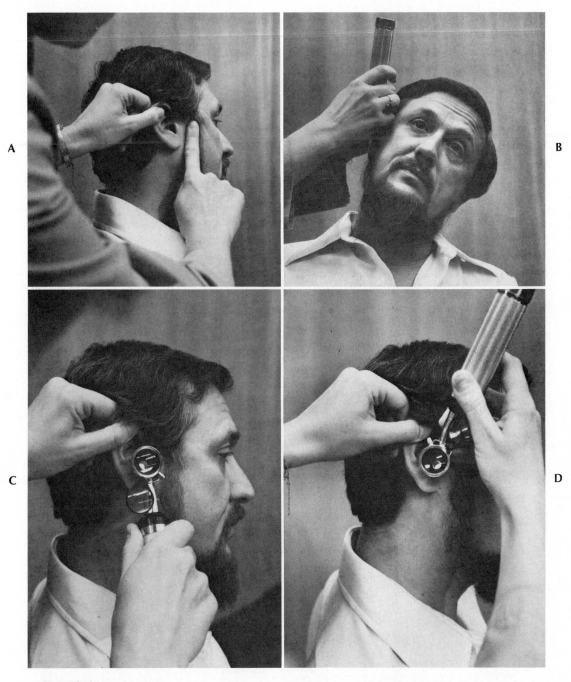

Fig. 10-4
Examination of the ear with the otoscope. **A,** Inspection of the meatus. **B,** Client's head is tipped toward the opposite shoulder. **C** and **D,** Two ways of holding the otoscope.

increases, and the membrane may bulge outward in one part, or the entire membrane may bulge, resulting in obliteration of some or all of the landmarks. The light reflex is usually lost, and the membrane appears dull.

Retraction of the tympanic membrane occurs when pressure is reduced resulting from obstruction of the eustachian tube, usually associated with an upper respiratory system infection. The retraction of the membrane causes the landmarks to be accentuated. The light reflex may appear less prominent.

Normal tympanic membranes vary to some extent in size, shape, and color. It is only by examining many normal, healthy membranes that the ability to recognize the abnormal membrane is acquired.

Testing of auditory function

Clinical testing of auditory function is a process that starts early in the physical examination of the client. Understanding the spoken word is the principal use of hearing, and it may become apparent during the interview that there is an impairment or loss of auditory function. The actual testing of auditory function should be delayed until the end of the examination, after obvious problems related to hearing may have been identified. A precise measurement of hearing requires the use of the audiometer, but a good estimate of hearing can be made during the physical examination with the use of the tests discussed in this section.

Simple assessment of auditory acuity requires that only one ear be tested at a time. Therefore, it is necessary to mask the hearing in the ear not being tested. The examiner may occlude one of the client's ears by placing a finger against the opening of the auditory canal and moving the finger rapidly but gently.

Voice tests are frequently used in estimating the client's hearing. The testing is begun with a very low whisper; the lips of the examiner should be 1 or 2 feet away from the unoccluded ear. The examiner exhales and softly whispers numbers that the client is to repeat. If necessary, the intensity of the voice is increased to a medium whisper, and then to a loud whisper; then to a soft, then medium, then loud voice. To prevent lipreading during the voice tests, the examiner may stand behind the client. If it is more convenient to be in front of the client, the client should be asked to close his eyes.

The watch tick is useful in testing but should not be used exclusively, because it provides only a high-frequency sound. The ticking watch is moved away from the ear until the client can no longer hear the sound.

Tuning fork tests are useful in determining whether the client has a conductive or a perceptive hearing loss. A fork with frequencies of 500 to 1,000 cps is used

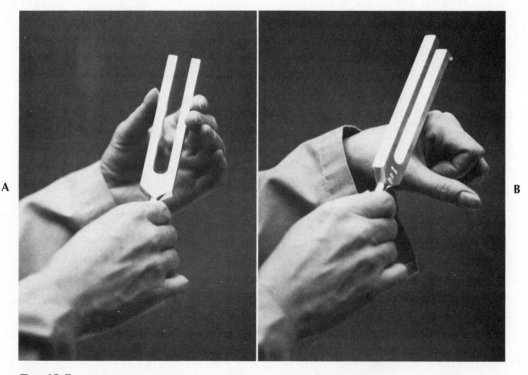

Fig. 10-5
Activating the tuning fork. **A,** Stroking the fork. **B,** Tapping the fork on the knuckle.

Table 10-1

Hearing tests using tuning forks

Hearing	Weber (bone conduction)	Rinne (air and bone conduction)
Normal	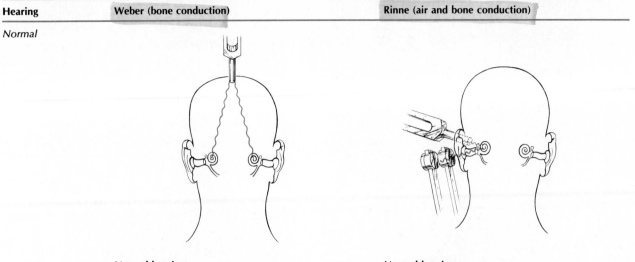	

Normal hearing

Sound does not lateralize to either side; heard equally well in both ears

Normal hearing

"Positive Rinne." Sound is heard twice as long by air conduction as by bone conduction

---

Conduction loss (problem of external or middle ear)

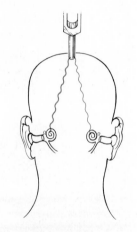

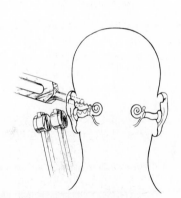

Conductive deafness in right ear

Sound lateralizes to defective ear as few extraneous sounds are carried through external or middle ear

Conductive deafness in right ear

"Negative Rinne." Sound heard longer by bone conduction than by air conduction

---

Sensorineural loss (perceptive problem of inner ear or nerve)

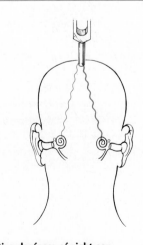

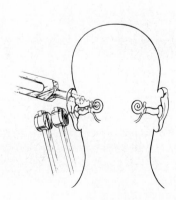

Perceptive deafness of right ear

Sound lateralizes to the better ear

Perceptive deafness of right ear

"Positive Rinne." Sound is heard longer by air conduction than by bone conduction

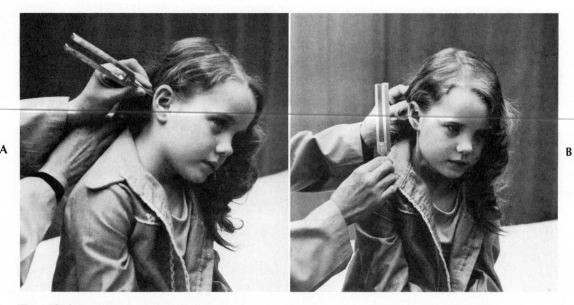

Fig. 10-6
Rinne test. **A,** Bone conduction. **B,** Air conduction.

because it can provide an estimate of hearing loss in the speech frequencies of roughly 500 to 2,000 cps. The tuning fork is held by the base without the fingers touching either of the two prongs. The sound vibrations are softened or stopped entirely when the prongs of the fork are touched or held. The fork is activated by gently stroking or tapping on the knuckles of the opposite hand (Fig. 10-5). It should be made to ring softly, not harshly.

The terms *bone conduction* and *air conduction* need to be clearly understood in the discussion of tuning fork tests. *Air conduction* implies the transmission of sound through the ear canal, tympanic membrane, and ossicular chain to the cochlea and auditory nerve. *Bone conduction* implies that sound is transmitted through the bones of the skull to the cochlea and auditory nerve. The client with normal auditory function will hear sound twice as long by air conduction, when the tuning fork is held opposite the external meatus, as he will by bone conduction, when the base of the tuning fork is placed on the mastoid bone.

The Rinne test makes use of air conduction and bone conduction. The tuning fork is used to compare the conduction of sound through the mastoid bone and the conduction of sound through the auditory meatus (Table 10-1). There are two different methods of performing the Rinne test, but the principle remains the same: the sound will be heard twice as long by air conduction as by bone conduction when there is no conductive hearing loss (Fig. 10-6). The most common method is to place the activated tuning fork against the

mastoid bone until the client can no longer hear the sound and then move the fork to a distance of ½ to 1 inch from the auditory meatus. The client with no conductive hearing loss will continue to hear the sound by air conduction.

The second method merely reverses the order. The activated tuning fork is held 1 inch from the auditory meatus and when the client can no longer hear the sound, the base of the fork is placed immediately on the mastoid bone. If the client cannot hear the sound when the fork is placed on the mastoid bone, his Rinne test is considered positive and he does not have a conductive hearing loss. If the opposite is true and the client can hear the sound better by bone conduction, his Rinne test is negative and there is a conductive hearing loss. A positive Rinne with *an overall reduction in the time* where the sound is heard and normal ratio of air conduction to bone conduction is maintained results when there is a sensorineural hearing loss. This demonstrates that the client does not hear well by either air conduction or bone conduction.

The *Weber test,* which makes use of bone conduction, is carried out by placing the base of the vibrating tuning fork on the vertex of the skull, on the forehead, or on the front teeth and asking the client if he hears the sound better in one ear or in the other (Fig. 10-7). In conductive deafness, the sound is referred to the deafer ear. This happens because the cochlea on that side will be undisturbed by extraneous sounds in the environment; these sounds are not transmitted, because of a problem or defect in the ear canal or

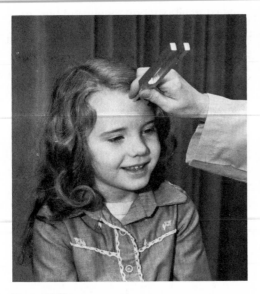

Fig. 10-7
Weber test.

middle ear. In perceptive deafness, the sound is referred to the better ear because the cochlea or auditory nerve is functioning more effectively.

Another test is the Schwabach test, which allows the examiner to compare the client's bone conduction with his own, presuming that the examiner has normal bone conduction. The tuning fork is moved back and forth and placed on the client's mastoid bone and then on the examiner's. Both should be able to hear the sound for an equal length of time if the client's hearing is normal. If the client has a conductive hearing loss, he will hear the sound longer. If the client has a sensorineural hearing loss, he will hear the sound for a shorter time.

The caloric tests that measure labyrinthine function of the inner ear are discussed in Chapter 24 on neurological assessment.

NOSE AND PARANASAL SINUSES
Anatomy and physiology

The nose is the sensory organ for smell. It also warms, moistens, and filters the air inspired into the respiratory system.

The functions of the paranasal sinuses are not definitely known, but they may perform the same functions as the nose—that of warming, moistening, and filtering air. They also aid in voice resonance.

The nose is divided into the external nose and the internal nose or nasal cavity (Fig. 10-8). The upper third of the nose is bone; the remainder of the nose is cartilage. The nasal cavity is divided by the septum into two narrow cavities. The cavities have two openings: the anterior cavity is the vestibule where the naris is located and is thickly lined with small hairs; the posterior opening, or choana, leads to the throat. The nasal septum forms the medial walls. The lateral walls are divided into the inferior, middle, and superior turbinate bones, which protrude into the nasal cavity. The turbinates are covered by a highly vascular mucous membrane. Below each turbinate is a meatus named according to the turbinate above it. The nasolacrimal duct drains into the inferior meatus, and most of the paranasal sinuses drain into the middle meatus. There is a plexus of blood vessels in the mucosa of the anterior nasal septum, which is a common site for epistaxis.

The receptors for smell are located in the olfactory area in the roof of the nasal cavity and upper third of the septum. The receptor cells, grouped as filaments, pass through openings of the cribriform plate, become the olfactory nerve (CN I), and transmit neural impulses for smell to the temporal lobe of the brain.

The paranasal sinuses are air-filled, paired extensions of the nasal cavities within the bones of the skull. They are the frontal, the maxillary, the ethmoidal, and the sphenoidal sinuses (Fig. 10-9). Their openings into the nasal cavity are narrow and easily obstructed. The frontal sinuses are located in the anterior part of the frontal bone. The maxillary sinuses, the largest of the paranasal sinuses, are located in the body of the maxilla. The ethmoidal sinuses are small and occupy the ethmoidal labyrinth between the orbit of the eye and the upper part of the cavity of the nose. The sphenoidal sinuses are found in the body of the sphenoid.

Examination

The external portion of the nose is inspected for any deviations in shape, size, or color; the nares are inspected for flaring or discharge (Fig. 10-10). The ridge and soft tissues of the nose are palpated for displacement of the bone and cartilage and for tenderness or masses.

Examination of the nasal function includes determination of the ability to smell and the patency of the nasal cavities. To determine if the nasal cavities are patent, the client is asked to close his mouth, exert pressure on one naris with a finger, and breathe through the opposite naris. The procedure is repeated to determine the potency of the opposite naris. To determine the adequacy of function of the olfactory nerve (CN I), the client is asked to close his eyes and occlude one naris again. The examiner places an aromatic substance, such as coffee or alcohol, close to the client's nose and asks the client to identify the odor. Each side is tested separately.

Color vision testing

Suspected defects in color vision, or screening for certain industrial or vehicle operation jobs, should include testing with color plates. These plates have numbers outlined in one color surrounded by confusion colors that are similar in color or intensity. The individual with a color vision deficiency is unable to see the number.

Ocular structures

The ocular structures to be examined include the eyelashes and eyelids, the conjunctiva, the cornea, the anterior chamber, the lacrimal apparatus, the sclera, the iris, the pupil, the lens, the vitreous body, and the retina.

Examination of outermost structures

Eyelids and eyelashes. The functions of the lids are to protect and lubricate the anterior portions of the globe. They are inspected for the ability to close completely, for position and color, and for any lesions, infection, or edema. When the lids do not close properly, drying of the cornea may result in serious damage.

The examiner observes for equality in the height of the palpebral fissures. The margins of the upper lids normally fall between the superior pupil margin and the superior limbus.

Raised yellow plaques, xanthelasma, may appear on the lids near the inner canthi; these grow slowly and may disappear spontaneously.

It is at this time that the position of the globe, whether it is normal, prominent, or sunken, can be most easily observed.

The distribution, condition, and position of the eyelashes are noted. The eyelashes should be evenly distributed and should curve outward.

Conjunctiva. The bulbar and palpebral portions of the conjunctiva are examined by separating the lids widely and having the client look up, down, and to each side. When separating the lids, the examiner should exert no pressure against the eyeball; rather, the examiner should hold the lids against the ridges of the bony orbit surrounding the eye (Fig. 11-11). The client is then instructed to direct his gaze upward and to each side. Many small blood vessels are normally visible through the clear conjunctiva. The white sclera is, of course, visible through the bulbar portion.

Although eversion of the upper lid is not a necessary part of the normal or screening examination, the beginning examiner should learn a careful technique for performing lid eversion when it is indicated. The entire procedure should be explained to the client before it is begun, and reassurance should be given during the process. In the absence of gentleness, carefulness, and reassurance, the client is very likely to become tense when the sensitive eye structures are manipulated, thereby making the examination much more difficult for both himself and the examiner.

Eversion of the upper eyelid is performed as follows (Fig. 11-12):

1. Ask the client to look down but to keep his eyes slightly open. This relaxes the levator muscle, whereas closing the eyes contracts the orbicularis muscle, preventing lid eversion.
2. Gently grasp the upper eyelashes and pull gently downward. Do not pull the lashes outward or upward; this, too, causes muscle contraction.
3. Place a cotton-tipped applicator about 1 cm above the lid margin on the upper tarsal border and push gently downward with the applicator while still holding the lashes. This everts the lid.
4. Hold the lashes of the everted lid against the upper ridge of the bony orbit, just beneath the eyebrow, never pushing against the eyeball.
5. Examine the lid for swelling, infection, a foreign object, and so on.
6. To return the lid to its normal position, move the lashes slightly forward and ask the client to look up and then to blink. The lid returns easily to a normal position.

Sclera. The sclera is easily observed during assessment of the conjunctiva. It is normally white, though some pigmented deposits are within the range of normal.

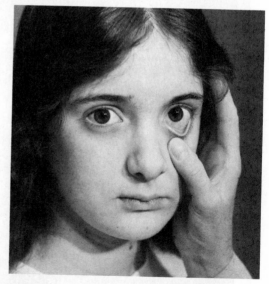

Fig. 11-11
The examiner inspects the conjunctiva by moving the lower lid downward over the bony orbit.

Cornea. The cornea is best observed by directing the light of a penlight at it obliquely from several positions. The cornea should be transparent, smooth, shiny, and bright. There should be no irregularities in the surface, and the features of the iris should be fully visible through the cornea. In older persons the appearance of arcus senilis is normal. Arcus senilis is a white ring located around the periphery of the cornea; it is composed of lipid deposits.

Testing of the corneal reflex may be reserved for later in the eye examination, after the observation of all external structures is complete, but is discussed here as part of the complete assessment of the cornea. Corneal sensitivity is tested by bringing a wisp of cotton from the lateral side of the eye and brushing it lightly across the corneal surface (Fig. 11-13). The normal response is lid closure of both eyes when either eye is brushed. A different wisp of cotton should be used for each eye.

Anterior chamber. The anterior chamber is easily observed in conjunction with the cornea. The technique of oblique illumination is also useful in assessing the anterior chamber. This, too, is a transparent structure. Any visible material in it is abnormal. The depth of the chamber should be noted by looking at the eye from the side instead of from directly in front. The depth is the distance between the cornea and the iris. From a side view, the iris should appear quite flat and should not be bulging forward (see Fig. 11-25, A).

Lacrimal apparatus. Of the various components of the lacrimal apparatus, including the lacrimal gland, the puncta, the lacrimal sac, and the nasolacrimal duct, only the puncta can normally be observed. These are located on the upper and lower nasal margins of the lids.

Blockage of the nasolacrimal duct can be checked by pressing against the lacrimal sac with the index finger or cotton-tipped applicator inside the lower inner orbital rim, not against the side of the nose (Fig. 11-14). In the presence of blockage, this will cause regurgitation of material through the puncta.

Iris. The iris should be observed for shape and coloration.

Pupils. Examination of the pupils involves several observations, including assessment of their size, shape, reaction to light, and accommodation.

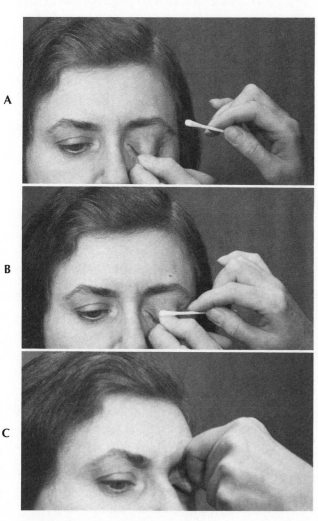

Fig. 11-12
Eversion of the upper eyelid. The examiner grasps the upper lid lashes, gently pulling downward and outward (**A**), then places the cotton-tipped applicator near the lower lid margin (**B**), and gently pulls the lashes upward over the applicator (**C**).

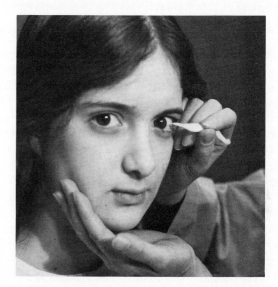

Fig. 11-13
Testing for corneal sensitivity, the examiner brings in a wisp of cotton from the side and lightly brushes it over the cornea.

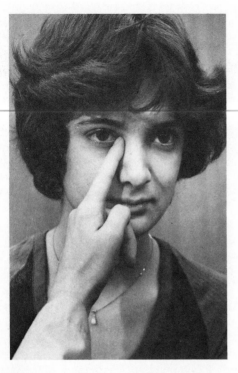

Fig. 11-14
To examine the lacrimal sac, the examiner presses with the index finger against the client's lower inner orbital rim, *not* against the nose.

The pupils are normally round in shape and equal in size. The pupillary response to light consists of both a direct and consensual reaction. The beam of a penlight is brought in from the side and directed on one eye at a time. The eye toward which the light is directed is observed for the direct response of constriction. Simultaneously, the other eye is observed for a consensual response of constriction. Each eye is observed for both the direct and consensual response. Normally, both responses are present; however, the rapidity with which the pupils respond does vary. A room that can be darkened to facilitate dilatation is helpful in assessing constriction in response to light; a sunny, well-lighted room can make the assessment of constriction responses very difficult.

The test for pupillary accommodation is the examination for change in pupillary size as the gaze is switched from a distant to a near object. It is performed by asking the client to stare at an object across the room. Visualization of a distant object normally causes pupillary dilatation. The client is then asked to fix his gaze on the examiner's index finger, which is placed 5 to 6 inches from the client's nose. The normal response is pupillary constriction and convergence of the eyes. The rapidity of the response in individuals varies; the response is slower in older persons.

The notation *PERRLA* stands for *pupils equal, round, react to light, and accommodate.*

Ophthalmoscopic examination

Examination of other ocular structures includes observation of the lens, the vitreous body, and the retinal structures and is performed with an ophthalmoscope. It is helpful to darken the room while performing the ophthalmoscopic examination, since this causes the pupils to dilate and thus facilitates the examination. If darkening the room does not adequately dilate the client's pupils, 10% phenylephrine hydrochloride, 0.5% Mydriacyl, or 1% Cyclogyl drops may be instilled in the client's eyes. Before using dilating drops, however, it is absolutely essential to rule out any suspicion of glaucoma. If the client wears corrective lenses, the examination may be done either with or without them. It is generally easier to perform the examination without the client's glasses on unless he has a high degree of astigmatism. Contact lenses may be left in place on the cornea. The examiner may choose to perform the retinal examination wearing or not wearing corrective lenses. Both ways should be tried to determine which is more satisfactory to the examiner.

Use of the ophthalmoscope (see also Chapter 1). The head of the ophthalmoscope is equipped with a series of lenses that are changed by moving the round, white wheel. The 0 lens is clear glass; the red, or negative, numbers focus farther away; and the black, or positive, numbers focus closer to the ophthalmoscope. Several apertures and filters for the light are built into most ophthalmoscopes; however, the round aperture with white light is best for most examinations. The examiner should read the manual accompanying the ophthalmoscope for information on other apertures and filters. The light should be turned to maximum brightness unless the client cannot tolerate it.

The client's cooperation is essential to the performance of this examination. The client is asked to stare directly ahead at some object across the room, such as the light switch or the corner of a picture. This assists in two ways: staring at a distant point encourages dilatation of the pupils, and staring at one fixed point helps to prevent the eyes from rotating and moving about so much that it is impossible for the examiner to focus on any of the retinal structures.

The client is told that he may blink from time to time during the examination. If the blinking becomes so frequent that it is difficult to visualize the retinal structures, the examiner may elevate the upper lid and hold it against the upper orbital rim.

The examiner holds the ophthalmoscope in the right hand and to the right eye to examine the client's right eye, and in the left hand and to the left eye to examine

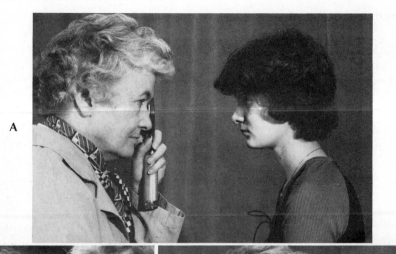

Fig. 11-15
A, The examiner uses the ophthalmoscope to inspect the lens and vitreous body from a distance of about 12 inches. The examiner uses the left eye and left hand to examine the client's left eye. **B,** The light from the ophthalmoscope is flashed on the eye through the pupil. **C,** Moving in closer to the client's eye, the examiner studies the retinal structures.

the client's left eye. The examiner initially sets the ophthalmoscope lens at 0, holds the viewing aperture directly in front of the eye with the top of the ophthalmoscope against the forehead, and begins about 12 inches away from the client's eye (Fig. 11-15, *A*). The index finger of the hand holding the ophthalmoscope rests on the lens wheel to permit focusing during the examination. The bright circle of light is flashed on the eye through the pupil (Fig. 11-15, *B*); a red glow, the red reflex, is visible through the pupil of the normal eye. While continuing to focus on the red reflex, the examiner moves close to the eye being examined (Fig. 11-15, *C*). If the examiner loses sight of the red reflex, it is usually because the light is no longer directed through the pupil and is resting instead on the iris or

sclera. If this occurs, it is easiest to relocate the red reflex by backing away several inches and redirecting the beam of light. As the examiner moves close to the eye, the lenses are rotated to the positive numbers (+15 to +20), which focus on the near objects. At this setting the anterior chamber and lens are examined for transparency; there should be no clouding or opacities.

Gradually rotating the lens back toward 0, the examiner also observes the vitreous body for transparency. At this setting the examiner begins to look for some retinal structure, such as a vessel or the disc. Once some structure is located, the lens wheel is rotated until it is brought into focus. In a myopic or nearsighted person, whose eyeball is more elongated than normal, the more negative lenses will be needed to focus farther back. In a farsighted client the lens wheel is rotated toward the positive numbers. Focusing is quite individual and does depend on the refractive status of both the client and the examiner.

Often, a vessel is detected first and can be followed in toward the optic disc. If the examiner directs the beam of light through the pupil in a slightly nasalward direction, the beam will fall on or near the optic disc initially.

Retinal structures. Examination of the various retinal structures should be performed in a consistent and orderly fashion. The following order is recommended: (1) optic disc, (2) retinal vessels, (3) retinal background, and (4) macular area.

The disc is examined for its size, shape, color, the distinctness of its margins, and the physiological cup. The disc is also used as a standard measurement device. The distance from the disc and the size of other findings are estimated in terms of disc diameters (DD); for example, an alteration slightly larger than the disc situated in the upper portion of the fundus may be described as being 1 × 2 DD in size and 3 DD away from the disc at 1:30 (clock position) in the left eye (Fig. 11-16).

The retinal vessels are examined for their color, the ratio in size of arterioles to veins is determined, arteriovenous crossings are examined for indentations, and the arterioles are examined for their light reflex. Each set of vessels should be followed out from the disc to the periphery. The retinal background is examined for its color and regularity of appearance and for any areas of light or dark color alterations. The more peripheral reaches of the vessels and retinal background can be examined by having the client direct his gaze upward, downward, and to each side. Observation of the macular area is reserved for last, because having a bright light directed at the center of acutest vision is very uncomfortable for the client. The macula is about 1 DD in size and is located 2 DD temporal to the optic disc. It appears as an avascular area with the bright spot of light reflected from its center, the fovea. This area can

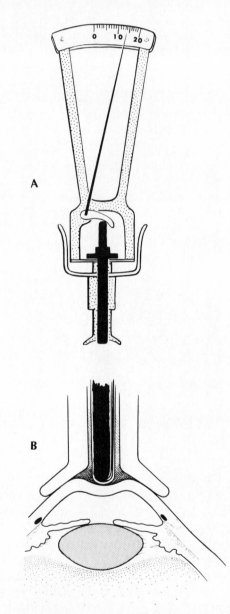

Fig. 11-17
A, Schiötz tonometer in which the plunger, in black, measures the ease of indentation of the cornea. **B,** Indentation of the anesthetized cornea by the plunger of the tonometer to measure ocular tension. (From Newell, F.W.: Ophthalmology: principles and concepts, ed. 5, St. Louis, 1982, The C.V. Mosby Co.)

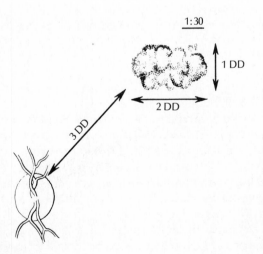

Fig. 11-16
Method of giving position and dimensions of a lesion in terms of disc diameters. (From Havener, W.H.: Synopsis of ophthalmology, ed. 6, St. Louis, 1984, The C.V. Mosby Co.)

be examined by having the client look directly at the examining light. When the client does so, the examiner is visualizing the macula. See color plate of eye.

Intraocular pressure

Screening for intraocular pressure is best accomplished by using the Schiötz tonometer (Fig. 11-17). Instructions accompanying the instrument on measurement and cleaning should be followed carefully.

For an accurate tonometry reading, the client should be in either a recumbent position or a reclining position in a chair. A tight collar or tie must be loosened to avoid an artificial increase in intraocular pressure caused by impeded venous return from the jugular system. If contact lenses are worn, they should be removed. Before proceeding, the examiner explains the procedure to the client. The cornea of each eye is then anesthetized by instilling a drop of a topical anesthetic such as proparacaine hydrochloride. Any tearing may be blotted with a tissue, but the eye should not be rubbed. The client is then asked to fix his gaze directly overhead and to breathe regularly. The examiner uses the thumb and index finger of one hand to hold the client's upper and lower lids against the bony orbital rim; with the other hand, the footplate of the vertically

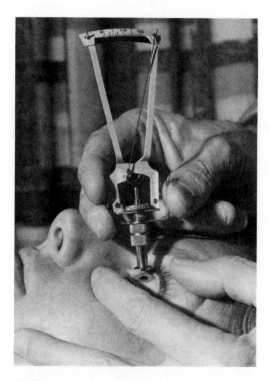

Fig. 11-18
Screening for intraocular pressure. (From Prior, J.A., Silberstein, J.S., and Stang, J.M.: Physical diagnosis: the history and examination of the patient, ed. 6, St. Louis, 1981, The C.V. Mosby Co.)

held tonometer is placed lightly on the center of the cornea (Fig. 11-18). The reading is taken, and the footplate is lifted, not slid, off the cornea. The lower the reading on the tonometer scale, the greater the pressure. The tonometer should be carefully cleaned after each prodecure.

The following conditions are contraindications to performing tonometry:
1. Any ocular infection or discharge
2. Recent ocular injury
3. Herpes on the face or eyelids
4. Corneal edema, distortion, thickening, or scarring
5. Marked nystagmus
6. Uncontrollable coughing
7. Significant apprehension or blepharospasm

It should be remembered that examination of the depth of the anterior chamber, assessment of the visual fields, and examination of the optic nerve head are also components of the examination for increased intraocular pressure, or glaucoma.

Intraocular pressure may be grossly estimated by touch. The client is asked to look down but to keep his eyes open; the examiner then palpates over the sclera with a gentle to-and-fro motion using both index fingers. This maneuver gives only a rough estimate and is much less valuable than tonometry for measurement of intraocular pressure. All persons over 40 years of age should be checked regularly by tonometry. Glaucoma is a major cause of blindness, and although it cannot be reversed, it can be halted.

PATHOLOGY
Visual acuity

Limited visual acuity may be an indication of a refractive error or of a more serious pathological condition. The determination of blindness cannot be made unless neither hand movements nor a bright beam of light can be perceived.

Visual fields

Visual field defects may be caused by lesions of the retina, by lesions at any point along the optic nerve or tract, or by lesions in the occipital lobes (Fig. 11-19). Damage to one optic nerve will affect the field of vision in that eye. Lesions occurring at the optic chiasm, at the optic tract, or in the brain usually affect the visual fields of both eyes because of the crossing of fibers at the chiasm. Lesions at the optic chiasm, as from a pituitary tumor, cause a loss of vision from the nasal portion of each retina, resulting in a loss of both temporal fields of vision. This condition is termed heteronymous or bitemporal hemianopia.

Since nerves from both eyes mingle behind the chiasm in the optic tracts and in the brain, lesions along

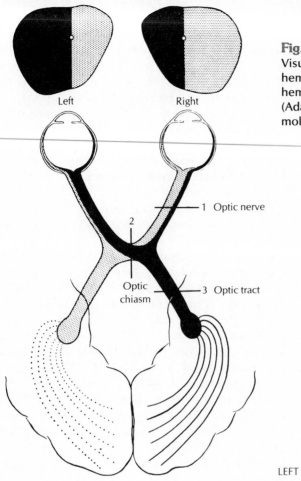

Left   Right

1 Optic nerve

2

Optic
chiasm

3 Optic tract

Fig. 11-19
Visual field defects. *1,* Blind right eye; *2,* bitemporal hemianopia—no temporal vision; *3,* left homonymous hemianopia—no vision in left field of either eye. (Adapted from Havener, W.H.: Synopsis of ophthalmology, ed. 6, 1984, The C.V. Mosby Co.)

Fig. 11-20
Visual fields showing optic nerve, optic chiasm, optic tracks, and optic radiations. Examples of various visual field defects. (From Rudy, E.B.: Advanced neurological and neurosurgical nursing, St. Louis, 1984, The C.V. Mosby Co.)

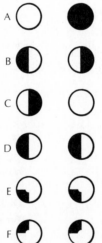

LEFT   RIGHT

A

B

C

D

E

F

A—Total blindness of right eye

B—Bitemporal hemianopsia

C—Left nasal hemianopsia

D—Left homonymous hemianopsia

E—Left homonymous hemianopsia inferior quadrant

F—Left homonymous hemianopsia superior quadrant

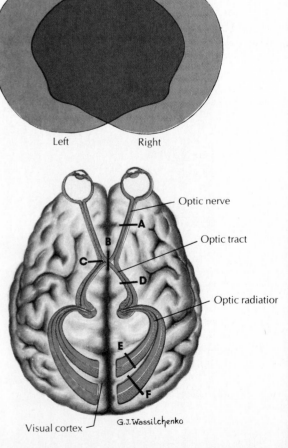

VISUAL FIELDS

Left   Right

Optic nerve

Optic tract

Optic radiation

Visual cortex

G.J.Wassilchenko

the optic tract or in the temporal parietal or occipital lobes will impair the same half of the field of vision in both eyes. For example, a lesion of the right optic tract or right side of the brain will result in visual field defects in the right nasal field and in the left temporal field. This condition is termed homonymous hemianopia and may be caused by occlusion of the middle cerebral artery. The effect of such lesions on the field of vision are illustrated in Fig. 11-20.

The location of disease on the retina determines the type of resultant visual field defects. Macular defects lead to a central blind area. Localized damage in other areas of the retina will cause a loss of vision corresponding to the involved area. A blind spot is known as a scotoma, that is, an area of blindness surrounded by an area of vision. Advanced diabetic retinopathy may cause macular damage, resulting in a loss of central vision. Glaucoma, or increased intraocular pressure, causes decreased peripheral vision because of the damage caused by the elevated pressure. As the disease advances, it may also cause a loss of central vision. A retinal detachment will cause loss of vision from that portion of the retina where the detachment occurs.

Extraocular neuromuscular function

An asymmetrical corneal light reflex, an inability of the eyes to move in parallel fashion to the six cardinal positions of gaze, or an abnormal cover test indicates a weakness or paralysis of one or more of the extraocular muscles or a defect in the nerve supplying it. Table 11-2 indicates the muscle and cranial nerve involved when the eye will not turn to one of these six positions.

Examples of the effects of nerve lesions are as follows:

1. *Oculomotor paralysis (CN III):* the eye turns down and out with drooping of the upper lid.
2. *Abducens paralysis (CN VI):* the eye turns in toward the nose because of unopposed action of the medial rectus.

Carrying the fixation point of the six cardinal positions out to the extremes will exaggerate a defect. A disparity of the anteroposterior axes of the eyes is called strabismus. Deviations in these axes may be detected during the cover test, which blocks the fusion reflex of the eyes. A mild weakness of the extraocular muscles is called phoria. If there is a weak tendency during the cover test, a definitely perceptible jerk of the eye is noted when the cover is removed. Tropia is a more pronounced imbalance producing a permanent disparity in the axes of the eyes. A mild outward deviation of the eye is called exophoria; an inward deviation is called esophoria. The rhythmical twitching motion of nystagmus may be normal at the end of the lateral position but is abnormal when the eyes are in any other position.

Ocular structures

Eyelids and eyelashes. Faulty positioning of the eyelids occurs in a variety of ways. The lid margins may fall above or below the middle part of the iris. A drooping lid margin (ptosis) that falls at the pupil or below may indicate an oculomotor nerve lesion or a congenital condition. If the lid margin falls above the limbus so that some sclera is visible, thyroid disease may be present. In the presence of thyroid disease the lid may lag behind the limbus as the gaze moves from an upward to a downward position (Fig. 11-21). Another type of faulty positioning of the lids is improper approximation of the lids to the eyeballs. The lids may be loose or lax and roll outward. This condition is called ectropion. Because the puncta cannot effectively drain the tears, epiphora (tearing) results. The lids may also roll inward because of lid spasm or the contraction of scar tissue. This condition is called entropion. Because the lashes are pulled inward, they may produce corneal irritation.

The tissues within the lids are loosely connected and collect excess fluid rather readily. Edema of the lids may be a manifestation of local or systemic disease. Examples of systemic problems that may cause lid edema include allergy, heart failure, nephrosis, and thyroid deficiency.

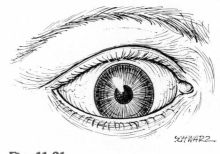

Table 11-2

Diagnostic clues to dysfunction of extraocular neuromuscular units

Position to which eye will not turn	Muscle	Cranial nerve
Straight nasal	Medial rectus	III
Up and nasal	Inferior oblique	III
Down and nasal	Superior oblique	IV
Straight temporal	Lateral rectus	VI
Up and temporal	Superior rectus	III
Down and temporal	Inferior rectus	III

Fig. 11-21
Lid lag.

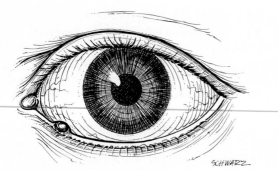

Fig. 11-22
Hordeolum or sty.

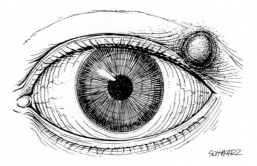

Fig. 11-23
Chalazion.

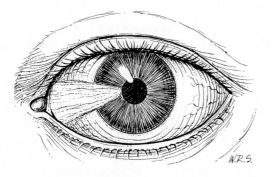

Fig. 11-24
Pterygium.

Fig. 11-25
A, Normal anterior chamber. **B,** Shallow anterior chamber. (From Havener, W.H.: Synopsis of ophthalmology, ed. 6, St. Louis, 1984, The C.V. Mosby Co.)

The glands of the lids may be sites of infection. A localized infection of the small glands around the eyelashes in the hair follicle at the lid margin is a hordeolum, or sty (Fig. 11-22). The meibomian glands lying within the posterior portion of the lid may develop an infection or a retention cyst, known as a chalazion (Fig. 11-23); crusting or scaling at the lid margins may occur as a result of staphylococcal infection or seborrheic dermatitis. If a lid infection is present or suspected, the lids may be gently palpated by moving the examining finger across the lid surface. Pressure should never be exerted over the eye in an effort to separate the lids. As mentioned earlier, the bony orbital rims should be used as points over which to slide the lids.

Xanthelasma, the raised yellow plaques that may appear on the lids, may have no pathological significance, or they may be associated with hypercholesterolemia.

Conjunctiva. Infectious disease of the conjunctiva typically produces engorgement of the conjunctival vessels and a discharge. The infected vessels are usually more pronounced at the fornices. Small subconjunctival hemorrhages may result from more severe involvement, although in some persons these may also result from sneezing, coughing, or lifting.

Sclera. Changes in the color of the sclera may be indicative of systemic disease. For example, jaundice manifests its presence in the eyes as a yellow discoloration, scleral icterus. Excessive bilirubinemia may be evident as scleral icterus before jaundice of the skin becomes apparent. In the presence of osteogenesis imperfecta the sclera is bluish.

Cornea. The cornea is a very sensitive structure, and pain and photophobia are common manifestations of corneal disease. Any dullness, irregularities, or opacities of the cornea are abnormal. Two of the more frequent abnormalities affecting the cornea are abrasions and opacities. Although an abrasion may cause the surface to look irregular or may cast a shadow on the iris, it may be invisible and detectable only with fluorescein stain. Suspected corneal abrasion should be referred to an ophthalmologist.

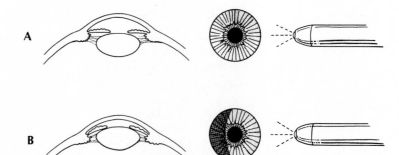

A

B

Abnormal growth of bulbar conjunctival tissue from the edge toward the center of the cornea, known as pterygium, may interfere with vision (Fig. 11-24).

Although the presence of arcus senilis is normal in elderly people, in younger individuals it may be associated with abnormal lipid metabolism.

Anterior chamber. Abnormalities observable in the anterior chamber are a decrease in depth and any foreign material interrupting the normal transparency. A shallow anterior chamber may be a sign of closed-angle glaucoma or may predispose the eye to glaucoma (Fig. 11-25). Symptoms typical of glaucoma include pain, redness, and seeing colored halos around lights. As the increased intraocular pressure causes the iris to become displaced anteriorly, there is less distance between the cornea and the iris. As a result of this anterior displacement, light directed obliquely from the temporal side will illuminate only the temporal side, and the nasal side will appear darker or shadowed. The presence of a shallow anterior chamber is a contraindication to the use of dilating drops for the ophthalmoscopic examination.

Any cloudiness of the aqueous fluid or accumulation of blood (hyphema) or purulent material (hypopyon) is abnormal. Hyphema may be caused by trauma or may result from spontaneous hemorrhage. If the hyphema is mild, the red blood cells settle out inferiorly by gravity to a height of a few millimeters. In severe hyphemas, the entire anterior chamber may be filled with blood.

Lacrimal apparatus. Both the lacrimal gland, which produces tears, and the system that drains the tears are subject to certain abnormalities. The lacrimal gland may be swollen as a result of infection or tumor. Infection with consequent blockage of the lacrimal sac or duct may occur with associated findings of swelling, redness, warmth, pain, and purulent discharge. The swelling tends to occur in the area below the inner canthus. The technique for examining for infection in the lacrimal sac is to press with the examining finger against the *inner* orbital rim (not against the nose), then to gently depress the lower lid over the lower orbital rim to observe for regurgitation of fluid through the puncta.

As mentioned earlier, ectropion may cause tearing because of inadequate drainage. Any unusual markings or growths should be noted. Persistent tearing of an infant's eye suggests either a blocked tear duct or congenital glaucoma.

Iris. Iritis, inflammation of the iris, results in throbbing pain and visual blurring and is associated with the findings of circumcorneal injection, a deep pinkish red flush about the cornea, and a constricted pupil. This is in contrast to conjunctivitis, wherein the infected vessels tend to extend from the periphery toward the cen-

ter. The iris may become inflamed because of bacterial infections, which may also lead to the production of a purulent exudate, as well as to diffuse congestion around the iris. If the lens has been removed, the normal support of the iris is absent and the iris will, with movements of the eye, have a tremulous, fluttering motion.

Pupils. Abnormalities of the pupils include alterations in size and in reflexes. Although a slight but noticeable difference in pupil size does occur in about 5% of the population, this finding should be regarded with suspicion because it can be an indication of central nervous system (CNS) disease. Inequality in the size of the pupils is known as anisocoria. Dyscoria is a congenital abnormality in the shape of the pupils.

Mydriasis, enlargement of the pupils, may result from emotional influences, recent or old local trauma, acute glaucoma, systemic reaction to parasympatholytic or sympathomimetic drugs, or the local use of dilating drops. A unilateral fixed enlarged pupil may be caused by local trauma to the eye or head injury. Fixed dilation of both eyes occurs with deep anesthesia, CNS injury, and circulatory arrest.

Miosis, constriction of the pupils, is associated with iritis, use of morphine, and glaucoma treatment by pilocarpine and is seen physiologically with sleep.

Any irregularity in pupil contour is abnormal and may result from iritis, trauma, CNS syphilis, or congenital defects.

Failure of the pupils to react to light with preservation of the accommodation reaction is another characteristic of CNS syphilis. This is known as the Argyll Robertson pupil.

In the case of monocular blindness, the blind eye and optic tract will transmit no response to light, and neither pupil will constrict. However, when the unaffected eye receives illumination, both pupils will constrict because the efferent pupil constriction stimuli are distributed evenly to both eyes.

Lens. Opacities in any of the clear portions of the eye (anterior chamber, lens, or vitreous body) will appear as dark shadows on black spots within the red reflex on ophthalmoscopic examination because they prevent light from being reflected back to the examiner's eye. An opacity within the lens is referred to as a cataract. These opacities vary in appearance; some look like pieces of coral, some look like various-shaped crystals, and others have a stellate, or starlike, appearance. Cataract formation may be associated with various systemic disorders, may occur as the complex of findings in various hereditary syndromes, or may result from senescent changes within the lens. In certain endocrine disorders, such as diabetes mellitus, the metabolic disturbance results in abnormal lens fiber formation and cataracts. Such cataracts typically attack young per-

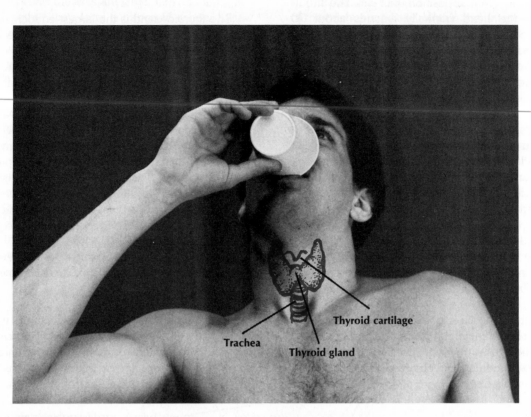

Fig. 12-7
Observation for the thyroid gland with the neck in slight extension. The structures of the thyroid gland are more distinct during swallowing.

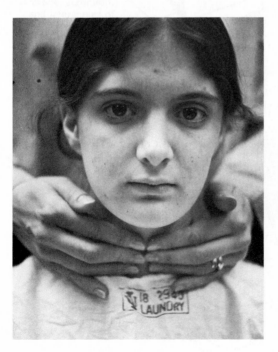

Fig. 12-8
Posterior approach to thyroid examination. Standing behind the client, the examiner palpates for the thyroid isthmus by placing the palmar aspects of the fingertips over the lower portion of the trachea.

cone shaped, each about 5 cm long, 3 cm in diameter, and 2 cm thick. The average weight of the total gland is about 25 g. The lobes curve posteriorly around the cartilages; the lateral portions are covered by the sternocleidomastoid muscles. Thyroid arteries supply the highly vascular thyroid tissue.

Examination

The techniques used to examine the thyroid gland include observation, palpation, and auscultation. Observation of thyroid function or possible dysfunction includes more than observation of the area where the thyroid gland is located. The effects of thyroid activity are widespread; therefore, observations of behavior, appearance, skin, eyes, hair, and cardiovascular status are important.

To inspect the thyroid gland, the examiner stands before the client and observes particularly the lower half of the neck first in normal position, next in slight extension, and then while the client swallows a sip of water (Fig. 12-7). The movements of the cartilages are easily observed. Any unusual bulging of thyroid tissue in the midline of the lobes or behind the sternocleidomastoid muscles should be noted; normally, none is seen. A good cross light is helpful for observing subtle neck movements or ascending masses.

Following observation, the neck is palpated for the presence of an enlarged thyroid, for consistency of the gland, and for any nodules. The normal thyroid gland is not palpable. However, in a thin neck, the isthmus is occasionally palpable; and in a short, stocky neck, even an enlarged gland may be difficult to palpate. Palpation may be done with the examiner standing either in front of or behind the client. Although there are several techniques used for palpation of the thyroid, the underlying principles for each technique include movement of the gland while the client swallows, adequate exposure of the gland by relaxation and manual displacement of surrounding structures, and comparison of one side of the gland with the other. The thyroid gland is fixed to the trachea and thus ascends during swallowing. This distinguishes thyroid structures from other neck masses.

Posterior approach. The client is seated on a chair or examining table while the examiner stands behind him. The client is requested to lower his chin to relax the neck muscles. The examining fingers are curved anteriorly, so that the tips rest on the lower half of the neck over the trachea (Fig. 12-8). The client is asked to swallow a sip of water while the examiner feels for any enlargement of the thyroid isthmus. To facilitate examination of each lobe, the client is asked to turn his head slightly toward the side to be examined with the chin still lowered. For example, to examine the right thyroid lobe, the examiner has the client lower his chin and turn his head slightly to the right. With the fingers of the left hand, the examiner displaces the thyroid cartilage slightly to the right while the fingers of the right hand palpate the area lateral to the cartilage where the thyroid lobe lies, for any enlargement (Fig. 12-9). The

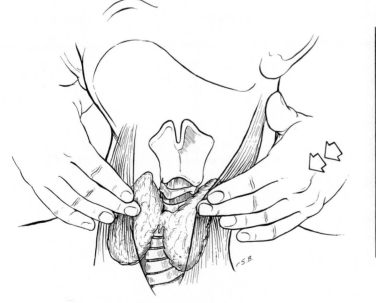

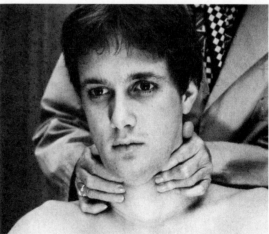

Fig. 12-9
Posterior approach to thyroid examination. To examine the right lobe of the thyroid gland, the examiner displaces the trachea slightly to the right with the fingers of the left hand and palpates for the right thyroid lobe with the fingers of the right hand.

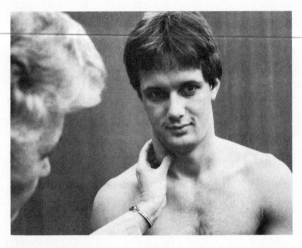

Fig. 12-10
Anterior approach to thyroid examination. Examining for an enlarged right thyroid lobe, the examiner grasps and palpates around and deep to the right sternoclei-domastoid muscle.

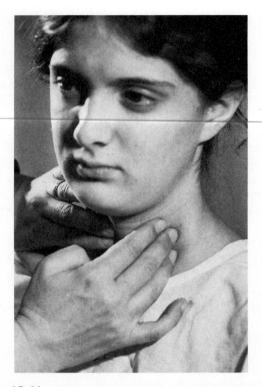

Fig. 12-11
Anterior approach to thyroid examination. Standing in front of the client, the examiner uses the fingers of the left hand to displace the trachea slightly to the left while the fingers of the right hand palpate for the left thyroid lobe.

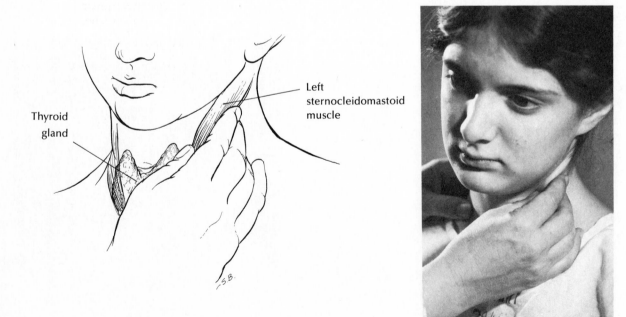

Left sternocleidomastoid muscle

Thyroid gland

Fig. 12-12
Anterior approach to thyroid examination. The examiner grasps around the left sternocleido-mastoid muscle with the right hand to palpate for an enlarged left thyroid lobe.

client is asked to swallow a sip of water as this procedure is being done. The examiner may also palpate for thyroid enlargement on the right side by placing the thumb deep to and behind the sternocleidomastoid muscle while the index and middle fingers are placed deep to and in front of the muscle (Fig. 12-10). This procedure is then repeated for the left lobe; the right hand displaces the cartilage, and the left hand palpates.

Anterior approach. The examiner stands in front of the client and with the palmar surfaces of the index and middle fingers palpates below the cricoid cartilage for the thyroid isthmus as the client swallows a sip of water. In a procedure similar to the one used with the posterior approach, the client is asked to flex his head and turn it slightly to one side and then the other. The examiner palpates for the left lobe by displacing the thyroid cartilage slightly to the left with the left hand and examining for thyroid enlargement with the right hand (Fig. 12-11). Again, the examiner palpates the area and hooks thumb and fingers around the sternocleidomastoid muscle (Fig. 12-12). The procedure is repeated for the right side.

If enlargement of the thyroid gland is detected or suspected, the area over the gland is auscultated for a bruit. In a hyperplastic thyroid gland, the blood flow through the thyroid arteries is accelerated and produces vibrations that may be heard with the bell of the stethoscope as a soft, rushing sound or bruit. (See Chapter 16, "Cardiovascular Assessment: the Heart and the Neck Vessels," for further discussion of bruits.)

The thyroid gland may incur diffuse or local enlargement. Diffuse enlargement may occur to varying degrees. Symmetrical thyroid enlargement is not uncommon in areas where there is a deficiency of dietary iodine. Localized or nodular enlargement may consist of one or more nodules and may occur in either lobe or in the isthmus. Solitary nodules are suggestive of carcinoma, particularly in younger people.

Thyroid tissue located in the retrosternal area may also become enlarged. This is not discernible by physical examination but should be considered if other physical findings are suggestive of thyroid dysfunction.

SUMMARY

I. Skull, scalp, and hair
   A. Observe size and shape of skull
   B. Observe scalp in several areas; inquire about injuries; palpate
   C. Observe condition of hair
II. Face
   A. Observe symmetry of structures, color, and condition of skin
   B. Test for facial sensation (CN V) and muscular function (CN VII)
   C. Palpate temporal artery
III. Neck
   A. Examine structure and function of neck muscles (CN XI)
   B. Palpate cervical vertebrae
   C. Palpate trachea
   D. Observe and palpate for thyroid gland
   E. Observe, palpate, and auscultate neck vessels, carotid arteries, and jugular veins (see Chapter 16)
   F. Palpate for cervical lymph nodes (see Chapter 13)

BIBLIOGRAPHY

DeGroot, L.J., and Stanbury, J.B.: The thyroid and its diseases, ed. 4, New York, 1975, John Wiley & Sons, Inc.

Hamburger, J.I.: Your thyroid gland—fact and fiction, ed. 2, Springfield, Ill., 1975, Charles C Thomas, Publisher.

Werner, S.C.: Physical examination. In Werner, S.C., and Ingbar, S.H., editors: The thyroid: a fundamental and clinical text, ed. 3, New York, 1971, Harper & Row, Publishers.

CHAPTER 13

ASSESSMENT OF THE LYMPHATIC SYSTEM

The technique of health assessment allows the detection of enlarged lymph nodes (lymphadenopathy) as an indicator of the function of the lymphatic system. Only the superficial lymph nodes (see Fig. 13-23) are accessible to palpation. Lymph nodes are not palpable in the normal individual except for occasional small (less than 1 cm), hard ("shotty") nodes usually in the inguinal region. The most common causes of lymphadenopathy are infection and neoplasm. An infectious condition that leads to a swollen lymph node, either an acute infectious process or a chronic granulomatous process, is the most common cause of a lump in a child's neck. To understand the findings of this system a discussion of the physiology of the lymphatic system follows.

The lymphatic capillary bed is very extensive. All tissues supplied with blood vessels also possess lymphatic vessels with the exception of the placenta. The lymphatic system is older in evolutionary history than the circulatory system. The function of the lymph is concerned with metabolic processes that have a slower pace than those of the blood circulatory system. The cardiovascular system was a phylogenetic development for a more active animal life wherein the transport of oxygen was necessary for the rapid processes of oxidation and reduction.

PHYSIOLOGY

The lymphatic system consists of a system of collecting ducts, the lymph fluid, and tissues; this tissue makes up the lymph nodes, the spleen, the thymus, the tonsils, and Peyer's patches in the intestines. Lymphoid aggregates are also found in bone marrow, in the lungs, and in gastric and appendiceal mucosa.

The lymphatic vessels originate as microscopic open-ended tubules termed capillaries. These capillaries merge to form larger collecting ducts, which drain to specific lymphatic tissue centers (nodes). Ducts from these lymph node centers eventually empty as trunks into the venous system at the subclavian veins (Fig. 13-1). The right subclavian vein receives the thin-walled lymphatic trunk, which drains from the right side of the head and neck, from the right arm, and from the right chest wall. The left subclavian vein is joined by the thoracic duct, which drains lymph from the remainder of the body. These vessels then return fluid and protein that has entered the lymphatic system from the interstitial space via the cardiovascular system.

Although the specific functions and properties of the lymphatic system are still imperfectly understood, the lymphocytic tissue has been ascribed responsibility for the immunological and various metabolic processes of the body and is implicated in the formation of corpuscular elements of the blood and in the extension of malignant disease.

Included in the functions of the lymphatic system are (1) the transport of lymph fluids, protein, and microorganisms for return to the cardiovascular system; (2) the production of lymphocytes in germinal centers of lymph nodes; (3) the production of antibodies (immune substances may be extracted from lymphocytes; lymphocytes contain at least one globulin identical with blood globulin); (4) phagocytosis by the reticuloendothelial cells lining the sinuses of the lymph nodes, the spleen, and the liver (Kupffer cells); (5) hemopoiesis in some pathological states; and (6) the absorption of fat and fat-soluble materials from the intestine.

Lymphatic tissue in human beings is calculated to be 2% to 3% of the total body weight. Lymphatic capillaries and collecting ducts are the transport ducts of the system. The lymph channel section of the lymphatic system consists of lymphatic capillaries, lymph node precollecting ducts, lymph node postcollecting ducts,

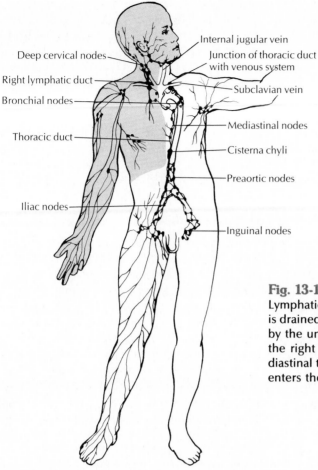

Deep cervical nodes

Right lymphatic duct

Bronchial nodes

Thoracic duct

Iliac nodes

Internal jugular vein

Junction of thoracic duct
with venous system

Subclavian vein

Mediastinal nodes

Cisterna chyli

Preaortic nodes

Inguinal nodes

Fig. 13-1
Lymphatic drainage pathways. Shaded area of the body
is drained via the right lymphatic duct, which is formed
by the union of three vessels: the right jugular trunk,
the right subclavian trunk, and the right bronchome-
diastinal trunk. Lymph from the remainder of the body
enters the venous system by way of the thoracic duct.

lymph nodes, and main lymphatic trunks. Lymphoid
tissue is organized in its biological architecture to form
nodes that are located at strategic points for filtering the
lymph. Structurally the lymph node consists of the capsule, the cortex, and the medulla. The lymph and any
substance that enters the lymph, including contrast
media injected for lymphography, are filtered by the
lymph nodes.

The lymph nodes are seldom found singly but are
usually arranged in chains or clusters called lymph centers. The lymph nodes are found either in the subcutaneous connective tissue (superficial lymph nodes) or
beneath the muscular fascia and in the cavities of the
body (deep lymph nodes). The nodes are dissemi-
nated along the course of the collecting ducts and are
usually round or oval, though they are often observed
as elongated and flattened to a cylindrical shape. Size
is variable from small (almost invisible) to the size of a
large pea or even an olive. Nodes found in children are
comparatively larger than those found in adults.

Lymphocytes are mobile, spherical, mononuclear
cells ($6\,\mu$ to $8\,\mu$ in diameter) derived from reticular cells
of the nodes. Lymphocytes may evolve in one of three
ways: (1) they may remain in lymphoid tissue and die

there; (2) they may differentiate in lymphoid tissue,
giving rise to other types of cells; or (3) they may leave
lymphoid tissue, entering the lymph and then the
blood and various organs.

Some of the processes carried on in this system have
been clarified by inspecting the ducts with a radi-
opaque dye (lymphography). Three stages of lymphography have been described. During the first stage
the afferent lymphatics, portions of the lymphoid
sinuses, and the efferent lymphatics are filled with the
contrast medium. The second stage is characterized by
phagocytosis by the reticuloendothelial cell of the lipid-
soluble contrast media, and the third stage is the period
during which the contrast media leaves the node. It can
be assumed that all substances entering the lymphatic
system undergo this fate.

Factors affecting the movement of lymph are (1)
remitting compression of the lymphatic vessels by surrounding structures, especially contracting muscles; (2)
respiratory movements that propel lymph from the cisterna chyli—origin of the thoracic duct in the lumbar
region—into the thoracic duct; (3) propulsive action of
the smooth muscles contained in the walls of the lymphatic vessels, lymph nodes, and collecting ducts; (4)

arterial pulsations (most of the lymphatic vessels course with the regional blood vessels; the deep lymphatic vessels accompany not only the veins but also the arteries, the pulsations of which can be transmitted to the lymphatic vessels); (5) negative pressure in the great vessels at the root of the neck, which determines the flow of lymph from the terminal parts of the jugular, subclavian, bronchial, mediastinal, and thoracic ducts into them; (6) peristaltic contractions of intestines; (7) capillary blood pressure; (8) force of gravity.

The formation and flow of lymph can be increased by the following processes: (1) an increase in capillary pressure resulting from increased venous pressure from venous stasis or obstruction; (2) an increase in permeability of the capillary walls resulting from an increase in temperature, a decrease in oxygen supply, or the administration of histamine; (3) increases in metabolic activity, the muscular pumping effect, or glandular activity (little lymph is formed when the client is given anesthesia or is on absolute bed rest); (4) passive movements and massage, which facilitate the flow of lymph through the lymphatic vessels; and (5) administration of hypertonic solutions, such as glucose and sodium chloride solutions.

PATHOPHYSIOLOGY

Pathological findings may be demonstrated for the lymphatic system as a result of (1) localized or systemic infection; (2) disorders in metabolism, particularly of lipids (storage-type adenopathy); (3) metastatic cancer; (4) infiltration of foreign substances; (5) primary hematopoietic disorders; and (6) hypersensitivity reactions.

The lymph nodes are the most significant parameters of the lymphatic system in physical diagnosis. The location and nature of involvement of diseased lymph nodes provide help in determining the site or origin of disease and the identity of the etiological agent.

The archaic term *swollen glands* is widely used by the lay populace. The early anatomists believed the lymph nodes were glands that functioned in a manner similar to true glands, such as the thyroid. Actual structure and function became apparent with the improved visualization afforded by light microscopy, but the continued use of the glandular reference will be apparent in both the chief complaint and the history.

Alterations in lymphatic flow patterns may also indicate disease.

Mechanical stasis of lymph

Any mechanical impediment to the flow of lymph results in deceleration or cessation of flow of lymph from that region. As a result of this impaired drainage, lymphatic vessels become dilated with the trapped lymphatic fluid. The valves become incompetent,

causing a backflow of lymph within the interstitial space. Because the lymphatic system functions to return protein to the blood supply, colloid osmotic pressure increases as the interstitial protein concentration rises. Consequently, even more fluid is drawn into the extracellular spaces from the capillaries. In the absence of effective intervention, the extracellular protein precipitates and a fibrin reticulum forms. Proliferation of fibrocytes is stimulated. Subsequently, elastic and collagen fibers are formed and accumulate to give the connective tissue the characteristics of the so-called brawny edema. This is followed by a fibrosclerotic end stage.

Lymphedema

Mechanical obstruction in the lymphatic system could result from extrinsic and intrinsic pressure, such as sclerosis, inflammation, neoplasm, surgical injuries, and functional lymphospasm. Compensating mechanisms are elicited that may result in complete or partial drainage of the lymph. The excess lymph of the dilated lymphatic vessels may be transuded back through the walls into the interstitial fluid and, as sufficient pressure builds up, back into the vascular system. Another compensating mechanism is the development of collateral anastomotic channels.

Lymphedema is the excessive accumulation of lymph in the interstitial spaces. Lymphedema results when the compensating mechanisms fail to provide drainage of all the lymph. Lymphedema is not accompanied by cyanosis, dilatation of veins, hyperpigmentation, or leathery indentation. It is usually firm and does not pit well. The more common pathological conditions leading to the formation of edema are inflammatory processes resulting from tuberculosis, syphilis or filariasis, thrombophlebitis, and trauma related to ionizing radiation or surgical operations.

Baseline measurement of edema should be as precise as possible. It is recommended that the circumference of the extremities be measured with a flexible measuring tape made of plastic or metal that will not stretch. It is important that the same reference point be used on subsequent measurements. This can be accomplished by measuring a certain number of inches or centimeters from a given point, such as the ankle or the knee. Some clinics have elected 10 cm as the distance always to be used in an effort to standardize these measurements.

Lymph nodes

In general, the lymph nodes closer to the center of the body are smaller. Thus, the axillary lymph nodes are larger than the supraclavicular lymph nodes, and the inguinal lymph nodes are larger than the iliac lymph nodes.

The number of lymph nodes varies from individual to individual; generally speaking, the smaller the nodes are, the more numerous they are. Some investigators have reported that the number of lymph nodes is diminished in older persons. Furthermore, the size of the lymph nodes decreases with aging because they lose some of their lymphoid elements. The nodes from older clients show fibrosis and fatty degeneration on sectioning.

The majority of cells in the lymph nodes are B lymphocytes, which are arranged in follicles. There are T lymphocytes in the paracortical areas, and the reticuloendothelial cells (macrophages) line the nodal sinuses. The function of lymphocytes is to respond to antigens. Lymphadenopathy may result from an increase in the number and size of the lymphocytes or reticuloendothelial cells or to an infiltration of the node by cells normally not present, such as metastatic carcinoma cells or polymorphonuclear white blood cells in lymphadenitis.

Whether a palpable node is clinically significant depends on its location, the client's age, and the living environment (including work) of the client. Children are more likely than adults to develop generalized lymphadenopathy. Children with mild infections of the respiratory tract and skin are frequently observed to have swollen nodes. Thus, lymphadenopathy in the adult is more frequently a sign of a serious disease (see boxed material below).

Normally, lymph nodes cannot be felt or seen. Thus, the size of the lymph nodes is an important diagnostic feature, and any increase is considered pathological. Usually, the greatest increases are found in acute and chronic inflammatory conditions and in systemic neoplastic disease. The size of the lymph nodes is almost never increased in cases of metastasis unless inflammatory reaction changes are also present. However, children with no other physical findings frequently have enlarged neck nodes, which may not have clinical significance.

Whereas in their normal state lymph nodes are round or oval, in pathological conditions their form may be greatly altered and they may assume an irregularly nodular (as in lymphadenitis) or horseshoe shape (as in senile involution).

The nodes of metastatic carcinoma are frequently described as stone hard, bound to surrounding tissue and thus immobile, and nontender. The characteristics of nodes resulting from acute infection are firm in texture, asymmetric and matted, and tender. The inflammation may extend to the skin, which may appear red and edematous.

However, in chronic infections the nodes are nontender and there is no edema. The nodes associated with lymphoma have been described as rubbery, firm, large, and movable.

EXAMINATION

The only equipment needed for the assessment of the lymphatic system is a ruler and a nonstretchable tape measure.

Clients' complaints of "swollen glands," "lumps," or "kernels" generally refer to enlarged lymph nodes. Examination of the lymphatic system is accomplished by incorporating the examination techniques into the regimen for each part of the body where lymph nodes are palpable. However, the information gained in these localized efforts must be integrated so that a general lymphadenopathy is not overlooked.

Inspection is the first step in regional lymph node examination. This is followed by palpation of the specific nodal regions for prominent nodes. Palpation of the lymph nodes is best accomplished through a gentle rotary motion of the palmar surface of the index and middle fingertips (Fig. 13-2). One should exercise enough pressure that the skin moves in concert with the fingers, but not so much that underlying nodes are obscured in the deeper soft tissues.

Detected nodes are described according to *location, size, regularity, consistency, tenderness, fixation to surrounding tissues,* and *discreteness* as opposed to *matting.* There may be no significance in a few discrete, mobile lymph nodes that measure less than 1 cm in diameter in any of the nodal sites; however, these nodes ought to move easily beneath the fingers. The fixed, immobile node may signify malignancy, whereas nodes that have coalesced may indicate infection. On judging a node to be normal, one must examine the

---

Conditions associated with lymphadenopathy

Neoplasm	Inflammation-immunological
Hematological	Infections
Lymphoma	Staphylococcus
Leukemia	Streptococcus
Histiocytosis	Salmonella
Carcinoma	Brucellosis
Head and neck	Tuberculosis
Lung	Syphilis
Breast	Infectious mononucleosis
Kidney	Histoplasmosis
	Coccidioidomycosis
	Acquired immune deficiency syndrome (AIDS)
	Connective tissue disease
	Systemic lupus erythematosus
	Rheumatoid arthritis
	Reactions to hydantoins

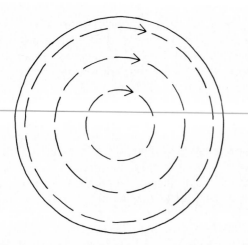

Fig. 13-2
Systematic circular movements of the palmar tips of the fingers are used for detection of superficial lymph nodes.

regions drained by this node for indications of infection or neoplasm. Furthermore, other lymph node regions should be investigated for the presence of enlarged nodes.

Characteristics assessed in examination of lymph nodes or masses

Location	Be specific in describing the site. Use imaginary body lines or axes and bony prominences to relate findings. Draw pictures where appropriate.
Size	Define the volume in centimeters from the three dimensions of length, width, and thickness. State the total volume. Describe the shape lucidly (round, cylindrical); if irregular, draw pictures.
Surface characteristics	Describe accurately as smooth, nodular, irregular.
Consistency	Describe as hard, firm, soft, resilient, spongy, cystic.
Symmetry	Use as a comparison with paired structures.
Fixation, mobility	Describe exact mobile parameters in centimeters. If mass is fixed in position, identify whether fixation is to underlying or overlying tissue by trying to move it with examining fingers.
Tenderness—pain	Describe whether present without stimulation or elicited by palpation or movement. Indicate whether direct, referred, or rebound.
Erythema	Describe extent of color change if present.
Heat	Describe extent if present.
Pulsatile nature	Describe pulsations when they are usually not palpable at this locus. Auscultate all pulsating masses for bruits.
Increased vascularity	Describe prominence of overlying veins or cyanosis of the area.

Transillumination	If pathological structure is in an anatomical area that can be transilluminated, such as the scrotum, describe the results of the procedure. The structure which can be transilluminated contains fluid. This is generally a cyst and not a lymph node.

Whether a primary cancer is found, the nodes draining the region must be examined, as well as those of known patterns of metastasis. Thus, the description of superficial lymph nodes (those close enough to the surface to be palpated) includes the origin of the collecting ducts entering the nodes and the destination of those ducts leaving the nodes. Matting of nodes may result from a superimposed infection or invasion of the lymph node capsule.

REGIONAL LYMPHATIC SYSTEMS— SUPERFICIAL NODES
Head and neck
Head

Lymphatic drainage from the integument of the head, ears, nose, cheeks, and lips is delivered by collecting ducts to the lymph centers of the head (Fig. 13-3).

The *suboccipital center* consists of three to six lymph nodes receiving the collecting ducts from the occipital region of the scalp and from the deep structures of the back of the neck. The efferent lymphatics from these lymph nodes reach the deep lymph nodes of the neck and spinal nerve chain.

The *postauricular,* or *mastoid, center* contains four or five lymph nodes over the outer surface of the mastoid process or under the sternocleidomastoid muscle. The afferent lymphatic vessels drain the parietal region of the head and part of the ear. Those vessels leaving these nodes reach the parotid substernocleidomastoid lymph nodes. These nodes are more likely to be palpated in young individuals and are frequently absent or atrophic in older persons.

The *preauricular center* is made up of one or two lymph nodes situated in front of the tragus. The afferent ducts are from the forehead and upper face (Fig. 13-4).

The nodes of the *parotid center* may be found on the surface of the gland, within the tissue of the gland, or under the parotid fascia. Those lying over the surface of the parotid gland are called preauricular parotid nodes, whereas those at the lower pole of the gland are called infraauricular parotid nodes. If they lie lower and outside the gland, they are a part of the external jugular chain. The infraauricular nodes are also known as superficial lateral cervical nodes. The nodes of both the preauricular and parotid centers receive collecting

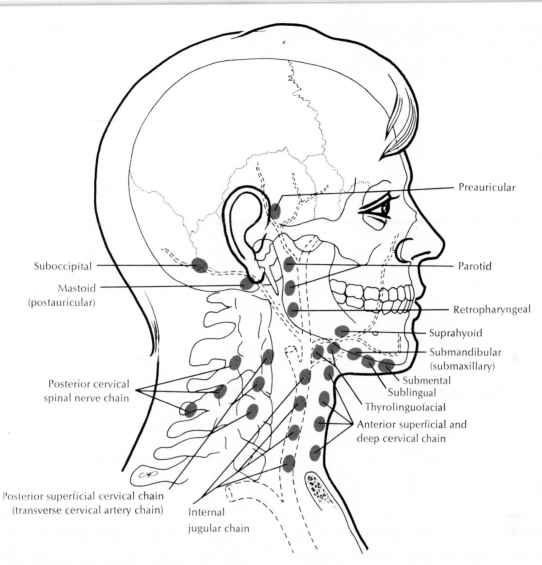

Preauricular

Suboccipital

Mastoid
(postauricular)

Parotid

Retropharyngeal

Suprahyoid

Submandibular
(submaxillary)

Submental

Sublingual

Thyrolinguofacial

Posterior cervical
spinal nerve chain

Anterior superficial and
deep cervical chain

Posterior superficial cervical chain
(transverse cervical artery chain)

Internal
jugular chain

Fig. 13-3
Lymphatic drainage system of the head and neck. If the group of nodes is commonly referred
to by another name, the second name appears in parentheses.

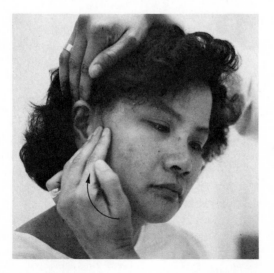

Fig. 13-4
Palpation of the preauricular lymph nodes.

ducts from the side of the head and the parotid gland, as well as from the forehead, cheek, eyelids, ear, nose, upper lip, and eustachian tube. These efferent ducts contribute to the lymph nodes of the internal jugular and subdigastric chains.

Nodes of the floor of the mouth. The *submandibular center* lies on the medial border of the mandible, following the mandibular branch of the facial nerve. This center receives collecting ducts from the chin, upper lip, cheek, nose, teeth, eyelids, part of the tongue, and floor of the mouth. The efferent vessels bring lymph to the internal jugular chain of the neck.

The nodes of the *retropharyngeal center* are found at the junction of the posterior and lateral walls of the pharynx near the location of the atlas. Lymph from the nasal cavity and lymph of the accessory sinuses of the nose, palate, epipharynx, and mesopharynx, and possibly of the middle ear, is delivered to these nodes; the lymph leaving this center reaches the internal jugular chain about at the level of the bifurcation of the carotid artery.

The *submental center* receives collecting ducts from the tongue. The submental nodes may number two to eight. They are located in the submental triangle between the platysma and mylohyoid muscles. These nodes receive ducts from the gums, the floor of the mouth, and the anterior third of the tongue.

The sublingual nodes are interrupted nodules along the collecting ducts of the tongue and sublingual salivary gland.

Neck

The lymph nodes of the neck receive the lymph from the head and from the structures of the neck itself. The nodes are grouped serially and are referred to as chains.

Anterior cervical chain. The *superficial cervical chain* of four to six lymph nodes is located over and anterior to the sternocleidomastoid muscle and near but deeper than the external jugular vein. The nodes are beneath the platysma muscle and superficial cervical fascia and receive lymph from the skin and neck.

The nodes of the *thyrolinguofacial chain* are found between the lower margins of the posterior head of the digastric muscle and the thyrolinguofacial venous trunk. Lymph draining to this group is from the parotid, submaxillary retrolaryngeal, prelaryngeal, pretracheal, and recurrent areas and from the tongue, palate, tonsils, thyroid and submaxillary glands, nose, pharynx, and outer and middle ear.

The *deep cervical chain* is made up of four chains of lymph nodes: (1) the prelaryngeal chain, located anterior to the larynx; (2) the prethyroid chain, situated anterior to the thyroid gland; (3) the pretracheal and

laterotracheal chain, located anterior and lateral to the trachea; and (4) recurrent chains, found along the course of the recurrent laryngeal nerve. These nodes receive lymph via the collecting ducts from the larynx, thyroid gland, trachea, and upper part of the esophagus. The efferent vessels go to the internal jugular chain, mediastinal lymph nodes, and the brachiocephalic trunk.

The finger must be bent or hooked around the sternocleidomastoid muscle to palpate the deep cervical nodes, which are frequently enlarged in rubella, infectious mononucleosis, and hepatitis.

Thus, the *internal jugular chain* is made up of many lymph nodes in contact with the jugular vein. The last of these nodes lie in contact with the thoracic duct.

The *chain of the spinal nerve* consists of four to twelve nodes and follows the external branch of the spinal nerve (CN IX). Collecting ducts from the posterior and lateral regions of the neck reach these nodes, as well as those of the occipital and mastoid regions of the head.

The posterior superficial cervical *transverse cervical artery chain* of six to eight lymph nodes follows the transverse cervical artery and vein (between the anterior scalene muscle and the carotid sheath). This chain terminates in the great lymphatic trunk on the right side and in the thoracic duct on the left side. Lymph from the subclavian, laterocervical, anterothoracic, and internal mammary regions reaches these nodes.

The entire neck is lightly palpated for nodes (Fig. 13-5).

The anterior border of the sternocleidomastoid muscle is the dividing line for the anterior and posterior triangles of the neck. Description of the locus of the pathological condition may be facilitated through the use of these triangles (Figs. 13-6 and 13-7).

Bending the client's head forward (Figs. 13-8 and 13-9) or to the side being examined (Figs. 13-10 and 13-11) will obviate tissue tension and permit more accurate palpation.

Examination

The following maneuvers may be helpful in examining specific lymph node chains of the head and neck.

The *submental, sublingual,* and *submandibular nodes* can be examined by facing the client and placing the fingertips under the mandible on the side nearest the palpating hand. The skin and subcutaneous tissue are pulled laterally over the ramus of the mandible, and enlarged nodes can be felt as they roll over the mandibular surface beneath the examining fingers.

Another technique for the examination of the submandibular nodes is accomplished by placing one index finger in the floor of the mouth and the other fingers below the ramus of the mandible. The tissue between the fingers is gently rotated.

Palpation of the supraclavicular or *scalene* region (Fig. 13-12) on the client's right side can be done by bending the left index finger over the clavicle and just lateral to the tendinous portion of the sternocleidomastoid muscle. Moving the bent or hooked index finger in a rotary manner should allow nodes in the scalene triangle to be felt. The index finger should probe deeply into the triangle. To facilitate this entry, bending the client's head forward with the right hand will promote relaxation of the sternocleidomastoid muscle. The hand maneuver is reversed for the client's left scalene area.

The client is encouraged to generally relax the musculature of the upper extremities so that the clavicles will be pulled down, allowing the supraclavicular area to be explored thoroughly.

Because of their location in proximity to the termination of the thoracic duct and other terminal lymphatic ducts, the supraclavicular nodes are frequently the sites of metastatic cancer. Virchow first described this phenomenon in 1849. Virchow's nodes are located in the left supraclavicular (scalene) region. However, mediastinal collecting ducts from the lungs go to both sides of the neck and thus may provide an avenue for metastasis of lung cancer to either supraclavicular region. The nodes from the supraclavicular region are frequently biopsied (scalene node biopsy) to search for occult metastases from the lung or esophagus and for gastric, pancreatic, or other abdominal structures. The supraclavicular nodes are the lowermost nodes of the internal jugular and posterior superficial cervical chains. The enlarged supraclavicular node connotes a serious prognosis. The supraclavicular node is less prone to infectious processes, especially those stemming from sinus infection, tonsillitis, and poor dental hygiene.

The posterior cervical nodes are examined from behind or while facing the client and by placing the dorsal surface of the fingertips along the anterior sur-

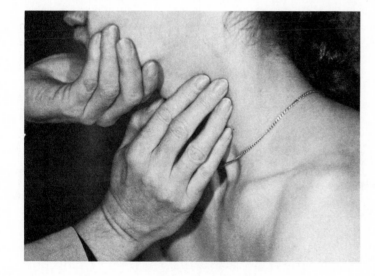

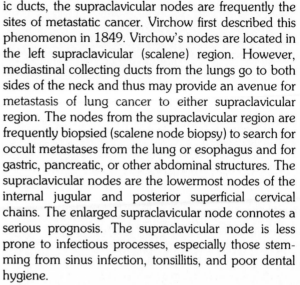

Fig. 13-5
The entire neck is lightly palpated for nodes. The anterior triangle is being palpated in this photograph.

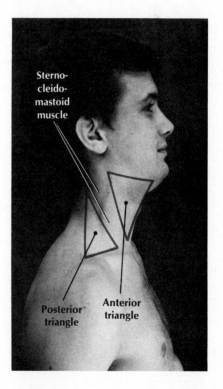

Fig. 13-6
The conception of the triangles of the neck is useful in defining the location of palpable lymph nodes. The sternocleidomastoid muscle is the division line between the anterior and posterior triangles. The trapezius muscle marks the posterior border of the posterior triangle. (Point of interest: this subject is executing a Valsalva's maneuver in an attempt not to laugh. Note the distention of the jugular vein as it passes over the sternocleidomastoid muscle.)

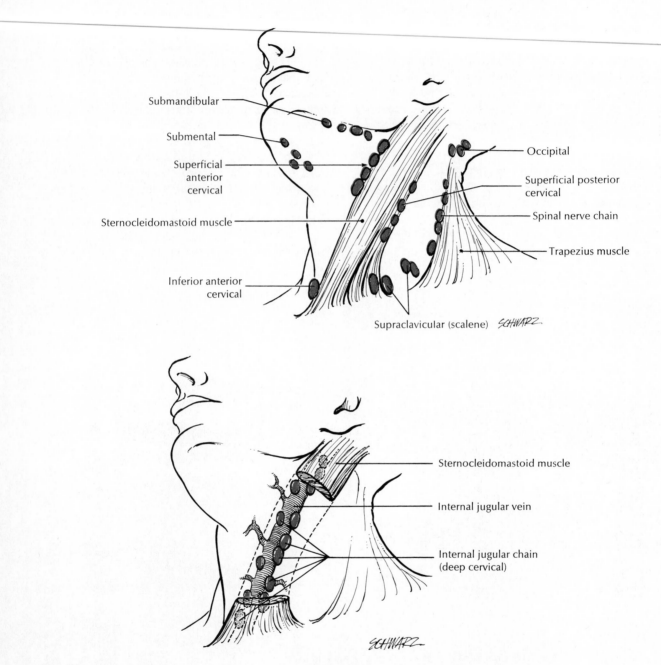

Submandibular

Submental

Superficial
anterior
cervical

Sternocleidomastoid muscle

Inferior anterior
cervical

Occipital

Superficial posterior
cervical

Spinal nerve chain

Trapezius muscle

Supraclavicular (scalene)   *SCHWARZ*

Sternocleidomastoid muscle

Internal jugular vein

Internal jugular chain
(deep cervical)

SCHWARZ

Fig. 13-7
The lymph nodes of the neck. Note relationship to the sternocleidomastoid muscle.

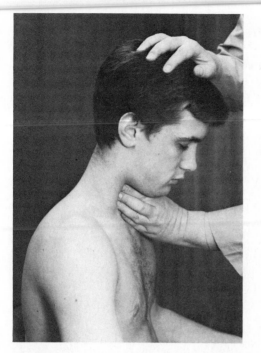

Fig. 13-8
Palpation of the anterior triangle.

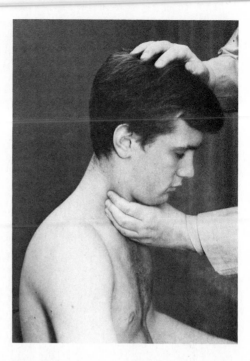

Fig. 13-9
Palpation of the posterior triangle.

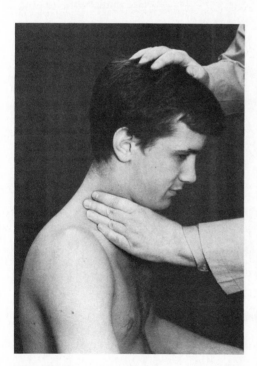

Fig. 13-10
Flexing the neck to obviate tissue tension.

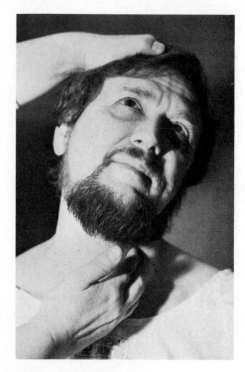

Fig. 13-11
Bending the head toward the side being examined to
relax muscles and soft tissue, allowing more accurate
palpation for lymph nodes.

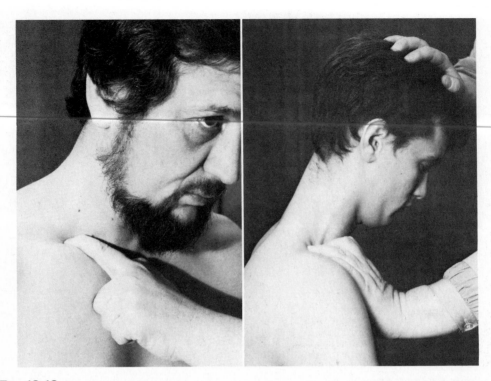

Fig. 13-12
Palpation of the scalene triangle for the supraclavicular lymph nodes. The client is encouraged to relax the musculature of the upper extemities, so that the clavicles are dropped. The examiner's free hand is used to flex the client's head forward to obtain relaxation of the soft tissues of the anterior neck. The left index finger is hooked over the clavicle lateral to the sternocleidomastoid muscle.

face of the trapezius muscle and moving them slowly forward in a circular motion against the posterior surface of the sternocleidomastoid muscle (Fig. 13-13).

In some cases it is possible to determine the source of an infection from a characteristic pattern of lymph node involvement. For instance, infections of the tongue might produce enlargement of the submental, submandibular, suprahyoid, thyrolinguofacial, and internal jugular nodes (Fig. 13-14).

Another example would be infections of the ear that typically involve the preauricular, mastoid, parotid retropharyngeal, and deep cervical nodes (Fig. 13-15).

Neck masses

Neck masses in clients over 35 are regarded as highly suspicious of malignancy. Almost all clients who have squamous cell carcinoma are heavy smokers. The curve of incidence of squamous cell carcinoma related to cigarette smoking starts to rise at one pack a day for 20 years. Other carcinogens related to neck masses are asbestos and leather tanning agents.

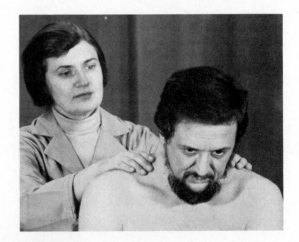

Fig. 13-13
Palpation of the posterior cervical nodes and spinal nerve chain. The dorsal surfaces (pads) of the fingertips are used to palpate along the anterior surface of the trapezius muscle and then moved slowly forward in a circular movement toward the posterior surface of the sternocleidomastoid muscle.

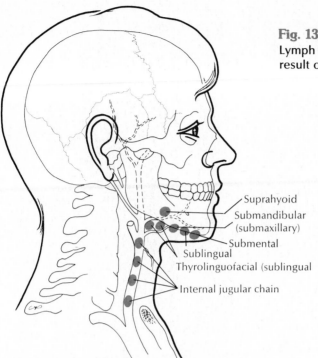

Fig. 13-14
Lymph nodes that may be potentially involved as a result of a pathological condition of the tongue.

Suprahyoid
Submandibular (submaxillary)
Submental
Sublingual
Thyrolinguofacial (sublingual
Internal jugular chain

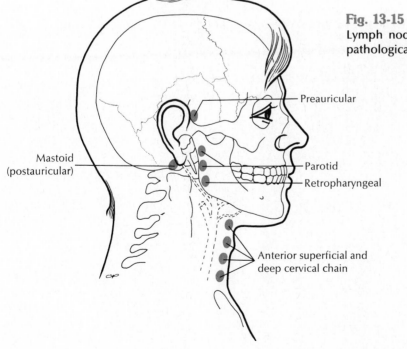

Fig. 13-15
Lymph nodes that may be involved as a result of a pathological condition of the ear.

Preauricular
Mastoid (postauricular)
Parotid
Retropharyngeal
Anterior superficial and deep cervical chain

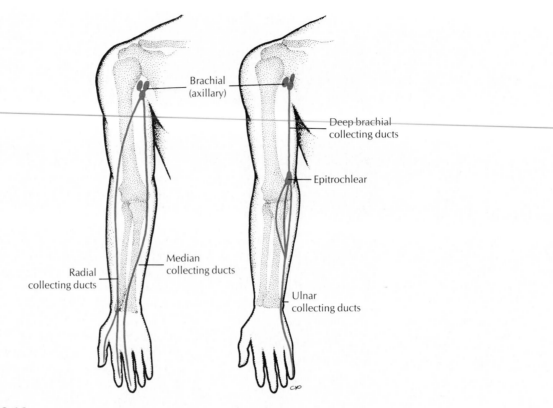

Fig. 13-16
System of deep and superficial collecting ducts, carrying the lymph from the upper extremity to the subclavian lymphatic trunk. The only peripheral lymph center is the epitrochlear, which receives some of the collecting ducts from the pathways of the ulnar and radial nerves.

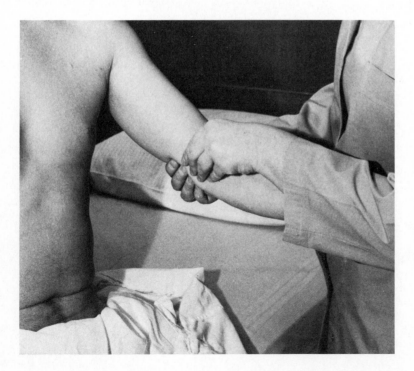

Fig. 13-17
Palpation for the epitrochlear lymph nodes is performed in the depression above and posterior to the medial condyle of the humerus.

A large posterior triangle node without any other enlarged nodes is most frequently from the oral cavity and anterior tongue. Metastases in nodes low in the neck most commonly originate from primary tumors below the clavicle, such as the lung, gastrointestinal tract pancreatic and colorectal tumors, prostate, and bladder.

Upper extremity

A system of superficial and deep collecting ducts carries the lymph from the upper extremity to the subclavian lymphatic trunk (Fig. 13-16). The only peripheral lymph center is the epitrochlear center, which receives some of the collecting ducts from the pathway of the ulnar artery and nerve and is located in a depression above and posterior to the medial condyle of the humerus (Fig. 13-17).

Enlargement of these nodes may be seen in secondary syphilis.

Lymphatics of the ulnar surface of the forearm, the little and ring fingers, and the medial surface of the middle finger drain into the epitrochlear nodes. Efferent ducts drain into the axillary or infraclavicular nodes, or both.

Axillary region

There are an average of fifty-three lymph nodes in the axillary fossa. Five groups of lymph nodes are distinguished in this area (Fig. 13-18).

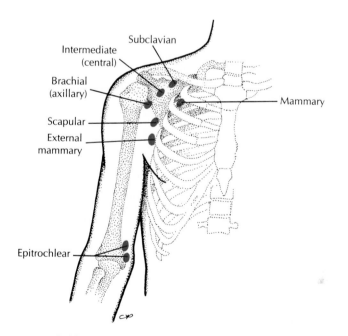

Fig. 13-18
Five groups of lymph nodes may be distinguished in the axillary fossa.

The *center of the axillary or brachial veins, or lateral group,* consists of two to seven nodes lying close to the axillary vein. These nodes receive collecting ducts from the upper extremity, deltoid region, and anterior wall of the chest, including the breast. Efferent ducts from this center terminate in the central lymph center, although some are known to connect with the subclavian lymph center.

The *scapular center,* or *posterior group,* consists of four or five nodes in contact with the inferior scapular vessels. The collecting ducts converging on these nodes are from the posterior wall of the chest and the posteroinferior neck. The efferent ducts drain to the central lymph center.

The *central* or *intermediate center* consists of eight to ten nodes and receives ducts from the brachial and scapular lymph centers and from the chest wall, breast, and arm. The ducts leaving these nodes go to the subclavian lymph center.

The *external mammary center,* or *anterior* or *pectoral group,* is a chain of nodes located along the course of the external mammary artery. A superior group of two or three nodes is found in the region of the third rib and the second and third intercostal spaces, and an inferior group is located over the fourth to sixth ribs. The ducts entering these nodes are from the breast and anterolateral chest wall and from the integument and muscles of the abdominal wall superior to the umbilicus. The efferent ducts from these nodes go to the subclavian center.

The *subclavian,* or *infraclavicular, center* may contain one to nine nodes situated in the tissues of the upper axilla. It receives lymph from all the other axillary centers, and ducts from this center empty into the venous junction of the jugular and subclavian veins.

Infections of the hand and arm may result in enlargement of these nodes.

Axillary examination is approached by regarding the area as a four-sided pyramid with its apex superior. The apex is located between the first rib and the clavicle. The apex in lay parlance is the armpit. The anterior border of the axilla is formed by the pectoral muscles; the posterior border is made up of back muscles, including the latissimus dorsi and subscapularis muscles; the medial border consists of the rib cage and serratus anterior muscle, and the lateral border, of the upper arm. Thus, the sides are anterior, posterior, medial, and lateral. Inspection and palpation must be done for each of the anatomical sides, first in a position of partial adduction of the subject's arms and then in abduction. The examination of the axillary area is accomplished by gently rolling the soft tissues against the chest wall and the muscles of the axilla (Fig. 13-19). Bimanual palpation is performed anteriorly to

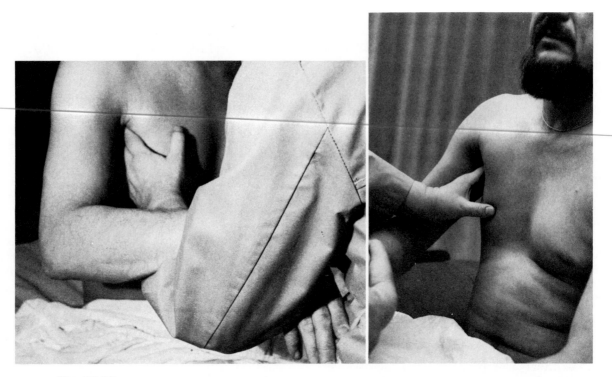

Fig. 13-19
The soft tissues of the axilla are gently rolled against the chest wall and the muscles surround-ing the axilla. Note two methods of supporting the client's arm.

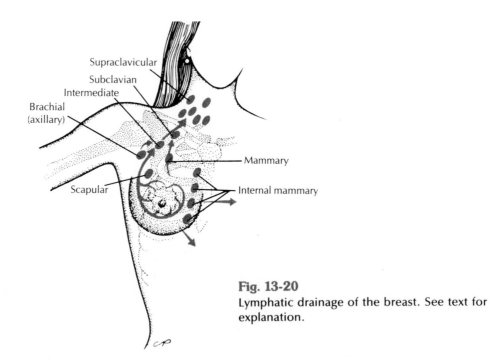

Fig. 13-20
Lymphatic drainage of the breast. See text for explanation.

encompass the pectoralis muscle, as well as the posterior wall to include the back muscles.

Breast

The lymphatic system of the breast is particularly abundant. The lymphatic vessels drain to two major sites: the axillary and the internal mammary centers (Fig. 13-20). Lymph from the lower outer quadrant of the breast drains to the lateroinferior lymph nodes. Lymph from the areolar area, the upper outer quadrant, and the tail of Spence drains to the mediosuperior axillary nodes. Lymph then courses through efferent ducts to the infraclavicular and supraclavicular nodes. The lymph from the inner aspect of the breast drains to the internal mammary nodes, which are three to four in number and inaccessible to palpation.

Lower extremity

As in the upper extremity, a system of superficial and deep collecting ducts drains the lymph from the leg (Fig. 13-21). Two or three nodes make up the *popliteal lymph center* in the back of the knee near the terminal portion of the saphenous vein. The afferent ducts to these nodes are, in fact, from the regions surrounding the external saphenous vein, that is, the heel and the outer aspect of the foot. However, the majority of the lymph is delivered to the inguinal nodes.

Superficial inguinal lymph center

A superior and inferior group of superficial inguinal nodes has been described.

The *inferior group* is a group of large lymph nodes that receive lymph from the superficial plexuses of the leg and foot (Fig. 13-22). They are the inguinal nodes below the junction of the saphenous and femoral veins. The superficial nodes lie along the course of the saphenous vein. The deep subinguinal nodes lie medial to the femoral vein and follow the vessel into the abdomen. Cloquet's gland, a node of this group, lies immediately above the saphenous opening. When this node is enlarged, incarcerated, or strangulated, femoral hernia may result.

The *superior group* is a center containing five or six nodes whose afferent ducts are from the abdominal wall inferior to the umbilicus, the buttocks, and the external genital organs, as well as the efferent vessels from the inferior center (Fig. 13-23). The superior group of nodes lies along and parallel to the inguinal ligament.

• • •

Fig. 13-24 is a diagrammatic summary of the areas where pathological lymph nodes may be identified by inspection and palpation. These are the sites to be assessed during the physical examination.

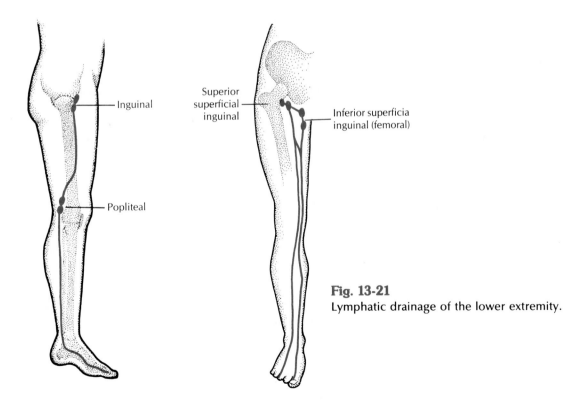

Inguinal

Popliteal

Superior superficial inguinal

Inferior superficial inguinal (femoral)

Fig. 13-21
Lymphatic drainage of the lower extremity.

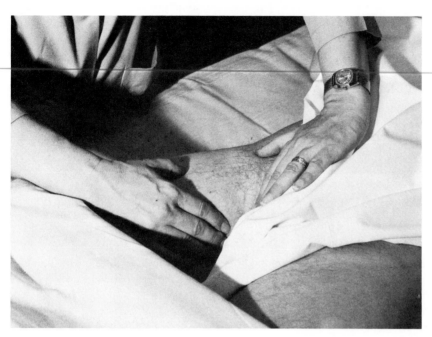

Fig. 13-22
Palpation of the inferior superficial inguinal (femoral) lymph nodes.

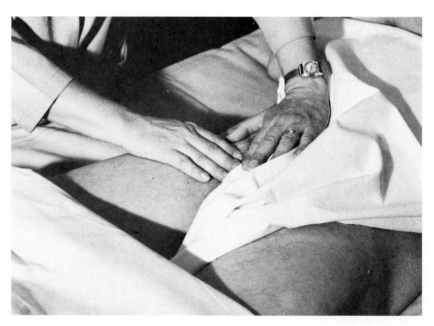

Fig. 13-23
Palpation of the superior superficial inguinal lymph nodes.

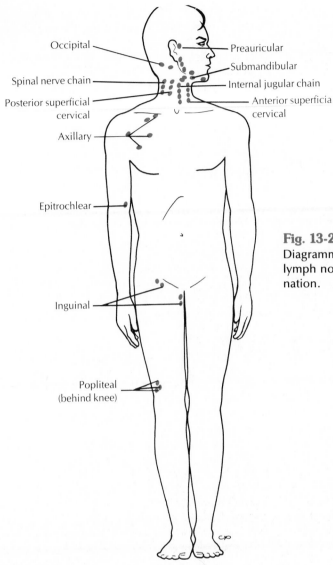

Occipital

Preauricular

Submandibular

Spinal nerve chain

Internal jugular chain

Posterior superficial cervical

Anterior superficia cervical

Axillary

Epitrochlear

Inguinal

Popliteal (behind knee)

Fig. 13-24
Diagrammatic summary of the areas to be examined for lymph nodes during the course of the physical examination.

PATHOLOGY
Common diseases related to lymph node characteristics

The assessment parameters of pathological lymph nodes may combine to establish the diagnosis of the disease process of the client. Some common findings related to specific diseases are described here.

Acute pyogenic infections. The nodes of acute infections are large, tender, and discrete. These alterations are accompanied by the classical signs of inflammation, which are *tumor* (swelling), *color* (redness and heat), and *dolor* (tenderness). The nodes may become confluent if the infection becomes chronic. The involvement may lead to limitation of motion.

Inflammatory nodes tend to be rather soft and somewhat tender, and they fluctuate in size during an episode of viral or bacterial infection.

Among the more common infections associated with enlarged nodes in the neck are viral exanthems of infectious mononucleosis (75% to 80%), cytomegalic inclusion disease (10% or less), and toxoplasmosis (1%). Other infectious diseases causing cervical adenopathy are mumps, other viruses, Rocky Mountain spotted fever, and cat-scratch fever, and the mycobacteria. Granulomatous processes may be a result of actinomycosis, coccidioidomycosis, and blastomycosis.

Individuals with a deficiency of secretory IgA may have adenopathy often associated with recurrent tonsillitis and upper respiratory infections. Lymphadenopathy is found with a higher than normal incidence in intravenous drug abusers. This must be considered in children as well, since addiction has been seen in small children (8 to 11 years of age). Lymphadenopathy is frequently seen in individuals with an acquired immune deficiency syndrome (AIDS) and is often observed early in the disease. The adenopathy is generalized rather than localized. Lymphadenopathy is commonly seen in children and adults (e.g., hemophiliacs) who are given blood products.

Tuberculosis. The lymph nodes of the tubercular client may be soft and matted together. The nodes are generally nontender to the client. Occasionally sinus formation is present.

Hodgkin's disease. Hodgkin's disease results in lymph node involvement in which the nodes are large, discrete, nontender, and of a firm, rubbery consistency.

Syphilis. A lymph node in the chain draining a syphilitic chancre is called a bubo. Characteristically, the nodes are enlarged, hard, nonfluctuant, and painless. Such a node in the inguinal chain should prompt the practitioner to inspect thoroughly for a genital chancre.

Metastatic cancer. Lymph nodes of metastatic cancer are described as discrete, nontender, of a firm to hard consistency, and unilateral in focus. They may be small or several centimeters in diameter.

Common disorders of lymphatic vessels

Acute lymphangitis. The chief complaint of the client may include pain in the affected extremity. Elevation of temperature may be present, and the client may complain of malaise.

Inspection of the affected limb may reveal redness along the course of lymphatic collecting ducts, which appear as fine lines. The tubules may be palpable. The source of infection is sought. In the lower extremity interdigital spaces are carefully examined for cracks, which are often the site of entry for epidermophytosis.

Lymphedema. Congenital lymphedema may result in swelling or distortion of the extremities caused by hypoplasia and maldevelopment of the system. Trauma to the ducts, allergy, infection, or tumor leading to blockage may result in lymphedema. This condition may be the result of surgery of the regional lymph nodes, as in radical mastectomy or groin dissection. Extension of cancer to the lymphatics may also result in stasis of lymph flow. Infection may also block lymphatic ducts.

Painless swelling of the involved extremity is the earliest and most common indication of lymphedema. Initially the swelling may subside at night, but as the process progresses and the subcutaneous tissue and skin become fibrotic, the swelling becomes permanent. Skin color and texture are generally normal early in the condition, but in late stages the skin becomes thickened and brown and multiple papillary projections (lymphostatic verrucosis) are seen.

The tissue involved in lymphedema pits only with difficulty. The tissue of the dorsa of the toes and feet are swollen with lymphedema of the lower extremity; this is uncommon in other causes of edema.

Elephantiasis. *Elephantiasis* is the term used for the massive accumulation of lymphedema. The condition may be the sequela of congenital or acquired forms of lymphedema. The marked lymphedema predisposes the client to further infection and episodes of cellulitis. Recurrent infectious involvement leads to marked fibrosis of the edematous tissues.

BIBLIOGRAPHY

Battezatti, M., and Donini, I.: The lymphatic system, New York, 1973, John Wiley & Sons, Inc.

Brady, L.W., and others: Differentiating neck masses in children, Patient Care **18:**12, 1984.

Brady, L.W., and others: Causes of neck masses in young adults, Patient Care **18:**30, 1984.

Brady, L.W., and others: When an older adult develops a neck mass, Patient Care **18:**56, 1984.

Brouse, N.L.: Response of lymphatics to sympathetic nerve stimulation, J. Physiol. **197:**25, 1968.

Haagensen, C.D., and others: The lymphatics in cancer, Philadelphia, 1972, W.B. Saunders Co.

Kinmonth, J.B.: The lymphatic disease: lymphography and surgery, Baltimore, 1972, Williams & Wilkins.

Mayerson, H.S.: Lymph and lymphatic system, Springfield, Ill., 1968, Charles C Thomas, Publisher.

Solnitzky, O.C., and Jeghers, H.: Lymphadenopathy and disorders of the lymphatic system. In McBride, C., and Blacklow, R., editors: Signs and symptoms: applied pathologic physiology and clinical interpretation, Philadelphia, 1970, J.B. Lippincott Co.

Yoffey, J.M., and Courtice, F.C.: Lymphatics: lymph and the lymphomyeloid complex, New York, 1970, Academic Press, Inc.

Zitelli, B.J.: Neck masses in children: adenopathy and malignant disease, Pediatr. Clin. North Am. **28:**813, 1981.

Zuelzer, W.W., and Kaplan, J.: The child with lymphadenopathy, Semin. Hematol. **12:**323, 1975.

CHAPTER 14

ASSESSMENT OF THE BREASTS

ANATOMY

The breast is a modified sebaceous gland that is paired and located on the anterior chest wall between the second and third ribs superiorly, the sixth and seventh costal cartilages inferiorly, the anterior axillary line laterally, and the sternal border medially.

The functional components of the breast consist of the acini or milk-producing glands, a ductal system, and a nipple (Fig. 14-1, A). The glandular tissue units are called lobes and are situated in circular, spokelike fashion around the nipple. There are fifteen to twenty-five lobes per breast. Each lobe is composed of twenty to forty lobules, each containing ten to 100 acini.

Much of the bulk of the breast is composed of subcutaneous and retromammary fat. The breast is fairly mobile but is supported by a layer of subcutaneous connective tissue and by Cooper's ligaments (Fig. 14-1, B). The latter are multiple fibrous bands that begin at the breast's subcutaneous connective tissue layer and run through the breast, attaching to muscle fascia.

Knowledge of the lymphatic drainage of the breast is critical because of the frequent dissemination of breast cancer through this system. There are three types of lymphatic drainage of the breast (Fig. 14-2).

Cutaneous lymphatic drainage is of lymph from the skin of the breast, excluding the areolar and nipple areas; this lymph flows into the ipsilateral axillary nodes (the mammary, scapular, brachial, and intermediate nodes). Lymph from the medial cutaneous breast area may flow to the opposite breast. Lymph from the inferior portion of the breast can reach the lymphatic plexus of the epigastric region and subsequently the liver and other abdominal regions and organs.

Areolar lymphatic drainage is of lymph formed in the areolar and nipple areas of the breast; this lymph flows into the anterior axillary group of nodes (the mammary nodes).

Deep lymphatic drainage is of lymph from the deep mammary tissues; this lymph flows into the anterior axillary nodes. Some of this lymph also flows into the apical, subclavian, infraclavicular, and supraclavicular nodes. Also, lymph from the retroareolar areas, medial glandular breast tissue areas, and lower glandular breast tissue areas communicate with lymphatic systems draining into the thorax and abdomen.

The largest portion of glandular breast tissue occurs in the upper lateral quadrant of each breast. From this quadrant there is an anatomical projection of breast tissue into the axilla. This projection is termed the axillary tail of Spence (Fig. 14-3). The majority of breast tumors are located in the upper lateral breast quadrant and in the tail of Spence.

On general appearance the normal breasts are reasonably symmetrical in size and shape, although not usually absolutely equal. This symmetry remains constant at rest and with movement. The skin of the breast is the same as that of the abdomen or back. There may be a small number of scattered hair follicles around the areola. In light-complected persons a horizontal or vertical vascular pattern may be observed. This pattern, when normally present, is symmetrical.

The areolae are pigmented areas surrounding the nipples. Their color varies from pink to brown, and their size varies greatly. Several or many sebaceous glands (termed Montgomery's tubercles or follicles) may be present on the areolar surface.

The nipples are round, hairless, pigmented, protuberant structures whose size and shape vary among women and in an individual woman depending on the state of contraction. Usually nipples are directed or "point" slightly upward and laterally.

Inversion of the nipple is an invagination or depression of its central portion. Inversion can occur congenitally or as a response to an invasive process.

During early embryonic development longitudinal

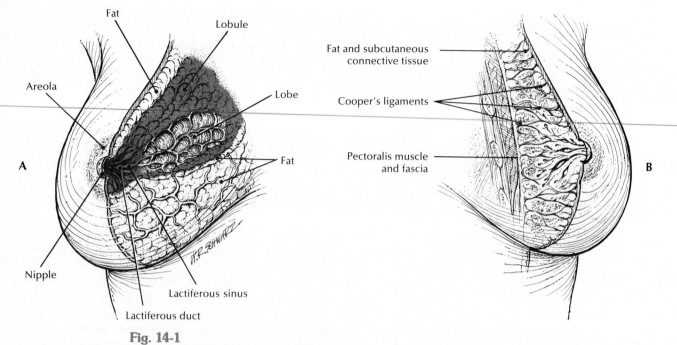

Fig. 14-1
Female breasts. **A,** Internal structures. **B,** Supportive tissue structures.

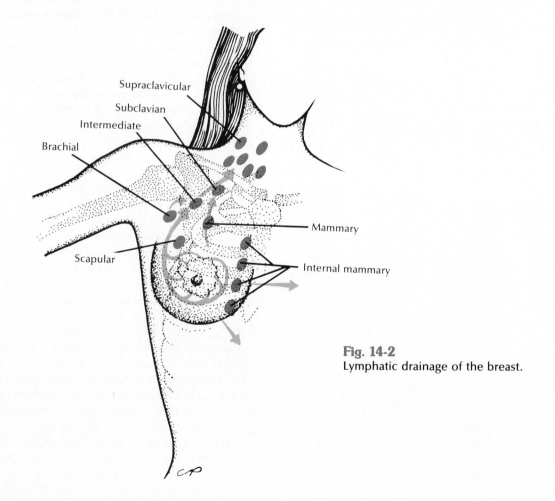

Fig. 14-2
Lymphatic drainage of the breast.

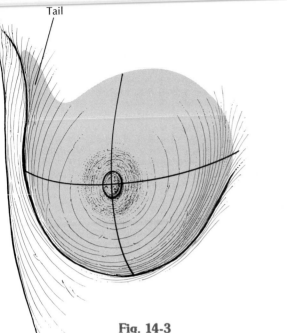

Fig. 14-3
Axillary tail of Spence.

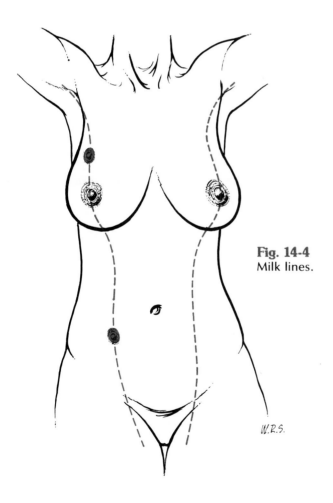

Fig. 14-4
Milk lines.

ridges exist, extending from the axilla to the groin. Called "milk lines" (Fig. 14-4), these ridges usually atrophy, except at the level of the pectoral muscles, where a breast will eventually develop. In some women the ridges do not entirely disappear, and portions of the milk lines persist. This existence is manifested in the presence of a nipple, a nipple and a breast, or glandular breast tissue only. This congenital anomaly is termed a supernumerary breast or nipple.

The gross appearance and size of the normal female breast vary both among individuals and for an individual at various phases of development. The following describes breast development through a woman's life span (Fig. 14-5):

1. *Appearance before age 10:* There is little difference in gross appearance between male and female breasts. The nipples are small and slightly elevated. There is no palpable glandular tissue or areolar pigmentation.

2. *Appearance between the ages of 10 and 14:* The mammary tissues adjacent to and beneath the areola grow, resulting in an increased diameter of the areola and the formation of a "mammary bud." The nipple and breast protrude as a single mound. Breast development may normally begin or progress unilaterally. Next the general mammary growth and increases in diameter and pigmentation of the areola continue, resulting in further elevation of the breasts. The separation of the nipple from the areola begins. Growth continues in the mammary tissues. The nipple and areola form a mound distinct from the globular shape of the rest of the breast.

3. *Appearance after age 14:* The shape of the adult female breast is gradually formed. The areola recedes into the general contour of the breast, and only the nipple protrudes. The size of the adult female breast is influenced by heredity, individual sensitivity to hormones, and nutrition.

4. *Appearance during the female reproductive years:* In response to hormonal changes during the menstrual cycle, there is a cyclic pattern of breast size change, along with nodularity and tenderness, that is maximal just before menses. The breast is smallest in days 4 through 7 of the menstrual cycle. During days 3 to 4 before the onset of menses, mammary tenseness, fullness, heaviness, tenderness, and pain are experienced by many women, and the total breast volume is significantly increased.

5. *Changes in pregnancy:* The breast increases in size, sometimes to as large as two or three times

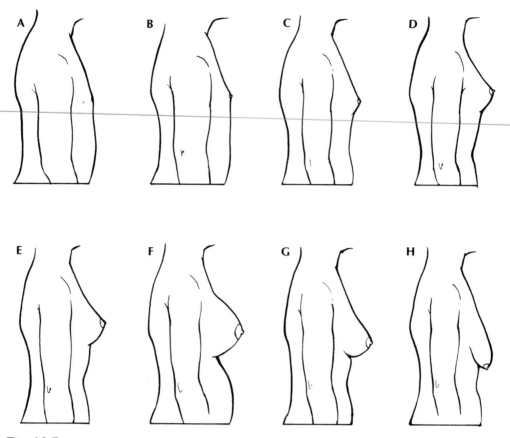

Fig. 14-5
Appearance of the female breast in various life periods. **A,** Appearance before age 10. **B** to **D,** Appearance between ages 10 through 14. **E,** Appearance of the nulliparous, adult, female breast. **F,** Appearance of the breast during pregnancy. **G,** Appearance of the breast in a woman who has had a pregnancy. **H,** Appearance of the breast after menopause.

the usual size. The areolae and nipples become more prominent and more deeply pigmented. The veins engorge, the Montgomery's glands become more apparent, and striae are often observed.

6. *Menopausal changes:* After menopause, the breast's glandular tissue gradually involutes, and fat is deposited in the breasts. Breast form becomes flabby and flattened.

The male breast contains a nipple and an areola. Beneath the nipple is a small amount of breast tissue, which usually cannot be clinically differentiated from the other subcutaneous tissues.

EXAMINATION
Approach to the examination

Some girls and women are embarrassed during the breast examination. The examiner should take care to assure privacy for the examination and to avoid unnecessary exposure of the breasts. Explanation of the

components of the examination can also assist to relieve discomfort.

During the health history preceding the physical examination, the examiner should assess the woman's level of knowledge and practice regarding breast self-examination. The examination provides an excellent opportunity for teaching self-examination and for reviewing the client's technique.

If the client has noticed a lump or change in one of the breasts, ask her to point out the area and to demonstrate the technique used to note the lump or change. The examiner can take special note of that area during the examination.

Many adolescent or adult male clients may not have had a breast examination previously and may be concerned that the examiner may have noticed a problem. Explanation to male clients that breast lesions are possible in men and that the breast examination is a routine component of a complete health assessment can decrease the possibility of worry and embarrassment.

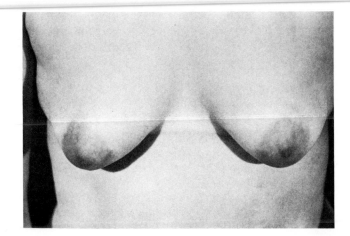

Fig. 14-6
Observation of the breasts. These breasts have several characteristics that are deviations within normal limits: (1) the left breast is slightly larger than the right; (2) the direction of the nipples is slightly different; and (3) there are two indentations in the outer right breast.

Often male clients have perspiration in the axilla and are embarrassed when a female examiner palpates the dampened area. A tissue may be offered to the male client to dry the area.

Inspection

Inspection and palpation are the techniques used in the examination of the breast. No special equipment is necessary. The client is uncovered to the waist and is seated on the side of the examining table. The breasts are observed for (1) symmetry of shape, color, size, and surface characteristics; (2) hyperpigmentation; (3) moles or nevi; (4) edema; (5) retraction or dimpling; (6) abnormal amount or distribution of hair; (7) presence of focal vascularity; and (8) lesions (Fig. 14-6).

Retraction, or dimpling, appears as a depression or pucker on the skin (Fig. 14-7, A). It usually is caused by the fibrotic shortening and immobilization of Cooper's ligament by an invasive process.

Whenever the skin of the breasts is stretched rapidly, damage to the elastic fibers or the dermis may occur and observable striae, or stretch marks, are produced. Newly created striae appear reddish; they become whitish with age.

Edema of the breasts produces exaggeration of the skin pores, creating an orange peel appearance of the breast, called peau d'orange (Fig. 14-7, B).

Vascular patterns should be diffuse and symmetrical. Focal or unilateral patterns are abnormal (Fig. 14-7, A).

The areolar area is inspected for size, shape, symmetry, color, surface characteristics, bulging, and lesions. As mentioned previously, size, shape, and col-

or can normally vary greatly. Any asymmetry, mass, or lesion should be considered abnormal.

If the breasts are symmetrical, both nipples should be pointing laterally in the same way. The nipple is observed for size, shape, ability to erect, color, discharge, and lesions. The nipples should be round, equal in size, homogeneous in color, and have convoluted surfaces, which give them a wrinkled appearance. Inversion of one or both nipples, if present from puberty, is normal; however, this condition may interfere with breastfeeding. Recent inversion of the nipple is probably retraction (Fig. 14-7, A) and should be investigated.

Paget's disease appears as a red glandular erosion of the nipple or as a nipple that is dry scaly, or friable. The areola may also be affected. Paget's disease is a malignant condition requiring prompt therapy.

Breast secretions are normal in pregnancy or lactation. Other causes of discharge are mechanical nipple stimulation, drug influence, hypothalamic and pituitary disorders, and malignant and benign breast lesions. The discharge can be milky, watery, purulent, serous, or bloody. The method for determining the site of discharge production is discussed under "Palpation."

There are four major sitting positions of the client used for breast inspection. Every client should be examined in each position:

1. The client is seated with her arms at her sides.
2. The client is seated with her arms abducted over her head.
3. The client is seated and is pushing her hands into her hips, simultaneously eliciting contraction of the pectoral muscles.

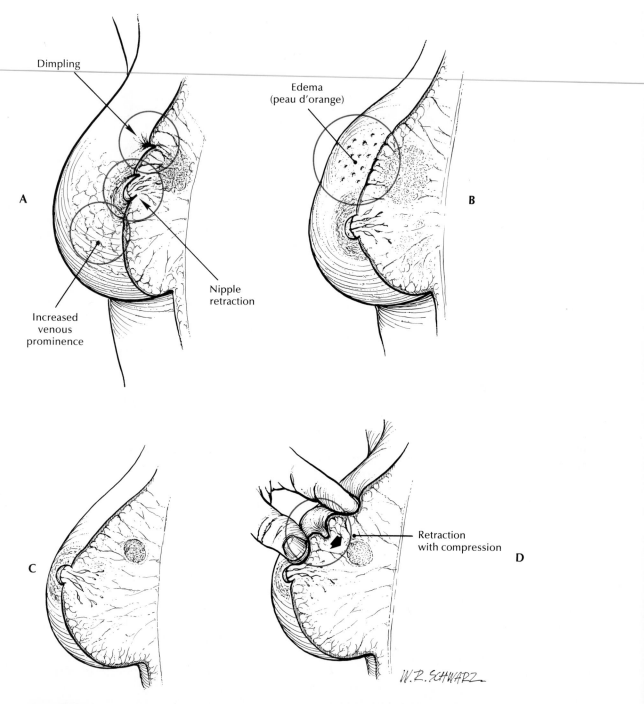

Fig. 14-7
Abnormalities of the breast. **A,** Breast with dimpling, nipple retraction, and increased venous prominence. **B,** Breast with edema (peau d'orange or pigskin appearance). **C,** Breast with tumor; no retraction is apparent. **D,** Breast with tumor; retraction is apparent with compression.

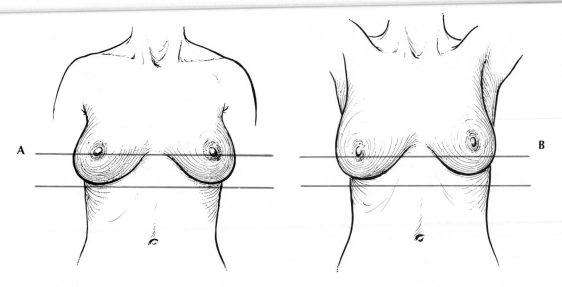

Fig. 14-8
A, Breasts appear symmetrical at rest. **B,** Breasts do not move symmetrically with arm elevation. The right breast is immobilized.

4. The client is seated and is leaning over while her
   examiner assists in supporting and balancing
   her.

While the client is performing these maneuvers, the
breasts are carefully observed for symmetry, bulging,
retraction, and fixation. An abnormality may not be
apparent in the breasts at rest (Fig. 14-8, *A*), but a mass
may cause the breasts, through invasion of suspensory
ligaments, to fix, preventing them from upward or forward movement in positions 2 (Fig. 14-8, *B*) and 4.
Position 3 specifically assists in eliciting dimpling if a
mass has infiltrated and shortened suspensory ligaments.

The breasts are also observed with the client lying
down, before the examiner palpates.

Palpation

The range of normal breast consistency is wide. The
normal breast feels granular. This granularity is generalized and becomes more prominent with age.

The breasts normally feel somewhat "lumpy." This
results from the configuration of the breast lobes, the
fat and connective tissue between and supporting the
lobes and other structures, and the irregular density of
lobules. Thus, the consistency of breasts is not uniform. However, this variation of consistency should be
noted uniformly through the breasts of an individual
client.

The breasts feel relatively homogeneous in the
young adolescent. The presence of progesterone in
pregnancy and premenstrually causes the breasts to

feel generally nodular. Hormonally induced nodularity
is bilateral and difuse.

The primary purpose for the palpation of breasts is
to discover masses. If a mass is discovered, it is assessed according to the following characteristics:

1. *Location:* Masses are designated according to the
   quadrant in which they lie: upper outer, lower
   outer, upper inner, or lower inner (Fig. 14-9, *A*).
   When describing the mass in the client's record,
   one may find it helpful to draw the mass within a
   diagram of the breast (Fig. 14-9, *B*). Another
   method of describing location is to visualize the
   breast as the face of a clock; the nipple is center.
   A mass can be designated, for example, as being
   "5 cm from the nipple in the 8 o'clock position."
2. *Size:* The size should be approximated in centimeters in all its planes. For example, a mass may
   be ovoid, 3 cm wide, 2 cm long, and 1 cm
   thick.
3. *Shape:* The shape may be round, ovoid, irregular, or matted. Matting occurs in the presence of
   multiple lesions.
4. *Consistency:* A breast may be soft or hard, solid
   or cystic.
5. *Discreteness:* The borders of the mass are assessed to determine if they are sharp and well
   defined or irregular.
6. *Mobility:* The examiner attempts to move the
   mass over the chest wall. It is noted as being freely movable, movable, or fixed.

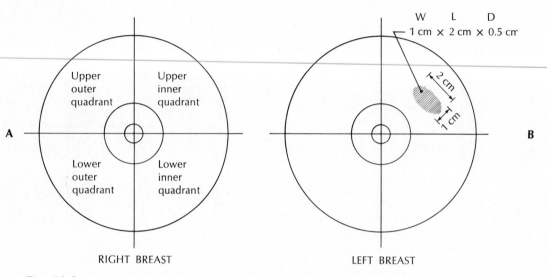

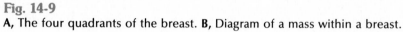

Fig. 14-9
A, The four quadrants of the breast. **B,** Diagram of a mass within a breast.

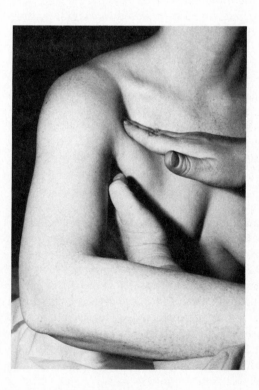

Fig. 14-10
Palpation of the axillary lymph nodes. (Note that the client's arm is supported on the arm of the examiner.)

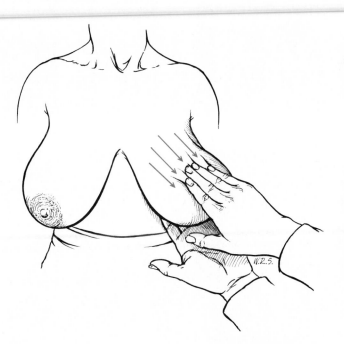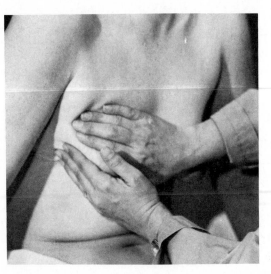

Fig. 14-11
Bimanual palpation of the breasts.

7. *Tenderness:* The client is questioned regarding any discomfort with palpation.
8. *Erythema:* The area of skin overlying the mass is inspected for erythema.
9. *Dimpling over the mass:* The tissue over the mass is compressed to determine if this maneuver produces dimpling (Fig. 14-7, *D*).

The palpation portion of the examination of the breast begins with palpation for axillary, subclavicular, and supraclavicular lymph nodes. This is most effectively performed with the client in a sitting position. The location and palpation of the axillary, subclavicular, and supraclavicular nodes are described in Chapter 13 on assessment of the lymphatic system. To emphasize the importance of an adequate axillary area examination with each breast examination, this procedure is reviewed here.

In examining the axilla, the tissues can be best appreciated if the area muscles are relaxed. Contracted muscles may obscure slightly enlarged nodes. To achieve this relaxation while at the same time abducting the arm, the examiner supports the ipsilateral arm (Fig. 14-10).

The examiner should visualize the axilla as a four-sided pyramid and thoroughly palpate the following areas: (1) the edge of the pectoralis major muscle for the mammary group of nodes, (2) the thoracic wall for the intermediate group of nodes, (3) the upper part of the humerus for the brachial axillary group of nodes,

and (4) the anterior edge of the latissimus dorsi muscle for the subscapular group of nodes.

The breasts are most effectively palpated with the client in a supine position. Because of time constraints on most physical examinations, it is not advised that all breasts be also palpated with the client in a sitting position. However, several groups of clients should also be examined in the sitting position: women with present or past complaints of breast masses, women at high risk of breast cancer, and women with pendulous breasts.

With the client in a sitting position, small breasts can be examined by using one hand to support the breast while the other hand palpates the tissue against the chest wall. Pendulous breasts are palpated using a bimanual technique (Fig. 14-11). The inferior portion of the breast is supported in one hand while the other palpates breast tissue against the supporting hand.

The client is then asked to lie down. The breasts are palpated while they are flattened against the rib cage. If the breasts are large, several mechanisms can be employed to enhance this flattening. A pillow can be placed under the ipsilateral shoulder, or the client can abduct the ipsilateral arm and place her hand under her neck. Both maneuvers shift the breast medially. The humerus should be at least slightly abducted to allow for thorough palpation of the tail of Spence.

The breasts are then thoroughly palpated (Fig. 14-12). The examiner should develop a system of breast

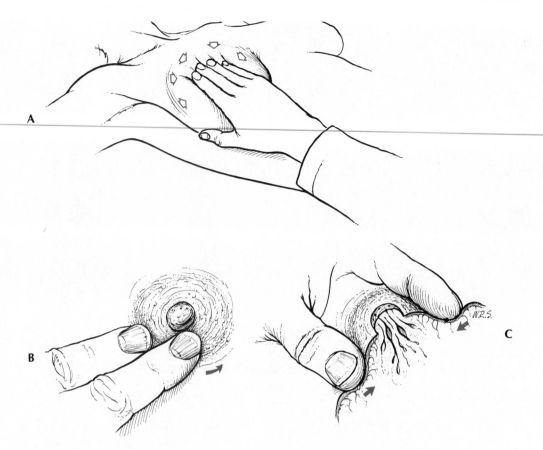

Fig. 14-12
Palpation of the breasts. **A**, Glandular area. **B**, Areolar area. **C**, Compression of the nipple.

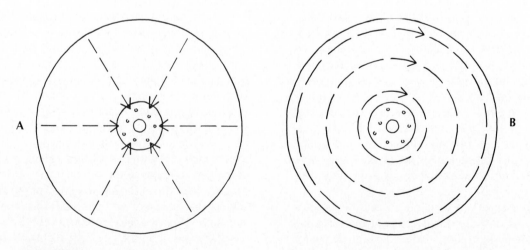

Fig. 14-13
Two methods of systematic breast palpation. **A**, Palpation in wedge sections from breast periphery to center. **B**, Palpation along concentric circles from periphery to center.

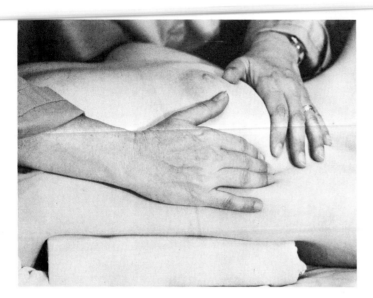

Fig. 14-14
Palpation of the axillary tail of Spence.

examination and habitually start and end at a fixed point on the breasts. The starting point is arbitrary. The breasts are palpated with the palmar surfaces of the fingers held together. The movements are smooth and back and forth or circular. The breast is visualized as a bicycle wheel with six or eight spokes, and palpation occurs along each spoke until the breast has been thoroughly surveyed (Fig. 14-13, *A*). Special attention is focused on the upper outer quadrant area and on the tail of Spence (Fig. 14-14).

An alternate method of breast palpation is to consider the breast as a group of concentric circles with the nipple as the center. Palpation occurs along the circumferences of the circle, starting at the outermost circle, until the total breast area is adequately surveyed (Fig. 14-13, *B*).

The areolar areas are carefully palpated to determine the presence of underlying masses. Each nipple is gently compressed to assess for the presence of masses or discharge (Fig. 14-12, *C*). If discharge is noted, the breast is milked along its radii to identify the lobe from which the discharge is originating. Compression of the discharge-producing lobe will cause discharge to exude from the nipple.

If a client reports a breast nodule, the "normal" breast is examined first so that the baseline consistency of that breast will serve as a control when the reportedly abnormal one is palpated.

Mammary folds, crescent-shaped ridges of breast tissue found at the inferior portions of very large or pendulous breasts, may be confused with breast masses but are nonpathological.

The sequence of the breast examination is illustrated in Fig. 14-15.

Despite improved mammographic techniques and their availability, a large portion of malignant breast lesions are found by women themselves. Therefore, the health-oriented examiner should assess each client's level of knowledge and practice related to breast self-examination. During the practitioner's examination of the breasts, the practitioner can describe the steps of the examination and the rationale for each step. A return demonstration by the client on her own breasts reinforces learning and memory of the procedure.

The following points should be emphasized in the teaching of breast self-examination:
1. The majority of breast lumps are not cancer.
2. The majority of cancerous breast lesions are curable.
3. Breasts should be examined each month between the fourth through the seventh day of the menstrual cycle, when the breasts are least congested.
4. Visual inspection and palpation should be done.
5. Visual inspection should be done in four arm positions and while the woman is stripped to her waist and looking at herself in a mirror. The four arm positions are: arms at rest, hands on hips and pressed into the hips contracting chest muscles, hands over the head, and torso leaning forward.
6. Many women prefer to do palpation in the shower when the soap and water assist the hands to glide easily over the skin. However, the examination of large breasts and the axilla are better done in a supine than a standing position. There-

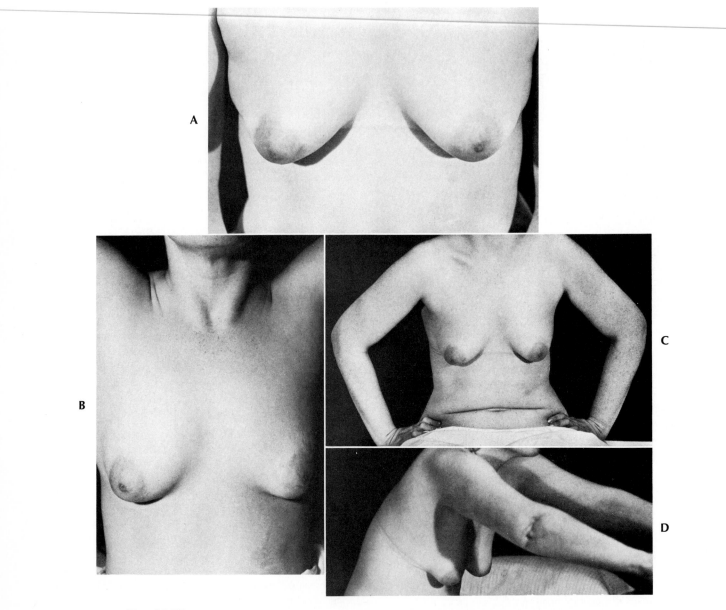

Fig. 14-15
Sequence of the breast examination. **A,** Observation of the breasts at rest. **B,** Observation with client's arms overhead. **C,** Observation with client contracting pectoral muscles. **D,** Observation with client leaning forward.

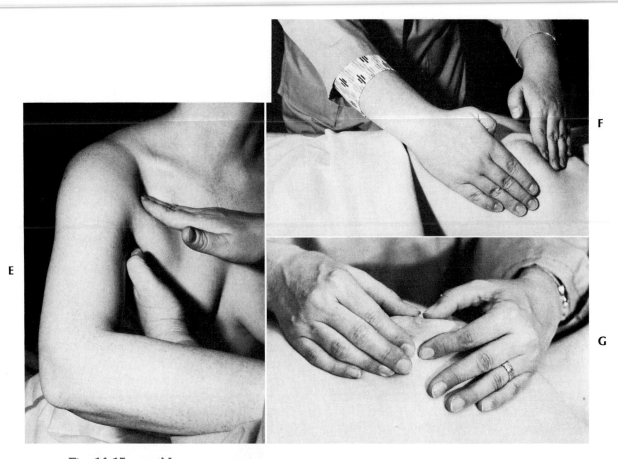

Fig. 14-15, cont'd
E, Palpation of axillary nodes. (Palpation of the supraclavicular and subclavicular areas is not illustrated.) **F,** Palpation of the glandular area. **G,** Palpation of the nipple and areolar area.

fore, supine examination is recommended, as well as the examination in the bath and shower.

7. The entire breast should be examined in a systematic way.
8. Specific examination of the nipple, through compression for discharge, and the areola, through palpation, should not be forgotten.
9. Any change should be reported to a health care provider as quickly as possible.

Special examination procedures

Further evaluation of breast masses is accomplished through the use of several recently developed techniques. These techniques are as follows:

1. *Mammography* is the technique of breast examination by the use of low-energy radiography.
2. *Xerography* is mammography using a xerographic plate instead of film. The advantages of this technique are that radiation doses are small-

er than with conventional mammography and the images produced are more distinct.

3. *Thermography* is a technique that measures temperature distribution of the breast. Malignant lesions appear as "hot spots" in the breast.

Mammographical techniques have been improved tremendously in terms of safety and effectiveness during the past 10 years. Mammography is the major method of detecting nonpalpable breast lesions. Nonpalpable lesions are generally early, small, and local. Therefore, survival rates are increased with early detection.

The taking and interpretation of mammograms require specialized skill. Often mammography is offered through a community-based screening program. A baseline mammogram is recommended for all women between the ages of 35 and 40, followed by mammograms every 2 years for asymptomatic women aged 40 to 49. Yearly mammograms are recommended for women over age 50.

PATHOLOGY
Breast cancer

Although certain breast lesions have characteristic findings on inspection and palpation, diagnosis is not made by clinical examination but by surgical procedures and laboratory examinations. The practitioner is encouraged to learn distinguishing characteristics of breast lesions but not to rely on them for diagnosis.

The lesions of breast cancer are often solitary, unilateral, solid, hard, irregular, poorly delineated, nonmobile, painless, nontender, and located in the upper outer quadrants.

Breast cancer is a leading cause of death in women in the United States and also a leading cause of cancer morbidity. On the average one out of every thirteen women will develop breast cancer. Knowledge of factors indicating that a woman is at a higher than usual risk of cancer can assist in making decisions about screening programs and the frequency of general physical examinations. The following groups of women are at higher than usual risk of breast cancer:

1. Women over 40
2. Women who have never been pregnant
3. Women whose first full-term pregnancy was at age 34 or older
4. Women with a history of an early menarche (before age 12) or late menopause (after age 50)
5. Women with a history of benign breast disease
6. Women of North American or European descent
7. Women with a previous breast cancer
8. Women with a strong family history of breast cancer
9. Women who have a wet type of cerumen

These women should be taught to perform self-examination and should receive a professional physical examination at least once a year.

The American Cancer Society (1983) recommends the following breast cancer screening test schedule for asymptomatic women:

1. All women over age 20 should perform breast self-examination monthly.
2. Women between the ages of 20 and 40 should have a breast examination by a qualified health care provider every 3 years, and women over age 40 should have an examination yearly.
3. All women should have a baseline mammogram between the ages of 35 and 40.
4. Asymptomatic women aged 40 to 49 should have a mammogram every 1 to 2 years.
5. All women over 50 should have a mammogram every year.

The male breast

Occurring most frequently in the areolar area, male breast cancer accounts for approximately 1% of all breast cancers. Every male client should be given a thorough breast examination with an adaptation of the technique used for female clients.

The male breast is observed with the man sitting. The various sitting positions used with the woman are unnecessary. Palpation of the breasts, nipple, and areolae can occur with the client supine. The palpation of the axillary nodes is an essential component of the examination of the male client.

Gynecomastia, enlargement of the male breast, is a frequently occurring multicausal condition. Causes include pubertal changes, hormonal administration, cirrhosis, leukemia, thyrotoxicosis, and drugs.

Benign lesions of the female breast

Benign lesions account for approximately 70% to 80% of breast operations. The most commonly seen benign breast lesions are fibrocystic disease and fibroadenomas.

Fibrocystic disease is an exaggeration of the normal changes in the breasts during the menstrual cycle and is eventually characterized by the formation of single or multiple cysts in the breasts. Fibrocystic disease develops in three stages:

1. The first stage is called *mazoplasia* and occurs in the late teens and early twenties. It is characterized by painful, tender, premenstrual breast swelling (chiefly in the axillary tails) that subsides after menses.
2. The second stage occurs in the late twenties and early thirties. The breasts exhibit multinodular changes, and sometimes a dominant mass can occur, which is usually described as a thickness rather than a lump.
3. Subsequently, cysts develop. The onset of cyst formation is often preceded by sudden dull pain, a full feeling, or a burning sensation in the breast.

The lesions of cystic disease are commonly bilateral, multiple, painful, tender, well delineated, and slightly mobile. The discomfort from and size of lesions increase premenstrually.

Fibroadenomas are benign lesions that contain both fibrous and glandular tissues. They are usually solitary and unilateral. They are generally palpated as mobile, solid, firm, rubbery, regular, well-delineated, nontender, painless lumps. Fibroadenomas are usually found in women between the ages of 15 and 35 and produce no premenstrual changes.

SUMMARY

I. Observation of breasts at rest
II. Observation of breasts in three additional positions
  A. Client with arms overhead
  B. Client contracting pectoral muscles
  C. Client leaning forward
III. Palpation of axillary node areas
IV. Palpation of supraclavicular and subclavicular areas
V. Palpation of breasts with client in a sitting position, if indicated
VI. Observation of breasts with client lying down and the breasts shifted medially
VII. Palpation of breasts
  A. Glandular tissue areas
  B. Areolar areas
  C. Nipples
  D. Tail of Spence areas

Every female client should be taught to examine her breasts and should be advised to do this each month on the completion of the menses.

BIBLIOGRAPHY

Dunphy, J.E., and Botsford, T.W.: Physical examination of the surgical patient, ed. 4, Philadelphia, 1975, W.B. Saunders Co.

Eggertsen, S.C., Berg, A.O., and Moe, R.E.: An evaluation of individual components of breast self-examination, J. Fam. Pract. **17**:921, 1983.

Evans, K.T., and Gravelle, I.H.: Mammography, thermography and ultrasonography in breast disease, Sevenoaks, Kent, 1973, Butterworth & Co., (Publishers) Ltd.

Fogel, C.I., and Woods, N.F.: Health care of women: a nursing perspective, St. Louis, 1981, The C.V. Mosby Co.

Gallagher, S., and others: The breast, St. Louis, 1978, The C.V. Mosby Co.

Kishner, R.: Breast cancer: a personal history and an investigative report, New York, 1975, Harcourt Brace Jovanovich, Inc.

Mahoney, L.J., Bird, B.L., and Cooke, G.M.: Annual clinical examination: the best available screening test for breast cancer, N. Engl. J. Med. **301**:315, 1979.

Mammography Guidelines 1983: Background statement and update of cancer-related check-up guidelines for breast cancer detection in asymptomatic women age 40 to 49, CA **33**:255, 1983.

Marty, P.J., McDermott, R.J., and Gold, R.S.: An assessment of three alternate formats for promoting breast self-examination, Cancer Nurs. **6**:207, 1983.

Memorial Hospital for Cancer and Associated Diseases: Breast Cancer Monograph, New York, 1973, Memorial Hospital.

Oberst, M.J.: Testing approaches to teaching breast self-examination, Cancer Nurs. **4**:246, 1981.

Papaioannou, A.N.: The etiology of human breast cancer, New York, 1974, Springer-Verlag New York, Inc.

Rush, B.: Breast. In Schwartz, S.I., editor: Principles of surgery, ed. 2, New York, 1969, McGraw-Hill Book Co.

Venet, L.: Self-examination and clinical examination of the breast, Cancer **46**:930, 1980.

Vorherr, H.: The breast, New York, 1974, Academic Press, Inc.

CHAPTER 15

ASSESSMENT OF THE RESPIRATORY SYSTEM

ANATOMY AND PHYSIOLOGY

The major purpose of the respiratory system is to supply the body with oxygen and eliminate carbon dioxide. This is accomplished through complex cooperation of many body systems that, in wellness, act in harmony. The actual transfer of oxygen and carbon dioxide between environmental gas and body liquid occurs in the alveoli, which are obviously not accessible to clinical examination. However, assessment of respiratory efficiency is accomplished by direct and indirect appraisal of structures supporting alveolar function.

The thoracic cage consists of a skeleton of twelve thoracic vertebrae, twelve pairs of ribs, the sternum, the diaphragm, and the intercostal muscles and is semirigid (Fig. 15-1). The skeletal parts of the thoracic cage consist of the ribs, the sternum, and the vertebrae. The ribs are paired. Anteriorly, the costal cartilages of the first seven ribs articulate with the body of the sternum, and the costal cartilages of the eighth to the tenth ribs are attached to the costal cartilages just above the ribs. The eleventh and twelfth ribs are termed "floating ribs" and are unattached anteriorly. The tip of the eleventh rib is located in the lateral thorax, and the tip of the twelfth rib is located in the posterior thorax. Posteriorly, all ribs articulate with the thoracic vertebrae.

The adult sternum measures approximately 17 cm in length and consists of three parts: the manubrium, the body, and the xiphoid process. The manubrium of the sternum articulates with and supports the clavicle. The manubrium and the body of the sternum articulate with the first seven ribs. None of the ribs articulates with the xiphoid. An anatomical landmark, the angle of Louis, is the junction of the manubrium and the body of the sternum. The second rib attaches to the sternum at the angle of Louis.

The spaces between the ribs are termed intercostal spaces (ICS). Intercostal spaces are named according to the rib immediately superior, e.g., the space between the second and third rib would be the second ICS.

The thoracic cage is perpetually moving in the inspiratory and expiratory phases of respiration (Fig. 15-2). During inspiration, the diaphragm descends and flattens and the intercostal muscles contract. These maneuvers produce differences in pressure among the areas of the mouth, the alveoli, and the pleural areas; and air moves into the lungs. The intrathoracic pressure is decreased, the lungs are expanded, and the ribs flare, increasing the diameter of the thorax. The second to the sixth ribs move around two axes in a motion commonly termed the "pump handle" movement. The lower ribs move in a "bucket handle" motion. Because of the length and positioning of the lower ribs and because the lower interspaces are wider, the amplitude of movement is greater in the lower thorax.

Inspiration is opposed by the elastic properties of the respiratory system. Expiration is a relatively passive phenomenon. At the completion of inspiration, the diaphragm relaxes and the elastic recoil properties of the lungs expel air and pull the diaphragm to its resting position.

The thoracic cavity is divided into two distinct right and left pleural cavities, separated by the mediastinum, containing the heart and the other structures that connect the head with the abdomen. The pleural cavities are lined by serous membranes, the parietal and visceral pleurae. The parietal pleura lines the chest wall and the diaphragm; the visceral pleura lines the outside of the lung. The space between the pleurae contains a lubricating fluid.

The lungs are paired, asymmetrical, conical organs

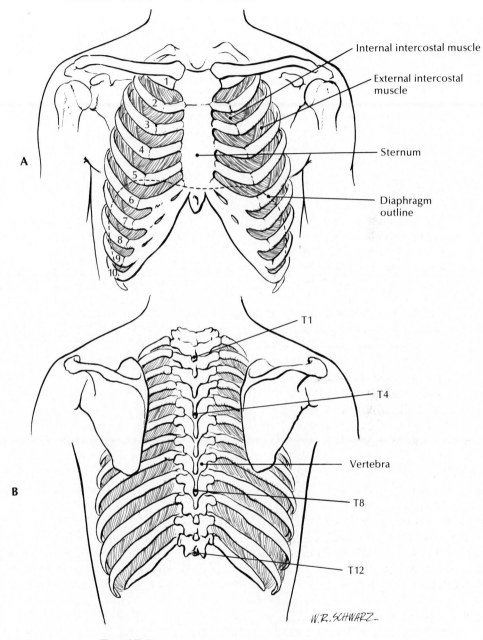

Fig. 15-1
Thoracic cage. **A,** Anterior thorax. **B,** Posterior thorax.

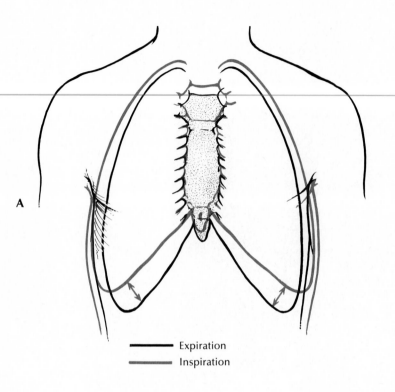

A

——— Expiration
——— Inspiration

Fig. 15-2
Movement of the thorax during respiration.
A, Anterior thorax. **B,** Lateral thorax.

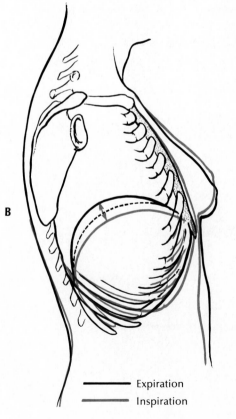

B

——— Expiration
——— Inspiration

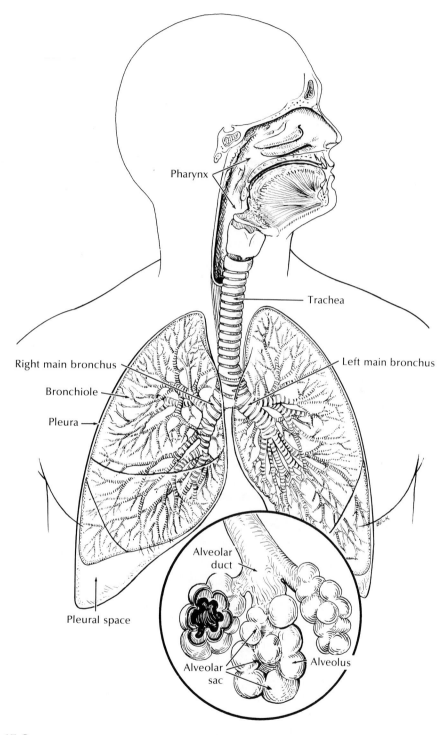

Fig. 15-3
Pharynx, trachea, and lungs. Alveolar sacs in inset. (From Anthony, C.P., and Thibodeau, G.A.: Textbook of anatomy and physiology, ed. 11, St. Louis, 1983, The C.V. Mosby Co.)

that conform to the thoracic cavity. The right lung contains three lobes, and the left lung contains two.

Air reaches the lungs via a system of flexible tubes. Air enters through the mouth or nose, traverses the respiratory portion of the larynx, and enters the trachea. The trachea begins at the lower border of the cricoid cartilage and divides into a left and right bronchus, usually at the level of T4 or T5 posteriorly and slightly below the manubriosternal joint anteriorly.

The right bronchus is shorter, wider, and more vertical than the left bronchus. The bronchial structures further subdivide into increasingly smaller bronchi and bronchioles. Each bronchiole opens into an alveolar duct from which multiple alveoli radiate (Fig. 15-3). Lungs in the adult contain approximately 300 million alveoli.

The bronchi have both transport and protective purposes. Their cavities contain mucus, which entraps for-

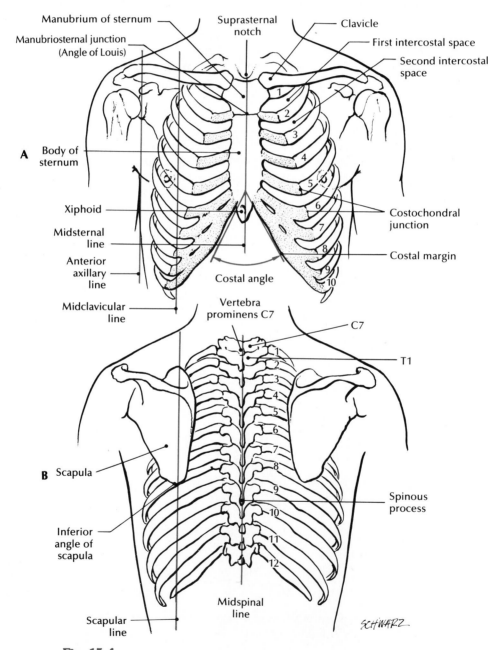

Fig. 15-4
Topographical landmarks. **A,** Anterior thorax. **B,** Posterior thorax.

eign particles and is continuously swept by ciliary action into the throat, where it can be eliminated.

Topographical anatomy

Topographical (surface) landmarks of the thorax assist the examiner in identifying the location of the internal, underlying structures and in describing the exact location of abnormalities (Fig. 15-4).

Manubriosternal junction (angle of Louis). The manubriosternal junction is the articulation between the manubrium and the body of the sternum and is an extremely useful aid in rib identification. This junction is named the angle of Louis. The angle of Louis is a visible and palpable angulation of the sternum.

The superior border of the second rib articulates with the sternum at the manubriosternal junction. The examiner can begin to palpate and count distal ribs and rib interspaces from this point. It should be reiterated that an ICS is numbered corresponding to the number of the rib immediately superior to the space. In palpation for rib identification, the examiner should palpate along the midclavicular line rather than at the sternal border because the rib cartilages are very close at the sternum and the cartilages of only the first seven ribs attach directly to the sternum.

Suprasternal notch. The suprasternal notch is the depression above the manubrium.

Costal angle. The costal angle is the angle formed by the intersection of the coastal margins.

Midsternal line. The midsternal line is an imaginary line drawn through the middle of the sternum.

Midclavicular lines. The midclavicular lines are left and right imaginary lines drawn through the midpoints of the clavicles and parallel to the midsternal line.

Anterior axillary lines. The anterior axillary lines are left and right imaginary lines drawn vertically from the anterior axillary folds, along the anterolateral chest, and parallel to the midsternal line.

Vertebra prominens (seventh cervical vertebra). When the client flexes his neck anteriorly and the posterior thorax is observed, a prominent spinous process can be observed and palpated. This is the spinous process of the seventh cervical vertebra. If two spinous processes are observed and palpated, the superior one is C7 and the inferior one is the spinous process of T1. The counting of ribs is more difficult on the posterior than on the anterior thorax. The spinous processes of the vertebrae can be counted relatively easily from C7 to T4. From T4 the spinous processes project obliquely, causing the spinous process of the vertebra not to lie over its correspondingly numbered rib but over the rib below it. For example, the spinous process of T5 lies over the body of T6 and is adjacent to the sixth rib.

Midspinal line. The midspinal line is an imaginary line that runs vertically along the posterior spinous processes of the vertebrae.

Scapular lines. The scapular lines are left and right imaginary lines that lie vertically and are parallel to the midspinal line. They pass through the inferior angles of the scapulae when the client stands erect with arms at his sides.

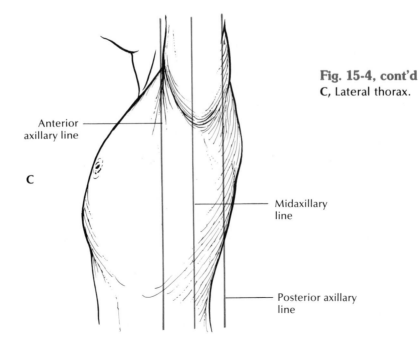

Fig. 15-4, cont'd
C, Lateral thorax.

Anterior axillary line

C

Midaxillary line

Posterior axillary line

Posterior axillary lines. The posterior axillary lines are imaginary left and right lines drawn vertically from the posterior axillary folds along the posterolateral wall of the thorax when the lateral arm is abducted directly from the lateral chest wall.

Midaxillary lines. The midaxillary lines are imaginary left and right lines drawn vertically from the apices of the axillae. They are approximately midway between the anterior and the posterior axillary lines and parallel to them.

• • •

The various landmarks and imaginary lines assist in determining the location of underlying structures and in describing the location of abnormal findings.

Underlying thoracic structures

When examining the respiratory system, the practitioner must maintain a mental image of the placement of organs and organ parts of the respiratory system and other systems sharing the thoracic area (Figs. 15-5 to 15-8).

Lung borders. In the anterior thorax, the apices of the lungs extend for approximately 2 to 4 cm above the clavicles. The inferior borders of the lungs cross the sixth rib at the midclavicular line. In the posterior thorax, the apices extend to T1. The lower borders vary with respiration and usually extend from the spinous process of T10 on expiration to the spinous process of T12 on deep inspiration. In the lateral thorax, the lung extends from the apex of the axilla to the eighth rib of the midaxillary line.

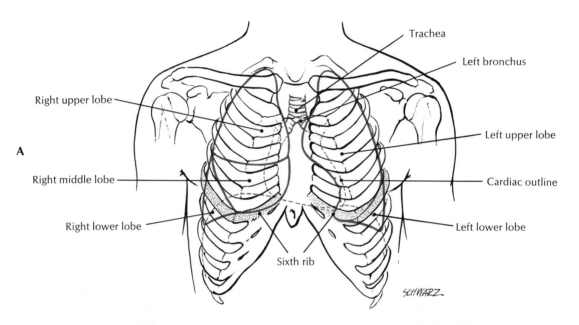

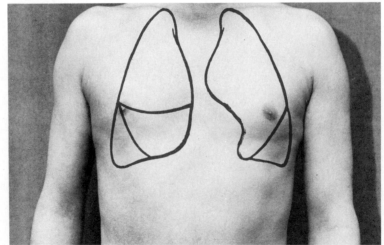

Fig. 15-5
Anterior thorax. **A,** Internal organs and structures. **B,** Lung borders.

Lung fissures. The right oblique (diagonal) fissure extends from the area of the spinous process of the third thoracic vertebra laterally and downward until it crosses the fifth rib at the right midaxillary line. It then continues anteriorly and medially to end at the sixth rib at the right and left midclavicular lines. The right horizontal fissure extends from the fifth rib slightly posterior to the right midaxillary line and runs horizontally to the area of the fourth rib at the right sternal border. The left oblique (diagonal) fissure extends from the spinous process of the third thoracic vertebra laterally and downward to the left midaxillary line at the fifth rib and continues anteriorly and medially until it terminates at the sixth rib in the left midclavicular line.

Border of the diaphragm. Anteriorly, on expiration, the right dome of the diaphragm is located at the level of the fifth rib at the midclavicular line and the left dome is at the level of the sixth rib. Posteriorly, on

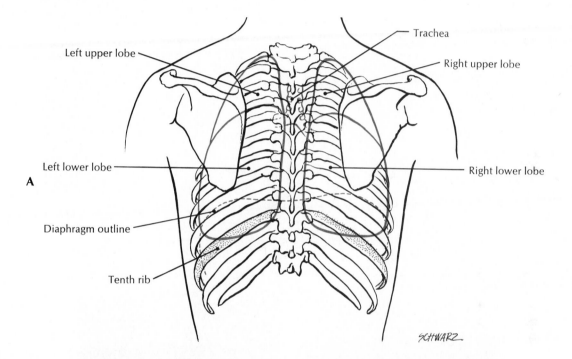

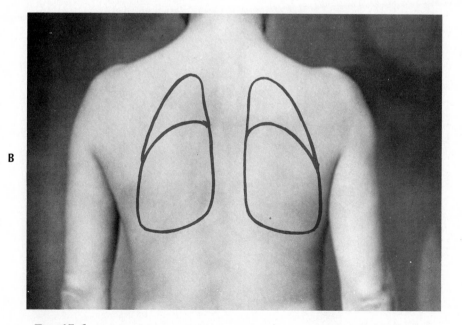

Fig. 15-6
Posterior thorax. **A,** Internal organs and structures. **B,** Lung borders.

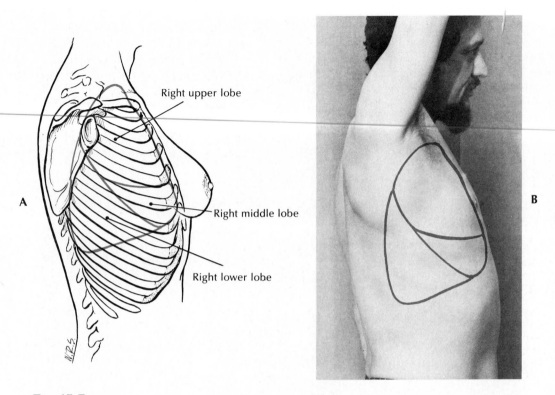

Right upper lobe

Right middle lobe

Right lower lobe

A

B

Fig. 15-7
Right lateral thorax. **A,** Internal organs and chest structures. (Note the relationship of the breast to chest organs and structures.) **B,** Lung borders.

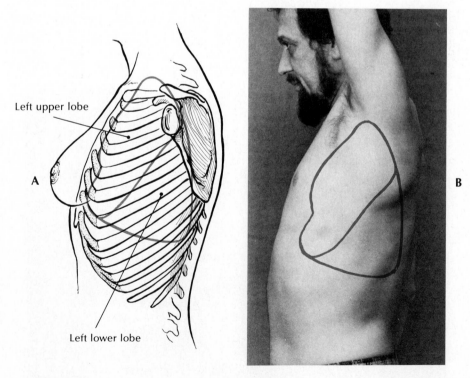

Left upper lobe

A

B

Left lower lobe

Fig. 15-8
Left lateral thorax. **A,** Internal organs and chest structures. **B,** Lung borders.

expiration, the diaphragm is at the level of the spinous process of T10; laterally, it is at the eighth rib at the midaxillary line. On inspiration the diaphragm moves approximately 1.5 cm downward with the right side being slightly higher than the left side.

Trachea. The bifurcation of the trachea occurs approximately just below the manubriosternal junction anteriorly and at the spinous process of T4 posteriorly.

EXAMINATION

Equipment needed for the respiratory system examination are a stethoscope, a marking pencil, and a centimeter ruler. The examination should be performed in a warm, quiet, well-illuminated area that allows for privacy.

Inspection

For adequate inspection of the thorax, the client should be sitting upright without support and uncovered to the waist. It is essential that the room lighting be adequate and that a mechanism for supplementary lighting be available for close inspection of small areas. It is critical that the client be warm and not observed by persons extraneous to the examination. The examiner first observes the general shape of the thorax and its symmetry. Although no individual is absolutely symmetrical in both body hemispheres, most individuals are reasonably similar side to side. Using the client as his own control whenever paired parts are examined is an excellent habit and will often yield significant findings.

Thoracic configuration. The anteroposterior diameter of the thorax in the normal adult is less than the transverse diameter at approximately a ratio of 1:2 to 5:7 (Fig. 15-9). In the normal infant, in some adults with pulmonary disease, and in aged adults the thorax is approximately round. This condition is called barrel chest. The barrel chest is characterized by horizontal ribs, slight kyphosis of the thoracic spine, and prominent sternal angle. The chest appears as though it were in continuous inspiratory position. Other observed abnormalities of thoracic shape might include the following:

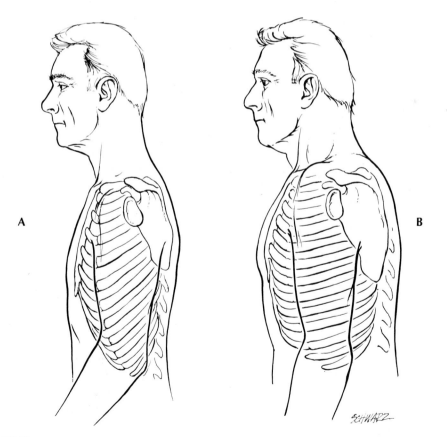

Fig. 15-9
A, Client with normal thoracic configuration. **B,** Client with increased anteroposterior diameter. Note contrasts in the angle of the slope of the ribs and the development of the accessory muscles of respiration in the neck.

1. Retraction of the thorax. The retraction is unilateral, or of one side.
2. Pigeon or chicken chest (pectus carinatum)—sternal protrusion anteriorly. The anteroposterior diameter of the chest is increased, and the resultant configuration resembles the thorax of a fowl.
3. Funnel chest (pectus excavatum)—depression of part or all of the sternum. If the depression is deep, it may interfere with both respiratory and cardiac function.
4. Spinal deformities. While the client is uncovered and the examiner is behind him, the spine should be examined for deformities. (See Chapter 22 on musculoskeletal assessment for the specific techniques of spinal examination.)

The approach to the physical examination is regional and integrated. The examination of systems is combined in body regions when appropriate. Since the client is uncovered to the waist during the examination, a large portion of skin and tissue is accessible to inspection. The observation of skin and underlying tissue provides the examiner with knowledge of the general nutrition of the patient. Common thoracic skin findings are the spider nevi associated with cirrhosis and seborrheic dermatitis (see Chapter 9 on skin assessment).

Ribs and interspaces. The reaction of interspaces on inspiration may be indicative of some obstruction of free air inflow. Bulging of interspaces on expiration occurs when there is obstruction to air outflow or may be the result of tumor, aneurysm, or cardiac enlargement. Normally, the costal angle is less than 90 degrees, and the ribs are inserted into the spine at about a 45-degree angle (see Fig. 15-1). In clients with obstructive lung diseases these angles are widened.

Pattern of respiration. Normally, men and children breathe diaphragmatically, and women breathe thoracically or costally. A change in this pattern might be significant. If the client appears to have labored respiration, the examiner observes for the use of the accessory muscles of respiration in the neck—the sternocleidomastoid, scalenus, and trapezius muscles—and for supraclavicular retraction. Impedance to air inflow is often accompanied by retraction of the intercostal spaces during inspiration. An excessively long expiratory phase of respiration accompanies outflow impedance and may be accompanied by the use of abdominal muscles to aid in expiration.

The normal adult resting respiratory rate is 12 to 20 breaths per minute and is regular. The ratio of respiratory rate to pulse rate normally is 1:4. Tachypnea is an adult respiratory rate of over 20 breaths per minute; bradypnea is an adult respiratory rate of less than 10 breaths per minute.

There are many abnormal patterns of respiration. Some of the commonly seen patterns are listed in Fig. 15-10. Dyspnea is a subjective phenomenon of inadequate or distressful respiration.

Lips and nails. Inspection in the respiratory system examination includes observation of lips and nail beds for color and observation of the nails for clubbing. These phenomena are discussed in Chapter 7 on general assessment and in Chapter 16 on cardiovascular assessment.

Palpation

Palpation is performed to (1) further assess abnormalities suggested by the history or observation, such as tenderness, pulsations, masses, or skin lesions; (2) assess the skin and subcutaneous structures; (3) assess the thoracic expansion; (4) assess vocal (tactile) fremitus; and (5) assess the tracheal position.

General palpation. The examiner should specifically palpate any areas of abnormality. The temperature and turgor of the skin should be generally assessed. The examiner then palpates the muscle mass and the thoracic skeleton. If the client has no complaints in relation to the respiratory system, a rapid, general survey of anterior, lateral, and posterior thoracic areas is sufficient. If the client does have complaints, all chest areas should be meticulously palpated for tenderness, bulges, or abnormal movements.

Assessment of thoracic expansion (Fig. 15-11). The degree of thoracic expansion can be assessed from the anterior or posterior chest. Anteriorly, the examiner's hands are placed over the anterolateral chest with the thumbs extended along the costal margin, pointing to the xiphoid process. Posteriorly, the thumbs are placed at the level of the tenth rib and the palms are placed on the posterolateral chest. The examiner feels the amount of the thoracic expansion during quiet and deep respiration and observes for divergence of the thumbs on expiration. Symmetry of respiration between the left and right hemithoraces should be felt as the thumbs are separated approximately 3 to 5 cm during deep inspiration.

Assessment of fremitus. Fremitus is vibration perceptible on palpation. Vocal or tactile fremitus is palpable vibration of the thoracic wall, produced by phonation.

The client is asked to repeat "one, two, three" or "ninety-nine" while the examiner systematically palpates the thorax (Fig. 15-12). The examiner can use the palmar bases of the fingers, the ulnar aspect of the hand, or the ulnar aspect of the closed fist. If one hand is used, it should be moved from one side of the chest to the corresponding area on the other side. If two hands are used for examination, they should be simul-

TYPE OF RESPIRATION	DIAGRAM	DISCUSSION
Normal		2-20/min in adults; regular in rhythm; ratio of respiratory rate to pulse rate is 1:4
Hyperventilation or Kussmaul's respiration		Increase in both rate and depth; hyperpnea is an increase in depth onl
Periodic respiration		Alternating hyperpnea, shallow respiration and apnea; sometimes called Cheyne-Stokes respiration; frequently occurs in the severely ill
Sighing respiration		Deep and audible; audible portion sounds like a sigh
Air trapping		Present in obstructive pulmonary diseases; air is trapped in the lungs; respiratory level rises, and breathing becomes shallow
Biot's breathing		Shallow breathing interrupte by apnea; seen in some CNS disorders and in healthy persons

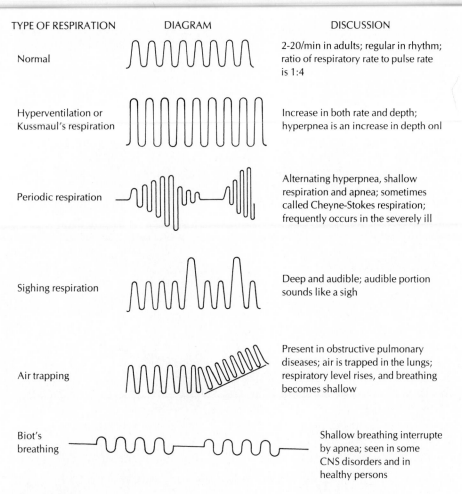

Fig. 15-10
Characteristics of commonly observed respiratory patterns.

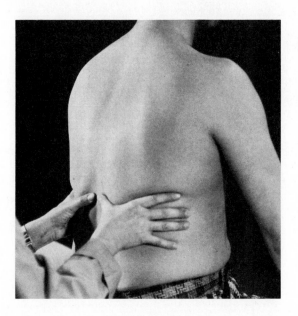

Fig. 15-11
Palpation for thoracic excursion.

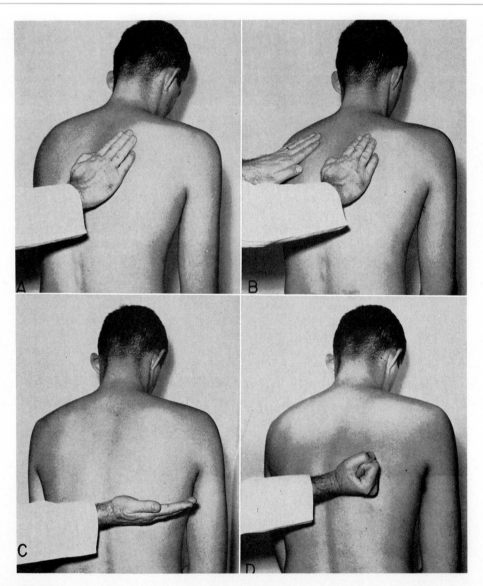

Fig. 15-12
Palpation for assessment of vocal fremitus. **A,** Use of palmar surface of fingertips. **B,** Simultaneous application of the fingertips of both hands. **C,** Use of ulnar aspect of the hand. **D,** Use of ulnar aspect of the closed fist. (From Prior, J.A., and Silberstein, J.S.: Physical diagnosis: the history and examination of the patient, ed. 4, St. Louis, 1973, The C.V. Mosby Co.)

taneously placed on the corresponding areas of each thoracic side. See Table 15-1 for types of fremitus.

When examining the thorax, the practitioner must be mindful of the four parts for examination: the posterior chest, the anterior chest, the right and left lateral thoracic areas, and the apices. The examiner should move from the area of one hemisphere to the corresponding area on the other (right to left, left to right) until all four major parts are surveyed. During palpation for assessing fremitus and all subsequent procedures for the examination of the respiratory system, all areas must be meticulously and systematically examined. Usually, the apices, posterior chest, and lateral areas can be examined with the practitioner standing behind the client.

Assessment of tracheal deviation. The trachea should be assessed by palpation for lateral deviation. The examiner places a finger on the trachea in the suprasternal notch then moves his finger laterally left and right in the spaces bordered by the upper edge of the clavicle, the inner aspect of the sternocleidomas-

toid muscle, and the trachea. These spaces should be equal on both sides. In diseases such as atelectasis and pulmonary fibrosis, the trachea may be deviated toward the abnormal side. The trachea may be deviated toward the normal side in conditions such as neck tumors, thyroid enlargement, enlarged lymph nodes, pleural effusion, unilateral emphysema, and tension pneumothorax.

Crepitations. In subcutaneous emphysema, the subcutaneous tissue contains fine beads of air. As this tissue is palpated, audible crackling sounds are heard. These sounds are termed *crepitations.*

Percussion

Percussion is the tapping of an object to set underlying structures in motion and consequently to produce a sound called a percussion note and a palpable vibration. Percussion penetrates to a depth of approximately 5 to 7 cm into the chest. Percussion is used in the thoracic examination to determine the relative amounts of air, liquid, or solid material in the underlying lung and to determine the positions and boundaries of organs. The techniques of percussion are discussed in Chapter 1, and the student is referred to that chapter for review.

Two techniques of percussion are immediate, or direct, percussion and mediate, or indirect, percussion. In *immediate,* or *direct, percussion,* the examiner strikes the area to be percussed directly with the palmar aspect of two, three, or four fingers held together or with the palmar aspect of the tip of the middle finger. The strikes are rapid and downward; movement of the hand from the wrist is in rapid strokes. This type of percussion is not normally used in thoracic examination. It is useful in the examination of the thorax in the infant and the sinuses in the adult. *Mediate,* or *indirect, percussion* is the striking of an object held against the area to be examined (Fig. 15-13). The middle finger of the examiner's left hand (if the examiner is right-handed) is the pleximeter. The distal phalanx and joint and the middle phalanx are placed firmly on the surface to be percussed. Although most practitioners usually find that the area of the interphalangeal joint is the most effective pleximeter point for percussion, the quality of the percussion sound and the comfort of the examiner should serve as criteria for the selection of a pleximeter point. The examiner may find that a point between the proximal and the distal interphalangeal joints is more effective and comfortable. This alteration of technique is acceptable. In all cases, the point struck by the plexor should be pressed as tightly as possible against the patient, with all other areas of that hand held off the client's skin. The plexor is the index finger of the examiner's right hand or the index and middle fingers held together. For position see Fig. 15-13.

Table 15-1

Characteristics of normal and abnormal tactile fremitus

Type of fremitus	Discussion of characteristics
Normal fremitus	Varies greatly from person to person and is dependent on the intensity and pitch of the voice, the position and distance of the bronchi in relation to the chest wall, and the thickness of the chest wall. Fremitus is most intense in the second intercostal spaces at the sternal border near the area of bronchial bifurcation.
Increased vocal fremitus	May occur in pneumonia, compressed lung, lung tumor, or pulmonary fibrosis. (A solid medium of uniform structure conducts vibrations with greater intensity than a porous medium.)
Decreased or absent vocal fremitus	Occurs when there is a diminshed production of sounds, a diminished transmission of sounds, or the addition of a medium through which sounds must pass before reaching the thoracic wall as, for example, in pleural effusion, pleural thickening, pneumothorax, bronchial obstruction, or emphysema.
Pleural friction rub	Vibration produced by inflamed pleural surfaces rubbing together. It is felt as a grating, is synchronous with respiratory movements, and is more commonly felt on inspiration.
Rhonchal fremitus	Coarse vibrations produced by the passage of air through thick exudates in the large air passages. These can be cleared or altered by coughing.

With the forearm and shoulder stationary and all movement at the wrist, the pleximeter is struck sharply with the plexor. The blow is aimed at the portion of the pleximeter that is exerting maximum pressure on the thoracic surface, usually the base of the terminal phalanx, the distal interphalangeal joint, or the middle phalanx. The blow is executed rapidly, and the plexor is immediately withdrawn. The plexor strikes with the tip of the finger at right angles to the pleximeter. One or two rapid blows are struck in each area. Bony areas are avoided; interspaces are used for percussion. The examiner compares one side of the thorax with the other.

With experience and study the practitioner will be able to differentiate among the five percussion tones commonly elicited on the human body. In the study of tones, the determination of four characteristics will assist in assessment and labeling:

1. *Intensity (amplitude):* the loudness or softness of the tone.
2. *Pitch (frequency):* relates to the number of vibrations per second. Rapid vibrations produce high-pitched tones; slow vibrations produce low-pitched tones. The greater the density of an object, the higher the frequency.
3. *Duration:* the amount of time a note is sustained.
4. *Quality:* a subjective phenomena relating to the innate characteristics of the object being percussed.

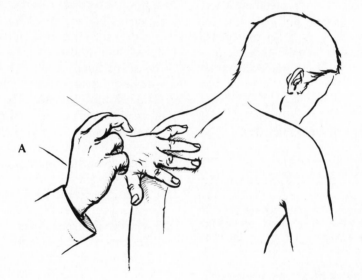

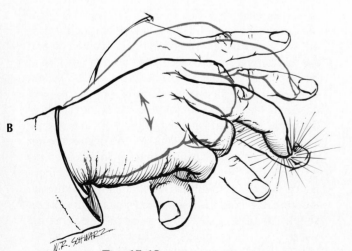

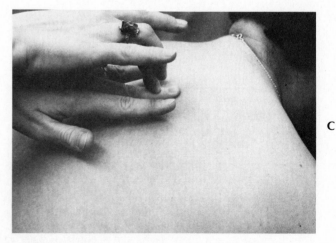

C

Fig. 15-13
Percussion. **A,** Positioning of the hands. **B,** Hand movement. **C,** Percussion of the posterior thorax.

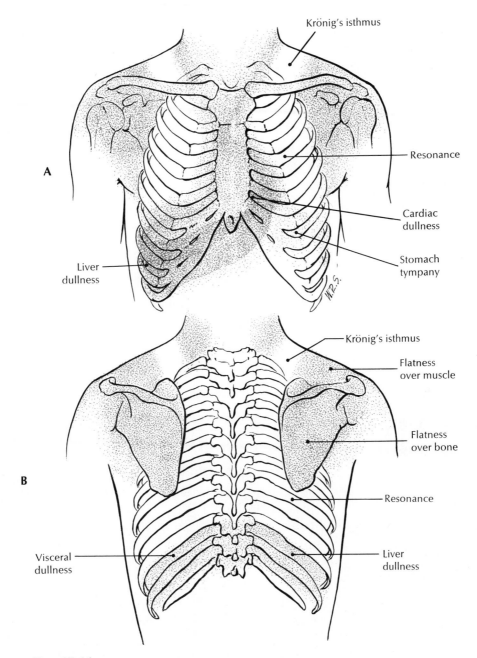

Fig. 15-14
Percussion areas. **A,** Normal anterior chest. **B,** Normal posterior chest.

Fig. 15-14 is a percussion map for the normal chest. The procedure for thoracic percussion is as follows:

1. Percuss the apices to determine if the normal 5 cm area of resonance is present between the neck and shoulder muscles (Fig. 15-14).
2. Position the client with his head bent and his arm folded over his chest (Fig. 15-15). With this maneuver, the scapulae move laterally and more lung area is accessible to examination.
3. On the posterior chest percuss systematically at about 5 cm intervals from the upper to lower chest, moving left to right, right to left, and avoiding scapular and other bony areas; percuss the lateral chest with the client's arms positioned over his head (Fig. 15-16).
4. Measure the diaphragmatic excursion. Instruct the client to inhale deeply and hold his breath in. Percuss along the scapular line on one side until the lower edge of the lung is identified. Sound will change from resonance to dullness. Mark the point of change on each side at the scapular line. Then instruct the client to take a few normal respirations. Next, instruct the client to exhale completely and hold his expiration. Proceed to percuss up from the marked point at the midscapular line to determine the diaphragmatic excursion in deep expiration. Repeat the procedure on the opposite side. Measure and record the distance

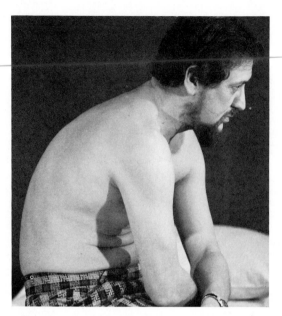

Fig. 15-15
Position of the client for examination of the posterior thorax.

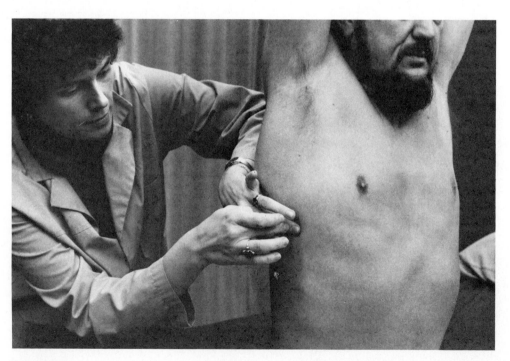

Fig. 15-16
Position of the client for percussion of the lateral thorax.

between the upper and lower points in centimeters on each side. The diaphragm is usually slightly higher on the right side, and excursion is normally 3 to 5 cm bilaterally. Diaphragmatic excursion is usually measured only on the posterior chest (Fig. 15-17).

In the actual examination, the practitioner would complete the examination of the apices and the posterior and lateral chest and would then percuss the anterior chest. A recommended sequence for the examination of the posterior, lateral, and anterior thoracic areas is illustrated in Fig. 15-18.

Auscultation

Through auscultation, the practitioner obtains information about the functioning of the respiratory system and about the presence of any obstruction in the passages. Auscultation of the lungs is accomplished by the use of a stethoscope. The diaphragm of the stethoscope is usually used for the thoracic examination because it covers a larger surface than the bell. The stethoscope is placed firmly, but not tightly, on the skin. Client or stethoscope movement is avoided because movements of muscle under the skin or movements of the stethoscope over hair will produce confusing extrinsic sounds.

Before beginning auscultation, the examiner should instruct the client to breathe through his mouth and more deeply and slowly than in usual respiration. The examiner systematically auscultates the apices and the posterior, lateral, and anterior chest (Fig. 15-18). At each application of the stethoscope, the examiner listens to at least one complete respiration. The examiner

should observe the client for signs of hyperventilation and stop the procedure if the client becomes lightheaded or faint. The process of auscultation includes (1) the analysis of breath sounds, (2) the detection of any abnormal sounds, and (3) the examination of the sounds produced by the spoken voice. As with percussion, the examiner should use a zigzag procedure, comparing the finding at each point with the corresponding point on the opposite hemithorax.

Breath sounds. Breath sounds are the sounds produced by the movement of air through the tracheobronchoalveolar system. These sounds are analyzed according to pitch, intensity, quality, and relative duration of inspiratory and expiratory phases. Table 15-2 outlines the types of sounds heard over the normal and the abnormal lung.

The sounds that are heard over normal lung parenchyma are called vesicular breath sounds. The inspiratory phase of the vesicular breath sound is heard better than the expiratory phase and is about 2.5 times longer. These sounds have a low pitch and soft intensity.

Bronchovesicular breath sounds are normally heard in the areas of the major bronchi, especially in the apex of the right lung and at the sternal borders. Bronchovesicular breath sounds are characterized by inspiratory and expiratory phases of equal duration, moderate pitch, and moderate intensity. When bronchovesicular breath sounds are heard over the peripheral lung, underlying pathology is likely.

Bronchial breath sounds are normally heard over the trachea and indicate a pathological condition if heard over lung tissue. They are high-pitched, loud

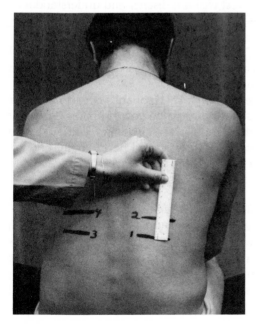

Fig. 15-17
Assessment of diaphragmatic excursion. The numbers indicate a suggested sequence of percussion.

lier (temporally, mitral valve opening is before ventricular filling), is sharper and higher pitched, and radiates more widely. In the pulmonic area, the opening snap must be differentiated from a split S_2. A split S_2 is best heard in the second left intercostal space, and an opening snap is best heard between the apex and the lower left sternal border. Whereas respiration affects the splitting of S_2, an opening snap is not affected by respiration and will remain at a fixed interval after the aortic component of S_2.

The loudness of the opening snap is affected by the pressure in the left atrium and by the flexibility of the mitral valve. Higher left atrial pressures increase the loudness of the opening snap. Marked fibrosis and calcification of the valve decrease the mobility, and consequently, the sound produced.

Ejection click. Semilunar valve changes may also be associated with an opening sound. This sound occurs early in systole at the end of isovolumic contraction when semilunar valves open (Fig. 16-14). The aortic ejection click, the more common of the two, is

heard both at the base and at the apex and does not change with respiration. Pulmonary ejection clicks are heard best at the second left interspace, radiate poorly, and change in intensity with respiration, increasing with expiration and decreasing with inspiration.

Pericardial friction rub. Inflammation of the pericardial sac causes the parietal and visceral surfaces of the roughened pericardium to rub against each other. This produces an extra cardiac sound of to-and-fro character with both systolic and diastolic components. One, two, or three components of a pericardial friction rub may be audible. A three-component rub indicates the presence of pericarditis and serves to distinguish a pericardial rub from a pleural friction rub, which ordinarily has two components. It resembles the sound of squeaky leather and is often described as grating, scratching, or rasping. The sound seems very close to the ear and may seem louder than or may even mask the other heart sounds. Friction rubs are usually best heard between the apex and sternum but may be widespread.

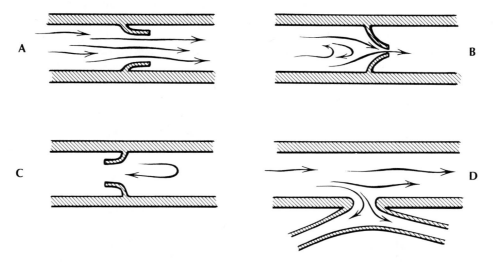

Fig. 16-15
Mechanisms of murmur production. **A,** Increased flow across a normal valve. **B,** Forward flow through a stenotic valve. **C,** Backflow through an incompetent valve. **D,** Flow through a septal defect or arteriovenous fistula.

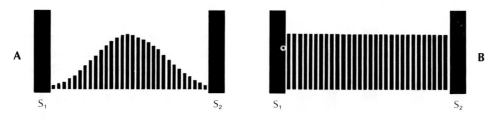

Fig. 16-16
Systolic murmurs. **A,** Crescendo-decrescendo systolic ejection murmur. **B,** Holosystolic regurgitant murmur.

Heart murmurs

A variety of conditions may result in the production of the more prolonged sound during systole or diastole known as a murmur. These are abnormal sounds produced by vibrations within the heart or in the walls of the large vessels. They tend to originate in the vicinity of the heart valve and are often best heard around the area of the valve responsible for their production.

Mechanisms of production. Three main factors related to murmur production are (1) increased flow rate of blood across normal valves; (2) forward flow through an irregular or constricted valve or into a dilated vessel or chamber; and (3) backflow, or regurgitant flow, through an incompetent or insufficient valve, a septal defect, or a patent ductus arteriosus (Fig. 16-15). In addition, a combination of these factors may prevail.

Murmurs are illustrated in a manner similar to the way in which they appear in a phonocardiogram, that is, with a series of vertical lines in systole between S_1 and S_2 or in diastole between S_2 and S_1. The lines are drawn in such a way as to indicate the level of, and increase or decrease in, intensity of the sound. For example, a midsystolic ejection murmur that is crescendo-decrescendo in nature is shown in Fig. 16-16, A; a holosystolic regurgitant murmur is shown in Fig. 16-16, B.

Valve alterations. The adequacy of opening and closure of the valves and of the orifice size determines many of the characteristics of murmurs. Heart valves that are functioning normally and competently permit the forward flow of blood and prevent backflow, or regurgitation. It is essential to understand the stations of the valves and flow patterns during systole and diastole. During ventricular systole, the mitral and tricuspid valves are closed, preventing backflow, and the aortic and pulmonic valves are open, permitting forward flow. During ventricular diastole, the mitral and tricuspid valves are open, permitting forward flow, and the aortic and pulmonic valves are closed, preventing backflow.

Stenotic valves prevent adequate forward flow; thus, a stenosed mitral or tricuspid valve interferes with normal flow during diastole, when the atrium empties blood into the ventricle. Mitral or tricuspid stenosis produces a diastolic murmur (Fig. 16-17, A). A stenosed aortic or pulmonic valve prevents adequate forward flow of blood during ventricular systole, when the blood is being forced from the ventricle into the aorta or pulmonary artery; thus, aortic (or pulmonic) stenosis produces a systolic murmur (Fig. 16-17, B). Blood flowing through such a narrowed orifice meets resistance and produces vibrations.

Incompetent or insufficient valves fail to close completely during that phase of the cardiac cycle when their leaflets should be firmly approximated; they leave an aperture through which blood flows inappropriately back from the ventricles to the atria or from the aorta or pulmonary artery back to the ventricles. This regurgitation, or backflow, of blood produces vibrations of the valve and of parts of the myocardium, producing a murmur. An incompetent mitral or tricuspid valve per-

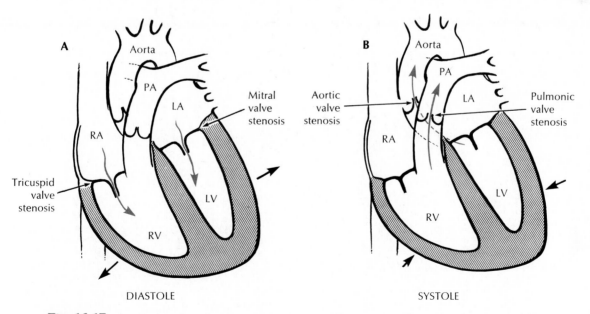

Fig. 16-17
A, Mitral or tricuspid valve stenosis produces a diastolic murmur. **B,** Aortic or pulmonic valve stenosis produces a systolic murmur.

mits the inappropriate backflow of blood from the ventricle to the atrium during ventricular systole, producing a systolic murmur (Fig. 16-18, A). An insufficient aortic or pulmonic valve permits the backflow of blood from the aorta or pulmonary artery to the ventricle during ventricular diastole, producing a diastolic murmur (Fig. 16-18, B).

Characteristics. Murmurs are classified and described according to several characteristics, including timing (systolic or diastolic), frequency, location, radiation, intensity, quality, and effects of respiration.

Timing. The timing of murmurs is according to their occurrence during either diastole or systole. At times, murmurs may occur during both phases of the cycle. The timing of the murmur may be further characterized as occurring during the entire phase of a cycle or, for instance, during early, mid-, or late systole. Murmurs that endure throughout systole are known as holosystolic or pansystolic murmurs; the same is true for diastolic murmurs. Early diastolic murmurs are known as protodiastolic, and late diastolic murmurs are called presystolic.

In general, systolic murmurs are caused by stenosed aortic or pulmonic valves or by incompetent mitral or tricuspid valves, and diastolic murmurs are produced by stenosed mitral or tricuspid valves or by incompetent aortic or pulmonic valves. It is important to remember, however, that not all murmurs result from valve defects; they may also be produced by alteration in the velocity of flow, by changes in the vessels, and by defects in the myocardium.

Frequency. The frequency, or pitch, of murmurs varies from high to low. The main determining factor is the velocity of blood flow. Generally, when the rate of flow is rapid, a high pitch results; when the velocity is slow, the pitch is low. The pitch of a murmur is described as high, medium, or low.

Location. A murmur is described by means of anatomical landmarks according to where it is best heard. Some are localized to small areas, whereas others are heard over large portions of the precordium. The location of a murmur is significant in terms of its site of production. The murmurs originating from valvular alterations are usually best heard in the area to which sounds from that valve are transmitted.

Radiation. Some murmurs radiate in the direction of the bloodstream by which they are produced. For example, the diastolic murmur of aortic insufficiency may be heard along the left sternal border. In this case, the blood leaks back from the aorta into the left ventricle. Other factors, such as the variation in sound transmission through various tissues, also influence radiation.

Intensity. The loudness of a murmur is described on a scale of one to six; one is the softest, and six is the loudest. The description of each level of loudness is as follows:

Grade I: Barely audible, very faint; can be heard only with special effort.

Grade II: Clearly audible but quiet.

Grade III: Moderately loud.

Grade IV: Loud.

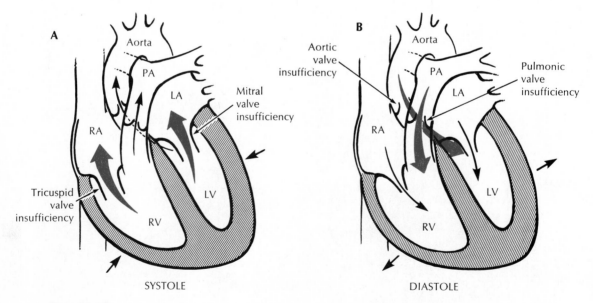

Fig. 16-18
A, Mitral or tricuspid valve insufficiency produces a systolic murmur. **B,** Aortic or pulmonic valve insufficiency produces a diastolic murmur.

Grade V: Very loud; may be heard with stethoscope partly off the chest.

Grade VI: Loudest possible; audible with the stethoscope just removed from contact with the chest wall.

It is important to note that although the grading of the loudness of a murmur is helpful, it is also a rather subjective description, dependent on the auditory acuity of the listener.

The terms *crescendo* and *decrescendo* are used to describe the pattern of intensity reflecting changes in the flow rate. A crescendo-decrescendo murmur, for example, increases from quiet to louder and then decreases again. In the case of aortic stenosis, for example, the flow rate increases, reaches a peak, and then decreases, producing a crescendo-decrescendo systolic murmur with a rather harsh quality. The diastolic murmur of aortic insufficiency is a decrescendo, high-pitched, blowing murmur. The flow rate of blood leaking back into the ventricle from the aorta is approximately proportional to the decreasing pressure gradient between the aorta and the ventricle. Although the patterns of the various murmurs may not be that easily determined with the stethoscope, the murmurs do appear that way on the phonocardiogram.

Quality. Several descriptive terms are often used to characterize a murmur; these include *musical, blowing, harsh,* and *rumbling.* For example, the murmur of aortic stenosis may be described as harsh; the murmur of mitral insufficiency may be described as a long, blowing sound; and the murmur of mitral stenosis tends to be of a low, rumbling quality.

Effects of respiration. As mentioned earlier in this chapter, certain events on the right side of the heart are affected by respiration as a result of intrathoracic pressure changes and right-sided filling changes. Murmurs that originate on the right side of the heart are also subject to influence by these factors. The murmur of tricuspid insufficiency, for example, may increase with inspiration.

Systolic murmurs. Murmurs occurring during ventricular systole are a result of increased flow rate across normal valves or abnormal blood flow patterns across (1) the inflow tract (the AV valves), (2) the outflow tract (the semilunar valves), or (3) ventricle to ventricle (ventricular septal defect). Incompetent or insufficient AV valves do not prevent backflow of blood from the ventricles to the atria during ventricular systole and thus produce systolic regurgitant murmurs. These murmurs may last during all or part of systole. Insufficient AV valves may be the result of rheumatic valvular disease or papillary muscle dysfunction. Stenotic aortic or pulmonic valves make it difficult for the blood to flow from the ventricles to the aorta and pulmonary arteries during ventricular systole and thus produce systolic

ejection murmurs. Because there is a short time interval between the closing of the AV valves (S_1) and the opening of the semilunar valves, systolic ejection murmurs will begin after the first heart sound, reflect the ejection of blood during systolic contraction, and end before the second heart sound. They are often called *midsystolic ejection murmurs.* Some systolic ejection murmurs are innocent, whereas others are pathological. The abnormalities that cause a turbulent flow across these semilunar valves may be the result of dilatation or narrowing of the pulmonary artery or aorta, aortic or pulmonic valvular or subvalvular stenosis, or high output states such as anemia, thyrotoxicosis, or pregnancy.

Innocent systolic ejection murmurs are commonly heard in children and adolescents. They occur within a normal cardiovascular system and are not the result of any recognizable heart abnormality. They reflect the contractile force of the heart that results in greater blood flow velocity during early or midsystole. Smaller chest measurements in the young also increase the audibility of these murmurs. Innocent systolic ejection murmurs may also occur with other high output states including pregnancy, anxiety, anemia, fever, and thyrotoxicosis.

Innocent systolic ejection murmurs are heard best with the bell held lightly against the chest in the pulmonic area (second left intercostal space) or around the lower left sternal border toward but not including the apex. They tend to be short, rarely extending through the entire systole, but begin shortly after the first heart sound and end well before the second heart sound (Fig. 16-19). They are softer than grade III, are of medium pitch, and have a blowing quality. They increase in held expiration, may change with position, and may be heard best when the client is in the recumbent position. The heart sounds remain unchanged.

These murmurs must be differentiated from pathological systolic ejection murmurs that may result from mild aortic or pulmonic stenosis or atrial or ventricular septal defects. A pansystolic or late systolic murmur indicates an organic problem.

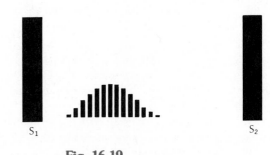

Fig. 16-19
Innocent systolic murmur.

Stenosis or obstruction of the aortic or pulmonic valves or deformity of the valves or adjacent vessels (the aorta and the pulmonary arteries) may cause *mid-systolic ejection murmurs*. The murmur of aortic valve stenosis or deformity begins after the first heart sound when the pressure in the ventricle is high enough to open the aortic and pulmonic valves, ends before the aortic and pulmonic valves close (S_2), and thus has a crescendo-decrescendo pattern (Fig. 16-16, *A*). With less aortic deformity present, the murmur reaches a peak earlier in systole. The murmur is medium pitched and harsh, may be faint to loud, and is best heard with the diaphragm at the first or second right intercostal spaces with the client sitting up and leaning forward with the breath held in expiration. If the murmur is loud, it may be heard over the entire thorax and is often accompanied by a thrill. (A thrill is a palpable vibration often associated with a very loud murmur; it usually signifies a pathological cardiac condition.) The existence of emphysema may cause the murmur to seem faint. Arrhythmias, shock, or heart failure causes the murmur to decrease in loudness.

The systolic murmur of aortic stenosis may be associated with a diminished second heart sound, an early ejection click, the sustained thrusting apical impulse of left ventricular hypertrophy, a slowly rising carotid pulse wave, and narrow pulse pressure. Rheumatic fever is the most common cause of aortic stenosis and valve deformity. Congenital deformities are another cause.

A basal systolic murmur associated with hypertension and arteriosclerotic roughening of the aorta and aortic valve are commonly heard in older people. This murmur is best heard at the second right intercostal space, is of medium pitch, has a rough quality, is usually not very loud, and is often transmitted to the apex. It is best heard with the client sitting up and leaning forward. Either the diaphragm or the bell may be used. The second heart sound is of normal or increased loudness.

Murmurs that occupy all of systole are called *holosystolic* or *pansystolic*. They are associated with turbulent blood flow from a high-pressure to a low-pressure area, such as occurs with regurgitation from a ventricular chamber to an atrial chamber across an incompetent AV valve, or with leakage from the left to the right ventricle through a ventricular septal defect. The murmur will continue as long as there is a sufficient pressure gradient across the incompetent orifice beginning with the first heart sound and lasting up to the second heart sound (Fig. 16-16, *B*).

Mitral regurgitation may result from malfunction of a number of structures including the valve ring or leaflets, the chordae tendineae, the papillary muscles, and the wall of the ventricle. This murmur is usually loudest at the apex; as the loudness increases, the sound may be transmitted to the axilla. It has a high pitch and a blowing quality and is best heard with the diaphragm of the stethoscope. If the murmur is faint, it may be heard better after exercise in the left lateral position or sitting up and leaning forward to the left. This murmur does not increase with inspiration. The first heart sound may be normal, increased, or decreased, depending on the condition of the mitral valve. The second sound may be normal or increased. A third heart sound may be present.

The murmur resulting from a ventricular septal defect is best heard at the fourth, fifth, and sixth interspaces at the left sternal border. It may radiate over the precordium but not to the axilla. It is high pitched and harsh and may be accompanied by a thrill. The size of the septal defect and the resistance in the pulmonary vessels determine the direction and velocity of flow during systole. With a small defect there may be greater resistance to pressure than with a larger defect, thus producing a louder holosystolic murmur.

Diastolic murmurs. Diastole is normally free of murmurs; therefore, a murmur heard during this portion of the cardiac cycle is almost always indicative of heart disease. Causes of diastolic murmurs include insufficiency of the aortic or pulmonic valves, permitting abnormal backflow from the aorta and pulmonary arteries, or stenosis of the mitral or tricuspid valves, preventing an adequate forward flow of blood.

Diastolic murmurs may occur in early, middle, or late diastole. Early diastolic murmurs are usually produced by aortic or pulmonic valvular insufficiency or dilatation of the valvular ring. Mid- and late diastolic murmurs are usually caused by narrowed, stenosed mitral or tricuspid valves that obstruct the inflow or by an increased flow rate across the valves.

Aortic valve insufficiency is associated with a diastolic regurgitant murmur that begins with the aortic component of the second heart sound at the time the aortic pressure exceeds the ventricular pressure. As the pressure in the aorta falls and the ventricles fill, the murmur decreases in intensity. This murmur begins loud in early diastole and then fades (Fig. 16-20), giving it a decrescendo character. It is high pitched and blowing and is best heard with the diaphragm with the client leaning forward in deep expiration. If the aorta is dilated, it may be loudest in the second right intercostal space. It may be accompanied by an aortic systolic murmur caused by increased flow, a third heart sound, a sustained thrusting apical impulse, and wide pulse pressure. The second heart sound may be increased or diminished depending on the condition of the aortic valve. This murmur is most commonly caused by rheumatic heart disease, but it may be caused by congenital valve disease.

Mitral stenosis is associated with a diastolic murmur that is produced by the flow of blood from the left atrium into the left ventricle and is most intense when that flow is greatest, that is, after the opening snap of the mitral valve. This is a middiastolic murmur. As the degree of stenosis increases, contraction of the auricle may force more blood across the valve and produce a presystolic accentuation of this diastolic murmur (Fig. 16-21). When faint or moderately loud, the murmur is low pitched and rumbling; as it becomes louder, it becomes more harsh. This murmur is generally heard only over a small area just medial to and above the apex or at the point of maximum impulse. It may be best heard when the client turns from the supine to the left lateral position. Exercise will increase the intensity of the murmur. The bell of the stethoscope should be held very lightly on the skin; heavy pressure on the bell may obliterate the sound of a faint middiastolic murmur.

Mitral stenosis is frequently associated with an increased first heart sound; there may also be an opening snap of the mitral valve. However, the first sound may be decreased and the opening snap absent if the valve and chordae tendineae are fibrosed or the mitral valve area is narrow in tight mitral stenosis.

The *venous hum* is a continuous low-pitched hum heard over the neck in many children and some adults. It is produced by turbulent blood flow in the internal jugular veins. The venous hum is best heard over the supraclavicular spaces, more commonly on the right. It is heard better with the client sitting up and is accentuated on the right by having the client turn his head to the left and slightly upward (Fig. 16-22). The hum is loudest in diastole. Because it is produced by blood flow in the jugular veins, it can be stopped by applying gentle pressure over the internal jugular vein in the neck between the trachea and the sternocleidomastoid muscle at about the level of the thyroid cartilage.

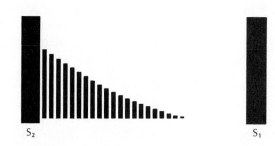

Fig. 16-20
The diastolic murmur of aortic valve insufficiency.

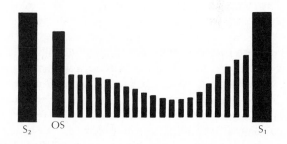

Fig. 16-21
The diastolic murmur of mitral stenosis with opening snap of mitral valve.

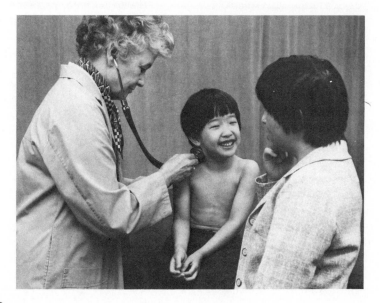

Fig. 16-22
Venous hum. The venous hum is a continuous, low-pitched hum heard over the neck in many children; it is often best heard over the right supraclavicular space.

EXAMINATION

The division of the cardiac examination into the techniques of inspection, palpation, and auscultation is useful. Because the findings of inspection and palpation are closely related and complementary to one another, these techniques are discussed together. Auscultation provides much valuable information about cardiac dynamics, but the practitioner must be cautious not to apply the stethoscope to the chest wall before performing the visual and palpatory examinations.

Several environmental considerations are basic to the cardiac examination. A quiet room is essential, because cardiac sounds are for the most part subtle and low pitched and are thus easily missed if outside noises prevail. A good light source that can be directed tangentially across the chest wall is important for adequate observation.

Examination of the precordium is most effectively performed with the examiner standing on the client's right side. The complete assessment requires that the client be examined in the sitting, supine, and left lateral recumbent positions. Whereas inspection and palpation are performed primarily with the client in the supine position, thorough auscultation should be performed with the client in all three positions. Both sitting forward and lying in the left lateral position bring various parts of the heart closer to the chest wall, thus enhancing certain auditory findings.

It is important to remember that examination of the peripheral pulses, including the radial, brachial, femoral, popliteal, dorsalis pedis, and posterior tibial, is an essential component in the assessment of the cardiovascular system. Also included are the assessment of the abdominal aorta and assessment of the blood pressure in the upper and lower extremities in the sitting, standing, and lying positions. These components may be assessed during this portion of the examination or integrated with other portions of the physical examination.

Inspection and palpation

Inspection and palpation of the precordium should be performed before the stethoscope is applied to the chest wall. It is sometimes tempting to use the stethoscope as the only means of assessing findings over the precordium, but much valuable information can be gained by using visual and tactile assessment procedures. These findings will enhance and may augment the auditory findings.

The purpose of both inspection and palpation is to determine the presence and extent of normal and abnormal pulsations over the precordium. These pulsations may be manifested as the apex beat (or apical impulse) or as heaves or lifts of the chest; they provide some reflection of myocardial and hemodynamic activity. Inspection and palpation together provide a useful method of assessing left, right, and combined ventricular hypertrophy. The visibility and palpability of those movements are affected by the thickness of the chest wall and by the type and amount of tissue through which the vibrations must travel.

Inspection

The chest wall and epigastrium are inspected while the client is in the supine position. A tangential light is helpful for observing subtle movements of the chest. The examiner stands to the client's right side and observes the chest for size and symmetry and then for any pulsations, retractions, heaves, or lifts. The location and timing of all impulses should be noted.

Apical impulse. The thrust of the contracting left ventricle may produce a visible pulsation in the area of the midclavicular line in the fifth left intercostal space. This is the normal apical impulse, and it is visibly evident in about half the normal adult population. It occurs nearly synchronously with the carotid impulse, and simultaneous palpation of a carotid artery is helpful in identifying it.

When visible, the apical impulse helps to identify an area very near the cardiac apex, thus giving some indication of cardiac size. In the case of left ventricular hypertrophy or dilatation, or both, as may occur with systemic hypertension, the apical impulse may be located more laterally or inferiorly, or both; for example, it may be located at the left anterior axillary line in the sixth left intercostal space.

Retractions. A slight retraction of the chest wall just medial to the midclavicular line in the fifth interspace is a normal finding. Marked or actual retraction of the rib is abnormal and may result from pericardial disease. Left ventricular hypertrophy is often accompanied by a systolic thrust, producing a "rocking" movement.

Heaves or lifts. When the work and forcefulness of the right ventricle is greatly increased, a diffuse lifting impulse is often produced along the left sternal border with each beat. This is referred to as a lift or heave; these terms are generally used interchangeably.

Palpation

The technique of palpation builds on and expands the findings gleaned from inspection. The entire precordium is palpated methodically, beginning at the apex, moving to the left sternal border, and then to the base of the heart (Fig. 16-23). Other areas may also be included if indicated, including the left axillary area, the epigastrium, and the right sternal border. During palpation the examiner is searching for the apical impulse at or near the apex and for any abnormal heaves, thrills, or retractions elsewhere on the precordium, indicating cardiac hypertrophy, dilatation, or murmurs. The abnormal flow of blood resulting in an audible murmur may also result in the palpatory sensation known as a thrill. It is rather like a rushing sensation beneath the fingers and has been likened to the feeling transmitted to the fingers placed over the larynx of a purring cat. As with inspection, the shape and thickness of the chest wall are important variables.

The client is in the supine position for this portion of the cardiac examination. The examiner should take adequate time to "tune in" or "warm up" to movements over the precordium, because many are faint and subtle and are perceived only after a "warming up" period. It is important to describe pulsations in relation to their timing in the cardiac cycle. This is facilitated by simultaneously palpating the carotid pulsation with the left hand while palpating the precordium with the right. All pulsations should be described in terms of their location in an interspace and their distance from the midsternal, midclavicular, or axillary lines.

Apical impulse. Although the thrust noted over the apex of the heart is sometimes referred to as the *point of maximum impulse* (PMI), this term is not recommended, because the actual point or area of maximum impulse may or may not be located over the apical area. The term *apical impulse* is preferred. The presence, location, size, and character of the apical impulse should be assessed. The apical impulse is palpable in about half the normal adult population.

Standing to the right of the client and using the fingertips and palmar aspect of the right hand, the examiner palpates first over the apex, particularly in the area of the fifth interspace in the midclavicular line. Normally, the apical impulse is palpable in or just medial to the midclavicular line and is felt as a faint, short-duration, localized tap less than 2 cm in diameter. On occasion the apical impulse may be normally located lateral to the midclavicular line, for example, in association with a high diaphragm, as occurs with pregnancy. The outward movement of the normal impulse is not excessively forceful and is palpable only during the first part of systole. The amplitude of the apical impulse may seem to be increased in normal individuals with thin chest walls. Turning the client to the left lateral position may cause a normal impulse to seem abnormal in both amplitude and duration, since the apex is brought closer to the chest wall, thus accentuating its activities. In obese persons or those with an increased anteroposterior chest diameter, the apical impulse is not likely to be palpable. Conditions such as anxiety, anemia, fever, and hyperthyroidism may produce an apical

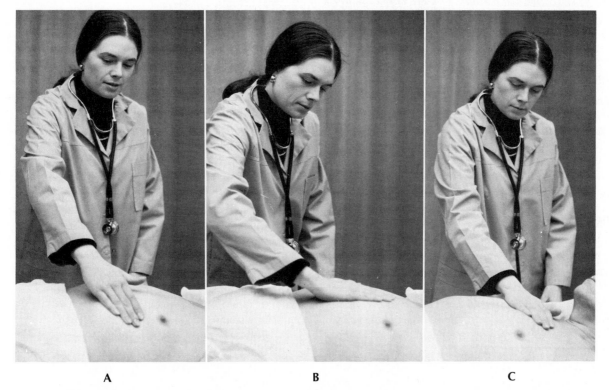

A   B   C

Fig. 16-23
Palpation of the precordium. The examiner palpates three areas of the precordium: **A,** over the apex; **B,** over the left sternal border; **C,** over the base of the heart.

impulse increased in force and duration. Normally, systolic ejection may be associated with a slight retraction of the lower left parasternal area.

Apex area: left ventricular hypertrophy. Hypertrophy of the left ventricle typically produces an abnormally forceful and sustained outward movement during ventricular systole. In addition, the apex impulse may be displaced laterally and downward and may be increased in size. For example, the apical impulse may be found 4 cm lateral to the midclavicular line in the sixth intercostal space and may be 4 cm in diameter.

Generally, the degree of displacement of the impulse correlates with the extent of cardiac enlargement. In addition to an alteration in location and size, the impulse may become more diffuse and palpable in more than one interspace; also, the amplitude or forcefulness may be increased. Displacement tends to be maximal when there is both dilatation and hypertrophy. Conditions associated with a volume overload, such as mitral and aortic regurgitation and left-to-right shunts, tend to produce such dilatation and hypertrophy. Hypertrophy of the left ventricle without dilatation, as may occur with aortic stenosis and systemic hypertension, results in an apical impulse that is increased in force and duration but not necessarily displaced laterally; it may still be located in the midclavicular line. In some persons with left ventricular hypertrophy, the increased force and prolonged duration of the apical impulse produces a lifting sensation under the examiner's fingers.

Left sternal border: right ventricular hypertrophy. Right ventricular hypertrophy is less common than left ventricular hypertrophy. It may be detected on palpation as a diffuse, lifting systolic impulse along the lower left sternal border. This finding may be associated with a systolic retraction at the apex, resulting from displacement and rotation of the left ventricle posteriorly by the enlarged right ventricle. A diffuse lift, or heave, along the lower left sternum is associated, for example, with pulmonary valve disease, pulmonary hypertension, and chronic lung disease. A thrill may also be palpated in this area and is associated with ventricular septal defects. The palmar aspect of the examiner's right hand is placed over the left sternal border.

Base of the heart. The examiner's right hand rests over the base of the heart at the second left and right intercostal spaces at the sternal borders and feels for pulsations, thrills, or the vibrations of semilunar valve closure. Normally, the base is fairly ''quiet'' to palpation.

Aortic stenosis may be associated with a thrill palpable in the first and third right interspaces, as well as in the second right interspace. In persons with systemic hypertension, it may be possible to palpate the accentuated vibration of aortic valve closure at the time of S_2.

Pulmonic valve stenosis may be associated with a thrill in the second and third left interspaces near the sternum. In persons with pulmonary hypertension, pulsations may be palpated in the same area. The most common causes of abnormal pulsations in the pulmonary artery area are increases in pressure or flow in the pulmonary artery, such as in pulmonary hypertension or atrial septal defect. In some normal people with thin chest walls, it is possible to palpate a brief, slight pulsation in this area. Conditions such as anemia, fever, exertion, and pregnancy would accentuate this pulsation.

Percussion

The technique of percussion is of limited value in cardiac assessment. In the past, percussion was used to determine the borders of cardiac dullness, but the actual size of the heart is much more accurately determined by a chest roentgenogram, and ventricular hypertrophy is better determined by combined inspection and palpation. Variations in chest wall configuration and the type and amount of interposed tissue, such as air or fat tissue, alter and limit the accuracy of this procedure. The value of percussion is further limited in the assessment of right ventricular enlargement, since this condition causes substernal and anteroposterior enlargement, which is not accessible to the percussion note.

Auscultation

The stethoscope is a device that gathers and slightly amplifies sound before it is transmitted to the ears. A comfortable and properly fitting stethoscope is essential for adequate auscultation. Although the selection of proper earpieces for comfort and the best sound transmission is a matter of individual preference, there are several general guidelines that are useful in making that selection. The earpieces should be large enough to provide a snug fit in the external canal and to block out extraneous room noises. Enough tension should be present to hold the earpieces tightly in place. The rigid metal tubing leading to the earpieces should be bent so as to angle in the same direction as the ear canal, that is, forward. The flexible tubing may be made of rubber or plastic, and it should be thick enough to keep out extraneous sounds; it should also be reasonably short, about 1 foot, because added length dampens the sound and decreases the efficiency of the stethoscope in transmitting higher frequencies.

The stethoscope chestpiece should be equipped with both a bell and a diaphragm, each of which selectively transmits different frequencies of sound. The valve facilitating a change between the two should be tight fitting, permitting a change without the admission of outside sound. The diaphragm accentuates the higher frequency sounds. It should be made of a fairly rigid substance and should be pressed firmly against the skin during auscultation, further enhancing faint, high-frequency sounds. In contrast to the diaphragm, the bell brings out the low-frequency sounds and filters out the high-frequency ones. It should be placed very lightly on the chest wall with just enough pressure applied to seal the edge. If greater pressure is applied to the bell against the chest wall, the skin becomes a relatively tight diaphragm, filtering out the lower pitched sounds. Alternating the application of light and heavy pressure to the bell may be a helpful maneuver when listening to low-pitched murmurs or filling sounds. Most low-pitched sounds are diastolic filling sounds or murmurs and are often best heard with the client lying down, since orthostatic pooling on standing may cause such sounds to diminish in intensity. Although heart sounds are referred to as being of "high" or "low" frequency, these terms are relative. All heart sounds are generally low pitched (low frequency) and are in a range ordinarily difficult for the human ear to hear. Thus, any technique that improves audibility should be carefully implemented.

Satisfactory auscultation requires a quiet room; mechanical and conversational noises must be minimized. The room should be comfortably warm for the client so that shivering and subsequent muscular noises are avoided. The anterior chest should be exposed to the waist. The examining table should be adequately large for the client to change positions from sitting to supine to left lateral recumbent with ease. Auscultation in only one position is not adequate.

A systematic method of auscultation is essential; all precordial areas and each sound and pause must be attended to. One recommended system is to begin at the apex and "inch" the stethoscope toward the left sternal border and up the sternal border to the second left and then to the second right intercostal space. Another method consists of beginning the examination at the base of the heart at the second right intercostal space, where S_2 is always the loudest of the two heart sounds. This is particularly helpful if the heart sounds are heard as nearly equal in intensity at the apex. Auscultation should be performed using both the bell and the diaphragm and should cover the entire precordium and areas of radiation, such as the axillary area or carotid arteries, when indicated.

In each area examined, the examiner listens selectively to each component of the cardiac cycle; as with palpation, this usually requires a period of "warming up" or "tuning in" to the various cardiac events. First, the examiner notes the rate and rhythm of the heartbeat. Then, at each auscultatory area, the examiner concentrates initially on S_1, noting its intensity and variations therein, possible duplication, and the effects of respiration. The examiner then selects out S_2 and focuses on the same characteristics. Next, he or she concentrates on systole, then on diastole, listening first for any extra sounds and then for murmurs. The examiner must listen selectively for each component; it is impossible to listen for everything at once.

If the initial part of the examination is performed while the client is lying in a supine position, the client is asked to roll to his left side; the examiner applies the bell lightly at the apex and listens for the presence or absence of low-frequency diastolic sounds, such as a filling sound or a mitral valve murmur (Fig. 16-24).

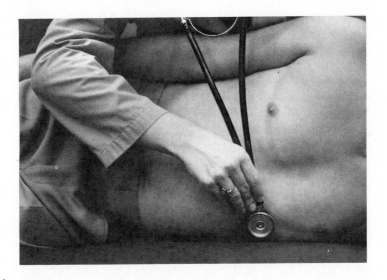

Fig. 16-24
With the client lying in the left lateral position, the examiner listens for low-pitched diastolic sounds using the bell of the stethoscope.

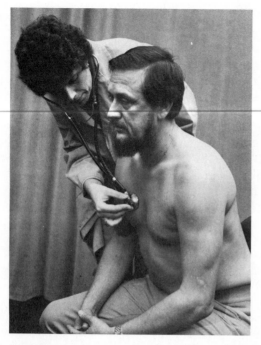

Fig. 16-25
Using the diaphragm of the stethoscope while the client leans forward and holds his breath in full expiration, the examiner listens for high-pitched murmurs at the base of the heart.

The client is then asked to sit up and lean slightly forward. Pressing the diaphragm firmly against the chest, the examiner listens at both the second left and the second right intercostal spaces at the sternal border to detect the presence or absence of high-pitched diastolic murmurs of aortic or pulmonic valve insufficiency (Fig. 16-25). Listening is done during normal respiration and then with the client's breath held in deep expiration.

NECK VESSELS

The vascular structures of the neck accessible for and included in the cardiovascular examination are the jugular veins and the carotid arteries. Examination of these vessels provides information on local states and also reflects the activity of the heart. The jugular veins are observed for pulse waves and pressure level; the carotid arteries are examined by inspection, palpation, and auscultation to assess the characteristics of their pulsations.

JUGULAR VEINS

Venous pulse waves and venous pressure are assessed at the external and internal jugular veins. The external jugular veins lie superficially and are visible above the clavicle close to the insertion of the sternocleidomastoid muscles. The internal jugular veins are larger and lie deep to the sternocleidomastoid muscles near the carotid arteries; reflection of their activity may be visible on the skin overlying these vessels. Blood from the jugular veins flows directly into the superior vena cava. Fig. 16-26 illustrates the location of the external and internal jugular veins.

Venous return and the filling volume are important determinants of cardiac performance. These cannot be directly assessed on physical examination, but a general estimate can be made from observation of the jugular veins. The veins leading to the right side of the heart may be thought of as a system of distensible tubes with partially competent valves. Therefore, some judgment of the filling pressure of the heart may be made by observing the pressure level and the waveforms transmitted from the heart. Observation of the two components of pressure level and pulse waves in the veins gives an indication of the dynamics of the right side of the heart.

When the normal person is in the sitting position, no jugular venous pulsations are visible; with the trunk elevated 45 degrees from horizontal, the jugular venous pulse does not rise more than 1 to 2 cm above the level of the manubrium. When the normal person is in the reclining position, the venous pulse becomes evident because gravity no longer prevents backflow from the heart and the veins become filled.

In the examination of the jugular veins the client is in the supine position. If this position is uncomfortable, the client's trunk may be elevated to a 45-degree angle. If the veins are very distended, it is best to examine them with the client in a sitting position. The veins or venous pulsations are more readily visible if the client's neck is slightly turned away from the side being examined, and the veins are observed with tangential lighting so that small shadows are cast. Clothing should be removed from the neck and upper thorax so that there is no constriction. The head and neck may rest comfortably on a pillow, but the neck should not be sharply flexed.

Jugular venous pulse

The normal venous pulse consists of three positive components—the a, c, and v waves—and two negative slopes—the x and y descents (Fig. 16-27). The a wave is frequently the highest part of the total pulse wave and is produced by atrial contraction. As the right atrium contracts, ejecting blood into the right ventricle, there is also a brief backflow of blood into the vena cava. This retrograde pulse wave is reflected in the jugular veins as the a wave. This wave occurs just before S_1; if an S_4 is present, it occurs at the peak of the a wave.

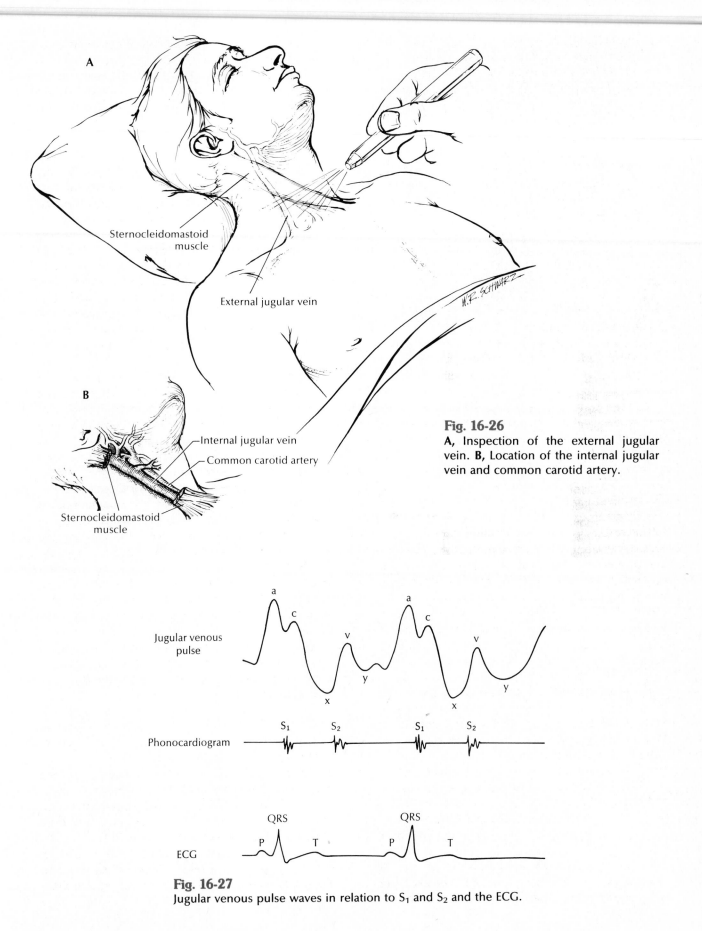

Sternocleidomastoid
muscle

External jugular vein

Internal jugular vein

Common carotid artery

Sternocleidomastoid
muscle

Fig. 16-26
A, Inspection of the external jugular vein. **B,** Location of the internal jugular vein and common carotid artery.

Jugular venous pulse

Phonocardiogram

ECG

Fig. 16-27
Jugular venous pulse waves in relation to S_1 and S_2 and the ECG.

Two simultaneous events contribute to the production of the c wave: the impact of the adjacent carotid artery pulsation and the retrograde transmission of a pulse wave, caused by right ventricular systole and bulging of the closed tricuspid valve. The c wave occurs at the end of S_1.

The tricuspid valve remains closed during ventricular systole while blood from the systemic circulation continues to fill the vena cava and the right atrium. The increased volume in these structures leads to a pressure increase reflected in the jugular veins as the v, or passive filling, wave. This wave reaches a peak during late ventricular systole. Following this, the pressure in the right atrium begins to fall as the bulging of the tricuspid valve decreases, first during relaxation of the right ventricle and then as the tricuspid valve opens.

The x descent following the c wave is produced by downward displacement of the base of the ventricles (including the tricuspid valve) during ventricular systole and by atrial diastole. The y descent following the v wave is produced by the opening of the tricuspid valve and the subsequent rapid flow of blood from the right atrium to the right ventricle.

It is usually possible to discern the three positive and two negative waves of the jugular venous pulse when the heart rate is below 90 beats per minute and the P-Q interval is normal. At more rapid heart rates, there is often a fusion or overlapping of some of the waves and analysis of the waveform is difficult.

Abnormalities of waves

The a wave. The a wave, which may be the highest or most pronounced of the three positive waves, is increased when it becomes more difficult for the contracting right atrium to empty into the right ventricle. For example, in tricuspid valve stenosis the a wave is more prominent. When there is right ventricular enlargement resulting from severe pulmonary stenosis or pulmonary hypertension and the right atrium must contract more forcefully to fill it, an enlarged a wave also results.

Irregularly enlarged a waves result from complete AV block. When the atrium contracts against a closed tricuspid valve, giant (cannon) a waves are produced. In ventricular tachycardia, the cannon waves may occur irregularly, since the cause of their production—simultaneous atrial and ventricular systole and a closed tricuspid valve—does not accompany each beat.

The x descent and c and v waves. When the tricuspid valve is insufficient, backflow of blood from the right ventricle to the right atrium occurs during ventricular systole. This causes the x slope to become obliterated or replaced by the positive waves, the c and v waves, which then form the c-v wave. Thus, with the obliteration of a negative slope and the accentuation of the two positive waves, a large jugular venous pulse wave is produced. The c-v wave may become so enlarged as to resemble exaggerated arterial pulsations. Tricuspid insufficiency may be organic, resulting from rheumatic heart disease; or it may be produced in clients with generalized cardiac failure, wherein the right ventricle becomes so dilated that the tricuspid ring is stretched and regurgitation ensues.

The y descent. The tricuspid valve opens shortly after S_2, and the rapid filling phase of ventricular diastole begins. The characteristics of the y descent depend on several factors, including pressure and volume circumstances in the great vessels, the right atrium, and the right ventricle, and resistance to flow across the tricuspid valve. Tricuspid stenosis, therefore, would produce a slow y descent because it presents obstruction to right atrial emptying. In clients with severe heart failure in which the venous pressure is extremely high, a sharp, exaggerated y wave is produced.

Differentiation from carotid arterial pulsations

Because the internal jugular vein lies deep to the sternocleidomastoid muscle and close to the carotid artery, its pulsations may be confused with those produced by the common carotid artery. There are several means of differentiating these pulsations.

Quality and character of the pulse. In normal sinus rhythm, the jugular venous pulse has three positive waves and the carotid pulse has one positive wave. Usually, the venous pulse waves are more undulating than the brisk arterial waves. The examiner may be assisted in differentiating the two by palpating the carotid pulse on one side of the neck and observing the jugular venous pulse on the other.

Effect of respiration. With normal inspiration, intrathoracic pressure decreases, blood flow into the right atrium increases, and the level of the pulse wave in the neck veins descends. The opposite occurs during expiration. Respiration does not have this effect on the carotid pulsations.

Effect of changing position. Pulsations in the neck veins become more prominent when the client assumes the recumbent position and less prominent when the client is in the sitting position. Carotid pulsations are not affected by posture.

Effect of venous compression. The pulsations of the jugular veins are rather easily eliminated by applying gentle pressure over the vein at the base of the neck above the clavicle. This blocks the retrograde transmission of the venous pulse wave, leaving only the arterial pulsations.

Effect of abdominal pressure. Pressure applied by the examiner's hand over the client's abdomen may cause an increased prominence of the venous pulsations. The examiner presses, using the palm of his hand and applying moderately firm pressure over the upper right quadrant of the abdomen for 30 to 60 seconds. In normal persons there is slight, if any, increase in the venous pulsations. However, if there is right-sided heart failure, the jugular venous pulsations and distention may markedly increase as venous return to the heart is increased. Normally this maneuver produces no change in the carotid pulsations.

Jugular venous pressure

The level of the column of blood in the jugular veins reflects the volume and pressure circumstances on the right side of the heart. Both the external and internal jugular veins can be assessed. Although other mechanical techniques are available for the evaluation of venous pressure, inspection on physical examination remains a useful and reliable maneuver.

In a normal client examined in the supine position, full neck veins are normally visible. When the normal person is examined with the thorax elevated to a 45-degree angle from horizontal, the venous pulses should ascend no more than a few centimeters above the clavicle. With markedly elevated venous pressure, the neck veins may be distended as high as the angle of the jaw, even when the person is in the upright sitting position. The height of venous pressure may be estimated by measuring the distance that the veins are distended above the manubrium sterni.

The examiner should inspect the veins on both sides of the neck. When the venous pressure is generally increased, distention is noted on both sides; unilateral distention may occur as a result of kinking in the left innominate vein in some older clients. It may be nec-

essary to change the position of the client to view the jugular venous pulse and pressure most clearly. The sternal angle, or angle of Louis, is used as a reference point. The vertical distance between the sternal angle and the highest level of the jugular pulsations is measured and recorded in centimeters (Fig. 16-28). The lower the client's head must be placed before the pulsations are visible, the lower the pressure; the higher the client's head must be placed before the upper level of the pulsations can be identified, the higher the venous pressure. Venous pressures greater than 3 to 4 cm above the sternal angle are abnormal. The level to which distention is observed and the position of the client should be noted.

Elevation of venous pressure may be an indication of congestive heart failure, constrictive pericarditis, or obstruction of the superior vena cava. The most common cause of elevated venous pressure is failure of the right ventricle resulting from left ventricular failure. As described earlier, the effect of applying increased abdominal pressure may increase the amount of venous distention in the presence of right-sided heart failure.

CAROTID ARTERIES

The techniques of inspection, palpation, and auscultation are used in examining the carotid arteries. The neck is observed for unusually large or bounding carotid pulses. The carotid arterial pulses are then palpated bilaterally, as are all the pulses, for rate, rhythm, equal-

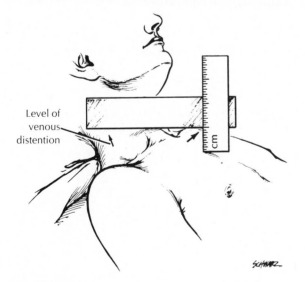

Fig. 16-28
Measurement of jugular venous pressure. The arrows indicate the height of the jugular venous pressure in centimeters.

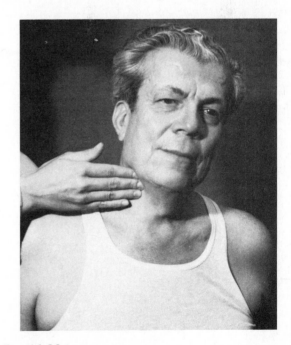
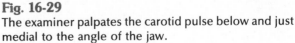

Fig. 16-29
The examiner palpates the carotid pulse below and just medial to the angle of the jaw.

ity, amplitude, and contour. The examiner palpates with his forefinger below and just medial to the angle of the jaw (Fig. 16-29). Only one side is examined at a time to avoid excessive carotid sinus massage, thus preventing unnecessary slowing of the pulse, and to avoid further embarrassment of borderline circulation in older clients. The head should be rotated slightly toward the side being examined to relax the sternocleidomastoid muscle. The heart sounds may be used as reference points, and simultaneous auscultation of the heart is then helpful. S_1 and the carotid impulse are very nearly simultaneous events. The carotid arteries are auscultated with the bell of the stethoscope for bruits indicating local obstruction or for the sound of transmitted cardiac murmurs.

Carotid arterial pulse

The carotid arteries are the best arteries in which to assess several characteristics of the arterial pulse, for example, whether the force is strong or weak, the rise and collapse rapid or slow, and the impulse double or single in nature.

The normal carotid pulse consists of a single positive wave followed by a dicrotic notch (Fig. 16-30). The upstroke is smooth and rapid, the summit is dome shaped, and the downstroke is less steep than the upstroke. The dicrotic notch on the downstroke may not be palpable or may be only slightly palpable. It is often definitely felt in the otherwise normal client during exercise, excitement, or fever.

The size or amplitude of the arterial pulse is determined by a variety of factors, including left ventricular stroke volume and ejection rate, peripheral resistance or distensibility, and pulse pressure. Clinically, abnormalities of the pulse size may be divided into two groups: exaggerated, or hyperkinetic, pulses and weak, or hypokinetic, pulses. During palpation, the examiner may gain an impression of the height of the pulse and the rate of change on the upstroke and downstroke.

Situations associated with a widened arterial pulse pressure—an increased stroke volume and decreased peripheral resistance—produce a hyperkinetic carotid pulse. The pulse may be large and strong with a normal contour (bounding pulse), or it may be characterized by a markedly high and rapid upstroke (waterhammer pulse) or by an extremely rapid downstroke (collapsing pulse). In the latter two cases, the peak of the pulse is short and rapid. The hyperkinetic pulse may be produced as the result of hyperdynamic or high-output states, such as occur with anxiety, exercise, fever, or pregnancy; as the result of hyperthyroidism or anemia; or as the result of abnormally rapid runoff of blood from the arterial system, such as occurs with abnormal shunting of blood (patent ductus arteriosus or septal defects) or with aortic insufficiency. Aortic insufficiency is a common organic cause of the hyperkinetic pulse in adults. With severe regurgitation, the pulse is described as water hammer and collapsing; a large volume of blood is rapidly ejected from and then returns to the left ventricle across the incompetent valve. Another cause of the hyperkinetic pulse in adults is a complete heart block with bradycardia and increased stroke volume.

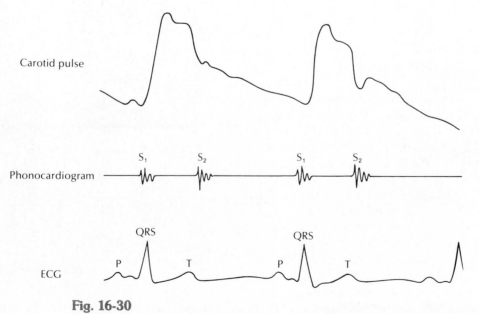

Fig. 16-30
The carotid pulse wave in relation to S_1 and S_2 and the ECG.

The hypokinetic carotid pulse is associated with conditions wherein there is a diminished stroke volume of the left ventricle, increased peripheral vascular resistance, a narrowed pulse pressure, or resistance to flow across the cardiac valves. Examples of causes of a hypokinetic pulse include left ventricular failure resulting from myocardial infarction, constrictive pericarditis, and moderate or severe valvular aortic stenosis. In aortic stenosis, the pulse may demonstrate a slow upstroke, a delayed peak, and a small volume.

Pulses with double, rather than single, pulsations may be produced by combined aortic stenosis and insufficiency (pulsus bisferiens) or by lowered peripheral resistance and lowered diastolic pressure (dicrotic pulse).

A pulse that occurs at regular intervals but varies in amplitude (pulsus alternans) is produced by alterations in left ventricular contractile force, as may occur with left ventricular failure. Premature ventricular contractions coupled with previous normal beats produce a bigeminal pulse; that is, every alternate beat is premature.

Auscultation

Several conditions may produce a palpable carotid thrill associated with an audible bruit. These conditions include local obstruction of a carotid artery, a jugular vein–carotid artery fistula, and high-output state, such as occurs with severe anemia and thyrotoxicosis. Aortic valvular stenosis may cause a thrill to be referred to the carotid arteries. The bruits are heard by placing the bell of the stethoscope on the skin overlying the carotid artery and listening while the client holds his breath (Fig. 16-31). The bell of the stethoscope is used because the bruits are low-pitched sounds.

Cardiovascular findings associated with hypertension

To assist the student clinician in organizing the examination around a prevalent cardiovascular problem, the various components of the history and physical examination of a client with elevated blood pressure, or hypertension, are presented here. Although approximately 90% of persons with hypertension have primary or essential hypertension, it is important to rule out potentially curable secondary causes; findings indicative of those causes are also included here.

Many persons with elevated blood pressure have no observable symptoms related to that abnormality, and it may be identified during a routine examination. Others, however, do describe one or several symptoms, most commonly a headache, which may be present on awakening and subside after the individual has been up for some time. Other early symptoms include light-headedness, dizziness, tinnitus, fatigue, weakness, nervousness, flushing sensations, and epistaxis. Later symptoms of hypertension are attributable to the effects of sustained high blood pressure on the heart, eyes, cerebral circulation, and kidneys. These symptoms may include, for example, dyspnea, orthopnea, paroxysmal nocturnal dyspnea, palpitations, chest pain, edema, eye fatigue, blurred vision, headache, weakness, numbness, tingling of the hands and feet, polyuria, nocturia, and flank pain.

The examiner should inquire about the presence of any of these symptoms. The client should also be asked about any family history of hypertension, the use of steroids, and, with women, the use of oral contraceptives or any previous hypertension associated with pregnancy.

Secondary causes of hypertension include coarctation of the aorta, primary hyperaldosteronism, Cushing's syndrome, pheochromocytoma, and renal vascular disease. Symptoms related to these causes include history of leg fatigue with coarctation of the aorta; episodes of muscular weakness, polyuria, nocturia, polydipsia, and intermittent paresthesias with primary aldosteronism; alteration of sexual function (amenorrhea, impotence), emotional lability, weakness, and backache with Cushing's syndrome; weight loss, palpitations, headache, nervousness, sweating, blanching,

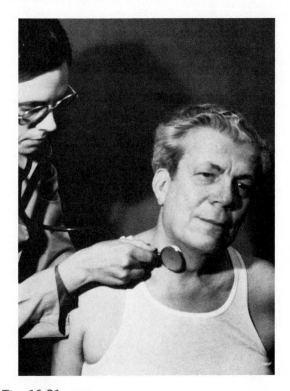

Fig. 16-31
The examiner listens with the bell of the stethoscope for bruits over the carotid artery.

coldness of skin, nausea, vomiting, and abdominal pain with pheochromocytoma; and flank pain and urinary tract infections and symptoms with renal and renal vascular disease. A careful history for any of these symptoms of secondary hypertension should be obtained.

The physical examination of a person with high blood pressure must include the following components:

1. Observation of general appearance—facial and body expression. Is nervousness, anxiety, or a plethoric expression apparent? Are the round face, head, neck, and trunk obesity, purple striae, or ecchymosis suggestive of Cushing's syndrome present?

2. Measurement of blood pressure in both arms in the sitting, lying, and standing positions and measurement of blood pressure in the lower extremities. A rise in the diastolic pressure when the client changes from the supine to the standing position suggests essential or renal arterial hypertension. Blood pressure that is lower in the legs than in the arms suggests coarctation of the aorta.

3. Examination of the retina. The status of the retina is one of the best indications of the duration and prognosis of the hypertension. Narrowing of the arterioles and an increased light reflex on them may be among the earliest manifestations of hypertension (see color plate of eye). Later, arteriovenous compression may be present. Small, well-defined exudates and isolated hemorrhages may accompany a more benign phase of hypertension. More hemorrhages and soft, poorly defined exudates indicate more severe hypertension. Papilledema (swelling of the optic nerve head) indicates a serious stage of the hypertension.

4. Palpation and auscultation of the carotid arteries for bruits, which give evidence of stenosis or occlusion.

5. Examination of the precordium for evidence of left ventricular hypertrophy, cardiac decompensation, or murmurs. Observe and palpate for lifts and heaves; auscultate for an increased second heart sound, for the presence of third and/or fourth heart sounds, and for murmurs. Coarctation of the aorta may give rise to a systolic murmur and it may be accompanied by aortic valvular disease that may be associated with an ejection click and murmurs of either aortic stenosis or regurgitation.

6. Examination of the lungs for evidence of congestion.

7. Examination of the abdomen by auscultation for bruits originating in stenotic renal arteries. These bruits may have both systolic and diastolic components and are best heard just to the right or left of the midline above the umbilicus. The abdomen should also be examined by palpation for pulsating abdominal aneurysm and for enlarged kidneys associated with polycystic renal disease.

8. Palpation of the femoral pulses. A decrease in amplitude and/or a delay in the pulse may accompany coarctation of the aorta.

9. Performance of a neurological examination to search for evidence of cerebrovascular disease (for specifics see Chapter 23 on the neurological examination).

SUMMARY

I. Measure blood pressure in both arms and, if indicated, legs

II. Examine heart
  A. Inspect anterior chest wall
  B. Palpate precordium
    1. Apex
    2. Left sternal border
    3. Base
    4. Other areas as indicated, e.g., right sternal border
  C. Auscultate heart sounds in sitting, supine, and left lateral recumbent positions
    1. Apex
    2. Along left sternal border
    3. Second left intercostal space
    4. Second right intercostal space

III. Examine neck vessels
  A. Jugular veins
    1. Observe jugular venous pulsations
    2. Observe jugular venous pressure
  B. Carotid arteries
    1. Observe carotid arterial pulsation
    2. Palpate carotid pulses, one at a time
    3. Auscultate carotid arteries

IV. Palpate peripheral pulses, including temporal, radial, femoral, popliteal, dorsalis pedis, and posterior tibial (Assessment of these pulses may be integrated with other portions of the physical examination.)

V. Palpate and auscultate the abdominal aorta

BIBLIOGRAPHY

Ayres, S.M., Gregory J.J., and Buehler, M.E., editors: Cardiology: a clinicophysiologic approach, New York, 1971, Appleton-Century-Crofts.

Burch, G.E.: A primer of cardiology, Philadelphia, 1971. Lea & Febiger.

Carson, P.: Cardiac diagnosis, New York, 1969, McGraw-Hill Book Co.

Examination of the heart (series of four), New York, 1967, American Heart Association.

Fowler, N.O.: Physical diagnosis of heart disease, New York, 1962, MacMillan, Inc.

Friedburg, C.K.: Diseases of the heart, ed. 3, Philadelphia, 1966, W.B. Saunders Co.

Goldberger, E.: Textbook of clinical cardiology, St. Louis, 1982, The C.V. Mosby Co.

Hurst, J.W., editor: The heart, ed. 3, New York, 1974, McGraw-Hill Book Co.

Ravin, A.: Auscultation of the heart, Chicago, 1958, Yearbook Medical Publishers, Inc.

Selzer, A.: Principles of clinical cardiology, Philadelphia, 1975, W.B. Saunders Co.

CHAPTER 17

ASSESSMENT OF THE ABDOMEN

Although physical assessment of the abdomen includes all the four methods of examination (inspection, auscultation, percussion, and palpation), palpation is the technique most useful in detecting abdominal pathological conditions. Inspection is done first, followed by auscultation, since the movement or stimulation by pressure on the bowel occasioned by palpation and percussion is known to alter the motility of the bowel and generally to heighten the sounds.

The only special equipment necessary for examination of the abdomen is a stethoscope; a metal, cloth, or plastic ruler or tape measure that will not stretch; a skin-marking pencil; examining table and light; small pillows; and drapes to cover the client.

POSITION

The position that the client assumes voluntarily is important to note. The individual with abdominal pain frequently draws up the knees to reduce tension on the abdominal muscles and to reduce intraabdominal pressure. The client with generalized peritonitis lies almost motionless with the knees flexed.

Marked restlessness has been associated with biliary and intestinal colic and intraperitoneal hemorrhage.

INSPECTION

Before positioning the client for the abdominal examination, the practitioner should be certain that the client has recently voided (the bladder is empty).

The optimum position of the client for inspection of the abdomen is supine with the abdominal muscles as relaxed as possible. Tension in the abdominal wall muscles is best avoided by placing the client's arms comfortably at his sides as opposed to extending them upward, as occurs in placing them behind the head. Contraction of the abdominal muscles may be further avoided by placing a small pillow beneath the knees to

aid in maintaining the legs in slight flexion. Also, a small pillow placed beneath the head may add to the comfort of the client.

The room should be sufficiently warm that the draped client does not shiver, thereby tensing the abdominal wall. A further advantage may be obtained by instructing the client to relax and to breathe quietly and slowly through the mouth. Explanation of the entire examination before beginning and support during the examination may help to ease tension.

The entire abdomen must be free of clothing. An examination gown may be folded up over the chest, or a small towel may be used to cover the breasts of women. A sheet may be folded downward to the level of the mons.

A single source of light is used in inspection of the abdomen (Fig. 17-1). The light may be directed at a right angle to the long axis of the client or may be focused lengthwise over him, shining from the foot to the head. The examiner assumes a sitting position, *generally at the right side of the client;* the examiner's head is only slightly higher than the client's abdomen. The resultant shadow will be high, so that even small changes in contour will be highlighted, thereby increasing the likelihood of detection of a pathological condition. The examiner should be familiar with the normal topography of the abdomen to avoid identifying normal contours as masses (see Fig. 17-8). The examiner should carefully focus attention on the abdomen to accurately describe the presence or absence of symmetry, distention, masses, visible peristaltic waves, and respiratory movements. If the presence of peristalsis is in question, the examiner should carefully study the abdomen for several minutes.

The client is instructed to take a deep breath, forcing the diaphragm downward and decreasing the size of the abdominal cavity. In this manner, masses such as enlarged liver or spleen are made more obvious. The

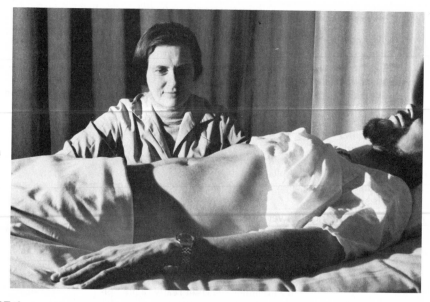

Fig. 17-1
Inspection of the abdomen with the examining light focused to provide the greatest amount of contrast for the abdominal terrain.

rectus muscles (Fig. 17-2) are prominent landmarks of the abdominal wall. Diastasis recti abdominis is a separation of rectus abdominis muscles. The separation may be palpated and may be observed as a ridge between the muscles when the intraabdominal pressure is increased by raising the head and shoulders. The defect does not pose a threat to the functions of the abdominal structures. Diastasis recti abdominis generally occurs as a result of pregnancy or marked obesity.

The examiner should then inspect the abdomen from a standing position at the foot of the bed or examining table. Asymmetry of the abdominal contour may be more readily detected from this position.

Anatomical mapping

Definitive description of signs and symptoms of the abdomen is facilitated through two commonly used methods of subdivision (Tables 17-1 to 17-4 and boxes on p. 361). The most frequently used method divides the abdomen into four quadrants (Fig. 17-3). An imaginary perpendicular line is dropped from the sternum to the pubic bone through the umbilicus, and a second line is dropped at a right angle to the first through the umbilicus.

For the most part, abdominal structures will be located in these quadrants as shown on p. 363.

Loops of the small bowel are found in all four quadrants. The bladder and the uterus are located at the lower midline.

Text continued on p. 365.

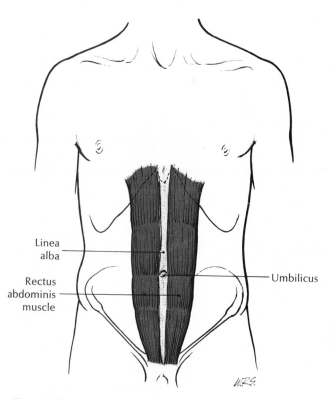

Linea alba

Rectus abdominis muscle

Umbilicus

Fig. 17-2
Rectus abdominis muscles. Separation of these muscles is called diastasis recti and may be detected by observation or palpation.

Percussion of liver dullness is important in detecting atrophy of the liver, such as might occur in acute fulminating hepatitis.

A less accurate sign of an enlarged liver is the percussion or palpation of the liver edge 2 or 3 cm below the costal margin in the midclavicular line because the upper border must be considered as well. The liver span is seen to be greater in men than in women and in the tall as opposed to the short individual. Error in estimating the liver span can occur when pleural effusion or lung consolidation obscures the upper liver border or when gas in the colon obscures the lower border.

On inspiration the diaphragm moves downward; thus, the span of liver dullness will normally be shifted inferiorly 2 to 3 cm. Pulmonary edema may also displace the liver caudally, whereas ascites, massive tumors, or pregnancy may push the liver upward. The liver assumes a more square configuration in cirrhosis of the liver, and the midclavicular and midsternal measurements may approach equality.

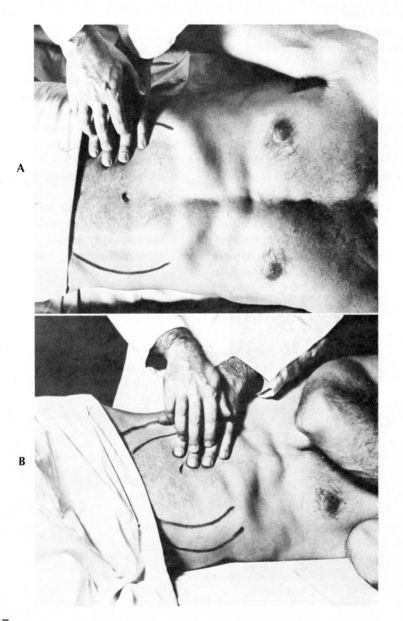

Fig. 17-17
Test for shifting dullness. **A,** With the client on his back, the line of dullness is marked in both flanks. **B,** The client is rotated on one side and then the other, and the new levels of dullness are marked each time. (From G.I. series: physical examination of the abdomen, Chapter 3, Percussion, Richmond, Va., 1981, A.H. Robins Co.)

Percussion for tympany and dullness

Spleen. Splenic dullness can be percussed from the level of the sixth or ninth to the eleventh rib just posterior to or at the midaxillary line on the left side.

Stomach. A lower-pitched tympany than that of the intestine is typical of the percussion note of the gastric air bubble. Percussion is performed in the area of the left lower anterior rib cage and in the left epigastric region to define the region occupied by the bubble. The percussion sounds of the stomach vary with the time the last meal was eaten.

Percussion for ascites (free fluid)

Test for shifting dullness. A technique for differentiating ascites from cysts or edema fluid in the abdominal wall is the percussion test for shifting dullness (Fig. 17-17).

The client is placed in the supine position, and fluid dullness is percussed laterally in the flank while the abdomen medial to the dullness is tympanitic as a result of the presence of gas within the bowel. The line of demarcation between the dull and tympanitic sounds is marked, and the client is instructed to lie on his side. The ascites fluid will flow via gravity to shift the line of dullness closer to the umbilicus on the same side as the client is lying. A new line is marked, and the change is measured in centimeters. Subsequently, the client is turned to the opposite side and the change recorded. The test enables the examiner to detect free fluid and make a rough estimate of the volume.

Knee-chest position. Percussion of the periumbilical region of a client in the knee-chest position enables the examiner to detect smaller amounts of fluid than is possible with the individual supine.

Puddle sign. After maintaining the client in the knee-elbow position for several minutes so that ascitic fluid puddles over the umbilicus by gravity, the examiner percusses the umbilical area for the dull notes of fluid (Fig. 17-18).

A volume of free fluid in the peritoneal cavity greater than 2 L can be detected by methods of shifting dullness. Ascites is caused by (1) diseases of the liver, such as cirrhosis and hepatitis; (2) diseases of the heart, such as congestive failure and constrictive pericarditis; (3) pancreatitis; (4) cancer, such as peritoneal metastases and ovarian tumors; (5) tuberculous peritonitis; and (6) hypoalbuminemia.

Fist percussion

Another use of percussion in the abdominal examination is the use of fist percussion to vibrate the tissue rather than produce sound (Fig. 17-19). The palm of the left hand is placed over the region of liver dullness and is struck a light blow by the fisted right hand. Tenderness elicited by this method is usually associated with hepatitis or cholecystitis. Fist percussion at the costovertebral junction is also useful in assessing renal tenderness. Fig. 17-20 demonstrates the relationship of the kidney to the costovertebral junction. The technique of direct fist costovertebral percussion is demonstrated in Fig. 17-21, and the indirect method is shown in Fig. 17-22.

Some disadvantage is recognized in the use of fist percussion to elicit renal tenderness. Even after warn-

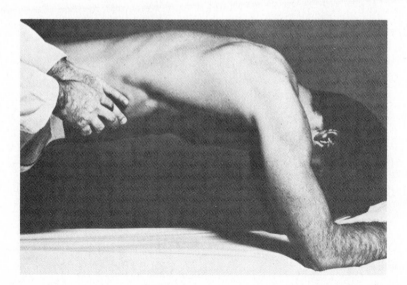

Fig. 17-18
Elicitation of the puddle sign. (From G.I. series: physical examination of the abdomen, Chapter 3, Percussion, Richmond, Va., 1981, A.H. Robins Co.)

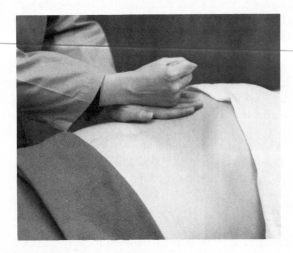

Fig. 17-19
Fist percussion of the liver. The palm of the hand is placed over the region of liver dullness and is struck a light blow with the fisted right hand. Tenderness elicited by this method is usually a result of hepatitis or cholecystitis. Fist percussion may be used over the costovertebral junction to elicit renal tenderness. (See text for alternate methods.)

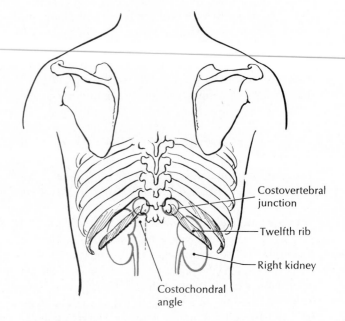

Costovertebral junction

Twelfth rib

Right kidney

Costochondral angle

Fig. 17-20
Relationship of the kidney to the twelfth rib. Note the costovertebral junction.

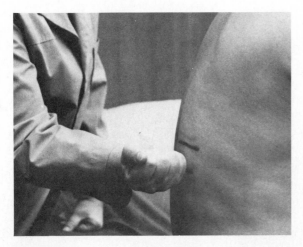

Fig. 17-21
Direct percussion of the costovertebral junction to elicit tenderness related to the kidney.

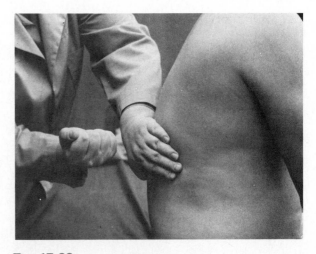

Fig. 17-22
Indirect percussion of the costovertebral junction to elicit tenderness related to the kidney.

ing the client, the blow sometimes startles him. Furthermore, the vibration may cause considerable pain and result in apprehension of further examination procedures. In addition, the examiner in standing behind the individual being examined is deprived of the opportunity to observe the client's response. Levinson (1982) has suggested the procedure of "flank lift" as a substitute for costovertebral fist percussion. With the client supine the examiner places both hands beneath the flanks, and gentle and quick lifting is applied. The person with renal inflammation will localize the pain. The stoical individual may only wince, but the presence of tenderness is confirmed. The lift can be graded in intensity, and there is less danger of hurting the client than with fist percussion.

PALPATION

Following careful visual scrutiny, auscultation, and percussion, palpation is used to substantiate findings and to further explore the abdomen. Palpation is used to evaluate the major organs of the abdomen; these organs are examined with respect to shape, position and mobility, size, consistency, and tension. Thorough and systematic screening is performed to detect areas of tenderness, muscular spasm, masses, or fluid.

The client's position is checked to make sure that maximum relaxation has been achieved. The examiner's hands should be warm, and the examiner should use techniques for enhancing bodily and psychological relaxation. Observation that the client does not relax

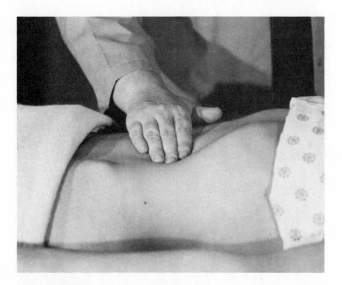

Fig. 17-23
Light palpation is performed with the hand parallel to the floor and the fingers approximated. The fingers depress the abdominal wall about 1 cm. This method of palpation is recommended for eliciting slight tenderness, large masses, and muscle guarding.

the abdominal muscles in spite of these maneuvers may justify the use of the technique in which the examiner exerts downward pressure on the lower sternum with his left hand while palpating with the other. The deeper inspiration that results inhibits abdominal muscle contraction. A suggestion for achieving relaxation in children is putting them into a tub of warm water, but this is not practical for a screening examination. The examiner is at the right side of the client, and the fingers of the examining hand are approximated. Measurements are more accurately recorded in centimeters. The older method of describing distance in finger breadths invites error, since the fingers of examiners are of varying diameters. The abdomen is explored in all four quadrants with both light and deep palpation. Light palpation is always done first.

Light palpation

Light palpation is gentle exploration performed while the client is in the supine position, with the examiner's hand parallel to the floor, the palm lying lightly on the abdomen, and the fingers approximated (Fig. 17-23). The fingers depress the abdominal wall approximately 1 cm without digging. This method of palpation is best for eliciting slight tenderness, large masses, and muscle guarding. Frequently, an enlarged or distended structure may be appreciated with this light touch as a sense of resistance.

Areas of tenderness or guarding, or both, defined by light palpation will alert the examiner to proceed with caution in the application of more vigorous manipulation of these structures during the remainder of the examination.

Tensing of the abdominal musculature may occur because (1) the examiner's hands are too cold or are pressed too vigorously or deeply into the abdomen; (2) the client is ticklish or guards involuntarily; or (3) there is a subjacent pathological condition, generally inflammatory. Rigidity is a boardlike hardness of the abdominal wall overlying peritoneal irritation. In generalized peritonitis, rigidity may be constant and hard.

• • •

Palpation should begin at a site distant from areas described as painful or that the examiner expects may be tender. Elicitation of pain may result in the client refusing further examination. The palms are rested gently on the abdomen, and the fingers are flexed, repetitively moving systematically from one quadrant to another.

Assessment of hypersensitivity

Zones of hypersensitivity of sensory nerve fibers of the skin have been described and are thought to reflect specific zones of peritoneal irritation. These are called

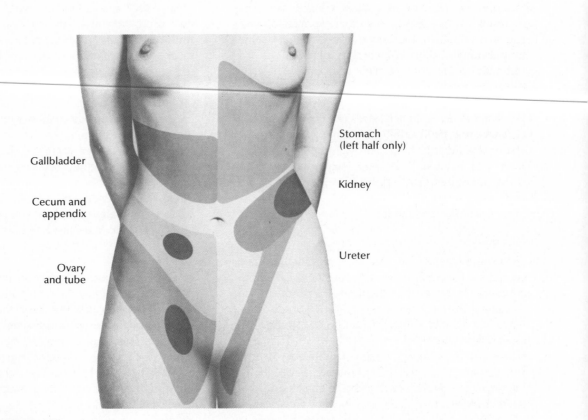

Gallbladder

Cecum and
appendix

Ovary
and tube

Stomach
(left half only)

Kidney

Ureter

Fig. 17-24
Head's zones of cutaneous hypersensitivity. (From G.I. series: physical examination of the abdomen, Chapter 2, Palpation, Richmond, Va., 1981, A.H. Robins Co.)

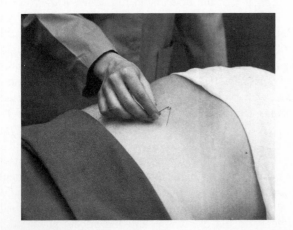

Fig. 17-25
Assessment of superficial pain sensation of the abdomen.

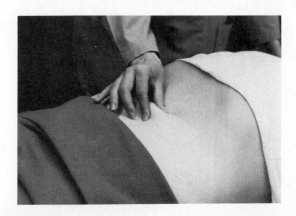

Fig. 17-26
Assessment of hypersensitivity by lifting a fold of skin away from the underlying musculature.

Head's zones of cutaneous hypersensitivity (Fig. 17-24). Although research has not provided proof for all the zones, clinical reliance has been demonstrated for the zone shown for the appendix in cases of appendicitis and for the midepigastrium in the individual with peptic ulcer.

Evaluation of this hypersensitivity may be achieved in two ways. One method is to stimulate gently with the sharp end of an open safety pin, a wisp of cotton, or the fingernail (Fig. 17-25). The second method is to gently lift a fold of skin away from the underlying musculature (Fig. 17-26). The alert client may be able to describe his reaction to this stimulation, or changes in facial expression (grimacing) may indicate the increased sensation the individual is experiencing.

Assessment of muscle spasticity

Involuntary muscle contraction or spasticity may indicate peritoneal irritation. Further palpation is done to determine whether the spasticity is unilateral or on both sides of the abdomen. Generalized and boardlike contraction is thought to be typical of peritonitis. Fur-

ther definition is achieved by asking the client to raise his trunk from a horizontal position without arm support. The experience of unilateral pain in response to this maneuver may further pinpoint the areas of spasticity. This mechanism may also help to differentiate muscle contraction from abdominal mass; as the head is raised, the hand would be moved away from an abdominal mass. Rigidity and tenderness over McBurney's point and in some cases over the entire right side are strongly suggestive of appendicitis. Acute cholecystitis is frequently accompanied by rigidity of the right hypochondrium.

Moderate palpation

The side of the hand rather than the fingertips is used in moderate palpation (Fig. 17-27). This method obviates the tendency to dig into the abdomen with the fingertips, as well as the resultant discomfort and involuntary guarding that may accompany such focal probing.

The sensation produced by palpating with the side of the hand is particularly useful in assessing organs that move with respiration, such as liver and the spleen. The organ is felt during normal breathing cycles and then as the client takes a deep breath. On inspiration the organ will be pushed downward against the examining hand.

Tenderness not elicited by gentle palpation may be perceived by the client on deeper pressure.

Deep palpation

Deep palpation is indentation of the abdomen performed by pressing the distal half of the palmar surfaces of the fingers into the abdominal wall (Fig. 17-28). The abdominal wall may slide back and forth while the fingers are moving back and forth over the organ being examined. Deeper structures, such as retroperitoneal organs (the kidneys), or masses may be felt with this method. Tenderness of organs not elicited by light or moderate palpation may be uncovered with this method. In the absence of disease, the pressure produced by deep palpation may produce tenderness over the cecum, the sigmoid colon, and the aorta.

The technique of deep palpation may help to give more specific information concerning a lesion or mass detected by lighter palpation.

Bimanual palpation

Superimposition of one hand. Bimanual palpation with superimposition of one hand may be used when additional pressure is necessary to overcome resistance or to examine a deep abdominal structure. In this method one hand is superimposed over the other, so that pressure is exerted by the upper hand while the

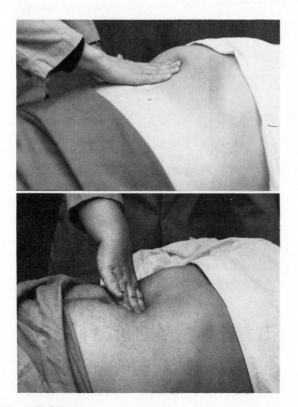

Fig. 17-27
Moderate palpation is performed with the side of the hand. This method of palpation is particularly useful in assessing organs that move with respiration, such as the liver and spleen.

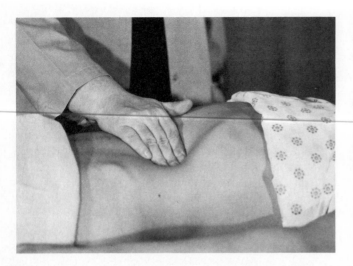

Fig. 17-28
Deep palpation is performed by pressing the distal half of the palmar surfaces of the fingers into the abdominal wall. Deep structures such as the retroperitoneal organs are assessed by deep palpation.

Fig. 17-29
Bimanual palpation with superimposition of one hand. Pressure is exerted by the upper hand while the lower hand remains relaxed and sensitive to tactile stimulation.

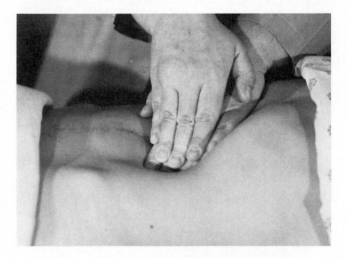

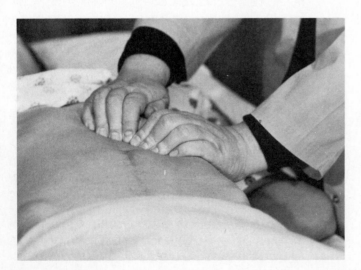

Fig. 17-30
Bimanual palpation with the hands side by side. Descent of the liver or spleen (as above) is often measured by hooking the fingers over the costal margin from above. This technique is called the Middleton technique and is used to examine the spleen.

lower hand remains relaxed and sensitive to the tactile sensation produced by the structure being examined. Generally, for the right-handed examiner the left hand is the lower, or examining, hand while the right hand applies pressure exerted by the tips of the left fingers on the terminal interphalangeal points of the examining fingers (Fig. 17-29). The technique is recommended because the palpating hand is less sensitive if it has to be used to exert pressure at the same time.

Trapping technique. Both hands may be used to establish the size of a mass. The mass is trapped between the examining hands for measurement.

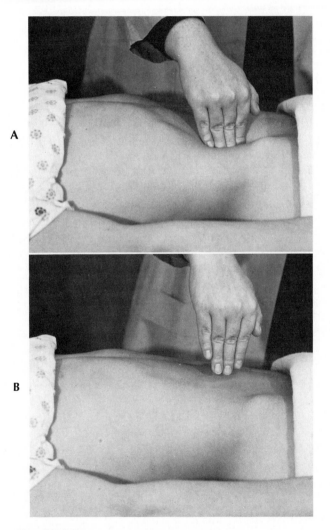

Fig. 17-31
Palpation to elicit rebound tenderness. **A,** Deep pressure is applied to the abdominal wall. **B,** On release of pressure, a sensation of pain would indicate peritoneal irritation. This is a test for appendicitis. In this case, the test for rebound tenderness is being performed over McBurney's point and may elicit tenderness related to appendicitis.

Detection of a pulsatile mass. Pulsation may be sensed in the fingertips of both hands as they are pushed apart as a pulsatile flow expands a structure such as the aorta; pulsation may also be felt in a mass held between the examining hands. This palpatory finding indicates that the structure being felt is pulsating rather than transmitting pulsation. The normal aorta is approximately 2.5 to 4 cm wide, whereas an aneurysm is a good deal broader. As noted previously, a bruit is generally heard over an aneurysm. The most common physical finding in clients with an abdominal aneurysm is the presence of an expansile, pulsating mass, more than 95% of which are located inferior to the renal arteries but generally at or above the umbilicus. Femoral pulses are usually present but are markedly damped in amplitude. More than half of clients with abdominal aneurysms are asymptomatic; thus, the mass might be discovered during a screening physical examination. Although more than 80% of abdominal aneurysms can be palpated, small aneurysms in the markedly obese client may not be felt.

Hands approximated (side by side). Minimum descent of the liver or spleen below the costal margin is occasionally detected by hooking the fingers over the costal margin from above while standing beside the thorax, facing the client's feet (Fig. 17-30). This procedure is called the Middleton technique and is used to examine the spleen.

The outline of a tubular structure such as the sigmoid colon or cecum can frequently be more specifically outlined with the hands side by side, rolling the fingers over the structure.

Palpation to elicit rebound tenderness

Rebound tenderness is a symptom of peritoneal irritation. To provoke rebound tenderness, the approximated fingers are pushed gently but deeply in a region remote from that suspected of tenderness and then rapidly removed. The maneuver as illustrated in Fig. 17-31 is being performed over McBurney's point and might elicit rebound tenderness related to appendicitis. The rebound of the structures indented by palpation causes a sharp stabbing sensation of pain on the side of the inflammation. This sensation of pain following the withdrawal of pressure is a sign of peritoneal irritation. The test may be repeated over to the side of the suspected disease. The test is best performed near the conclusion of the examination, since the production of severe pain or muscle spasm may interfere with subsequent examination. Voluntary coughing by the client may produce the same results.

Many examiners consider the elicitation of rebound tenderness by palpation as a crude and painful technique. The resultant severe pain and muscle spasm not

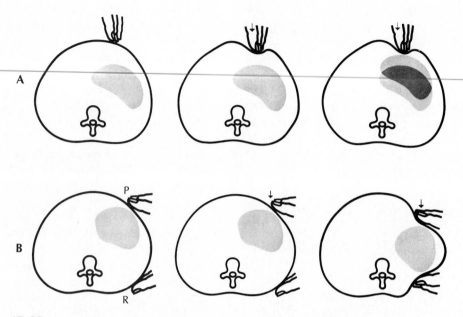

Fig. 17-32

Ballottement. **A,** Single-handed ballottement. **B,** Bimanual ballottement: *P,* pushing hand; *R,* receiving hand. (From G.I. series: physical examination of the abdomen, Chapter 2, Palpation, Richmond, Va., 1981, A.H. Robins Co.)

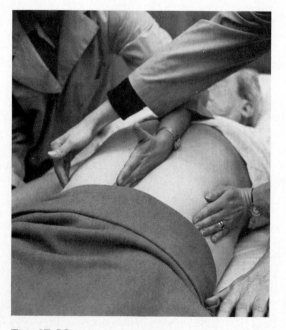

Fig. 17-33

Test for presence of a fluid wave.

Table 17-5

Characteristics of abdominal masses related to common pathological conditions

Description of mass	Possible pathological condition
Descends on inspiration	Liver, spleen, or kidney mass
Pulsatile mass	Abdominal aneurysm, tortuous aorta
Movable from side to side, not head to foot	Mesenteric or small bowel mass
Complete fixation	Tumor of pancreatic or retroperitoneal origin

only interfere with subsequent examination but may interfere with trust in the client-clinician relationship. Light percussion can be used to produce vibration, which produces a mildly uncomfortable response in the presence of peritoneal inflammation. The technique is reputed to be able to localize very small areas of peritoneal inflammation, in some cases as small as a quarter.

Ballottement (Fig. 17-32)

Ballottement is a palpation technique used to assess a floating object. Fluid-filled tissue is pushed toward the examining hand so that the object will float against the examining fingers. This is the technique used to determine by abdominal palpation whether the head or the breech of the fetus is in the fundus of the uterus.

Single-handed ballottement. Single-handed ballottement is performed with the fingers extended in a straight line with the forearm and at a right angle to the abdomen. The fingers are moved quickly toward the mass or organ to be examined and held there. As fluid or other structures are displaced, the mass will move upward and be felt at the fingertips. Some examiners prefer this technique for examination of the spleen.

Bimanual ballottement. Bimanual ballottement is accomplished by using one hand to push on the anterior abdominal wall to displace contents to the flank while the other receives the mass or structure pushed against it and feels the dimensions.

Demonstration of ascites by palpation

The presence of large amounts of fluid within the peritoneal cavity allows the elicitation of a fluid wave (Fig. 17-33). To test for the presence of a fluid wave, the client is placed in a supine position. The examiner places the palmar surface of one hand firmly against the lateral abdominal wall and taps the contralateral wall with the other hand. An assistant places the edge of one hand and lower arm firmly in the vertical midline of the client's abdomen to damp vibrations that might otherwise be transmitted through the tissues of the anterior abdominal wall.

Palpation for abdominal masses

All the quadrants of the abdomen are examined systematically by palpation. For the most part, bimanual examination with the hands superimposed is the technique most useful. Initially, light palpation is used; the examiner then proceeds to deep palpation.

The characteristics of an abdominal mass are carefully described. Of particular importance are consistency, regularity of contour movement with respiration, and mobility (Table 17-5). A sketch of the anterior

abdominal wall with all its bony landmarks and the umbilicus may be the most efficient way to convey location, shape, and size.

Difficulties in determining that a palpable mass is in the anterior abdominal wall rather than in an intraabdominal position may be resolved by asking the client to flex the abdominal muscles. Masses in the subcutaneous tissue will continue to be palpable, whereas those in the peritoneal cavity will be more difficult to feel or will be pushed out of reach altogether.

Normal abdominal structures occasionally mistaken for masses are:

1. Lateral borders of the rectus abdominis muscles
2. Uterus
3. Feces-filled ascending colon
4. Feces-filled descending colon and sigmoid colon
5. Aorta
6. Common iliac artery
7. Sacral promontory

Palpable bowel segments. The presence of feces within the bowel frequently contributes to the examiner's ability to palpate the cecum, the ascending colon, the descending colon, and the sigmoid colon. The feces-filled cecum and ascending colon produce a sensation suggestive of a soft, boggy, rounded mass. The client may complain of cramps resulting from stimulation of the bowel by the movements of palpation.

EXAMINATION OF THE SPECIFIC ABDOMINAL STRUCTURES

Palpation is a useful technique for identification and assessment of the specific abdominal structures. A systematic approach, always beginning at the same area, is suggested so that the examiner not skip any part of the abdomen. Since most examiners approach the client from the right, the liver may prove to be the most convenient structure to palpate first.

Liver

Two types of bimanual palpation are recommended for palpation of the liver. The first of these is superimposition of the right hand over the left hand. The client is asked to breathe normally for two or three breaths. Then he is asked to breathe deeply. The diaphragm is exerted downward in inspiration and will push the liver toward the examining hand. The liver usually cannot be palpated in the normal adult. However, in extremely thin but otherwise well individuals, it may be felt at the costal margin. When the normal liver margin is palpated, it feels regular in contour and somewhat sharp. Descriptions of the abnormal liver are listed in Table 17-6.

Table 17-6

Characteristics of hepatomegaly related to common pathological conditions

Description of liver	Possible pathological condition
Smooth, nontender	Portal cirrhosis
	Lymphoma
	Passive congestion of the liver
	Portal obstruction
	Obstruction of the vena cava
	Lymphocytic leukemia
	Rickets
	Amyloidosis
	Schistosomiasis
Smooth, tender	Acute hepatitis
	Amebic hepatitis or abscess
	Early congestive cardiac failure
Nodular	Late portal cirrhosis
	Tertiary syphilis
	Metastatic carcinoma
Hard	Carcinomatosis

In the second technique, the left hand is placed beneath the client at the level of the eleventh and twelfth ribs and upward pressure applied to throw the liver forward toward the examining right hand. The palmar surface of the examiner's right hand is placed parallel to the right costal margin. As the client inspires, the liver may be felt to slip beneath the examining fingers.

Tenderness over the liver may be demonstrated by placing the palm of one hand over the lateral costal margin and delivering a blow to that hand with the ulnar surface of the other hand, which has been curled into a fist (see Fig. 17-19).

Whichever technique is chosen, the initial attempt to palpate the liver should be done slowly, carefully, and gently so that the liver margin is not missed.

Gallbladder

Whereas the normal gallbladder cannot be felt, a distended gallbladder may be palpated below the liver margin at the lateral border of the rectus muscle. The cystic nature of the mass helps in the identification of the gallbladder. There is, however, a good deal of variation in the location of the left border; it may be found either more medially or more laterally.

An enlarged, tender gallbladder is indicative of cholecystitis, whereas a large but nontender gallbladder portends of obstruction of the common bile duct.

Murphy's sign: inspiratory arrest. Murphy's sign is helpful in determining the presence of cholecystitis through bimanual examination. While performing deep palpation, the examiner asks the client to take a deep breath. As the descending liver brings the gallbladder in contact with the examining hand, the client with cholecystitis will experience pain and stop the inspiratory movement. Pain may also occur in the client with hepatitis.

Spleen

The spleen is generally not palpable in the normal adult. Since the spleen is normally soft and is located retroperitoneally, it is frequently difficult to palpate. Turning the client on his right side (to gain gravitational advantage) brings the spleen downward and forward and thus closer to the abdominal wall and is often employed in the examination.

With the client in the supine position, three techniques of palpation are useful. In the first technique, the right hand is placed flat on the client's abdomen in the upper left quadrant with the fingers delving beneath the costal margin and toward the anterior axillary line (Fig. 17-34). The left hand is stretched over the client's abdomen and brought posterior to the client in the flank below the costal margin. This hand is used to exert an upward pressure that will displace the spleen anteriorly.

The Middleton technique for examination of the spleen is performed with the examiner standing on the client's left side, facing the client's feet. The fingers are hooked over the costal margin, pressing upward and inward at the anterior axillary line (see Fig. 17-30). On inspiration the spleen may be felt at the fingertips. The client may assist by placing his left fist under the left eleventh rib.

Either of these techniques may be used while the client lies on the right side to throw the spleen forward and flexes the knees to relax the abdomen. Some authorities recommend that the client lie on the left side during splenic palpation; they propose that lying on the left side more effectively relaxes the musculature of the abdomen.

The technique of one hand superimposed over the other may also be used to palpate the spleen. Again, the examiner stands at the client's left side, facing the client's feet. The fingers are hooked over the costal margin, and the uppermost hand is used to apply pressure while the lower hand is used as a sensing device. Again, the client is asked to breathe in and out while the examiner focuses on the inspiratory phase in an attempt to feel the contour of the spleen.

Splenic enlargement is described by the number of centimeters the spleen extends below the costal margin: (1) slight is 1 to 4 cm below the costal margin, (2) moderate is 4 to 8 cm below the costal margin, and (3) great is more than 8 cm below the costal margin.

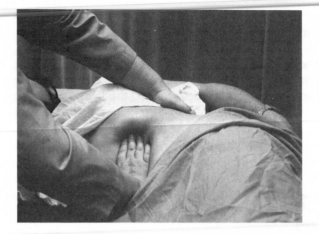

Fig. 17-34
Assessment of the spleen.

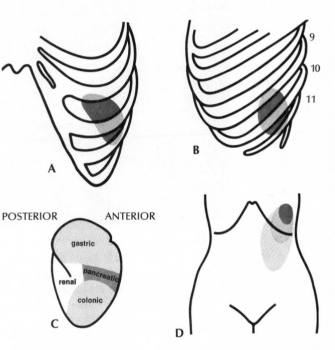

Fig. 17-35
Normal (**A, B, C**) and enlarged (**D**) spleen. **A,** Anterior view. **B,** Left lateral view. **C,** Regions of spleen (anterior view) that touch other viscera. **D,** Directions of splenic enlargement. (From G.I. series: physical examination of the abdomen, Chapter 2, Palpation, Richmond, Va., 1981, A.H. Robins Co.)

The spleen may also be percussed. Normally, splenic dullness may be percussed from the sixth or the ninth to the eleventh rib in the midaxillary line or posterior to the line. The span of normal splenic dullness does not exceed 7 cm.

A practical technique is to begin percussion at the tenth rib just posterior to the midaxillary line and to percuss in several directions from dull to resonance or tympany to outline the edges of the spleen.

When the spleen has normal dimensions, resonance may be percussed over the lowest left intercostal space between the anterior and midaxillary lines both during inspiration and expiration. However, a finding of resonance on expiration and dullness on inspiration probably denotes splenic hypertrophy. It is important to note that a full stomach or a colon packed with feces may percuss dull and therefore mimic splenic enlargement.

Enlargement of the spleen may best be described by a drawing of the anterior abdomen indicating the relative site and shape of the spleen in relation to the costal border and the umbilicus (Fig. 17-35).

Pancreas

The pancreas cannot be palpated in the normal client because of its small size and retroperitoneal position. However, a mass of the pancreas may occasionally be felt as a vague sensation of fullness in the epigastrium.

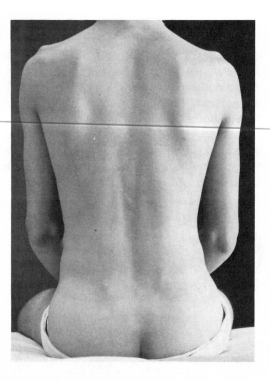

Fig. 17-43
Inspection of the back with the client in the sitting position is the final step in the abdominal examination.

Back

The final step in the abdominal examination is inspection of the back with the client in the sitting position (Fig. 17-43). The flanks in the normal individual are symmetrical. Fullness or asymmetry may be a result of renal disorders. Ecchymoses of the flanks (Grey Turner's sign) are associated with retroperitoneal bleeding and may be associated with hemorrhagic pancreatitis. Unilateral flank pain or tenderness suggests renal or ureteral disease such as stone, tumor, infection, or infarct.

The costovertebral margin is percussed for tenderness (see "Fist percussion").

SUMMARY

I. Inspection
  A. Contour
  B. Symmetry
  C. Condition of umbilicus
  D. Musculature
  E. Dilated veins
  F. Skin
    1. Pigmentation
    2. Lesions
    3. Striae
    4. Scars
  G. Respiratory movement
  H. Abnormal movements

II. Auscultation
  A. Peristaltic sounds
  B. Bruits
III. Percussion
  A. Liver span
  B. Spleen
  C. Stomach
  D. Masses
IV. Palpation
  A. Tone of abdominal wall
    1. Resistance—distention
    2. Muscle tone
  B. Tenderness
  C. Masses
  D. Hernia
V. Organ examination
  A. Liver
    1. Palpation
      a. Size, contour, and character of edge
      b. Tenderness
    2. Percussion—midclavicular diameter
  B. Spleen
    1. Palpation
    2. Percussion
  C. Kidneys
    1. Palpation
      a. Location
      b. Mobility
      c. Costovertebral tenderness
    2. Percussion

BIBLIOGRAPHY

Brooks, F.P., editor: Gastrointestinal pathophysiology, New York, 1974, Oxford University Press, Inc.

Castell, D.O.: The spleen percussion sign: a useful diagnostic technique, Ann. Intern. Med. **67:**1265, 1967.

Castell, D.O.: Abdominal examination: role of percussion and auscultation, Postgrad. Med. **62:**131, 1977.

Castell, D.O., and others: Estimation of liver size by percussion in normal individuals, Ann. Intern. Med. **70:**1183, 1969.

Chalmers, T.C.: Centimeters, even inches, but no fingers, N. Engl. J. Med. **282:**397, 1970.

Cope, Z.: The early diagnosis of acute abdomen, ed. 14, New York, 1972, Oxford University Press, Inc.

Dunphy, J., and Botsford, T.: Physical examination of the surgical patient: an introduction to clinical surgery, Philadelphia, 1975, W.B. Saunders Co.

Dworken, H.J.: The alimentary tract, Philadelphia, 1974, W.B. Saunders Co.

Gelin, L., Nyhus, L., and Condon, R.: Abdominal pain: a guide to rapid diagnosis, Philadelphia, 1969, J.B. Lippincott Co.

Levinson, D.: Personal communications, 1982.

Silen, W.: Cope's early diagnosis of the acute abdomen, ed. 15, New York, 1979, Oxford University Press.

Sullivan S., Krasner, N., and Williams, R.: The clinical estimates of liver size: a comparison of techniques and analysis of sources of error, Br. Med. J. **2:**1042, 1976.

CHAPTER 18

ASSESSMENT OF THE ANUS AND RECTOSIGMOID REGION

The terminal gastrointestinal tract is a distal section that may be termed the rectosigmoid region and includes the anus, the rectum, and the caudal portion of the sigmoid colon.

ANATOMY

The anal canal is the final segment of the colon; it is 2.5 to 4 cm in length and opens into the perineum (Fig. 18-1). The tract is surrounded by the external and internal sphincters, which keep it closed except when flatus and feces are passed. These sphincters are laid down in concentric layers. The striated external muscular ring is under voluntary control, whereas the internal, smooth muscle sphincter is under autonomic control. The internal sphincter is innervated from the pelvic plexus; sympathetic stimulation contracts the sphincter; parasympathetic stimulation relaxes it. The distal portion of the external sphincter extends past the internal sphincter and may be palpated by the examining finger. The stratified squamous epithelial lining of the anus is visible to inspection, since it extends beyond the sphincters, where it merges with the skin. The junction is characterized by pigmentation and the presence of hair. From an internal view of the anal canal, columns of mucosal tissue, which extend from the rectum and terminate in papillae, may be identified; these anal columns, or columns of Morgagni, fuse to form the pectinate, or dentate, line. Spaces between these columns are called crypts. The anal columns are invested with cross channels of anastomosing veins, which form mucosal folds known as anal valves. These anastomosing veins form a ring known as the zona hemorrhoidalis. When dilated, these veins are called internal hemorrhoids. The lower section of the anal canal contains a venous plexus, which has only minor connection with the zona hemorrhoidalis and drains downward into the inferior rectal veins. Varicosed veins of this plexus are known as external hemorrhoids. Thus, internal hemorrhoids are encountered superior to the pectinate line and are characterized by the moist, red epithelium of the rectum, whereas external hemorrhoids are located inferior to the pectinate line and have the squamous epithelium of the anal canal or skin as their surface tissue.

The rectum is encountered as the portion of the gastrointestinal tract rostral to the anal canal. It is approximately 12 cm in length and is lined with columnar epithelium. Superiorly, the rectum has its origin at the third sacral vertebra and is continuous with the sigmoid colon. Its distal end dilates to form the rectal ampulla, which contains flatus and feces. Four semilunar transverse folds (valves of Houston) extend across half the circumference of the rectal lumen. The purpose of the valves is not clear. It has been suggested that the valves serve to support feces while allowing flatus to pass. The rectum ends where the muscle coats are replaced by the sphincters of the anal canal.

The sigmoid colon has its origin at the iliac flexure of the descending colon and terminates in the rectum. It is approximately 40 cm in length. It is accessible to examination via the sigmoidoscope, and examination is limited by the length of the scope. Recently, flexible fiberoptic instruments have made possible inspection of the mucosal surfaces of the entire sigmoid colon and of the other portions of the colon.

EXAMINATION

The rectal examination is an important procedure in the physical examination; it is particularly significant when the client's chief complaint includes anal pain or spasm, itching or burning, and a history of black, tarry stools (melena).

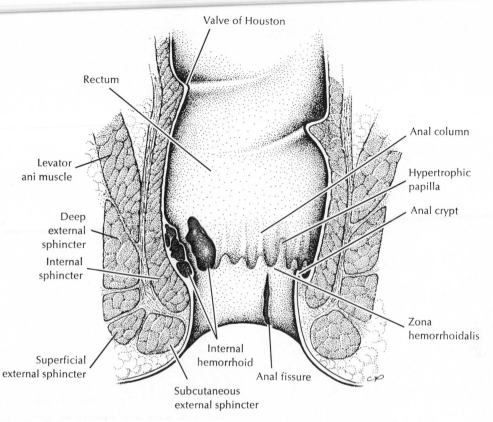

Fig. 18-1
Anorectal structures and common pathological conditions. (Adapted from Dunphy, J.E.:
Arch. Surg. 57:791, 1948.)

The client may give some indication of a problem by his movements; for example, shifting from one buttock to the other often alleviates the discomfort of a thrombosed hemorrhoid.

The purposes of the rectal examination include assessment of anorectal status, assessment of the male prostate gland and seminal vessels (see Chapter 19 for assessment of the male genitalia and assessment of the inguinal area for hernias), and assessment of the accessible pelvic viscera.

Since most clients experience a good deal of embarrassment and fear of discomfort at the prospect of the rectal examination, the procedure should be preceded by an explanation and assurance that the examiner will proceed with gentleness. The client should be draped to avoid undue exposure and helped to assume the desired position. The client may be examined in several positions:

1. *Left lateral* or *Sims' position:* The client lies on his left side with the superior thigh and knee flexed, bringing the knee close to the chest. The rectal ampulla is pushed down and posteriorly in this position and thus is advantageously aligned for the detection of rectal masses. However, the upper rectum and pelvic structure tend to fall away in this position, and a pathological condition of these structures may be overlooked.

2. *Knee-chest position:* The client is on his knees with his shoulders and head in contact with the examining table. The knees are positioned more widely apart than the hips. The angle at the hip is 75 to 80 degrees. Assessment of the size of the prostate gland is best done in this position.

3. *Standing position:* The client's hips are flexed, and the trunk is resting on a bed or table. Prostate evaluation is facilitated in this position. This is the most commonly used position for examination of the prostate gland.

4. *Lithotomy position:* With the client supine, both knees are drawn up as far as possible toward the chest. It is convenient to perform the rectal examination in the female client immediately following the pelvic examination while her feet remain in stirrups.

5. *Squatting position:* Rectal prolapse may frequently be brought out in this position. Lesions of the rectosigmoid region and pelvis may be felt in this position only.

The equipment needed is a small penlight to facilitate inspection of the perianal and anal area, a finger cot or disposable glove, lubricating jelly, and a guaiac testing kit.

The methods of the rectal examination include inspection and palpation.

Inspection

The buttocks are carefully spread with both hands to examine the anus and the tissue immediately around the anus. This skin is more pigmented and coarse than the surrounding perianal skin and is also moist and hairless. The examiner visually assesses the perianal region for skin tags, lesions, scars or inflammation, perirectal abscesses, fissures, sentinel piles from rectal fissures, external hemorrhoids or fistula openings, con-

dyloma acuminatum (viral warts), tumors, and rectal prolapse.

Valsalva's maneuver. The client is asked to strain downward as though defecating, so that with slight pressure on the skin, rectal fissures, rectal prolapse, polyps, or internal hemorrhoids might be identified. Abnormal findings are described by locating them in terms of a clock, with the 12 o'clock position toward the symphysis pubis in the midline of the back over the lower sacrum or coccyx.

The sacrococcygeal area is inspected for pilonidal cyst or sinus. The pilonidal area is inspected for dimples (at the tip of the coccyx), sinus openings, or the presence of inflammation. The pilonidal area is felt for tenderness, induration, or swelling.

The skin of the pilonidal sinus may have abundant

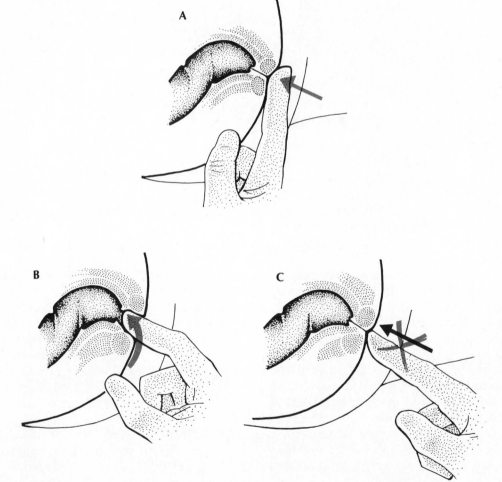

Fig. 18-2
A, Digital pressure is applied against the anal verge until the external sphincter is felt to yield. **B,** The gloved, lubricated finger is slowly introduced in the direction of the umbilicus. **C,** Avoid discomfort for the client by this incorrect approach at a right angle to the sphincter and without promoting relaxation. (Adapted from Dunphy, J.E., and Botsford, T.W.: Physical examination of the surgical patient: an introduction to clinical surgery, ed. 4, Philadelphia, 1975, W.B. Saunders Co.)

hair growth. The accumulation of secretions often leads to infection, which is generally accompanied by a foul-smelling discharge and local tenderness. The sinus may be simply blocked up by secretion, so that a tumescence is observed, which is tender to palpation.

Palpation

The nondominant hand of the examiner is used to spread the buttocks apart. In the event the sphincter tightens, reassurance should be given to the client and when the sphincter relaxes, the examination continued. Painful lesions or bleeding may prevent completion of the examination.

While the client strains downward, the pad of the lubricated, gloved index finger is gently placed against the anal verge; firm pressure is exerted until the sphincter begins to yield, and the finger is then slowly inserted in the direction of the umbilicus as the rectal sphincter

relaxes (Fig. 18-2). The client is asked to tighten the sphincter around the examining finger to provide a measurement of muscle strength of the anal sphincter. Hypertonicity of the external sphincter may occur with anxious, voluntary or involuntary contraction or as a result of an anal fissure or other local pathological condition. A relaxed or hypotonic sphincter is seen occasionally after rectal surgery or may be a result of a neurological deficiency. The subcutaneous portion of the external sphincter is palpated on the inner aspect of the anal verge. The palpating finger is rotated to examine the entire muscular ring. The intersphincteric line is marked by a palpable indentation. Palpation of the deep external sphincter is performed through the lower part of the internal sphincter, which it surrounds. Assessment of the levator ani muscle is accomplished by palpating laterally and posteriorly where the muscle is attached to the rectal wall on one side and then the other (Fig. 18-3).

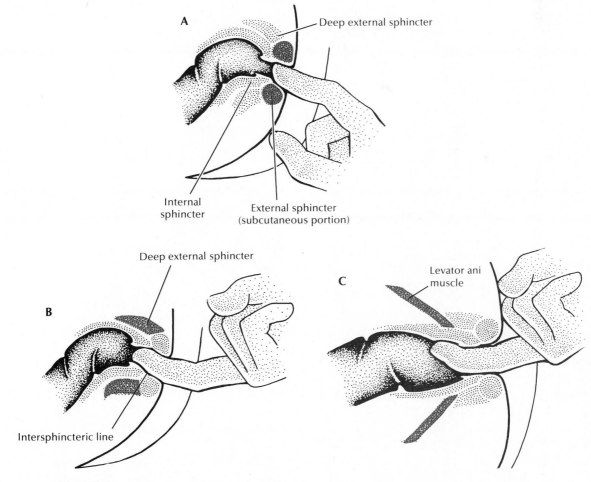

Fig. 18-3
The subcutaneous portion of the external sphincter is palpated, **A,** followed by digital exploration of the deep external sphincter, **B. C,** Palpation of the levator ani muscle. (Adapted from Dunphy, J.E., and Botsford, T.W.: Physical examination of the surgical patient: an introduction to clinical surgery, ed. 4, Philadelphia, 1975, W.B. Saunders Co.)

The posterior wall of the rectum follows the curve of the coccyx and sacrum and feels smooth to the palpating finger. The mucosa of the anal canal is palpated for tumor or polyps. The coccyx is palpated to determine mobility and sensitivity.

The examining finger is able to palpate a distance of 6 to 10 cm of the rectal canal. A bidigital palpation of the sphincter area may yield more information than would be obtained by probing with the index finger alone. This is accomplished by pressing the thumb of the examining hand against the perianal tissue and moving the examining index finger toward it. This is a useful technique for detecting a perianal abscess and for palpating the bulbourethral (Cowper's) glands.

Rectal valves may be misinterpreted as protruding intrarectal masses, especially when they are well developed.

The lateral walls of the rectum may be palpated by rotating the index finger along the sides of the rectum. The ischial spines and sacrotuberous ligaments may be identified through palpation.

The prostate gland is situated anterior to the rectum; therefore, palpation through the mucosa of the anterior wall of the rectum allows the examiner to assess the size, shape, and consistency of the prostate gland. The client is asked to bear down so that a mass not otherwise reached might be pushed downward into the range of the examining finger.

The prostate gland, a bilobed structure, has a normal diameter of approximately 4 cm. The palpating finger identifies the smooth lateral lobes separated by a central groove. The prostate is approximately 2.5 cm in length, and the presence of nodules is noted. The prostate should feel firm and smooth. The client should be asked to report tenderness to touch. (See Chapter 19 for assesment of male genitalia.)

The normal cervix can be felt as a small round mass through the anterior wall of the rectum. (See Chapter 20 for assessment of the female genitalia.)

Examination of the stool

On withdrawal of the examining finger, the nature of any feces clinging to the glove should be examined (Table 18-1). The presence of pus or blood is noted. Bright red blood in small or large amounts may be from the large intestine, the sigmoid colon, the rectum, or the anus. However, the stool may be burgundy in color if the bleeding occurred in the ascending colon. Colonic bleeding may be suspected when blood is mixed with the feces, whereas rectal bleeding is probably occurring when the blood is observed on the surface of the stool. The presence of a good deal of blood in the stool may be associated with marked malodor.

Table 18-1

Characteristics of the stool related to the possible pathological conditions

Description of the stool	Possible pathological condition
Light tan, gray	Absence of bile pigments—obstructive jaundice
Greasy, pale, and yellow; increased fat content (steatorrhea, sprue)	Malabsorption syndromes
Tarry, black (melena)	Gastrointestinal tract bleeding; ingestion of iron compounds or bismuth preparations
Small flakes of jellylike mucus mixed with stool	Inflammation

A black, tarry stool (melena) results from bleeding in the stomach or small intestine; the blood is partially digested during its passage to the rectum. On the other hand, the black color may result from ingested iron compounds and bismuth preparations.

A small quantity of the feces is subjected to a chemical test for the presence of occult blood. Minimum abrasions of the gastrointestinal tract are thought to be responsible for blood loss of 1 to 3 ml daily in the feces. The loss of more than 50 ml from the upper gastrointestinal tract will produce melena. To detect quantities less than 50 ml or to determine whether black stools actually do contain blood, several reagents may be used.

The guaiac test is the most frequently used test for routine screening. The gum guaiac solution can identify 0.5% to 1% of hemoglobin in aqueous solution. The procedure involves wiping the gloved examining finger on a piece of filter paper and then adding 1 to 2 drops of guaiac solution, glacial acetic acid, and hydrogen peroxide. A positive reaction is denoted by the solution turning blue or dark green within 30 seconds (Fig. 18-4). Orthotolidine is also useful in the detection of occult blood and is more sensitive than guaiac solution (it detects 0.01% to 0.1% of hemoglobin in aqueous solution).

The most common cause of occult bleeding is cancer of the colon.

Endoscopic procedures

The presence of a pathological condition detected by the digital examination is further explored by endoscopy.

Anoscopy. The Hirshman or Brincker-Hoff anoscope may be used for a more complete examination of the anal canal and internal hemorrhoidal zone.

Proctoscopy. Direct visualization of anal or lower rectal pathological conditions (or 9 to 15 cm of the

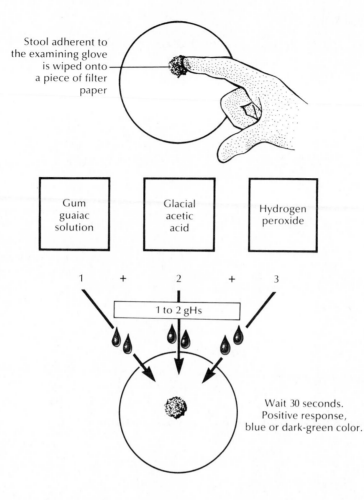

Fig. 18-4
Procedure for the guaiac assessment for occult blood. (Adapted from Dunphy, J.E., and Botsford, T.W.: Physical examination of the surgical patient: an introduction to clinical surgery, ed. 4, Philadelphia, 1975, W.B. Saunders Co.)

lower gastrointestinal tract) is possible with a proctoscope. The position most frequently used for this procedure is the knee-chest position. The warmed and lubricated instrument is passed with the obturator in place to its full length. The obturator is removed, and the proctoscope is removed slowly while the examiner observes for ulcers, inflammation, strictures, or the cause of a palpable mass. Biopsy may be performed through the tube.

Sigmoidoscopy. Visual examination of the upper portion of the rectum that cannot be felt with the examining finger is possible with a sigmoidoscope; it allows direct visualization of the lower 24 cm of the gastrointestinal tract. This examination is particularly important, since one half of all carcinomas occur in the rectum and colon. The early detection of polyps and malignant lesions may result in early and successful treatment of an otherwise fatal disease.

Careful explanation of the procedure and gentle manipulation of the client's tissue allow the examination to take place with little discomfort to the client.

The procedure is effective for the identification of proctitis, polyps, and carcinoma. Sigmoidoscopy is also helpful in the identification of diarrhea of colonic origin. The mucous membrane may be inspected, and scrapings may be taken for microscopic examination.

PATHOLOGY
Pilonidal cyst or sinus

Pilonidal sinus is generally first diagnosed between the ages of 15 and 30, even though it is thought to be a congenital lesion. It is located superficial to the coccyx or lower sacrum. The sinus opening may look like a dimple, with another very small opening in the midline. In other cases a cyst is observed and may be palpated; in more advanced conditions a sinus tract may be palpated. The area may become erythematous, and a tuft of hair may be observed. The ingrowth of the hairs is probably the cause of infection, cyst, and fistula formation.

Pruritus ani

Excoriated, thickened, and pigmented skin may result from chronic inflammation of pruritus ani. The itching and burning of the rectal area are most often traceable to pinworms in children and to fungal infections in adults. Diabetic clients are particularly vulnerable to fungal infections. A dull, grayish pink color of the perianal skin is a characteristic of fungal infections. The radiating folds of skin may appear enlarged, and the skin may be cracked or fissured. Pruritus ani characterized by dry and brittle skin is thought to be related to psychosomatic disease.

Rectal tenesmus

Rectal tenesmus is the painful straining at stool associated with spasm of anal and rectal muscles; the client complains of a distressing feeling of urgency. The client is questioned concerning the nature of the stool. A hard, dry stool is indicative of constipation. A bloody, diarrheal stool might be indicative of ulcerative colitis. Rectal fissure may be the cause of tenesmus with normally constituted stools.

Tenesmus may also be a symptom experienced by the client with a perirectal inflammation, such as prostatitis.

The client who complains of constant rectal pain is examined carefully for thrombosed rectal hemorrhoids.

Fecal impaction

Fecal impaction is the accumulation and dehydration of fecal material in the rectum. When motility of the rectum is inhibited, the normal progression of feces does not occur and more water is reabsorbed through the bowel wall. The feces become hard and difficult to pass and may lead to complete obstruction. Fecal impaction is observed in individuals with chronic constipation and in individuals who have retained barium following gastrointestinal x-ray examination. The client complains of a sense of rectal fullness or urgency. Frequent small, liquid-to-loose stools may occur in incomplete obstruction. The dehydrated fecal mass is easily felt on palpation.

Anal fissure

A thin tear of the superficial anal mucosa, generally weeping, may be identified by asking the client to perform Valsalva's maneuver. The fissure is most commonly (more than 90%) found in the posterior midline of the anal mucosa and less frequently in the anterior midline.

Anal fissure is generally the result of the trauma associated with the passage of a large, hard stool. The client may complain of local pain, itching, or bleeding. Pain generally accompanies the passage of stool, and blood may be observed on the stool or on the toilet tissue. The inspection findings may include a sentinel skin tag or ulcer through which the muscles of the internal sphincter may be visible at the base. Because the examination is painful to the client, making it difficult to relax the anal muscles, local anesthesia may be necessary.

Fistula in ano

A tract from an anal fissure or infection that terminates in the perianal skin or other tissue is termed an anorectal fistula; it usually has its origin from local crypt abscesses. The fistula is a chronically inflamed tube made up of fibrous tissue surrounding granulation tissue and may frequently be palpated. The external opening is generally visible as a red elevation of granulation tissue. Local compression may result in the expression of serosanguinous or purulent drainage. Palpation (bidigital) is best accomplished with a finger in the anorectal cavity compressing the tissue against the thumb on the skin surface. The fistulous tract feels like an indurated cord.

The site from which drainage from an anal infection occurs can be identified by relating the location of the external opening of the fissure to the anus (Table 18-2 and Fig. 18-5).

Hemorrhoids

Hemorrhoids are dilated congested veins of the hemorrhoidal group. The swelling is associated with increased hydrostatic pressure in the portal venous system. The pressure associated with hemorrhoids correlates highly with pregnancy, straining at stool, chron-

Table 18-2
Location of fissure site related to the external opening

	External opening	Location in the anus
Goodsell's rule	Posterior to a line between the ischial tuberosities	Posterior
	Radial from the drainage site	Anterior
Salmon's law	Posterior to the anus or more than 2.5 anterior or lateral	Posterior
	Anterior or less than 2.5 cm lateral	Anterior

ic liver disease, and sudden increases in intraabdominal pressure. Bowel habits also play a role in that hemorrhoids frequently occur with diarrhea or incomplete bowel emptying. Local factors such as abscess or tumor may also contribute to venous stasis.

Hemorrhoidal skin tags are ragged, flaccid, skin sacs located around the anus. These skin tags cover connective tissue sacs and are the locus of resolved external hemorrhoids. Clients describe these tags as painless. Internal hemorrhoids occur proximal to the pectinate line, whereas external hemorrhoids are those that are seen distal to this boundary. External hemorrhoids are covered by skin or anal squamous tissue.

External hemorrhoids are often accompanied by pain, particularly if the skin is stretched by a sudden increase in mass; since the mass is located near the sphincter muscles, spasm is not uncommon. External hemorrhoids often cause itching and bleeding on defecation. These dilated veins may not be apparent at rest, but may appear as bluish, swollen areas at the anal verge when thrombosed. A thrombosed hemorrhoid is one in which blood has clotted, both within and outside the vein.

Internal hemorrhoids generally do not contribute to pain sensation unless they are complicated by thrombosis, infection, or erosion of overlying mucosal surfaces. Discomfort is increased if the hemorrhoids prolapse through the anal opening. Bleeding may occur from the internal hemorrhoids with or without defecation. Proctoscopy is generally necessary for their identification.

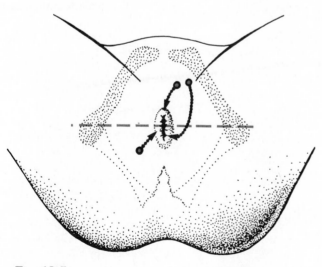

Fig. 18-5

Salmon's law. Fissure location related to the aperture of the fistula. (Adapted from Dunphy, J.E., and Botsford, T.W.: Physical examination of the surgical patient: an introduction to clinical surgery, ed. 4, Philadelphia, 1975, W.B. Saunders Co.)

Rectal polyps

Rectal polyps, which feel like soft nodules, are encountered frequently. They may be pedunculated (on a stalk) or sessile (irregularly moundlike, growing from a relatively broad base, and closely adherent to the mucosal wall). Because of their soft consistency, they may be difficult or impossible to identify by palpation. Proctoscopy is usually necessary for identification, and a biopsy is performed to identify malignant lesions.

A pedunculated rectal polyp occasionally prolapses through the anal ring.

Rectal prolapse

Internal hemorrhoids are the type most commonly identified because of mucosal tissue prolapsing through the anal ring. The pink-colored mucosa is described as appearing like a doughnut or rosette. In the older client, however, protruding mucosa may herald eversion or prolapse of the rectum. Incomplete prolapse involves only mucosa, whereas complete rectal prolapse involves the sphincters.

The prolapse of tissue through the anal ring is described by the client as occurring on exercise or while straining at stool. Frequently, the client describes being able to push the mass back in with digital pressure. Inspection reveals a red, bulging, mucosal mass protruding through the anal ring.

Anal incontinence

The loss of the voluntary ability to control defecation is called incontinence. The loss may range from the involuntary passage of flatus to complete loss of sphincter tone. The loss of fecal gases or liquids may also occur in the presence of a normal sphincter in hyperdynamic bowel states.

Abscesses or masses

Abscesses of the lower gastrointestinal tract that may be identified by physical examination (Fig. 18-6) include:

1. *Perirectal abscess:* This abscess may be palpated as a tender mass adjacent to the anal canal. The increased temperature of the mass may be helpful in the identification of the inflammatory process.
2. *Ischiorectal abscess:* This abscess may be palpated as a tender mass protruding into the lateral wall of the anal canal.
3. *Supra–levator ani muscle abscess:* This abscess may be felt by the examining finger as a tender mass in the lateral rectal wall.

The presence of a mass in the rectum deserves special attention, since nearly half those discovered are

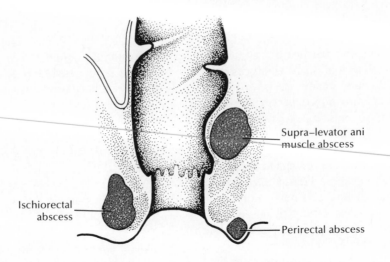

Supra–levator ani muscle abscess

Ischiorectal abscess

Perirectal abscess

Fig. 18-6
Common sites of abscess formation of the lower gastrointestinal tract. (Adapted from Dunphy, J.E., and Botsford, T.W.: Physical examination of the surgical patient: an introduction to clinical surgery, ed. 4, Philadelphia, 1975, W.B. Saunders Co.)

malignant. The client frequently denies pain or other symptoms. Early lesions are felt as small elevations or nodules with a firm base. Ulceration of the center of the lesion results in a crater that may be palpated. An ulcerated carcinoma may be identified through palpation by its firm, nodular, rolled edge. The lesion of carcinoma is described by including annular or tubular shape, degree of fixation, and distance from the anus. The consistency of the malignant mass is often stony and hard, and the contour is irregular. Extension of metastatic carcinoma from the peritoneum to the pelvic floor is described as a rectal shelf. It is palpated as a hard, nodular ridge.

SUMMARY

I. Inspection of perianal skin and perineum
  A. Pilonidal sinus
  B. Pruritus ani
  C. Fissure
  D. Fistula in ano
  E. Hemorrhoids
  F. Prolapse
II. Palpation
  A. Sphincter tone
  B. Prostate evaluation
    1. Size
    2. Shape
    3. Consistency
  C. Seminal vesicles
  D. Polyp

  E. Abscess
  F. Tumor
    1. Nature of mass
    2. Rectal shelf
III. Inspection of stool
  A. Pus
  B. Blood
  C. Guaiac test for occult blood

BIBLIOGRAPHY

Brooks, F.P., editor: Gastrointestinal pathophysiology, New York, 1974, Oxford University Press, Inc.

Deyhle, P., and Demlingi, L.: Colonoscopy: technic, results and indications, Endoscopy **3:**143, 1971.

Dunphy, J.E., and Botsford, T.W.: Physical examination of the surgical patient: an introduction to clinical surgery, Philadelphia, 1975, W.B. Saunders Co.

Dworken, H.J.: The alimentary tract, Philadelphia, 1974, W.B. Saunders Co.

Ganchrow, M.I., Bowman, E., and Clark, J.F.: Thrombosed hemorrhoids: a clinicopathologic study, Dis. Colon Rectum **14:**331, 1971.

Graham-Stewart, C.W.: The etiology and treatment of fissure in ano, Int. Abstr. Surg. **115:**511, 1962.

Mazier, W.P.: The treatment and care of anal fistulas: a study of 1000 patients, Dis. Colon Rectum **14:**134, 1971.

Ostrow, J.D., and others: Sensitivity and reproducibility of chemical tests for fecal occult blood with an emphasis on false positive reactions, Am. J. Dig. Dis. **18:**930, 1973.

Schrock, T.R.: Diseases of the anorectum. In Sleisenger, M.H., and Fordtran, J.S., editors: Gastrointestinal disease, ed. 2, Philadelphia, 1978, W.B. Saunders Co.

CHAPTER 19

ASSESSMENT OF THE MALE GENITALIA AND ASSESSMENT OF THE INGUINAL AREA FOR HERNIAS

MALE GENITALIA

The examination of the genital organs of any client is usually perceived by both the client and the practitioner as being different from the examination of other body parts. Culturally, male gynecologists have been accepted and sometimes even preferred by female clients. This chapter discusses the approach of the female practitioner to the examination of the male client's genital system.

First, the female practitioner should feel emotionally comfortable with the examination. If she does not, she should routinely refer this part of the physical examination to a male practitioner. Next, if she is comfortable with the examination, she must accept the possibility of the male client's reluctance to having his genitalia examined by a woman. Cajoling a client into an uncomfortable procedure may destroy further rapport; his wishes in the situation should be respected. In most clinical settings, there is a male practitioner present who would be available for a few minutes to examine the male genitalia. Our experience has been that most male clients are agreeable to examination by a woman; if there is discomfort, it is usually on the part of the examiner. It is therefore recommended that the beginning female examiner critically analyze her own feelings, fears, and beliefs; attempt male genital examination under supervision and with several cooperative clients; and then reexamine her feelings.

A male client will occasionally have an erection during examination of the genitalia regardless of the sex of the examiner. If this does occur, the most appropriate response is to reassure the client that an erection sometimes occurs and that the examiner is not offended and to proceed with the examination.

Characteristically the genital and rectal examinations are the last portions of the physical assessment. The examination should be preceded by a thorough history of the urinary system and a history of sexual functioning. As with the female client, questioning about sexual activity or performance while the genitalia are being handled may be perceived by the client as evaluative or provocative.

ANATOMY

The following is a review of the anatomy of the male genitalia (Fig. 19-1).

The shaft of the penis is formed by three columns of erectile tissue bound together by heavy fibrous tissue to form a cylinder. The dorsolateral columns are called the corpora cavernosa; the ventromedial column is called the corpus spongiosum, and this column contains the urethra. Distally the penis terminates in a cone-shaped entity called the glans penis. The glans penis is formed by an extension and expansion of the corpus spongiosum penis, which fits over the blunt ends of the corpora cavernosa penis. The corona is the prominence formed where the glans joins the shaft. The urethra traverses the corpus spongiosum, and the external urethral orifice is a slitlike opening located slightly ventrally on the tip of the glans.

The skin of the penis is thin, hairless, dark, and only loosely connected to the internal parts of the organ. At the area of the corona, the skin forms a free fold, called the prepuce or foreskin. When allowed to remain, this flap covers the glans to a variable extent. Often the prepuce is surgically removed in circumcision (Fig. 19-2).

The scrotum is a deeply pigmented cutaneous

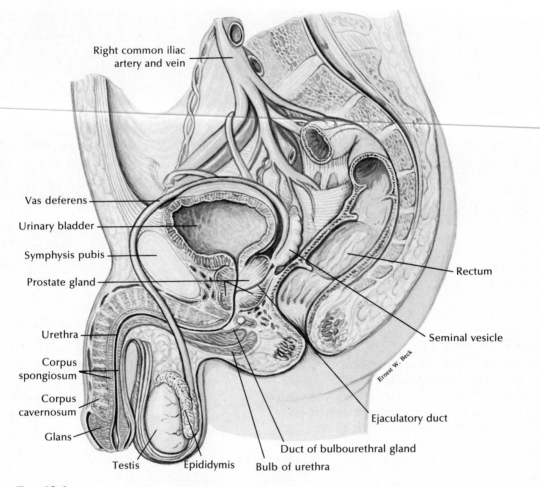

Right common iliac artery and vein

Vas deferens

Urinary bladder

Symphysis pubis

Prostate gland

Urethra

Corpus spongiosum

Corpus cavernosum

Glans

Testis

Epididymis

Bulb of urethra

Duct of bulbourethral gland

Ejaculatory duct

Seminal vesicle

Rectum

Ernest W. Beck

Fig. 19-1
Male pelvic organs. (From Anthony, C.P., and Thibodeau, G.A.: Anatomy and physiology, ed. 11, St. Louis, 1983, The C.V. Mosby Co.)

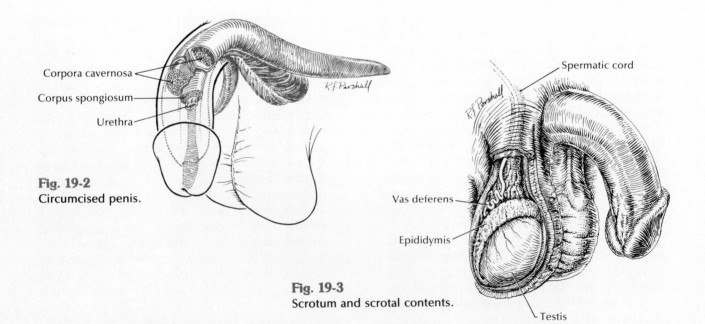

Corpora cavernosa

Corpus spongiosum

Urethra

R.f. Parshall

Fig. 19-2
Circumcised penis.

Spermatic cord

R.f. Parshall

Vas deferens

Epididymis

Testis

Fig. 19-3
Scrotum and scrotal contents.

pouch, containing the testes and parts of the spermatic cords (Fig. 19-3). The sac is formed by an outer layer of thin, rugous skin overlying a tight muscle layer. The left side of the scrotum is often lower than the right side because the left spermatic cord is usually longer. Internally the scrotum is divided into halves by a septum; each half contains a testis and its epididymis and part of the spermatic cord. The testes are ovoid and are suspended vertically, slightly forward; they lean slightly laterally in the scrotum. The mediolateral surfaces are flattened. Each is approximately 4 to 5 cm long, 3 cm wide, and 2 cm thick.

The epididymis is a comma-shaped structure that is curved over the posterolateral surface and upper end of the testis; it creates a visual bulge on the posterolateral surface of the testis. The ductus deferens (or vas deferens) begins at the tail of the epididymis, ascends the spermatic cord, travels through the inguinal canal, and eventually descends on the fundus of the bladder (see Fig. 19-1).

The prostate, a slightly conical gland, lies under the bladder, surrounds the urethra, and measures approximately 4 cm at its base or uppermost part, 3 cm vertically, and 2 cm in its anteroposterior diameter. The prostate gland has been compared to the chestnut in size and shape. It has three lobes, left and right lateral lobes and a median lobe. These lobes are not well demarcated from each other. The median lobe is the part of the prostate that projects inward from the upper, posterior area toward the urethra. It is the enlargement of this lobe that causes urinary obstruction in benign prostatic hypertrophy.

The posterior surface of the prostate is in close contact with the rectal wall and is the only portion of the gland accessible to examination. Its posterior surface is slightly convex; a shallow median furrow divides all except the upper portions of the posterior surface into right and left lateral lobes.

The seminal vesicles are a pair of convoluted pouches, 5 to 10 cm long, which lie along the lower posterior surface of the bladder, anterior to the rectum (Fig. 19-4).

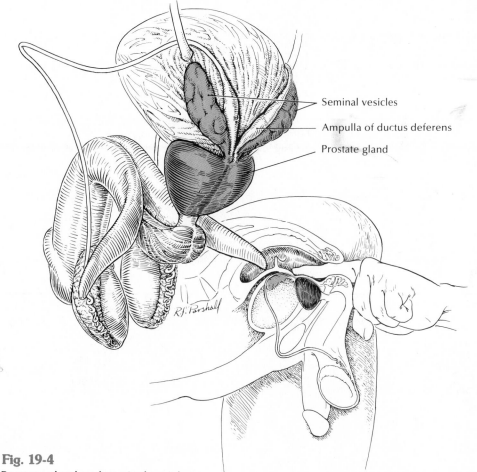

Seminal vesicles

Ampulla of ductus deferens

Prostate gland

Fig. 19-4
Prostate gland and seminal vesicles.

EXAMINATION

The techniques of inspection and palpation are used to examine the male genitalia. The examination occurs with the client standing, facing the examiner who is seated. After the inguinal and genital areas are exposed, the skin, hair, and gross appearance of the penis and scrotum are inspected. Examination of the skin, nodes, and hair distribution are discussed elsewhere in this text. The size of the penis and the secondary sex characteristics are assessed in relationship to the client's age and general development. If inflammation or lesions are observed or suspected, gloves are used for the examination.

The onset of the appearance of adult sexual characteristics is extremely variable. Pubic hair appears and the testes enlarge between the ages of 12 and 16 years. Penile enlargement and the onset of seminal emission normally occurs between the ages of 13 and 17 years. Table 19-1 contains a summary of developmental changes in the male genital system.

Table 19-1

Developmental changes in the appearance of the male genital organs

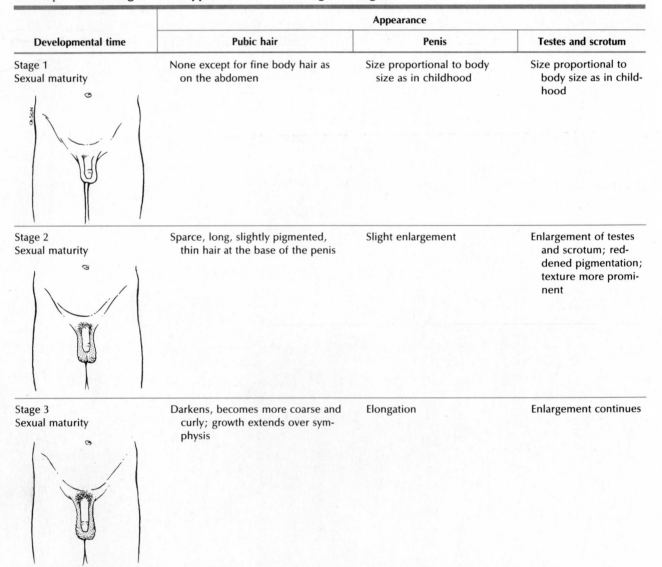

Developmental time	Appearance		
	Pubic hair	**Penis**	**Testes and scrotum**
Stage 1 Sexual maturity	None except for fine body hair as on the abdomen	Size proportional to body size as in childhood	Size proportional to body size as in childhood
Stage 2 Sexual maturity	Sparce, long, slightly pigmented, thin hair at the base of the penis	Slight enlargement	Enlargement of testes and scrotum; reddened pigmentation; texture more prominent
Stage 3 Sexual maturity	Darkens, becomes more coarse and curly; growth extends over symphysis	Elongation	Enlargement continues

Illustrations adapted from Tanner, J.M.: Growth at Adolescence, ed. 2, Oxford, 1962, Blackwell Scientific Publications.

Penis

The color of the penis ranges from pink to light brown in whites, and from light brown to dark brown in blacks. The penis is observed for lesions nodules, swelling, inflammation, and discharge. If the client is uncircumcised, he is requested to retract the prepuce from the glans and the glans and foreskin are examined carefully. If the uncircumcised client has been asked to retract the foreskin for examination of the glans, he is reminded to return the foreskin to its usual position after the inspection of the glans. The client is next asked to compress the glans anteroposteriorly. This opens the distal end of the urethra for inspection. The examiner observes for evidence of neoplastic lesions or inflammatory processes.

If any discharge is present, a smear and culture for gonorrhea are obtained (see Chapter 20 on assessment of the female genitalia and procedures for smears and cultures). If the client has reported a discharge, he is requested to milk the penis from the base to the

Table 19-1

Developmental changes in the appearance of the male genital organs—cont'd

Developmental time	Appearance		
	Pubic hair	Penis	Testes and scrotum
Stage 4 Sexual maturity 	Continues to darken, thicken, and become coarser and more curly; growth extends	Breadth and length increase; glans develops	Enlargement continues; skin pigmentation darkens
Stage 5 Sexual maturity 	Adult distribution and appearance; growth extends to inner thighs	Adult appearance	Adult appearance
Elderly clients 	Hair sparce and gray	Decrease in size	Testes hang low in scrotum; scrotum appears pendulous

urethra; if a discharge is present, a culture should then be made.

Among the more common penile lesions are syphilitic chancre, condylomata acuminata, and cancer. The syphilitic chancre is the primary lesion of syphilis. It begins as a single papule that eventually erodes into an oval or round red ulcer with an indurated base that discharges serous material. It is usually painless.

Condylomata acuminata are wart-appearing growths. They are caused by a venereal infection and may be seen occurring singly or in multiple, cauliflower-like patches.

Carcinoma of the penis occurs most frequently on the glans and on the inner lip of the prepuce. It may appear dry and scaly, ulcerated, or nodular. It is usually painless.

The urethral meatus should be positioned rather centrally on the glans. When the distal urethral ostium occurs on the ventral corona or at a more proximal and ventral site on the penis or perineum, the condition is called hypospadias (Fig. 19-5). A similar malposition-

ing of the urethral meatus in the dorsal area is called epispadias.

When hypospadias or epispadias is noted, the location of the urethral meatus should be described as precisely as possible. Hypospadias can be classified as being glandular, penile, penoscrotal, or perineal. Epispadias can be classified as being glandular, penile, or complete. Glandular refers to a location somewhere between the normal position and the junction of the glans with the body of the penis. Penile refers to a location on the penile shaft. Penoscrotal hypospadias indicates a positioning of the meatus along the anterior margin of the scrotum. Hypospadias is described as perineal when the urethral orifice is on the perineum. In the latter condition, the scrotum is bifid. Epispadias is described as complete when the urethral orifice is located anterior to and off the penis.

The prepuce should be easily retractable from the glans and returnable to its original position. Phimosis exists when retraction cannot occur (Fig. 19-6). This condition presents problems with cleanliness and pre-

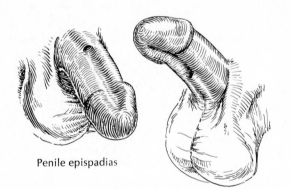

Penile epispadias

Penile hypospadias

Fig. 19-5
Malpositioning of the urethral meatus.

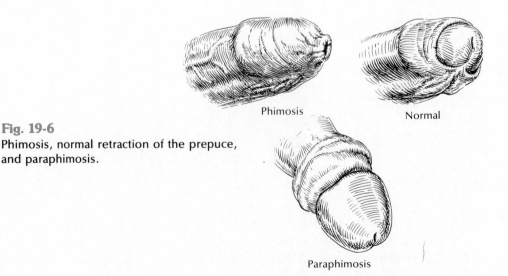

Phimosis

Normal

Paraphimosis

Fig. 19-6
Phimosis, normal retraction of the prepuce, and paraphimosis.

vents observation of the glans and interior surfaces of the prepuce. If the foreskin has been partially retracted but has impinged on the penis, so that it cannot be returned to its usual position, the condition is called paraphimosis.

The penile shaft should be carefully palpated with the thumb and the first two fingers of the examining hand. The penis should feel smooth and semifirm in consistency. The overlying skin appears slightly wrinkled and feels slightly movable over the underlying structures. Swelling, nodules, and induration are noted as possibly abnormal findings. Occasionally, hard, nontender subcutaneous plaques are palpated on the dorsomedial surface. The client with this condition, called Peyronie's disease, may report penile bending with erection and painful intercourse.

Scrotum

The client is instructed to hold the penis out of the way, and the examiner observes the general size, superficial appearance, and symmetry of the scrotum. The scrotum may normally appear asymmetrical because the left testis is generally lower than the right testis. Also, the tone of the dartos muscle determines the size of the scrotum; it contracts when the area is cold and relaxes when the area is warm. In advanced age, the dartos muscle is somewhat atonic and the scrotum may appear pendulous.

When the scrotal skin is being observed, its rugated surface should be spread. Also, the examiner should remember to inspect the posterior and posterolateral and anterior and anterolateral skin areas. A common abnormality, occurring as a single lesion or as multiple lesions, is that of sebaceous cysts. These are firm, yellow to white, nontender cutaneous lesions measuring up to 1 cm in diameter.

The scrotum may become edematous, and palpation may produce pitting. This may occur in any condition that causes edema in the lower trunk, for example, cardiovascular disease.

The contents of each half of the scrotal sac are palpated. Both testes should be present in the scrotum at birth; if not present, their location should be determined by retracing their course of descent back into the abdomen.

Both testes are palpated simultaneously between the thumb and the first two fingers. Their consistency, size, shape, and response to pressure are determined. They should be smooth, homogeneous in consistency, regular, equal in size, freely movable, and slightly sensitive to compression.

Next, each epididymis is palpated. The epididymides are located in the posterolateral area of the testes in 93% of the male population. In approximately

7% they are in the anterolateral or anterior areas. They are palpated, and their size, shape, consistency, and tenderness are noted. Then each of the spermatic cords is palpated by bilaterally grasping each between the thumb and the forefinger, starting at the base of the epididymis and continuing to the inguinal canal. The vas deferentia feel like smooth cords and are movable; the arteries, veins, lymph vessels, and nerves feel like indefinite threads along the side of the vas.

If swelling, irregularity, or nodularity is noted in the scrotum, attempts are made to transilluminate it by darkening the room and placing a lit flashlight behind the scrotal contents. Transillumination is a red glow. Serous fluid will transilluminate; tissue and blood will not. The more commonly occurring abnormalities of the scrotum are described and illustrated in Table 19-2.

All scrotal masses should be described by their placement, size, shape, consistency, tenderness, and whether they transilluminate.

Prostate gland

With an ambulatory client it is most satisfactory to execute the rectal and prostate examination with the client standing, hips flexed, toes pointed toward each other, and upper body resting on the examining table. This position flattens the buttocks, deters gluteal contraction, and makes the anus and rectum more accessible to evaluation. A debilitated client may be examined in the left lateral or lithotomy position. In the left lateral position he is reminded to flex his right knee and hip and to have his buttocks close to the edge of the examining table. The general procedure for the anal and rectal examination is described in Chapters 17 and 18 on assessment of the abdomen and rectosigmoid region. The general rectal examination is performed first; then the prostate gland and seminal vesicles are palpated (see Fig. 19-4). The pad of the index finger is used for palpation. The prostate gland is located on the anterior rectal wall but should not be protruding into the rectal lumen.

Prostatic enlargement is protrusion of the prostate gland into the rectal lumen and is commonly described in grades:

Grade I: Encroaches less than 1 cm into the rectal lumen

Grade II: Encroaches 1 to 2 cm into the rectal lumen

Grade III: Encroaches 2 to 3 cm into the rectal lumen

Grade IV: Encroaches more than 3 cm into the rectal lumen

The gland should be approximately 3 cm in length, symmetrical, movable, and of a rubbery consistency.

Table 19-2
Description of scrotal abnormalities

Abnormality	Definition/causation	Basis for diagnosis
Hydrocele	An accumulation of serous fluid between the visceral and parietal layers of the tunica vaginalis	Transilluminates; fingers can get above the mass
Scrotal hernia	A hernia within the scrotum	Bowel sounds auscultated; does not transilluminate; fingers cannot get above the mass
Varicocele	Abnormal dilatation and tortuosity of the veins of the pampiniform plexus; often described as a "bag of worms" in the scrotum*	Complaints of a dragging sensation or dull pain in the scrotal area; feels like a soft bag of worms; collapses when the scrotum is elevated and increases when the scrotum is dependent; more commonly present on the left side; usually appears at puberty
Spermatocele	An epididymal cyst resulting from a partial obstruction of the spermatic tubules*	Transilluminates; round mass, feels like a third testis; painless

*Betesh, S., editor: Diseases of the urinary tract and male genital organs, Geneva, 1974, Council for Internal Organizations for Medical Sciences, pp. 86-90.

Table 19-2
Description of scrotal abnormalities—cont'd

Abnormality	Definition/causation	Basis for diagnosis
Epididymal mass or nodularity	May be a result of benign or malignant neoplasms, syphilis, or tuberculosis	Nodules are not tender; in tuberculosis lesions, vas deferens often feels beaded
Epididymitis	An inflammation of the epididymis, usually resulting from *Escherichia coli*, *Neisseria gonorrhoeae*, or *Mycobacterium tuberculosis* organisms*	Spermatic cord often thickened and indurated; pain relieved by elevation
Torsion of the spermatic cord	Axial rotation or volvulus of the spermatic cord, resulting in infarction of the testicle	Elevated mass; pain not relieved by further elevation; more common in childhood or adolescence; history of extreme pain and tenderness of the testis, followed by hyperemic swelling and hydrocele
Testicular tumor	Multiple causes	Usually not painful; hydroceles may develop as a result of a tumor—if a testis cannot be palpated, fluid may need to be aspirated so that the testis can be accurately evaluated.

Its median sulcus normally can be felt. The lateral margins of the prostate gland should be discrete, and a moderate degree of mobility can be noted when the tip of the index finger is hooked over the upper border of the gland and the gland is pulled down. The proximal portions of the seminal vesicles can sometimes be palpated as corrugated structures above the lateral to the midpoint of the gland. Normally they are too soft to be palpated. The examiner should attempt to examine all available surfaces of the prostate gland and seminal vesicles. Significant abnormalities of the prostate gland or seminal vesicles include protrusion into the rectal lumen; hard, nodular areas; bogginess; tenderness; and asymmetry.

The examiner should mentally consider the following questions about these structures:

Surface: Smooth or nodular?

Consistency: Rubbery, hard, boggy, soft, or fluctuant?

Shape: Rounded or flat?

Size: Normal, enlarged, or atrophied?

Sensitivity: Tender or not?

Movability: Movable or fixed?

A hard, single or multiple lesion on a firm and fixed prostate gland may indicate cancer. The initial lesion of carcinoma is frequently on the posterior lobe and can be easily identified during the rectal examination. A soft, symmetrical, boggy, nontender prostate gland may indicate benign prostatic hypertrophy, a condition very common in men over 50 years of age. In the later stages of this condition, the median sulcus may be obliterated. A boggy, fluctuant, or tender prostate gland may indicate acute or chronic prostatitis.

The prostate gland can be massaged centrally from its lateral edges to force secretions into the urethra. The method of prostate massage is indicated in Fig. 19-7. The prostate is stroked from its distal to proximal areas using the order of strokes indicated in the figure. Secretion at the urethral opening can be examined and cultured.

SCROTAL SELF-EXAMINATION

Testicular self-examination is a means of early identification of scrotal cancer. Malignant scrotal tumors are the most common neoplasms in men aged 20 to 34. In addition to age, the following are risk factors for scrotal cancer: (1) history of undescended testes; (2) white race; (3) history of maternal use of oral contraceptives or diethylstilbestrol during early pregnancy; (4) history of maternal abdominal or pelvic x-ray examination during pregnancy; (5) higher social class; and (6) never married or late marriage.

The health-oriented practitioner should assess the male client's level of knowledge about testicular self-examination, reinforce the importance of a monthly self-examination, and provide instruction for the examination. The following outline can be used for the health teaching along with pictures of the anatomy of the male genitalia:

1. Examine the testicles once a month.
2. Do the self-examination following a shower or warm bath when the testes are descended and accessible for palpation.
3. Hold the scrotum in the palms of the hands.
4. Use the thumbs and the index and middle fingers for examination.
5. Identify the structures in the scrotum, the testes, the epididymides, and the vas deferentia. All the surfaces of each testes should be examined individually, using a small amount of pressure. The testes normally feel rubbery and have a smooth surface. The epididymis feels softer than the testes and is located on the back and side of each testis. The vas deferens extends from the bottom of the epididymis to the groin and is a firm, smooth cord.
6. The examination should not be painful, unless the pressure is too hard or there is some problem. A small amount of tenderness may be noticed during the palpation of the testes and epididymides and is normal.

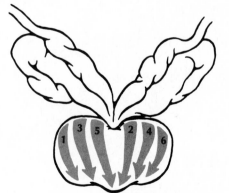

Fig. 19-7

Prostatic massage. The arrows indicate the areas of the prostate that are massaged and the sequence and direction of the massage. It is important that all areas of the prostate available to the palpating fingers be massaged.

7. Any lump or change in texture, whether painful or not, should be reported to and assessed by a health care provider as soon as possible.

INGUINAL AREA: ASSESSMENT FOR HERNIAS

If a client has an inguinal or groin area hernia, he (or she) will probably complain of a swelling or bulging in that area, especially during abdominal straining. All clients should be screened for inguinal and femoral hernias, even if they do not complain of groin swelling, as part of the routine physical examination.

No special equipment is needed for the examination.

ANATOMY

The following is a review of the anatomy of the inguinal area (Fig. 19-8).

The inguinal (Poupart's) ligament extends from the anterosuperior spine of the ilium to the pubic tubercle.

The inguinal canal is a flattened tunnel between two layers of abdominal muscle, measuring approximately 4 to 6 cm in the adult. Its internal ring is located 1 to 2 cm above the midpoint of the inguinal ligament. The spermatic cord traverses through this internal ring, passes through the canal, exits the canal at its external (subcutaneous) ring, and then moves up and over the inguinal ligament and into the scrotum.

Hesselbach's triangle is the region superior to the inguinal canal, medial to the inferior epigastric artery, and lateral to the margin of the rectus muscle.

The femoral canal is a potential space just inferior to the inguinal ligament and 3 cm medial and parallel to the femoral artery. If the examiner's right hand is placed on the client's right anterior thigh with the index finger over the femoral artery, the femoral canal will be under the ring finger.

The three main types of pelvic area hernias are shown in Fig. 19-9. In the *indirect inguinal hernia*, the hernial sac enters the internal inguinal canal and its tip is located somewhere in the inguinal canal or beyond

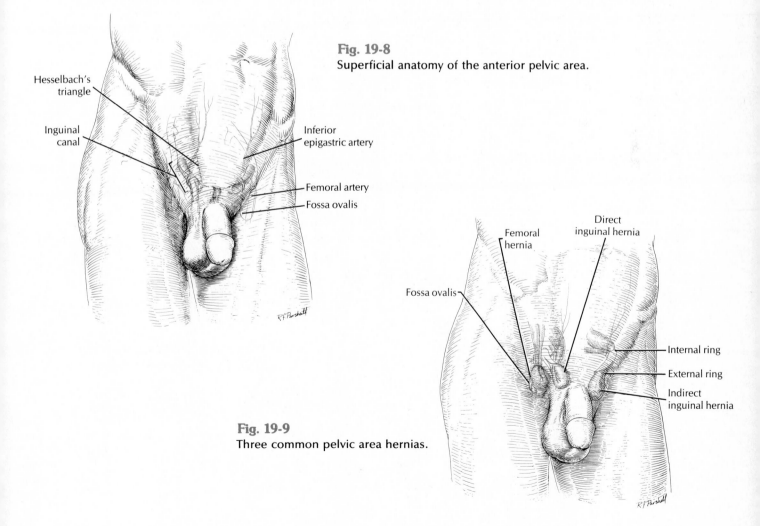

Fig. 19-8
Superficial anatomy of the anterior pelvic area.

Fig. 19-9
Three common pelvic area hernias.

Table 19-3
Comparison of inguinal and femoral hernias

	Inguinal hernia		Femoral hernia
	Indirect	**Direct**	
Course	Sac emerges through the internal inguinal ring, lateral to the inferior epigastric artery; can remain in the canal, exit the external ring, or pass into the scrotum	Sac emerges directly from behind and through the external inguinal ring; located in the region of Hesselbach's triangle	Sac emerges through the femoral ring, the femoral canal, and the fossa ovalis; observed lateral to the femoral vein
Incidence	More common in infants under 1 year and in young men 16 to 20 years; more common in men than in women at a ratio of approximately 4:1; 60% of all hernias	Most often observed in men over 40 years of age; rarer than the indirect hernia	Less common than inguinal hernias; seldom seen in children; more common in women; 4% of all hernias
Cause	Congenital or acquired	Congenital weakness exacerbated by (1) lifting, (2) atrophy of abdominal muscles, (3) ascites, (4) chronic cough, or (5) obesity	Acquired; may be caused by (1) stooping frequently, (2) increased abdominal pressure, or (3) loss of muscle substance
Clinical symptoms and signs	Soft swelling in the region of the internal inguinal ring—swelling increases when client stands or strains, is sometimes reduced when client reclines; pain during straining	Abdominal bulge in the area of Hesselbach's triangle, usually in the area of the internal ring; usually painless; easily reduced when client reclines; rarely enters scrotum	Right side more commonly affected; pain may be severe; strangulation frequent; sac may extend into the scrotum, into the labium, or along the saphenous vein

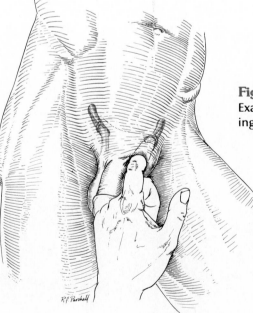

Fig. 19-10
Examination of a male client for indirect inguinal hernia.

the canal. In men, indirect inguinal hernias may descend into the scrotum. The *direct inguinal hernia* emerges directly from behind and through the external inguinal ring. The *femoral hernia* emerges through the femoral ring, the femoral canal, and the fossa ovalis.

A comparison of the three main types of hernias is presented in Table 19-3.

EXAMINATION

Inspection and palpation are the techniques used. Whenever possible, the examination for hernias is performed with the client standing. However, if the client is debilitated or especially tense, the examination may be performed while the client is lying down on a flat surface.

First, the areas of inguinal and femoral hernias are exposed and observed with the client at rest and while the client holds his breath and exerts abdominal pressure with the diaphragm. Straining is preferred to coughing because a more sustained pressure is elicited. Sometimes the impulse of coughing can be confused with the impulse of a hernia. Often, small hernias in women and children are more easily observed than felt because of the fatty tissue in the area.

The examiner palpates for a direct inguinal hernia by placing two fingers over each external inguinal ring and instructing the client to bear down. The presence of a hernia will produce a palpable bulge in the area.

To determine the presence of an indirect inguinal hernia, the client is asked to flex the ipsilateral knee slightly while the examiner attempts to direct his index or little finger into the path of the inguinal canal. When the finger has traversed as far as possible, the client is asked to strain. A hernia will be felt as a mass of tissue meeting the finger and then withdrawing. The left index or little finger, hand with palm side out, is used to examine the client's left side. The right hand in turn is used for the client's right side. In women, the canal is narrow, and the finger cannot be inserted far, if at all. In men, the finger invaginates scrotal skin into the inguinal canal (Fig. 19-10).

In both men and women, each fossa ovalis area is palpated while the client is straining. The femoral hernia will be felt as a soft tumor at the fossa, below the inguinal ligament and lateral to the pubic tubercle.

Occasionally, the client may complain of the symptoms of hernia, but none can be palpated. In such cases a load test is suggested. The client lifts a heavy object while the inguinal area is being observed. A previously unobserved bulge may become prominent.

SUMMARY

I. Equipment needed
   A. Gloves
   B. Lubricant
   C. Flashlight
II. Examination of male genitalia
   A. General inspection
      1. Skin characteristics
      2. Hair
         a. Distribution
         b. Parasites
      3. Inguinal area
         a. Swelling—at rest and with straining
         b. Inflammation
   B. Inspection of the penis
      1. Size relative to age and development
      2. Color
      3. Discharge
      4. Skin and surface characteristics
      5. Urethral meatus
         a. Location
         b. Discharge
         c. Lesions
      6. Glans
         a. Color
         b. Lesions
      7. Foreskin
         a. Presence or absence
         b. Mobility, if present
   C. Palpation of the penis
      1. Tenderness
      2. Consistency
      3. Presence of nodules
   D. Palpation of inguinal nodes
      1. Swelling
      2. Tenderness
   E. Inspection of the scrotum
      1. Color
      2. Surface characteristics
      3. Size
      4. Symmetry
   F. Palpation of the scrotum
      1. Testes
         a. Presence
         b. Size
         c. Tenderness
         d. Contour
         e. Mobility
         f. Symmetry
      2. Epididymides
         a. Tenderness
         b. Location
         c. Consistency
         d. Shape
         e. Surface characteristics

3. Vas deferentia
    a. Tenderness
    b. Mobility
    c. Surface characteristics
G. Transillumination of any swelling or masses
III. Examination of the inguinal area
    A. Palpation of inguinal rings for direct inguinal hernias
    B. Palpation into external inguinal rings for indirect inguinal hernias
    C. Palpation for femoral hernias
IV. Rectal examination
    A. Observation of the anus
    B. Rectal examination
    C. Palpation of the prostate and seminal vesicles
        1. Size
        2. Contour
        3. Consistency
        4. Surface characteristics
        5. Tenderness

BIBLIOGRAPHY

Bedenoch, A.W.: Manual of urology, ed. 2, London, 1974, William Heinemann Medical Books, Ltd.

Bodner, H.: Diagnostic and therapeutic aids in urology, Springfield, Ill., 1974, Charles C Thomas, Publishers.

Brandes, D., editor: Male accesory sex organs, New York, 1974, Academic Press, Inc.

Btesh, S., editor: Disease of the urinary tract and male genital organs, Geneva, 1974, Council for International Organizations for Medical Sciences.

Calman, C.H.: Atlas of hernia repair, St. Louis, 1966, The C.V. Mosby Co.

Haggerty, B.J.: Prevention and differential of scrotal cancer, Nurse Pract. **8:**45, 1983.

Harrison, J.H., and others: Campbell's urology, Philadelphia, 1978, W.B. Saunders Co.

Johnson, D.E., editor: Testicular tumors, Flushing, N.Y., 1972, Medical Examination Publishing Co., Inc.

Maingot, R., editor: Abdominal operation, ed. 6, New York, 1974, Appleton-Century-Crofts.

Ravitch, M.M.: Repairs of hernias, Chicago, 1969, Year Book Medical Publishers, Inc.

Scott, R., editor: Current controversies in urologic management, Philadelphia, 1972, W.B. Saunders Co.

Smith, D.R.: General urology, Los Altos, Calif., 1981, Lange Medical Publications.

Zornow, D.H., and Landes, R.R.: Scrotal palpation, Am. Fam. Physician **23:**150, 1981.

CHAPTER 20

ASSESSMENT OF THE FEMALE GENITALIA AND PROCEDURES FOR SMEARS AND CULTURES

FEMALE GENITALIA

Most female clients perceive the examination of their reproductive organs as being different from the examination of other body parts. Past admonitions of "do not touch" and "keep it covered" have created a population of anatomically unaware and sometimes inappropriately "modest" women who are often unnecessarily difficult to examine. Most practitioners believe that a great amount of information about a female client can be obtained by examining the genital area and performing screening tests; but because of their experience with the fearful and tense reactions of many clients, practitioners have sometimes routinely omitted the examination of the genital organs or have referred their clients to gynecological specialists for routine examinations.

One cause of the female client's tenseness during an examination of the genital area may be fear of discovery. During the history the practitioner investigates areas of anatomical and physiological function and dysfunction. The review of systems on all clients should include a sexual history. If this portion of the history is accomplished skillfully and if the client has been cooperative, she should not be apprehensive about the possible discovery of sexual "secrets."

Other causes of tenseness during the pelvic examination include fear of discovery of disease and the memory of previous, uncomfortable pelvic examinations.

Also, many clients are not knowledgeable regarding the anatomy of the pelvic area. The practitioner should determine the client's need for basic information regarding the structure of the genital organs and provide this instruction before the pelvic examination,

along with a demonstration of the instruments and an explanation of the procedure. The client should be shown the speculum and the mechanism used to open and close it. The client should be advised regarding the clicking sounds normally made by a speculum as it is opened and closed. If a relatively short amount of time were taken to inform and orient all female clients at the time of their first examination, practitioners and clients would reap the benefits of enhanced mutual cooperation.

Teaching the client a relaxation technique will often make an examination shorter or even possible. One relaxation technique that has been successful is the following: the client is instructed to place her hands on her chest at about the level of the diaphragm, breathe deeply and slowly through her mouth, concentrate on the rhythm of breathing, and relax all body muscles with each exhalation. The tense client is apt to hold her breath and tighten. Even the coached client may forget and hold her breath; a gentle reminder, advising her to keep breathing, usually enables the client to maintain relaxation. This technique is particularly helpful in the adolescent or virginal client, whose introitus may be especially tight.

Another relaxation or, more specifically, distraction technique that has been used by some practitioners is the placement of a sign or mobile above the examining table. Clients appreciate having something to look at, and their attention is constructively diverted from the activities of the examiner.

For most clients it is distressing to attempt to converse while in a lithotomy position. Most clients appreciate an explanation and reassurance from the examiner but prefer not to have to respond to questions until

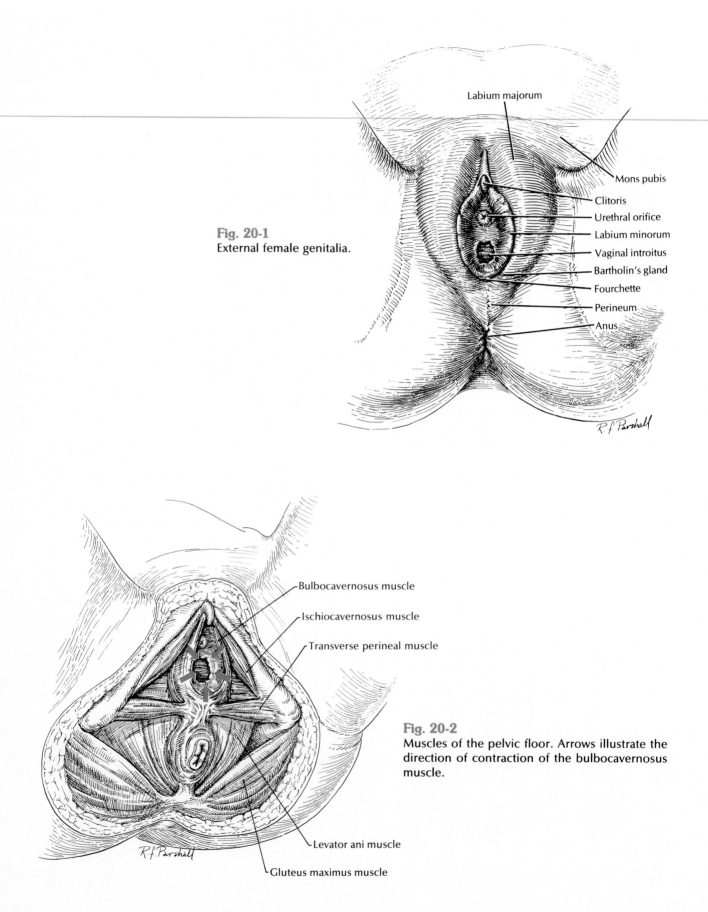

Fig. 20-1
External female genitalia.

Labium majorum

Mons pubis

Clitoris

Urethral orifice

Labium minorum

Vaginal introitus

Bartholin's gland

Fourchette

Perineum

Anus

Bulbocavernosus muscle

Ischiocavernosus muscle

Transverse perineal muscle

Fig. 20-2
Muscles of the pelvic floor. Arrows illustrate the direction of contraction of the bulbocavernosus muscle.

Levator ani muscle

Gluteus maximus muscle

they are again upright and at eye level with the examiner. Questioning a client during the pelvic examination is apt to make her tense.

Environmental conditions are also important in enhancing cooperation during the examination of the genital area. The environment and the client should be warm. The examining area should be private and safe from unexpected intrusion. The room, the examiner's hands, and all materials touching the client should be warm.

ANATOMY AND PHYSIOLOGY
External genitalia

The external female genitalia are termed the vulva or pudendum (Fig. 20-1). The symphysis pubis is covered by a pad of fat called the mons pubis or mons veneris. In the postpubertal female the mons is covered by a patch of coarse, curly hair that extends to the lower abdomen. The abdominal portion of the female escutcheon is flat and forms the base of an inverted triangle of hair.

The labia majora are two bilobate folds of adipose tissue extending from the mons to the perineum. After puberty, their outer surfaces are covered with hair and their inner surfaces are smooth and hairless. The labia minora are two folds of skin that are thinner and darker in color than the labia majora. The labia minora lie within the labia majora and extend from the clitoris to the fourchette. Anteriorly, each labium minus divides into a medial and a lateral part. The lateral parts join posteriorly to form the prepuce of the clitoris, and the medial parts join anterior to the clitoris to form the frenulum of the clitoris. The clitoris is composed of erectile

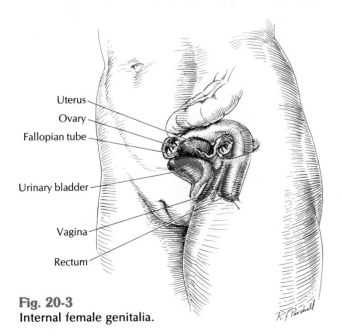

Fig. 20-3
Internal female genitalia.

Labels: Uterus, Ovary, Fallopian tube, Urinary bladder, Vagina, Rectum

tissue and is homologous to the corpora cavernosa of the penis. Its body is normally about 2.5 cm in total length; the length of its visible portion is 2 cm or less.

The vestibule is the boat-shaped anatomical region between the labia minora. It contains the urethral and vaginal orifices. The urethral orifice is located approximately 2.5 cm posterior to the clitoris and is visualized as an irregular, vertical slit. The vaginal orifice, or introitus, lies immediately behind the urethral orifice and can be observed as a thin vertical slit or as a large orifice with irregular skin edges, depending on the condition of the hymen. The hymen is a membranous, annular, or crescentic fold at the vaginal opening. When unperforated, it is usually a continuous membrane but on occasion may be cribriform. After perforation small rounded fragments of hymen attach to the introital margins; these are called hymenal caruncles.

The ducts of two types of glands open on the vulva. Skene's glands are multiple, tiny organs located in the paraurethral area. Their ducts, numbering approximately 6 to 31, lie inside and just outside of the urethral orifice and are usually not visible. These ducts open laterally and slightly posterior to the urethral orifice in approximately the 5 and 7 o'clock positions; the urethral orifice is the center of the clock. Bartholin's glands are small, ovoid organs located lateral and slightly posterior to the vaginal orifice, partially behind the bulb of the vestibule. Their ducts are approximately 2 cm long and open in the groove between the labia minora and the hymen in approximately the 5 and 7 o'clock positions. These ducts are also usually not visible.

The perineum consists of the tissues between the introitus and the anus.

The pelvic floor consists of a group of muscles attached to points on the bony pelvis (Fig. 20-2). These muscles form a suspended sling that assists in holding the pelvic contents in place. The muscles are pierced by the urethral, vaginal, and rectal orifices and function both passively as a pelvic support and actively in voluntary contraction of the vaginal and anal orifices.

Internal genitalia

Fig. 20-3 illustrates the internal genitalia.

The vagina is a pink, transversely rugated, collapsed tube that in the adult is approximately 9 cm long posteriorly and 6 to 7 cm long anteriorly. It inclines posteriorly at approximately a 45-degree angle with the vertical plane of the body. The vagina is highly dilatable, especially in its superior portion and anteroposterior dimension. When collapsed, it is roughly H shaped in transverse section. Superiorly and usually anteriorly, the vagina is pierced by the uterine cervix. The recess between the portion of the vagina adjacent to the cervix and the cervix is called the vaginal fornix. Although it is actually continuous, the fornix is anatomically divided into anterior, posterior, and lateral fornices.

The uterus is an inverted, pear-shaped, muscular organ that is flattened anteroposteriorly. It is usually found inclined forward 45 degrees from the vertical plane of the erect body and is approximately 5.5 to 8 cm long, 3.5 to 4 cm wide, and 2 to 2.5 cm thick. The uterus of the parous client may be normally enlarged an additional 2 to 3 cm in any of the three dimensions. The uterus is divided into two main parts: the body and the cervix. The body in turn is composed of three parts: the fundus, the prominence above the insertion of the fallopian tubes; the body, or main portion, of the uterus; and the isthmus, the constricted lower portion of the uterus, which is adjacent to the cervix. The cervix extends from the isthmus and into the vagina.

The uterine cavity communicates with the vagina via an ostium, the cervical os. The os is a small, depressed, circular opening in the nulliparous client. In women who have borne children the os is enlarged and irregularly shaped. The position of the uterus is not fixed; it is a relatively movable organ. The uterus may be anteverted, anteflexed, retroverted, or retroflexed in position; or it may be in midposition. In the normal adult with an empty bladder the uterus is usually anteverted and slightly anteflexed in position.

The ovaries are a pair of oval organs; each is approximately 3 cm long, 2 cm wide, and 1 cm thick. They are usually located near the lateral pelvic wall, at the level of the anterosuperior iliac spine. The two uterine tubes insert in the upper portion of the uterus, are supported loosely by the broad ligament, and run laterally to the ovaries. Each tube is approximately 10 cm long.

The uterus, ovaries, and tubes are supported by four pairs of ligaments: the cardinal, uterosacral, round, and broad ligaments (Fig. 20-4).

The rectouterine pouch, or Douglas' cul-de-sac, is a deep recess formed by the peritoneum as it passes over the intestinal surface of the rectum. It is the lowest point in the abdominal cavity.

EXAMINATION
Preparation

Clients should be advised not to douche during the 24 hours preceding the pelvic examination and reminded to empty their bladders immediately before the examination.

Materials needed for the examination should be assembled and readily available before the client is put in the lithotomy position. Materials needed for the examination minimally include:

    Rubber gloves
    Speculums of various sizes
    Culture plates for gonorrhea screening
    Glass slides
    Glass cover slides
    Ayre spatula
    Sterile cotton swabs
    Lubricant on a piece of paper or gauze*
    Cotton balls
    Sponge forceps
    Cytology fixative
    Source of light
    Hand mirror

---

*An amount of lubricant, sufficient for the examination, should be placed on a piece of paper or gauze. The examiner should avoid handling the whole tube of lubricant during the examination, since it might be contaminated during handling and become a source of cross-contamination of infection between clients.

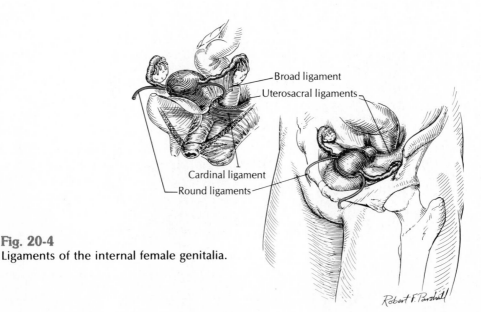

Fig. 20-4
Ligaments of the internal female genitalia.

Broad ligament
Uterosacral ligaments
Cardinal ligament
Round ligaments

Robert F. Parshall

Some clients have difficulty assuming the lithotomy position, especially moving their buttocks sufficiently downward to the edge of the table. The practitioner can assist the client by asking the client to raise her buttocks (while the client is lying on the table with heels in the stirrups) and by guiding the client's buttocks downward from a position at the client's side or from a position at the foot of the table. Clients usually feel more comfortable wearing shoes when their feet are in the stirrups, rather than supporting their weight with bare heels against the hard, cold stirrups.

Components of the examination

The regional examination of the female genital system consists of (1) the abdominal examination, (2) inspection of the external genitalia, (3) palpation of the external genitalia, (4) the speculum examination, (5) obtaining specimens, (6) the bimanual vaginal examination, and (7) the rectovaginal examination.

The client and the examiner assume several positions for the examination. For the abdominal examination, the client is lying on the examination table and the examiner is facing the client's right side. For the inspection and palpation of the external genitalia and the speculum examination, the client is in the lithotomy position and the examiner is seated on a stool, facing the client's genitalia (Fig. 20-5, A). For the bimanual examination and the rectovaginal examination, the client remains in the lithotomy position and the examiner is standing (Fig. 20-5, B).

The abdominal examination is discussed in Chapter 17 on assessment of the abdomen. The examination of the female genital system should be preceded by a thorough examination of the abdomen.

It is recommended that the examiner wear two gloves for the genital area examination. This will allow for a thorough external examination and complete spreading of the labia and also will protect subsequent clients from the possible transfer of infection.

Inspection of the external genitalia. The examiner is seated on a stool, facing the external genitalia. First, the skin and hair distribution are observed. Hair distribution should be approximately shaped as an inverse triangle. Some abdominal hair is normal and may be hereditary. Male hair distribution patterns in women are abnormal.

In the adolescent client, sexual maturity is assessed by observation of breast growth and pubic hair growth. Table 20-1 outlines and illustrates sexual maturity ratings for the appearance of the female genitalia. Along with changes in pubic hair, the following also occur:
1. Increase in prominence in labia majora
2. Enlargement of the labia minora
3. Increase in size of the clitoris
4. Increase in elasticity of vaginal tissue
5. Enlargement of vagina and ovaries

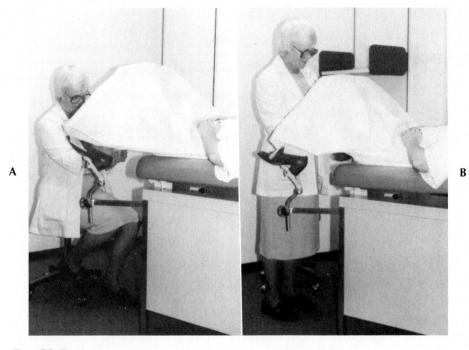

Fig. 20-5
Examination of the female genital system. **A,** Examiner seated. **B,** Examiner standing.

The total skin area is inspected for lesions and parasites. The gloved fingers should be used to spread the hair and labia so that all skin surfaces can be adequately visualized. The area of the clitoris particularly is a common site for chancres of syphilis in the younger client and for cancerous lesions in the older client.

The labia are flat in childhood and atrophic in old age. Estrogen influences fat deposition, which causes a round, full appearance of the labia. The labia majora of the nulliparous client will be in close approximation, covering the labia minora and the vestibule area. After a vaginal delivery, the labia may be slightly shriveled and gaping in appearance.

The skin of the vulvar area is a slightly darker pigment than the skin of the rest of the body. The mucous membranes are normally dark pink in color and moist in appearance.

Common abnormalities of the skin and labia include parasites, skin lesions of all types, areas of leukoplakia, varicosities, hyperpigmentation erythema, depigmentation, and swelling. Leukoplakia appears as white, adherent patches on the skin; it may be likened to spots of dried white paint.

The clitoris is examined for size; the visible portion of the clitoris should not *exceed* 2 cm in length and 1 cm in width.

Table 20-1
Developmental changes in the general appearance of female genitalia

Developmental stage	Description	Developmental stage	Description
Stage 1 sexual maturity (preadolescence)	No pubic hair, except for fine body hair	Stage 4 sexual maturity	Texture and curl of pubic hair as in adult but not as thick and not spread over the thighs (usually seen between ages 13 and 14)
Stage 2 sexual maturity	Sparce growth of long, slightly pigmented, fine pubic hair, which is slightly curly and located along the labia (usually seen at ages 11 to 12)	Stage 5 sexual maturity	Adult appearance in quality and quantity of pubic hair; growth is spread onto the inner aspect of the upper thighs
Stage 3 sexual maturity	Pubic hair becomes darker, curlier, and spreads over the symphysis (usually seen at ages 12 to 13)	Elderly	Pubic hair is thin, sparce, brittle, and gray

The urethral orifice normally appears slitlike or stellate and is of the same color as the membranes surrounding it. The openings of the paraurethral (Skene's) glands are not usually visible. Erythema or a polyp located in this area or a discharge from the urethra or gland ducts is abnormal.

The examiner next observes the area of Bartholin's glands and their ducts for swelling, erythema, duct enlargement, or discharge. The presence of any of these conditions is abnormal.

The perineum is inspected for evidence of an episiotomy and its healing. The anus is also inspected at this time (see Chapter 17 on assessment of the abdomen).

Palpation of the external genitalia. Although the client knows she will be touched, she may startle when the fingers are placed on the genitalia for the initiation of the palpation. In an anxious client, touching the client's inner thigh with the back of a hand might prevent excess tensing of pelvic muscles.

Any areas of observed abnormality are palpated to determine the size, shape, consistency, and tenderness of the mass or lesion. The labia are palpated. They should feel soft, and the texture should be homogeneous.

The index finger and the middle finger are inserted into the vagina. First, the urethra and area of Skene's duct openings are gently milked from about the level of 4 cm in on the anterior vaginal wall down to the orifice (Fig. 20-6). This procedure should not normally cause pain or discharge. If a discharge is present, a specimen is inoculated onto a Thayer-Martin culture plate. Then the area of Bartholin's glands and their ducts are pal-

pated for swelling or tenderness (Fig. 20-7). Normally Bartholin's glands are not palpable.

While the examiner's fingers are in the vagina, several maneuvers are performed to assess the integrity of the pelvic musculature. First, the perineal area is palpated between the fingers inside the vagina and the thumb of that same hand. In the nulliparous client the perineum is felt as a firm, muscular body. After an episiotomy has healed, the perineum feels thinner and more rigid because of scarring. If this area is very thin and if the palpating fingers can almost approximate, the client should be questioned again about bowel or sexual problems.

The client is then asked to constrict her vaginal orifice around the examiner's fingers while they are still placed in the vagina. A nulliparous client will demonstrate a high degree of tone and a multiparous client, less tone.

In the third maneuver the index and middle fingers remain in the vagina; they are spread laterally, and the client is asked to push down against them. The presence of urinary stress incontinence, cystocele, rectocele, enterocele, or uterine prolapse can be observed if present.

Cystocele is the prolapse into the vagina of the anterior vaginal wall and the bladder. Clinically, a pouching would be seen on the anterior wall as the client strains.

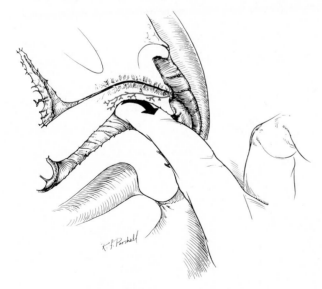

Fig. 20-6
Palpation of Skene's glands.

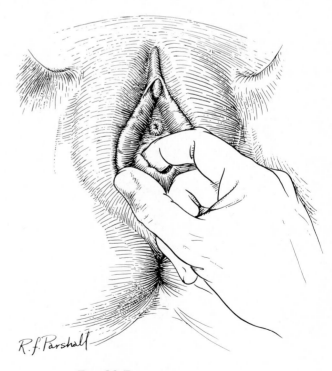

Fig. 20-7
Palpation of Bartholin's glands.

Rectocele is the prolapse into the vagina of the posterior vaginal wall and the rectum. Clinically, a pouching would be seen on the posterior wall as the client strains.

Enterocele is a hernia of the pouch of Douglas into the vagina. Clinically, a bulge would be seen emerging from the posterior fornix. If this is observed, the client should be additionally examined by assessing the effect of straining (1) during the speculum examination with the speculum inserted, half opened, three fourths of its length into the vagina; and (2) during the bimanual examination with the intravaginal fingers in the posterior fornix.

There are three degrees of *uterine prolapse*. In first-degree prolapse, the cervix appears at the introitus when the client strains. In second-degree prolapse, the cervix is outside of the introitus when the client strains. In third-degree prolapse, the whole uterus is outside the introitus and the vagina is essentially turned inside out when the client strains.

Speculum examination. The examiner will have obtained clues regarding the most appropriate type and size of speculum to use in the speculum examination through the history and inspection of the external genitalia. There are two basic types of speculums, the Graves speculum and the Pederson speculum (Fig. 20-8). The Graves speculum is one of the most commonly used in the examination of the adult female client. It is available in lengths varying from 3½ to 5 inches and in widths from ¾ to 1½ inches. The Pederson speculum is both narrower and flatter than the Graves speculum and is used with virgins, nulliparous clients, or clients whose vaginal orifices have contracted postmenopausally.

A metal speculum needs to be warmed before insertion. An effective way to do this is by running warm water over it. Lubricant is bacteriostatic and also distorts cells on Papanicolaou (Pap) smears; thus, it cannot be used if a culture or smear is to be obtained. The warm water also assists in lubricating both the metal and plastic speculums and may be used if cultures and smears are to be taken.

The index finger and middle finger of one hand are placed 1 inch into the vagina. The fingers are then spread, and pressure is exerted toward the posterior vaginal wall. The client is advised that she will feel intravaginal pressure. The speculum is held in the opposite hand with the blades between the index and middle fingers. The client is asked to bear down. This maneuver helps to additionally open the vaginal orifice and to relax perineal muscles (Fig. 20-9).

The speculum blades are inserted obliquely, taking advantage of the H configuration of the relaxed vagina (Fig. 20-9, *B*). They are inserted at a plane parallel to

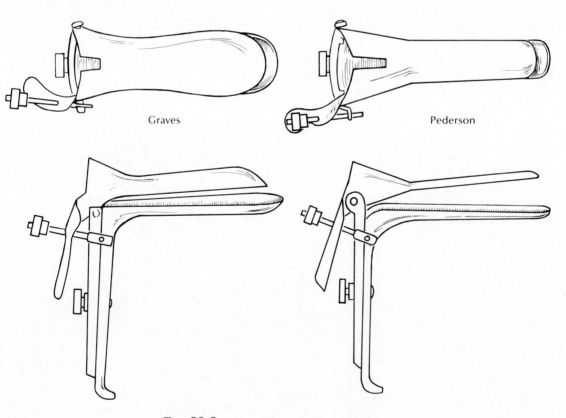

Graves

Pederson

Fig. 20-8
Graves speculum and Pederson speculum.

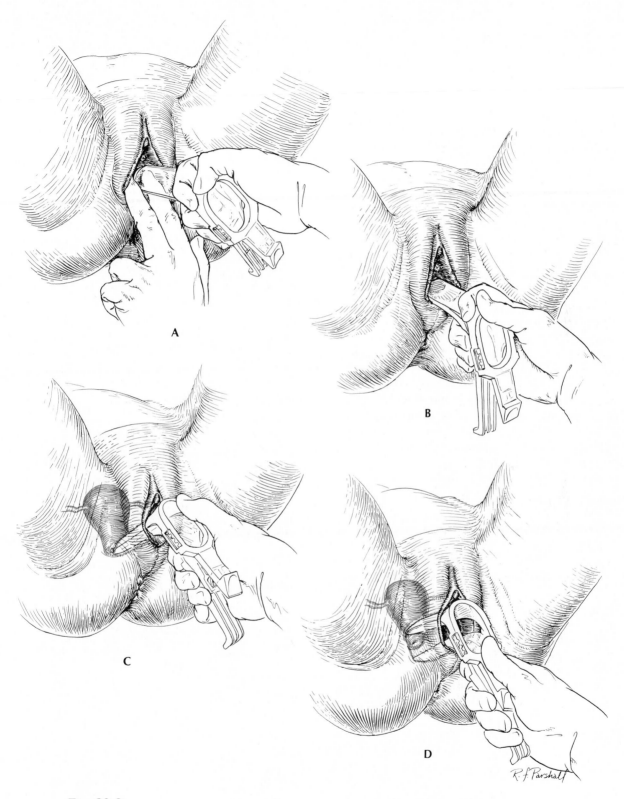

Fig. 20-9
Procedure for vaginal examination. **A,** Opening of the introitus. **B,** Oblique insertion of the speculum. **C,** Final insertion of the speculum. **D,** Opening of the speculum blades.

the examining table until the end of the speculum has reached the tips of the fingers in the vagina.

The speculum is then rotated to a transverse position, and the plane is altered in adaptation to the plane of the vagina, approximately one of a 45-degree angle with the examining table (Fig. 20-9, C). The intravaginal fingers are simultaneously withdrawn, and the speculum is inserted until it touches the end of the vagina. The lever of the speculum is then depressed; this opens the blades and allows visualization. Ideally, the cervix is seen between the blades (Fig. 20-9, D). Sometimes, however, especially for the beginning examiner, it is not. In such cases the speculum is either anterior (usually the situation) or posterior to the cervix. If this occurs, the speculum is withdrawn halfway and reinserted in a different plane. After the entire cervix is in view of the examiner, the depressed lever is fixed in an open position.

If the client is tense and is resisting the insertion of the speculum, the examiner should not withdraw the speculum but stop the insertion and leave the speculum in its position, remind the client to use relaxation techniques, and continue the examination when relaxation has occurred.

The appearance of the normal cervix has already been described. The cervix is observed for color, position, size, projection into the vaginal vault, shape, general symmetry, surface characteristics, shape and patency of the os, and discharge:

1. *Color:* The color of the cervix is normally pale after menopause and cyanotic in pregnancy. Cyanosis can occur with any condition that causes systemic hypoxia or regional venous congestion. Hyperemia may be an indication of inflammation. An additional cause of pallor is anemia.
2. *Position:* A cervix projecting more deeply than 3 cm into the vaginal vault may indicate uterine prolapse. A cervix situated on a lateral vaginal wall may indicate tumor or adhesion of a superior structure.
3. *Size:* A cervix larger than 4 cm in diameter is hypertrophied, and the presence of inflammation or tumor should be considered.
4. *Surface characteristics:* Lesions and polyps are commonly seen on the cervix and require more than visual assessment to determine if pathology exists. Any irregularity or nodularity of the cervical surface should be considered possibly abnormal (Fig. 20-10). One relatively benign condition is the presence of nabothian cysts, which appear as smooth, round, small (less than 1 cm in diameter) yellow lesions. Nabothian cysts are caused by obstruction of the cervical gland ducts.

When the squamocolumnar junction is on the ectocervix, the columnar epithelium will appear as a red, relatively symmetrical circle around the os. This condition may be a normal variation of the placement of the squamocolumnar junction or may be caused by the separation by speculum blades of a cervix whose external os has been altered and enlarged by childbirth. This condition is termed eversion or ectropion. Erosions appear similar to eversions. However, erosions are usually irregular, rough, and friable. Erosions frequently indicate pathology and require further assessment and treatment. Because of the occasional presence of the squamocolumnar junction on the ectocervix, the differential assessment of normal cervix from abnormal cervix using inspection alone is impossible.

Diffuse punctate hemorrhages, colloquially termed "strawberry spots," are occasionally observed in association with trichomonal infections.

5. *Discharge:* The character of the normal cervical mucus varies in the menstrual cycle. It is always odorless and nonirritating. Its color and consistency may vary from clear to white and from thin to thick and stringy. Colored or purulent dis-

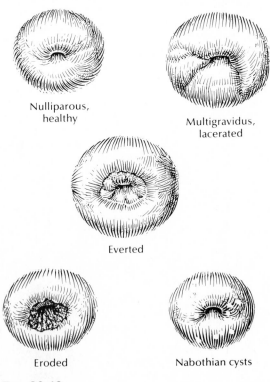

Nulliparous, healthy

Multigravidus, lacerated

Everted

Eroded

Nabothian cysts

Fig. 20-10
Common appearances and lesions of the cervix.

charges exuding from the os or present in the area of the cervix are probably abnormal.

6. *Shape of the os:* The cervical os of the nulliparous client is small and evenly round. The cervical os of a parous client shows the effects of the stretching and laceration of childbirth and is irregular in shape.

Many clients have not seen their cervices. The client should be asked if she wishes to see her cervix. This visualization can easily be accomplished through the use of a hand mirror.

After the cervix is inspected, a Pap smear, culture for gonorrhea, and hanging drop specimen may be obtained if indicated. The procedures for these are described at the end of this chapter. The vagina is then inspected. This is done during speculum insertion, while the speculum is open, and during its removal. The color and condition of the vaginal mucosa and the color, odor, consistency, and appearance of vaginal secretions are noted. Pallor, cyanosis, and hyperemia may be present for the same reasons as described for the cervix. Leukoplakia may also occur on vaginal mucosa.

As with cervical discharge, vaginal discharge is normally odorless, nonirritating, thin or mucoid, and clear or cloudy. Also, the presence of some whitish, creamy material is normal. Any other vaginal discharge should be described according to its color, odor, consistency, amount, and appearance. Three basic types of vaginal infections produce observable discharge: monilial infections, characterized by thick, white, curdy exudates that appear as adherent patches and free discharge; trichomonal infections, characterized by a profuse watery, gray or green, frothy, odorous discharge; and bacterial infections, characterized by an odorous, gray, homogeneous discharge of moderate amount.

After the inspection of the vaginal area, the speculum is slowly withdrawn. As it is withdrawn, the nut, or catch, is loosened and the lever is again controlled by the thumb. The blades are slowly closed as they are removed, and the speculum is carefully rotated so that all areas of vaginal tissue are inspected. As the blades are closed, caution is taken to prevent pinching of tissue or the catching of hairs in the blades.

The speculum is inspected for odors and is either discarded or placed in a soaking solution.

Bimanual vaginal examination. The purpose of the bimanual examination is the palpation of the pelvic contents between the examiner's two hands (Figs. 20-11 and 20-12). Examiners vary in their preference of the placement of the dominant, more sensitive hand. The beginning examiner should attempt alternating hands for examinations and then decide on a routine that is most workable.

The client remains in the lithotomy position. The examiner stands between the client's legs. The vaginal examining hand assumes the obstetrical position: index and middle fingers extended and together, thumb abducted, and fourth and little fingers folded on the palm of the hand. The vaginal examining fingers

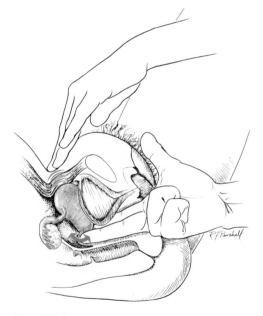

Fig. 20-11
Bimanual palpation of the uterus.

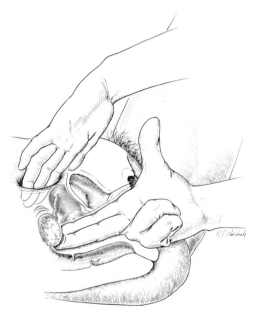

Fig. 20-12
Bimanual palpation of the adnexa.

uterus is not straight but is bent upon itself, the uterus is said to be flexed. Thus, the anteverted or retroverted uterus can be flexed, or bent upon itself, to produce two additional variations of position: anteflexion and retroflexion.

The position of the cervix provides the examiner with clues of the uterine position. A cervix on the anterior wall may indicate an antepositioned or retroflexed uterus; a centrally located cervix probably indicates a uterus in midposition; and a cervix on the posterior vaginal wall implies a uterus in retroposition.

Approximately 85% of uteri are in anteposition; therefore, palpation is first attempted anteriorly. The intravaginal fingers are placed in the anterior fornix. The hand on the abdomen is placed flat on the midline and in a position approximately halfway between the symphysis pubis and the umbilicus. This hand acts as a resistance against which the pelvic organs are palpated by the intravaginal fingers. The fingers in the anterior fornix gently lift the tissues against the hand on the abdomen. If the uterus is in anteposition, it will be palpated between the hands. If the uterus is not palpated anteriorly, the fingers are placed in the posterior fornix and again raised forward toward the hand on the abdomen. If the uterus is in retroversion, only the isth-

mus will be felt between the hands and the corpus may be felt with the backs of the intravaginal fingers. A retroverted uterus is felt best during the rectovaginal examination.

If the uterus is identified as being in anteposition or midposition, an attempt is made to palpate all its anterior and posterior surfaces by maneuvering its position and by "walking up" its surface with the intravaginal fingers. After the uterus is palpated, the adnexal areas are examined. The structures in these areas are of a size, consistency, and position that they may not be specifically palpated. If the examiner has appropriately examined the area and no masses larger than the normal-size ovaries are identified, it is assumed that no masses are present.

Each of the adnexal areas, left and right, is palpated. The index and middle finger of the intravaginal hand are placed in one of the lateral fornices; the hand on the abdomen is placed on the ipsilateral iliac crest; and the hands are brought together and moved in an inferior and medial direction, allowing the tissues lying between the two hands to slip between them (see Fig. 20-12). The hand on the abdomen acts as resistance, and the intravaginal hand palpates the organs between the hands. Frequently, no specific organ is palpated in

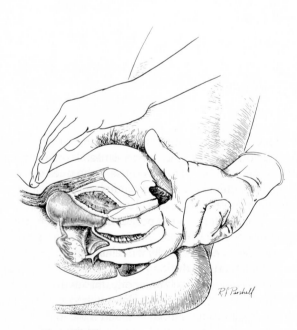

Fig. 20-13
Rectovaginal palpation.

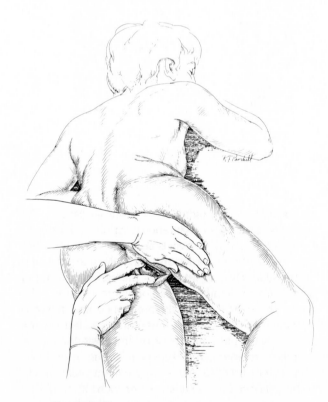

Fig. 20-14
Left lateral position for genital examination.

this maneuver. If normal ovaries are palpated, they are smooth, firm, slightly flattened, ovoid, and no larger than 4 to 6 cm in their largest dimension. Ovaries of prepubertal girls or postmenopausal women are normally smaller than 4 cm in their largest dimension. The ovaries are sensitive to touch but are not tender. They are highly movable and will easily slip between the palpating hands.

Normal fallopian tubes are not palpable. One clue to an ectopic pregnancy is the presence of arterial pulses in the adnexal areas.

Cordlike structures that are sometimes palpable are round ligaments.

Rectovaginal examination. After the completion of the vaginal examination, the hands are withdrawn, and the glove on the internal examining hand is changed to prevent the possible transfer of infection from the vagina to the rectum. The index finger is placed into the vagina, and the middle finger is placed into the rectum. The intravaginal finger remains on the cervix, identifying it, lest it be mistaken for a mass by the intrarectal finger.

The uterine position is confirmed by the rectal examination. If the uterus is retroverted, its body and fundus are now palpated. In addition, the adnexal areas are reassessed. The procedure is the same as that described with the vaginal examination (Fig. 20-13).

The area of the rectovaginal septum and cul-de-sac is palpated. The rectovaginal septum should be palpated as a firm, thin, smooth, pliable structure. The posterior cul-de-sac is a potential space. The normal pelvic organs are palpated through it. Often, abnormal masses and normal ovaries are discovered in the cul-de-sac.

Uterosacral ligaments may be palpable.

The rectal examination is completed (see Chapter 18 on assessment of the anus and rectosigmoid region), and the client is helped to sit up.

Examination of clients who are unable to assume the lithotomy position

The lithotomy position is the optimum one for a pelvic examination. However, it may be difficult for a very ill or debilitated client to assume and maintain a lithotomy position. An alternative position for the female genital examination is a left lateral or Sims' position (Fig. 20-14). The client's buttocks should be close to the edge of the examining table as safety allows. The right leg is positioned on top of or over the left leg and bent and abducted. The examiner stands behind and at the side of the client. All the examination procedures described previously in this chapter can be performed with the client in this position.

PROCEDURES FOR SMEARS AND CULTURES

CERVICAL PAPANICOLAOU SMEAR

The client is in the lithotomy position, and the speculum has been inserted. All materials listed earlier in the chapter are assembled. If a cervical mucous plug is present, it can be removed with a cotton ball held with forceps. There are many variations among laboratories regarding the areas from which cell samples are to be obtained, the mixing of cells from two or more areas, and the fixing of cells. One procedure is described here. However, variations are acceptable, and the practitioner should consult with the cytopathologist reading the smears for locally recommended procedures.

Endocervical smear

Fig. 20-15 illustrates the procedure for an endocervical smear:

1. A sterile applicator is inserted approximately 0.5 cm into the cervical os. It is rotated 360 degrees and left in 10 to 20 seconds to ensure saturation.
2. The endocervical smear is spread on the portion of the slide marked E. The swab is rotated so that all sampled areas are smeared on the slide. The smear should not contain thick areas that would be difficult to visualize microscopically.

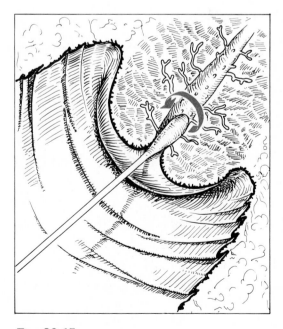

Fig. 20-15
Endocervical smear.

Cervical smear

Fig. 20-16 illustrates the procedure for a cervical smear:

1. The larger humped end of the Ayre spatula is inserted into the cervical os, so that the cervix fits comfortably into the groove created by the two humps. With moderate pressure, the spatula is rotated 360 degrees, scraping the entire cervical surface and the squamocolumnar junction.
2. The material from both sides of the spatula is spread on the portion of the slide marked C.

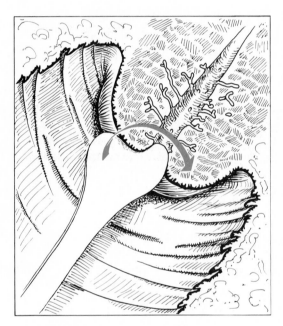

Fig. 20-16
Cervical smear.

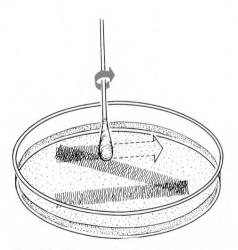

Fig. 20-17
Inoculation of the Thayer-Martin culture.

Vaginal pool smear

1. With the paddle or handle end of the Ayre spatula, the area of the posterior fornix is scraped.
2. The material on the spatula is spread in the area marked V.
3. The slide is fixed immediately by spraying or immersion into a fixative solution.

GONORRHEAL CULTURE

The female client is in the lithotomy position. The male client can be seated when a urethral specimen is to be taken. If a rectal culture is also to be taken, the male client may assume the Sims' position or bend over an examining table with buttocks exposed, feet spread, and toes pointing inward. An oropharyngeal culture is sometimes indicated.

Endocervical culture

1. A specimen from the endocervical canal is obtained with a sterile cotton applicator. The technique is the same as that described for the Pap smear.
2. The Thayer-Martin culture plate is inoculated. With the medium at room temperature, the swab is rolled in a large Z pattern on the culture plate; the swab is simultaneously rotated as it is creating the Z, so that all swab surfaces will be inoculated (Fig. 20-17).
3. The culture plate is incubated within 15 minutes of its inoculation in a warm, anaerobic environment. The culture plate is placed medium side up in a

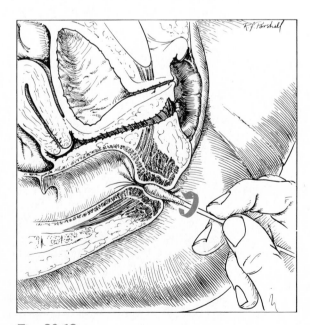

Fig. 20-18
Anal smear.

candle jar, the candle is lit, the cover of the jar is tightly secured, and the jar is left in a warm area until specimens can be placed in an incubator. In some clinic situations, the inoculation is immediately cross-streaked with a sterile wire loop. Usually, however, this is done in the laboratory, not in the examining room.

Anal culture: female or male client

Fig. 20-18 illustrates the procedure for an anal culture:

1. A sterile cotton-tipped applicator is inserted into the anal canal. The applicator is rotated 360 degrees and moved from side to side. It is left in for a total of 10 to 30 seconds to allow for absorption of secretion and organisms. If the swab contains feces, it is discarded and another specimen taken.
2. The culture plate is inoculated and incubated as described previously, using a separate culture plate.

Urethral culture: male client

1. A urethral culture is obtained. A sterile bacteriological loop is inserted into the urethra for 1 to 2 cm, and the mucosa is gently scraped.
2. The culture medium is inoculated and incubated.

Oropharyngeal culture

1. A specimen of secretion from the oropharynx is obtained with a sterile swab.
2. The medium is inoculated and incubated as described for endocervical specimens.

SMEARS FOR VAGINAL INFECTIONS

1. A specimen of vaginal secretions is obtained directly from the vagina or from material in the inferior speculum blade. For *Trichomonas vaginalis,* the secretions are mixed with a drop of normal saline solution on a glass slide. For *Candida albicans,* the secretions are mixed with a drop of 10% potassium hydroxide solution on a slide. For *Hemophilus vaginalis,* the secretions are not mixed with any solution.
2. A cover glass is placed on the slide.
3. The slide is immediately observed under a microscope (Fig. 20-19). If positive for *T. vaginalis,* trichomonads will be seen. These are single-cell flagellates about the size of a white blood cell. If positive for *C. albicans,* mycelia and spores are seen. If positive for *H. vaginalis,* characteristic "cue cells" are seen.

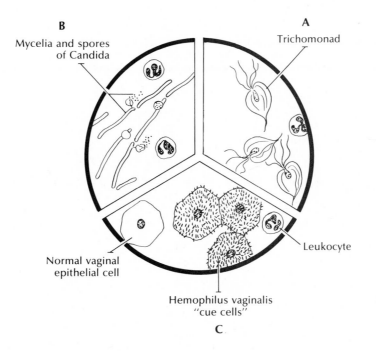

Fig. 20-19
Microscopic appearance of vaginal microorganisms. **A,** Trichomonads. **B,** Mycelia and spores. **C,** Epithelial cells stippled by *Hemophilus vaginalis* bacteria.

SUMMARY

I. External genitalia
  A. Inspection
    1. Hair distribution
    2. Skin
    3. Labia
    4. Clitoris
    5. Urethral orifice
    6. Bartholin's glands
    7. Perineum
  B. Palpation
    1. Skene's glands
    2. Bartholin's glands
II. Muscular integrity
  A. Strength of the bulbocavernosus muscle, that is, general vaginal tone
  B. Observation for bladder, rectal, uterine, and intestinal prolapse
III. Speculum examination
  A. Inspection of the cervix
  B. Inspection of vaginal mucosa
IV. Collection of any needed specimens
V. Bimanual vaginal palpation
  A. Cervix
  B. Uterus
  C. Cul-de-sac area
  D. Adnexal area
    1. Ovaries
    2. Fallopian tubes
VI. Rectovaginal palpation
  A. Uterus
  B. Adnexal area
  C. Cul-de-sac area
  D. Rectovaginal septum
  E. Rectum

BIBLIOGRAPHY

Barr, W.: Clinical gynecology, Edinburgh, 1972, Churchill Livingstone.

Burghardt, E.: Early histological diagnosis of cervical cancer, Philadelphia, 1973, W.B. Saunders Co.

Fogel, C.I., and Woods, N.F.: Health care of women: a nursing perspective, St. Louis, 1981, The C.V. Mosby Co.

Frankfort, E.: Vaginal politics, New York, 1972, Quadrangle Books.

Garrey, M.M., and others: Obstetrics illustrated, ed. 12, Edinburgh, 1974, Churchill Livingstone.

Greenhill, J.P.: Office gynecology, Chicago, 1971, Year Book Medical Publishers, Inc.

Greenhill, J.P., and Friedman, E.A.: Biological principles and modern practices of obstetrics, Philadelphia, 1974, W.B. Saunders Co.

Howkins, J., and Bourne, G.: Shaw's textbook of gynecology, Edinburgh, 1971, Churchill Livingstone.

Hughes, E.C., editor: Obstetric-gynecologic terminology, Philadelphia, 1972, W.B. Saunders Co.

Kistner, R.W.: Gynecology: principles and practice, ed. 2, Chicago, 1971, Year Book Medical Publishers, Inc.

Novak, E.R., Jones, G.S., and Jones, H.W., Jr.: Textbook of gynecology, ed. 9, Baltimore, 1975, Williams & Wilkins.

Tanner, J.M.: Growth of adolescence, ed. 2, Oxford, 1962, Blackwell Scientific Publications.

Tunnadine, P.: The role of genital examination in psychosexual medicine, Clin. Obstet. Gynecol. **7**:283, 1980.

U.S. Department of Health, Education, and Welfare: Criteria and techniques for the diagnosis of gonorrhea, Atlanta, 1974, U.S. Public Health Service.

Willson, R.J., Carrington, E.R., and Ledger, W.J.: Obstetrics and gynecology, ed. 7, St. Louis, 1983, The C.V. Mosby Co.

CHAPTER 21

HEALTH ASSESSMENT OF THE PRENATAL CLIENT

In this chapter the physical changes that occur in normal pregnancy are presented, as well as the adaptation of the health history and the physical examination for the pregnant client. The student practitioner should either know or review the performance of the female genital examination presented in Chapter 20 because it is a component of the assessment of the prenatal client. That assessment procedure will not be repeated here except as the examination or findings may change in pregnancy.

PHYSICAL CHANGES IN PREGNANCY
Hormonal changes

All the physiological changes of pregnancy are directly or indirectly initiated by the hormones produced by the fetal chorionic tissues and placenta. In early pregnancy, the fetal trophoblast produces large amounts of human chorionic gonadotropic hormone (HCG) that provides the basis for biological pregnancy testing. HCG is present in detectable amounts by immunological tests 8 to 10 days after conception.

Large amounts of estrogens and progesterone are produced during pregnancy. Estriol, an estrogen, is produced in large amounts during middle and late pregnancy and is the basis for biological tests of placental and fetal well-being because a well-functioning placenta, a healthy fetus, and intact fetal circulation are prerequisites for the continuous production of this hormone. The estrogens and progesterone maintain the decidua of pregnancy and cause the growth and hyperemia of the uterus, other pelvic organs, and the breasts.

The thyroid gland is enlarged in over 50% of prenatal clients as a result of hyperplasia of glandular tissue, new follicle formation, and increased vascularity. The basal metabolic rate is increased largely because of increased growth and oxygen consumption by the pregnant uterus, the fetus, and the placenta.

Changes in the uterus, cervix, and vagina

Changes in the uterus include the development of the decidua, hypertrophy of muscle cells, increased vascularity, formation of the lower uterine segment, and softening of the cervix. The overall size of the uterus increases five to six times, the weight increases about twenty times, and the capacity increases from approximately 2 to 5,000 ml.

Hormones supply the initial stimulus for uterine hypertrophy. During the first 6 to 8 weeks of pregnancy, the uterus will increase in size whether the pregnancy is uterine or extrauterine. In early pregnancy, the uterus is a pelvic organ and only internally palpable. At about 10 to 12 weeks' gestation, the growing uterus is double its nonpregnant size and reaches the top of the symphysis, where it is palpable abdominally. The uterine fundus is about halfway between the symphysis and umbilicus at about 16 weeks and is at the umbilicus at about 20 to 22 weeks' gestation. After the twentieth week, the average upward growth of the uterus is about 3.75 cm per month. At approximately 36 weeks' gestation, the uterus reaches the xiphisternum. In the last month of pregnancy, the fundus of the uterus may drop several centimeters if the fetal head descends deeply into the pelvis.

The position of the uterus changes during gestation. In early gestation an exaggerated anteflexion is common. As the uterus ascends into the abdomen, a slight dextrorotation develops. The uterus changes from a flattened pear shape to a globular shape in early pregnancy. This globular shape continues until approximately 20 to 24 weeks, when a definite ovoid shape develops and continues until delivery.

In about the sixth to eighth week of gestation, the uterine isthmus becomes softened and easily compressible, to the extent that the cervix, on palpation, seems almost detached from the uterine fundus. At about the eighth week of gestation, the entire uterus softens in consistency.

During pregnancy the uterus contracts intermittently. These painless contractions, called Braxton Hicks contractions, begin in early pregnancy and are first noted by the client and examiner at about 24 weeks' gestation. They can be stimulated by palpation of the uterus. If a contraction occurs during abdominal examination, the examiner should wait until the contraction ends to continue palpation and subsequently palpate more gently.

Three major changes occur in the cervix: (1) hypertrophy of the glands in the cervical canal, (2) softening of the cervix, and (3) bluish discoloration. These changes begin early in pregnancy—at about the sixth week of gestation. Because of changes in the cervical epithelium, commonly a portion of the squamous epithelium is replaced by an outward extension of the columnar epithelium, producing an observable cervical ectropion or eversion of the cervical canal. This condition usually persists throughout pregnancy but disappears soon after.

The increase in pelvic vascularity causes a bluish discoloration of the cervix, vagina, and vulva at about 6 to 8 weeks. In addition, the vaginal mucosa thickens, the connective tissue becomes less dense, and the muscular areas hypertrophy. These changes are reflected in palpatory findings of softening and relaxation. The hypertrophied glands secrete more mucus; the total vaginal discharge is increased and is more acid in reaction.

Changes in the breasts

Breast changes begin at about the eighth week of pregnancy with the enlargement of the breasts. Shortly afterward, the nipples become larger and more erectile, the areolae become more darkly pigmented, and the sebaceous glands (Montgomery's tubercles) in the areolae hypertrophy. Sometimes an irregular secondary areola develops, extending from the primary areola. Hypertrophy of the breasts often causes a slight tenderness. In women with well-developed axillary breast tissue, the hypertrophy may produce symptomatic lumps in the armpits. Colostrum can be expressed from the breasts at about the twenty-fourth week of pregnancy. The colostrum appears clear and yellowish at first, but it becomes cloudy later.

Stretching of the skin on the breasts may produce striae, and increased vascular supply may visibly engorge superficial breast veins.

Abdominal changes

The muscles of the abdominal wall stretch to accommodate the growing uterus, and the umbilicus becomes flattened or protrudes. The rapid stretching of abdominal skin may cause the formation of striae gravidarum, which appear pink or red during pregnancy and become silvery white after delivery. In the third trimester of pregnancy, the rectus abdominis muscles are under considerable stress, and their tone is diminished. A wide, permanent separation of these muscles, called diastasis recti abdominis, may occur. This condition allows abdominal contents to protrude in the midline of the abdomen.

In pregnancy, peristaltic activity is reduced, resulting in decreased bowel sounds. Smooth muscle relaxation or atony contributes to a variety of changes in gastrointestinal function. These include a high incidence of pregnancy-associated nausea and vomiting, heartburn, and constipation. In addition, the increased regional blood flow to the pelvis and venous pressure contribute to hemorrhoids—a source of discomfort in late pregnancy. Nausea and vomiting should not persist beyond the third month, but heartburn, constipation, and hemorrhoids are more characteristic and troublesome in late pregnancy.

Less frequently noted gastrointestinal symptoms include ptyalism or excessive salivation, and pica, a craving for substances of little or no food value. Pica is often an expression of the folkways of some cultural groups and is a common concern when it interferes with good nutrition.

The enlarging uterus displaces the colon laterally, upward, and posteriorly. This changes the anatomical situation of the appendix, and signs of appendicitis during pregnancy are not localized in McBurney's area of the right lower quadrant.

Skin, mucous membrane, and hair changes

The melanocytes in all portions of the skin are extremely active in pregnancy. There is a tendency toward generalized darkening of all skin, especially in skin hyperpigmented in the nonpregnant state. In some women a brownish black pigmented streak may appear in the midline of the abdomen. This line of pigmentation is called the linea nigra. Some women develop a dark, pigmented configuration on the face that has been characteristically called the "mask of pregnancy," or chloasma. Scars and moles may also darken during pregnancy from the influence of melanocyte-stimulating hormone (MSH). Palmar erythema and spider nevi on the face and upper trunk may accompany pregnancy.

Many women observe hypertrophy of gums or epulis resulting from hormones and increased vascularity.

The hair of pregnant women may straighten and change in oiliness. Some women experience hair loss, especially in frontal and parietal areas. Occasionally, increases in facial and abdominal hair resulting from increased androgen and corticotropic hormone are noted.

Cardiovascular system changes

Many changes—too numerous to adequately discuss here—occur in the maternal circulatory system during pregnancy. Several of those changes that alter physical examination findings are mentioned.

Blood volume is increased up to 45% and cardiac output is increased up to 30% in pregnancy as compared to the prepregnant state. Blood volume and cardiac output changes contribute to auscultatory changes common in pregnancy. There is accentuation of the heart sounds, and a low-grade systolic murmur (usually grade II) is often noted.

As pregnancy advances, the heart is displaced upward and laterally. The point of maximum impulse (PMI) is displaced to a point 1 to 1.5 cm lateral to that of the nonpregnant client. The pulse rate increases up to about 10 beats per minute more than prepregnant rates and palpitations may be noticed during pregnancy. The blood pressure is unchanged or sometimes decreased in the second trimester.

There is a progesterone-induced generalized relaxation of the smooth muscle, arteriolar dilatation, and increased capacity of the vascular compartment. Systolic blood pressure remains the same or slightly lower during midpregnancy. There is no change in venous pressure in the upper body, but venous pressure increases in the lower extremities when the woman is supine, sitting, or standing. This predisposes the woman to varicosities of the legs and vulva, to edema, and to faintness from hypotensive effects. Hypotensive tendencies are aggravated by a supine position, and approximately 10% to 20% of gravida develop the supine hypotensive syndrome, manifested by dizziness, diaphoresis, nausea, and hypotension when they are lying on their backs.

Respiratory system changes

During pregnancy, tidal volume increases and there is a slight increase in respiratory rate. Alveolar ventilation is increased and a more efficient exchange of lung gases occurs in the alveoli. Oxygen consumption rises by almost 20%, and plasma carbon dioxide content is decreased.

As the uterus enlarges, the thoracic cage and diaphragm are pushed upward and the thorax is widened at the base. A change in respiration from abdominal to costal may be noted on physical examination. Also, dyspnea is a common complaint, especially in the last trimester, and deep respirations and sighing may be more frequent.

The tissue of the respiratory tract and nasopharynx manifests hyperemia and edema. This may contribute to engorgement of the turbinates, nasal stuffiness, and mouth breathing. Some women note increased nasal and sinus secretion and nosebleeds. Vocal cord edema may cause voice changes. Increased vascularity of the tympanic membranes and blockage of the eustachian tubes may contribute to decreased hearing, a sense of fullness in the ears, or earaches.

Musculoskeletal system changes

The pelvic joints exhibit slight relaxation in pregnancy resulting from some unknown mechanism. This relaxation is maximum from about the seventh month onward. Because the gravid uterus has caused the pregnant client's weight to be thrust forward, the muscles of the spine are used to achieve a temporary new balance. The pregnant woman throws her shoulders back and straightens her head and neck. The lower vertebral column is hyperextended.

The musculoskeletal changes are often reflected in postural and gait changes, lower backache, and fatigue. Often the pregnant woman's gait is described as waddling.

PRENATAL HEALTH HISTORY

The health history is important in pregnancy because information derived from the history assists the practitioner in differentiating the client who is essentially normal and who will be expected to deliver a full-term, healthy baby from the high-risk expectant mother whose pregnancy is likely to negatively affect her own health or who may not deliver a full-term or healthy baby. High-risk clients are given special care in most health care systems. The early identification and referral of the high-risk client enable the special program to achieve maximum benefit for the mother and baby.

The health history for the obstetrical client follows the same basic protocol as that presented for all adults in Chapter 3. However, in prenatal care, the following areas of history-taking should receive special and complete attention:

I. Age
II. Race
III. Marital status
IV. Parity
A four-number code is often used to summarize parity information. The first digit in the code is used to denote the number of full-term births; the second, the number of preterm births; the third, the number

of abortions; and the fourth, the number of living children. Thus, for example, the parity of 2-1-1-3 indicates that the client has three living children, two of whom were delivered after full-term gestation and one of whom was premature, and has had one abortion.

V. Past obstetrical history, including the following for each pregnancy:
   A. Date of delivery
   B. Duration of gestation
   C. Significant problems
   D. Manner in which labor started, specifically whether labor was spontaneous or induced; if induced, the reason for induction should be noted. Abortion should be described as being spontaneous (S) or induced (I).
   E. Length of labor
   F. Complications of labor
   G. Presentation of infant at delivery
   H. Type of delivery—vaginal or cesarean; if cesarean, the reason
   I. Type of anesthesia used at delivery
   J. Condition of infant(s) at birth and birth weight
   K. Postpartum problems, especially infections, hemorrhage, or thrombophlebitis
   L. Problems of the infant, especially jaundice, respiratory distress, infection, or congenital anomalies
   M. Type of infant feeding
   N. Current health of child

VI. Present obstetrical history
   A. Last normal menstrual period (LNMP)
      An important task during the prenatal history is the estimation of the expected date of confinement (EDC). Because the exact date of conception is unknown for the majority of prenatal clients, the EDC is calculated according to the first day of the last normal menstrual period (LNMP). The EDC is determined by counting backwards 3 calendar months from the LNMP and adding 7 days (Nägele's rule). The year, of course, may change. For example, if the LNMP were 10-15-84, the EDC would be 7-22-85. If the client has a history of irregular menses, the EDC would be more accurately estimated by physical examination than by using the LNMP. Critical features that aid in determination or validation of the EDC are the date of quickening, when the mother first notices fetal movement (at about 18 weeks), and the time at which the fetal heart tones can be auscultated (at about 20 weeks' gestation). Because of the variation that characterizes these events, ultrasonic measurement of fetal size and growth is being used more frequently to "date" pregnancy and assess fetal growth, along with measurement of the progressive enlargement of the uterus.
   B. Symptoms of pregnancy
   C. Feelings about pregnancy, especially determination if pregnancy was planned or unplanned

   D. Bleeding since last normal menstrual period
   E. Date when fetal movements were first felt
   F. Fetal exposure to infections, x-ray, and drugs

VII. Current and past medical and gynecological history
   A. Urinary and venereal infections
   B. Bacterial and viral infections during pregnancy
   C. Diabetes
   D. Hypertension
   E. Heart disease
   F. Endocrine disorders
   G. Anemia
   H. Genital tract history, especially:
      1. Anomaly
      2. Cervical incompetence
      3. Myomas
      4. Contracted pelvis
      5. Ovarian mass
      6. Vaginal infections
      7. Surgery
      8. Abnormal Pap test results
      9. Use of hormones (for example, birth control pills)
      10. Menstrual history and functioning
      11. Endometriosis
   I. Medication history
   J. Habitual use of alcohol, tobacco, or mood-altering drugs

VIII. Family history
   Features of the family history that have special significance in pregnancy include diabetes, renal or hematological disorders, hypertension, multiple pregnancy, and congenital defects or retardation. It is important to learn if the primigravida's mother had preeclampsia or high blood pressure with her pregnancies, especially if she convulsed. A woman with a family history of hypertension during pregnancy is three times more likely to develop hypertension with her pregnancy (24% incidence) than most other primigravida (7% to 8% incidence of preeclampsia, or pregnancy-induced hypertension).

IX. Emotional, psychological, and developmental status
   Pregnancy is an important developmental event in the life of a woman. Development involves the achievement-relevant tasks, and the developmental tasks of pregnancy are incorporation, differentiation, and, eventually, separation from the fetus. These tasks roughly coincide with the three trimesters of pregnancy.
   During the first trimester, the gravida is involved with the process of accepting the fetus as a fact and a part of her body. Most women initially experience some ambivalence about their pregnancy with a resultant increase in anxiety. Many body changes occur that cause increased somatic awareness and inward focus. Relationships with key persons, especially the baby's father and the gravida's mother, become especially important. Unresolved feelings and conflicts undergo reexamination. Feelings of dependency and vulnerability occur and can be additional causes of anxiety.

In the second trimester, the fetus develops a separate identity. The gravida has had some time to become accustomed to her bodily changes and often feels better because the nausea has ceased. The baby's movements are an important event, confirming the presence of the fetus and reminding the woman of the independence of the fetal movements from her control. She begins to daydream about the baby and their future. Worries about the possibility of producing an abnormal baby are common.

In the last trimester of pregnancy, the gravida prepares her separation from the fetus and entrance into a new relationship with the newborn. This time is occupied with preparatory activities such as attending parents' classes and buying clothing and equipment for the newborn. Concerns about labor and delivery and physical discomforts of late pregnancy contribute to the woman's readiness for separation from the fetus and movement to the tasks of parenthood.

X. Social, economic, and cultural status

Because pregnancy and birth are important events in the development of any family and because the quality of the family has impact on the health of the infant, an assessment of the circumstances relating to the pregnancy and the family environment is essential. The following are several important areas of exploration in the social history.

A. Client's desire for and feelings about this pregnancy

B. Feelings of significant others regarding this pregnancy

C. Client's personal and culturally derived health beliefs about pregnancy

D. Client's knowledge regarding pregnancy and parenting

E. Amount of support and assistance provided by family and significant others

F. Economic burdens imposed on client and/or family by pregnancy

G. Condition of the family's physical and emotional environment

PRENATAL RISK FACTORS

The following is a list of factors that have been associated with increased morbidity and mortality of mothers and infants. Special note should be taken of these factors during the health history interview and its recording:

Maternal characteristics
Age: less than 18 or over 35
Poverty
Unmarried
Family disorganization
Conflict about pregnancy
Height less than 5 feet
20% overweight or underweight
Inadequate diet
Nonwhite race

Reproductive history
More than one previous abortion
Gravidity over 8
Stillbirth
Neonatal death
Infant less than 2,500 g
Infant over 4,000 g
Infant with isoimmunization or ABO incompatibility
Infant with major congenital or perinatal disease
Preeclampsia or eclampsia
Antepartal hemorrhage
Cesarean section
Difficult midforceps delivery
Genital tract anomaly
Myomas
Ovarian masses

Medical problems
Hypertension
Renal disease
Diabetes mellitus
Heart disease
Sickle cell disease
Anemia
Pulmonary disease
Endocrine disorder

Present pregnancy
Bleeding after 20 weeks' gestation
Premature rupture of membranes
Anemia
No prenatal care
Preeclampsia or eclampsia
Hydramnios
Multiple pregnancy
Low or excessive weight gain
Hypertension (blood pressure greater than 140/90, a 30 mm Hg systolic increase, or a 15 mm Hg diastolic increase)
Abnormal fasting blood sugar
Rh-negative sensitized
Exposure to teratogens
Viral infections
Syphilis
Bacterial infections
Protozoal infections
Postmaturity
Abnormal presentation

PHYSICAL ASSESSMENT DURING PREGNANCY
General physical examination

A complete physical examination should be made on the first prenatal visit because (1) the examination may reveal problems that need special or immediate attention, and (2) initial data serve as a baseline against which changes later in pregnancy can be compared. The initial, general physical examination of the prenatal client is the same as that for other clients, except for special emphasis on the diagnosis of pregnancy, the assessment of the adequacy of the pelvis, and the assessment of the growth and well-being of the fetus.

A number of nonreproductive system signs may be normally altered in pregnancy. Such alterations of physical findings include:

Respiratory system
Change in breathing from abdominal to costal
Shortening and widening at the base of the thoracic cage
Elevation of the diaphragm
Increase in respiratory rate

Cardiovascular system
Displacement of the point of maximum impulse laterally 1 to 1.5 cm
Grade II systolic murmur
Increase in pulse rate
Slight fall in blood pressure in the second trimester

Musculoskeletal system
Slight instability of pelvis
Alteration of standing posture and gait to accommodate for gravid uterus

Abdominal region
Contour changes because of gravid uterus
Striae gravidarum
Decrease in muscle tone
Linea nigra
Reduced peristaltic activity

Skin and mucous membranes
Chloasma
Linea nigra
Hyperpigmentation of skin and bony prominences
Palmar erythema
Spider nevi on face and upper trunk
Striae gravidarum on breasts and abdomen
Gum hypertrophy

Breasts
Enlargement
Large, erect nipples
Darkening of areolar pigment
Development of a secondary areola
Hypertrophy of sebaceous glands in the areola
Formation of colostrum
Tenderness on palpation
Striae gravidarum
Engorgement of superficial veins

Other alterations
Straightening of hair
Loss of hair over frontal and parietal regions
Enlarged thyroid

Diagnosis of pregnancy

The diagnosis of pregnancy is made from the history of subjective symptoms noticed by the woman together with objective signs noted by the examiner. In addition, laboratory tests are especially helpful in confirming early pregnancy.

Traditionally, the signs and symptoms of pregnancy have been categorized as presumptive symptoms, probable signs, and positive signs.

Presumptive symptoms are those concerns that the prenatal client identifies in the present illness and chief complaint portions of the history and several additional general physical signs. They include the subjective data that may have led the client to seek confirmation of pregnancy. Presumptive symptoms include (1) absence of menses 10 or more days after the expected date of onset, (2) morning nausea or appetite change, (3) frequent urination, (4) soreness or a tingling sensation in the breasts, (5) Braxton Hicks contractions, (6) quickening, (7) abdominal enlargement, and (8) bluish discoloration of the vagina.

The following are probable signs of pregnancy: (1) progressive enlargement of the uterus, (2) softening of the uterine isthmus (Hegar's sign), (3) asymmetrical, soft enlargement of one uterine cornu (Piskacek's sign), (4) bluish or cyanotic color of the cervix and upper vagina (Chadwick's sign), (5) softening of the cervix (Goodell's sign), (6) internal ballottement, (7) palpation of fetal parts, and (8) positive test results for HCG in urine or serum. These signs are termed "probable" because clinical conditions other than pregnancy can cause any of these signs. However, if they occur together, a strong case can be made for the presence of a pregnancy.

In pregnancy, uterine enlargement can be noted on pelvic examination about 6 to 8 weeks after the last normal menses. The uterus first enlarges in the pelvis, and by 12 weeks' gestation it can be palpated abdominally just above the symphysis pubis. In addition to enlarging, the uterus becomes globular and then ovoid in shape.

The uterus softens in pregnancy because of increased vascularity. The isthmus of the uterus is the first part to soften. At about 6 to 8 weeks' gestation, the softened isthmus produces a dramatic palpatory finding. On palpation, the enlarged, globular uterus feels almost detached from the still not completely softened cervix because the isthmus feels so indistinct (Fig. 21-1). This phenomenon is called Hegar's sign. By 7 or 8 weeks the cervix and uterus can be easily flexed at their junction (McDonald's sign).

Cyanosis of the cervix is noted on speculum examination as early as 6 to 8 weeks' gestation and results from the increased vascularity in the area.

Often uterine enlargement does not progress symmetrically. Rather, the area of placental development enlarges more rapidly. This produces a palpatory asymmetrical enlargement of one uterine cornu, called Piskacek's sign (Fig. 21-2).

Immunological tests for the presence of HCG are commonly used to assist in the diagnosis of pregnancy.

The commonly used immunological tests are the hemagglutination inhibition test and the latex agglutination test. These tests depend on an antigen-antibody reaction between HCG and an antiserum obtained from rabbits immunized against this antigen. These tests are available for use by both health professionals and women themselves and are very sensitive. Most commercial tests use standardized anti-HCG rabbit serum and dead cells or standardized latex particles coated with HCG. Anti-HCG serum is mixed first with a sample of the client's urine, then HCG-coated red blood cells or particles are added. The lack of agglutination is a positive test because urine containing HCG has neutralized the HCG antibodies. If the urine sample contains no HCG, agglutination would occur, indicating a negative test for pregnancy.

Pregnancy tests based on the presence of HCG in the urine can be reliably made in the period from 2 weeks after the first missed menses through 16 weeks' gestation. During this period of time, the production of HCG is at its peak.

The positive signs of pregnancy are those that prove the presence of a fetus. These signs are (1) documentation of a fetal heartbeat by auscultation, electrocardiogram, or Doppler instrument; (2) palpation of active fetal movements; and (3) the radiological or ultrasonographical demonstration of fetal parts. Ultrasonographical techniques can demonstrate the presence of a gestational sac as early as the sixth week of gestation. Doppler instruments can detect a fetal heartbeat as early as 10 to 12 weeks.

Currently, clinical diagnosis of pregnancy is more

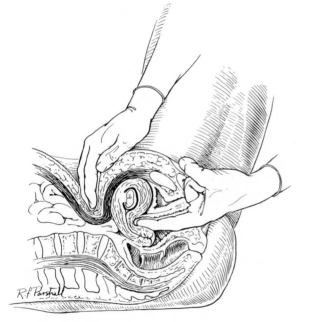

Fig. 21-1
Hegar's sign, softening of the lower uterine segment.

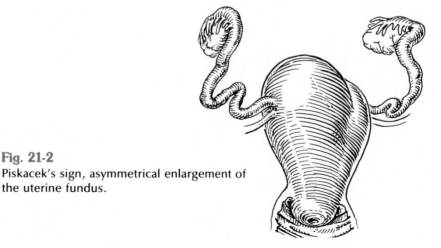

Fig. 21-2
Piskacek's sign, asymmetrical enlargement of the uterine fundus.

Table 21-1
The physical signs of pregnancy and corresponding stage of fetal development

Sign	Approximate gestation (weeks since last menses)		Fetal development
Amenorrhea.	2	0-4	Fertilization occurs. Blastocyst implants. Placental circulation established. Organogenesis initiated. Development of nervous system and vital organs initiated. Anatomical structures and systems are in rudimentary form. Size: 0.25 inch by fourth week.
Softening of cervix (Goodell's sign).	4-6		
Softening of cervicouterine junction (Ladin's sign).	5-6	5-8	All major organs in rudimentary form.
Gestational sac may be noted by ultrasonography.	6		Fingers are present.
Compressibility of the lower uterine segment (Hegar's sign).	6-8		Ears and eyes are formed. Heart complete and functioning.
Dilatation of breast veins.			Development of muscles is initiated.
Pulsation of uterine arteries in lateral fornices (Oslander's sign).			Size: 1.25 inch by eighth week.
Flexing of fundus of cervix (McDonald's sign).	7-8		
Asymmetrical softening and enlarging of uterus (Piskacek's sign).			
Uterus changes from pear to globular shape.			
Bluish coloration of the vagina and cervix (Chadwick's sign).	8-12	9-12	Organs forming and growing. Swallowing and sucking reflexes present.
Detection of fetal heart beats with a Doppler instrument.	10-12		Body movements increase. Size: 3 inches, 0.5 ounce by twelfth week.
Uterus palpable just above symphysis pubis.	12	13-16	Circulatory system is established.
Ballottement of fetus possible by abdominal and vaginal examination.	16		Size: 6 inches, 4 ounces by sixteenth week.
Uterus palpable halfway between symphysis and umbilicus.			
Fetal movements noted by mother (quickening).	16-20	17-20	Rapid growth.
Pigment changes may occur.			Size: 8 inches, 8 ounces by twentieth week.
Uterine fundus at lower border of umbilicus.	20	21-24	Meconium present in intestines.
Fetal heart beat auscultated with fetoscope.			Size: 11 inches, 1-1.5 pounds by twenty-fourth week.
Fetus palpable.	24		
Mother begins to notice Braxton Hicks contractions.	24-26	25-28	Nervous system can control breathing and temperature.
Uterus changes from globular to ovoid shape.			Size: 12 inches, 2-3 pounds by twenty-eighth week.
Fetus easily palpable, very mobile, and may be found in any lie, presentation, or position.	28	29-32	Fat deposits under skin. Size: 13 inches, 3-5 pounds by thirty-second week.
Uterus is approximately half the distance from the umbilicus to the xiphoid.			
Fetus usually lies longitudinally with a vertex presentation.	32	33-36	Primitive reflexes are present. Size: 14 inches, 5-6 pounds by thirty-sixth week.
Uterine fundus is approximately two thirds the distance between the umbilicus and the xiphoid.			
Uterine fundus is just below the xiphoid.	34		
Vertex presentation may engage in the pelvis.	36-40	37-40	Less active because of crowding. Size: 19-21 inches, 6-8 pounds by fortieth week.

dependent on the probable signs than the presumptive symptoms and positive signs of pregnancy. However, with new developments in immunological blood testing, radioimmunoassay, and more available ultrasonographical technology, the methods of pregnancy diagnosis may change.

The radioimmunoassay test that is specific for the B subunit of the HCG molecule at very low concentrations is also considered a positive test for pregnancy. With this test there is no cross-reaction with luteinizing hormone as with other immunological tests and thus it is more accurate for HCG itself.

The timetable for physical signs of pregnancy is presented in Table 21-1. Table 21-1 also includes an outline of fetal development during pregnancy. During prenatal assessments, both the mother and the developing fetus are being examined.

PRENATAL EXAMINATIONS

After the initial assessment, the prenatal client is examined at regular intervals. Reexamination schedules vary for clients, but the schedule includes examination approximately every 3 to 4 weeks during the first 28 weeks of pregnancy and every 1 to 2 weeks during the final 12 weeks.

At each prenatal revisit, the following assessments are usually made:

1. Weight
2. Blood pressure
3. Urine screening for glucose and protein
4. Determination of the presence of edema
5. Abdominal assessment
   a. Determination of fundal height
   b. Determination of fetal presentation and position
   c. Measurement of fetal heart rate

Weight gain

Optimum weight gain during pregnancy based on the lowest rate of complications and low birth weight infants is 24 to 27.5 pounds (a wider range is 20 to 30 pounds). High prepregnancy weight correlates significantly with an increased risk of preeclampsia. Women with low prepregnancy weight who gain little weight during pregnancy are more likely to have low birth weight babies (that is, babies weighing 2,500 g or less). Sudden weight gain, especially in the third trimester, usually means fluid retention and is evaluated in conjunction with maternal blood pressure. Apart from this transient cause of weight gain, many women tend to add to their body fat stores during pregnancy, and this weight gain may not be entirely lost after delivery. The gain in weight should occur gradually, averaging 1½ to 2 pounds per month during the first 24 weeks and ½ to 1 pound a week during the remainder of pregnancy.

Blood pressure

Mean systolic blood pressure and mean diastolic blood pressure are essentially unchanged during pregnancy except, as indicated, for a mild and transient decrease during the middle trimester. Hypertension, however, contributes significantly to prenatal morbidity and mortality, and pregnancy-induced hypertension is a disease peculiar to pregnancy. This disorder typically develops after the twenty-fourth week of pregnancy and is characterized by the following:

1. A systolic blood pressure of at least 140 mm Hg or a rise of 30 mm Hg or more above the usual level in two readings 6 hours apart
2. A diastolic pressure of 90 mm Hg or more or a rise of 15 mm Hg above the usual level in two readings 6 hours apart
3. Proteinuria
4. Edema of the face or hands

Clinicians have described what has come to be known as the Roll Over Test to detect gravidas who are likely to develop hypertension in late pregnancy. Such women have an increased vascular reactivity and have lost their resistance to vasopressor substances that characterize normal pregnancy. This sensitivity or vascular reactivity is exhibited by an increase of 20 mm Hg in diastolic pressure when a woman of 28 to 32 weeks' gestation turns from her side to her back. This increase is termed a positive Roll Over Test, and such a woman requires closer monitoring of her blood pressure during the latter portion of her pregnancy because she is much more likely to develop the classical signs and symptoms of preeclampsia.

Assessment of edema and the extremities

Ankle swelling and edema of the lower extremities occur in two thirds of women in late pregnancy. Women notice this swelling later in the day after standing for a period of time. Sodium and water retention caused by steroid hormones, an increased hydrophilic property of intracellular connective tissue, and increased venous pressure in the lower extremities during pregnancy contribute to this edema. Assessment includes palpation of the ankles and pretibial areas to determine the extent of the edema and observation for hand, face, or generalized edema. Generalized edema may be manifested by pitting in the sacral area or by the appearance of a depression on the gravid abdomen from the rim of the fetoscope after it has been pressed against the abdomen to auscultate the fetal heart rate.

In addition to assessment for edema formation, examination of the legs includes inspection for varicose veins and dorsiflexion of the foot with the legs extended to check for Homans' sign and thrombophlebitis. In the presence of an elevated or a borderline elevated blood pressure, deep tendon reflexes are assessed. Hyperreflexia and clonus, combined with other signs, can indicate preeclampsia.

Leg cramps during pregnancy may accompany extension of the foot and sudden shortening of leg muscles. This may be caused by an elevation of serum phosphorus with a diet that includes a large quantity of milk.

A variety of discomforts and sensations in the legs are attributed to compression of nerves from the pressure of the enlarging uterus. This includes numbness in the lateral femoral area, resulting from compression of that nerve beneath the inguinal ligament. Medial thigh sensation may result from the compression of the obturator nerve against the side walls of the pelvis. Periodic numbness of the fingers is reported to occur in at least 5% of gravidas. This is apparently caused by a brachial plexus traction syndrome from drooping shoulders. This drooping is associated with the increased weight of the breasts as pregnancy advances. Movement of fingers may be impaired by compression of the median nerve in the arm and hand caused by physiological changes in fascia, tendons, and connective tissue during pregnancy. This is known as carpal tunnel syndrome and is characterized by a paroxysm of pain, numbness, tingling, or burning in the sides of the hands and fingers—particularly the thumb, second, and third fingers and the side of the fifth finger.

Abdominal examination

As pregnancy progresses, the uterus enlarges steadily. The height of the fundus serves as a rough guide to fetal gestation and overall fetal growth. Fig. 21-3 displays the expected fundal height at various gestational ages. At the twelfth week of pregnancy, the fundus is palpable just above the symphysis. At 16 weeks, the fundus is approximately halfway between the symphysis and umbilicus. At the twentieth gestational week, the fundus usually reaches the lower border of the umbilicus. After the twentieth week, the uterus increases in height at approximately 3.75 cm per month or around 1 cm per week until weeks 34 to 36, when the fundus almost reaches the xiphoid. Then, in approximately 65% of gravidas, the fetal head drops further into the pelvis with lightening. If this occurs, the fundal measurement at 36 weeks may be greater than that later in pregnancy.

Unless the fetal head drops into the pelvis, the fundal height between weeks 37 and 40 will stay the same. During this period the fetus is increasing in size, but the amount of amniotic fluid decreases.

The routine procedure for abdominal reevaluation during pregnancy is (1) inspection, (2) palpation and measurement, and (3) auscultation.

In addition to the observations the practitioner makes when observing the abdomen (for example, skin and scars), for the pregnant client, the examiner also observes the size and configuration of the enlarging uterus.

Normally, the uterine size should relate to the estimated gestational age. Any discrepancy between observed size and estimated gestational age should be further explored. A uterus larger than expected may indicate incorrect gestational age estimation or multiple pregnancy; a smaller uterus may indicate a poorly growing fetus or gestational miscalculation.

Abdominal assessment

Observation of the abdomen may provide the first clues to the presentation and position of the fetus. Asymmetrical appearance or distention in width versus longitudinal enlargement may suggest a transverse or oblique lie of the fetus that can be verified by palpation. After about week 28 fetal movements may be seen.

The uterus is palpated to determine the top, or height, of the fundus. The examiner stands at the right side of the supine client. The ulnar surface of the examiner's left hand is placed approximately 3 to 4 cm above where the fundal apex is expected to be located in the midline of the abdomen. This hand palpates downward in small progressive steps until the examiner can differentiate between the softness of the abdomen generally and the firm, round fundal edge (Fig. 21-4). The use of only the palmar surface of the middle finger of the examining hand can assist in locating the precise level of fundal height.

When the fundal edge is located, its distance from the symphysis is estimated. When the fundus is below the umbilicus, the measurement in centimeters above the symphysis or below the umbilicus can be estimated or measured with a tape.

When the fundus is above the umbilicus, measurement with a measuring tape is recommended. The examiner places the zero point of the tape at the top of the symphysis and measures the distance to the top of the fundus (Fig. 21-5). Various methods exist for estimating fundal height. Methods that avoid the measurement of the fundal curve and abdominal adipose tissue are more accurate estimations of actual fundal growth. The practitioner should choose one method and use it consistently. This measurement is approximate, and estimates of fundal height measurement may vary 1 to 2 cm among examiners. However, measurement is more reliable than visual estimation beyond 20 weeks and, if it is practiced consistently by one examiner, should provide an excellent picture of fetal growth with each visit.

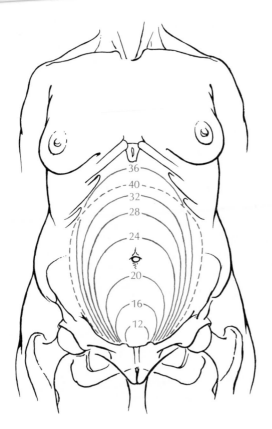

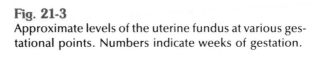

Fig. 21-3
Approximate levels of the uterine fundus at various gestational points. Numbers indicate weeks of gestation.

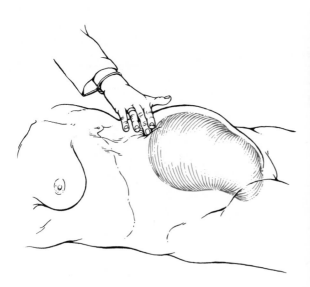

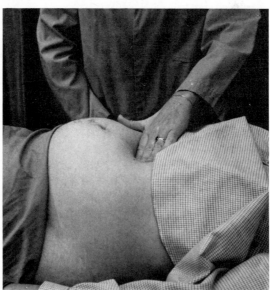

Fig. 21-4
Palpation to determine the height of the uterine fundus.

The examiner next palpates the abdomen to determine fetal lie, presentation, position, attitude, and size.

The lie is the relationship of the long axis of the fetus to the long axis of the uterus. The lie can be longitudinal, oblique, or transverse (Fig. 21-6).

The presentation of the fetus is that fetal part that is most dependent. The presentation can be vertex, brow, face, shoulder, or breech (Fig. 21-7).

The position is the relationship of a specified part of the fetal presentation, the denominator, to a particular part of the maternal pelvis (Fig. 21-8). The denomina-

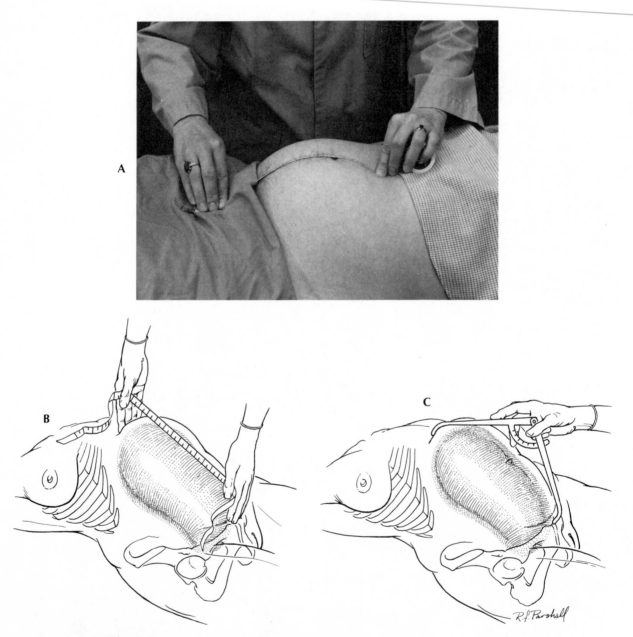

Fig. 21-5
Various methods of measuring the height of the fundus. **A,** Measurement accounting for some of the fundal curve. **B,** Measurement avoiding the fundal curve. **C,** Measurement using obstetrical calipers. This method also avoids measuring the fundal curve.

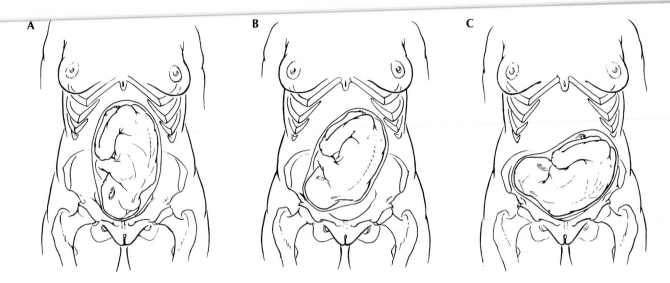

Fig. 21-6
Examples of fetal lie. **A,** Longitudinal lie. **B,** Oblique lie. **C,** Transverse lie.

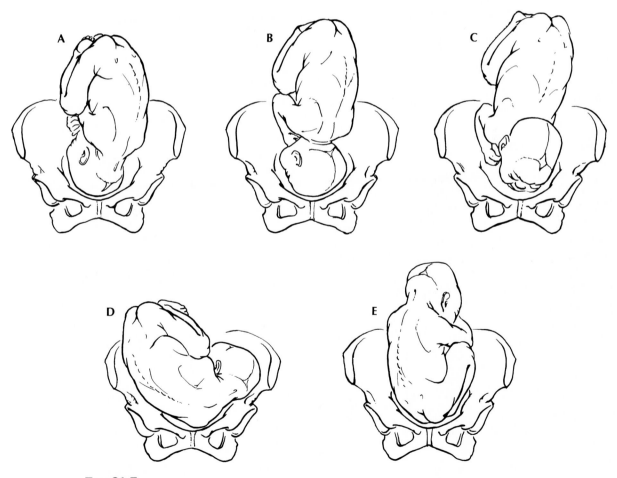

Fig. 21-7
Examples of fetal presentation. **A,** Vertex. **B,** Brow. **C,** Face. **D,** Shoulder. **E,** Breech.

of the top of the fundus has already been described. Usually the buttocks of the fetus will be in the fundus and felt as a soft, irregular, and slightly movable mass. The lower limbs are felt adjacent to the buttocks. If the head is in the fundus, it is felt as smooth, round, hard, and ballottable. The groove of the neck is felt between the trunk and the upper limbs. The head is freely movable in contrast to the buttocks, which can only move sideways and with the trunk.

Lateral palpation

For Leopold's second maneuver (Fig. 21-12), the examiner, while still facing the client's head, moves both hands to either side of the uterus to determine which side the fetal back is on. The examiner supports the fetus with one hand while the other hand palpates the fetus. The examiner then reverses the procedure to palpate each side of the uterus. The fetal back is felt as a continuous, smooth, firm object, whereas the fetal

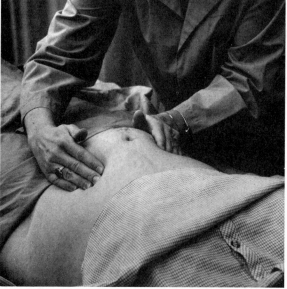

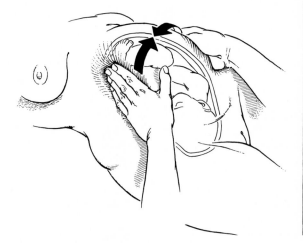

Fig. 21-12
Palpation of lateral uterine fundus to determine the position of the back and extremities of the fetus.

Fig. 21-13
Pawlik palpation to determine fetal presenting part.

limbs, or small parts, are felt as small, irregular, sometimes moving objects. On each side, the examiner palpates the flank to the midline, making special note of the edge of the fetal back as a landmark in determining the fetal position.

Pawlik palpation

This procedure is done with the right hand only to determine what fetal part lies over the pelvic inlet. The right hand is placed over the symphysis so that the fingers are on the left side of the uterus and the thumb is on the right side (Fig. 21-13). The hand should be approximately around the fetal presenting part, usually the head. The presenting part is gently palpated to determine its form and consistency and grasped and gently moved sideways to determine its movability. This palpation confirms impressions about the presenting part and determines if the presenting part (if the fetal head) might be engaged. If the fetal head is movable above the symphysis, it is not engaged. If the head is not movable, it may be engaged. Engagement can only be confirmed by pelvic examination to determine if the biparietal diameter of the fetal head is level with the ischial spines.

Deep pelvic palpation

The examiner changes position (Fig. 21-14). The examiner remains on the right side of the client but is turned so that she or he is facing the woman's feet. A hand is placed on each side of the uterus near the pelvic brim. The client is asked to take a deep breath and to exhale slowly. As she does, the examining fin-

gers are allowed to sink deeply above the pubic bones to palpate the presenting part and to determine which side the cephalic prominence is on. If the presenting part is the head, the location of the cephalic prominence, that is, the forehead, assists in determining the fetus' position and attitude. If the head is flexed, the occiput lies deeper in the pelvis, is flatter, and is less defined than the forehead, which is more prominent and on the same side as the small parts. If the head is not well flexed, the cephalic and occipital prominences will be palpated at the same level, and the occipital portion may feel more prominent and is on the same side as the back.

Throughout these maneuvers the examiner assesses the congruence of the size of the fetus with the gestational age.

In summary to this section on abdominal assessment, a series of questions the examiner mentally asks about each client are listed with an indication of the procedures that assist in answering the questions.

Question	Methods of obtaining evidence to answer the question
What is the fetal lie?	Abdominal inspection Lateral abdominal palpation
What is the fetal presentation?	Fundal palpation Pawlik palpation Deep pelvic palpation
What is the fetal position?	Lateral palpation Deep pelvic palpation
What is the fetal attitude?	Deep pelvic palpation
Is the fetal growth congruent with gestational age?	Fundal height measurement All of Leopold's maneuvers

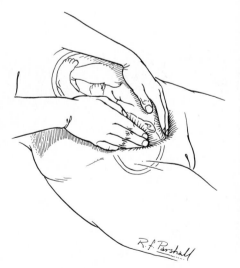
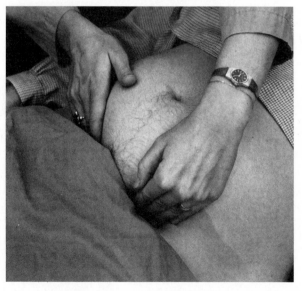

Fig. 21-14
Deep pelvic palpation to determine the attitude and descent of the fetus.

Auscultation

The fetal heart rate is an indicator of the health status of the fetus and is monitored throughout pregnancy. Auscultation of the fetal heart rate is accomplished by use of a special stethoscope, or fetoscope, or a Doppler instrument. With the Doppler instrument, the fetal heart rate can be monitored after about 10 weeks' gestation. Using a fetoscope, the examiner can first hear the fetal heart rate between the sixteenth and twentieth weeks of gestation.

The use of the fetoscope is demonstrated in Fig. 21-15. The fetal heart rate is rapid and soft. The use of a fetoscope avoids noises produced by fingers on the stethoscope and makes use of the benefits of both air and bone conduction. The bell of an ordinary stethoscope can be used but is less effective than a fetoscope in listening to fetal heartbeats, especially around 20 weeks.

The fetal heart rate is normally between 120 and 160 beats per minute, and the heartbeats resemble a watch tick heard through a pillow. They are best heard through the fetal back. When the fetus is large enough for its position to be determined, the bell of the fetoscope or the Doppler head is placed at the back of the fetal thorax. When the fetus is under 20 weeks' gestation, the heart rate is often best heard at the midline, just above the pubic hairline.

The fetal heart rate is counted for at least 15 seconds and is recorded in number of beats per minute. The fetal heart rate is normally much faster than the maternal heart rate and thus can usually be well differentiated from it. Moreover, the fetal and maternal heart rates are not synchronous, and the maternal rate can be differentiated by palpating the mother's pulse while auscultating the abdomen.

Blood rushing through the placenta can be heard as a uterine souffle. The uterine souffle is a soft, blowing sound that is synchronous with the maternal pulse. The intensity of the souffle has been interpreted as an indicator of uterine blood flow and placental function. A loud uterine souffle has been associated with high urinary estriol levels and soft or absent souffle with lower estriol levels. Thus, a soft or absent uterine souffle may indicate poor uterine blood flow and placental function, particularly in late pregnancy.

Examination of the bony pelvis

The purpose of the examination of the bony pelvis is to determine if the pelvic cavity is of adequate size to allow for the passage of a full-term infant. This exam-

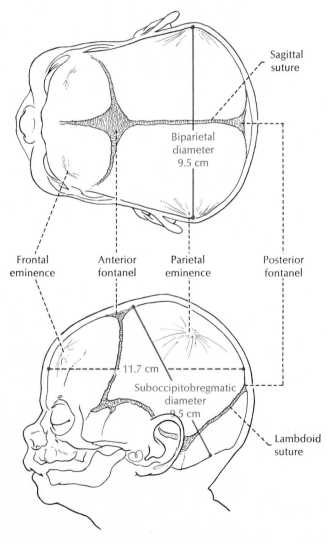

Fig. 21-16
Various diameters of the fetal head at term.

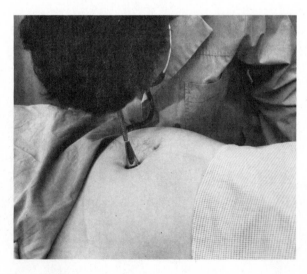

Fig. 21-15
Use of the fetoscope to auscultate the fetal heartbeat.

ination is performed on the initial prenatal evaluation and need not be repeated if the pelvis is of adequate size. However, if findings indicate that the pelvis is of borderline adequacy or if the examination could not be done on the initial visit because of client tenseness and subsequent muscular contraction, the examination should be repeated between 32 to 36 weeks' gestation. In the third trimester of pregnancy, there is a relaxation of pelvic joints and ligaments, and the client is more accustomed to examination. Thus, the examination of the bony pelvis can be more thoroughly and accurately accomplished then.

The examination of the bony pelvis is done not so much to diagnose the type of pelvis but to determine its configuration and size. Because the examiner does not have direct access to the bony structures and because the bones are covered with variable amounts of soft tissue, estimates are approximate. Precise bony pelvis measurements can be determined using roentgenogram examination. However, roentgenogram examinations are not needed or indicated for the vast majority of prenatal clients.

The assessment of the bony pelvis needs to be put in the perspective of the capacity needed to accommodate a full-term fetus. When the head of a full-term fetus is well flexed, the two largest presenting diameters are the biparietal and the suboccipitobregmatic, each measuring approximately 9.5 cm (Fig. 21-16).

The pelvis consists of four bones: the two innominate bones, the sacrum, and the coccyx. Each innominate bone consists of three bones that fuse after puberty. These three bones are the ilium, the ischium, and the os pubis (Fig. 21-17). The innominate bones form the anterior and lateral portions of the pelvis.

The sacrum and coccyx form the posterior portion of the pelvis. The sacrum is composed of five fused vertebrae. Its upper anterior portion is termed the sacral promontory, which forms the posterior margin of the pelvic brim. The coccyx is composed of three to five fused vertebrae and articulates with the sacrum.

The pelvis is divided by the brim into two parts: the false pelvis and the true pelvis. The false pelvis is that part above the brim and is of no obstetrical interest.

The true pelvis is that portion of the pelvis that includes the brim and the area below. The true pelvis is divided into three parts: the inlet or brim, the midpelvis or cavity, and the outlet. The inlet is formed anteriorly by the upper margins of the pubic bones, laterally by the iliopectineal lines, and posteriorly by the anterior upper margin of the sacrum, the sacral promontory. The cavity is formed anteriorly by the posterior aspect of the symphysis pubis, laterally by the inner surfaces of the ischial and iliac bones, and posteriorly by the anterior surface of the sacrum. The outlet is diamond-shaped and is formed anteriorly by the inferior rami of the pubic and ischial bones, laterally by the ischial tuberosities, and posteriorly by the inferior edge of the sacrum, if the coccyx is movable.

Each of the pelvic portions can be imagined as a series of planes: the plane of the brim, or pelvic inlet;

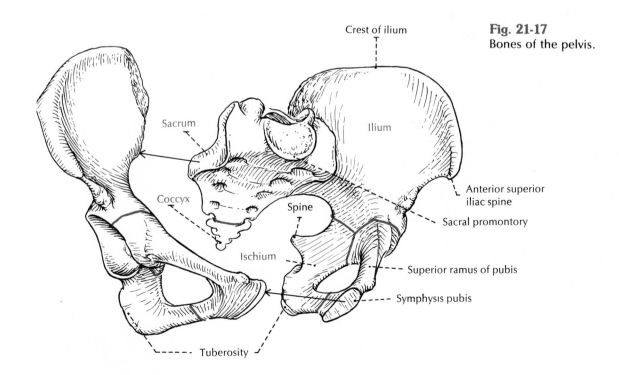

Fig. 21-17
Bones of the pelvis.

Crest of ilium

Sacrum

Ilium

Coccyx

Spine

Anterior superior iliac spine

Sacral promontory

Ischium

Superior ramus of pubis

Symphysis pubis

Tuberosity

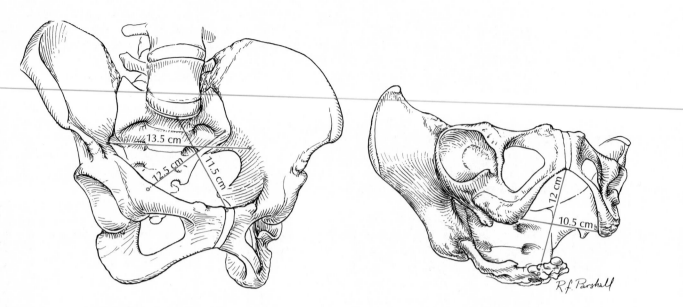

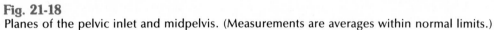

Fig. 21-18
Planes of the pelvic inlet and midpelvis. (Measurements are averages within normal limits.)

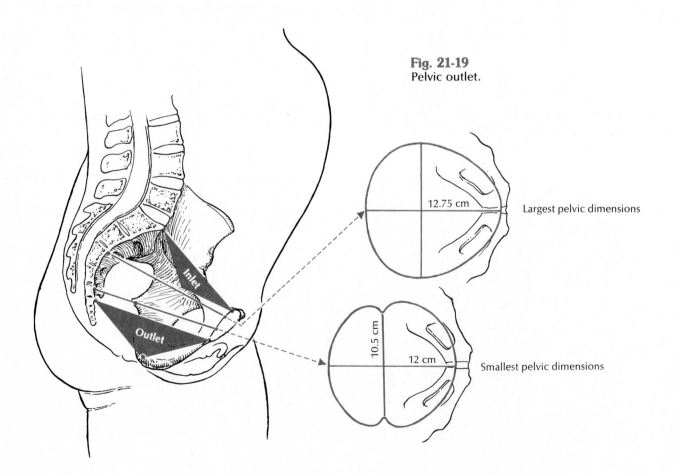

Fig. 21-19
Pelvic outlet.

the planes of the midpelvis; and the plane of the outlet. These planes are illustrated in Fig. 21-18.

The plane of the inlet in an average female pelvis measures approximately 11 to 13 cm in the anteroposterior diameter and 13 to 14 cm in the transverse diameter. The anteroposterior diameter of the inlet measured from the middle of the sacral promontory to the superior posterior margin of the symphysis pubis is called the true conjugate and is an important obstetrical measurement. However, it cannot be assessed directly, except by radiographic methods. An estimate of the true conjugate is made by measuring the diagonal conjugate, which is the distance between the inferior border of the symphysis pubis and the sacral promontory. The diagonal conjugate is about 1 to 2 cm longer than the true conjugate, depending on the height and inclination of the symphysis. The clinical measurement of the diagonal conjugate, the most valuable single measurement of pelvic adequacy, will be discussed later in this section.

The midpelvis contains the planes of greatest and least pelvic dimensions. The plane of least pelvic dimensions is bounded by the junction of the fourth and fifth sacral vertebrae, the symphysis, and the ischial spines. The average dimensions of this plane are 12 cm (anteroposterior diameter) and 10.5 cm (transverse diameter). The transverse diameter is the distance between the ischial spines.

The pelvic outlet is composed of two triangular planes, having a common base in the most inferior portion of the transverse diameter between the ischial tuberosities. The obstetrical anteroposterior diameter of the outlet is the distance between the inferior edge of the symphysis pubis and the edge of the sacrum, if the coccyx is movable. This measurement is usually 11.5 cm.

The transverse diameter of the outlet is the distance between the inner surfaces of the ischial tuberosities and usually measures about 11 cm (Fig. 21-19).

Although there is a characteristic shape of the adult female pelvis that is different from the characteristically male pelvis, a female client may have any one of four types of human pelves or a mixture of these types. In addition, the shape of the pelvis may have been distorted congenitally or by disease.

The four basic pelvic types as classified by Caldwell, Moloy, and Swenson (1939) are (1) gynecoid, (2) android, (3) anthropoid, and (4) platypelloid.

The typical female pelvis is the gynecoid pelvis, which is found in approximately 40% to 50% of adult women. This pelvis is characterized by a rounded inlet, except for a slight projection of the sacral promontory; a deep posterior half made possible by a wide sacrosciatic notch and concave sacrum, and a wide anterior half made possible by a wide, subpubic angle.

The android pelvis is found in approximately 15% to 20% of adult women. This pelvic type is roughly wedge- or heart-shaped with the transverse diameter of the inlet approximately equal to the anteroposterior diameter but with the widest transverse diameter located closer to the sacrum. Other characteristics of the android pelvis include the following:

1. Narrow subpubic arch
2. Convergent side walls
3. Large encroaching spines
4. Short sacrosciatic notch and sacrospinous ligament
5. Short interspinous diameter
6. Straight sacrum
7. Short intertuberous diameter

The anthropoid pelvis has an elongated anteroposterior diameter and is found in approximately 25% to 35% of women. It is characterized by the following:

1. Narrow subpubic arch
2. Prominent ischial spines
3. Wide sacrosciatic notch and long sacrospinous ligaments
4. Deeply curved sacrum

The platypelloid pelvis has a flattened anteroposterior dimension with a relative widening of the transverse diameter. This pelvic type is seen in approximately 5% of women. The platypelloid pelvis is characterized by the following:

1. Wide subpubic arch
2. Flat ischial spines
3. Wide sacrosciatic notch and long sacrospinous ligaments
4. Straight sacrum

The various dimensions of the four basic pelvic types are compared and contrasted in Fig. 21-20. Pure pelvic types are unusual; most pelves are admixtures of two pelvic types, with the characteristics of one type predominating.

The examination of the bony pelvis can be uncomfortable for the client, and it should be done after the internal examination of the soft pelvic organs. Therefore, the preparation of the client should include the explanation of the procedure, the client's emptying of her bladder, and instructions to the client for relaxation.

A routine standard procedure is recommended for the bony pelvis examination, beginning with the examination of the anterior pelvis, proceeding to lateral examination on one side, comparing the initially examined side with the opposite side, and concluding with the examination of the posterior and inferior portions.

The following bony pelvis parts and landmarks are especially important in examining the pelvis:

examined. The spine is assessed as being blunt, prominent, or encroaching. The sacrosciatic notch is outlined with palpating fingers, if possible, and its width is determined in centimeters or finger breadths. Often the examiner cannot trace the entire notch, and the sacrospinous ligament is useful in estimating the width of the notch (Fig. 21-23).

The other side of the pelvis is then examined in the manner previously described to determine overall pelvic symmetry. The examiner should attempt to do this part of the examination with the palm of the hand up, rather than rotating the hand so that the palm is down.

The interspinous diameter is an important obstetrical measurement. This diameter is estimated by moving the examining fingers in a straight line from one spine across to the other (Fig. 21-24). The hand may need to be pronated for this estimation. The estimate is calculated in centimeters. The usual measurement is 10.5 cm. Special calipers are available to measure the interspinous diameter, but these are not often used in clinical practice.

Next the sacrum and coccyx are examined. The fingers are swept down the sacrum, noting whether it is straight, curved, or hollow and if its inclination is forward or backward. The coccyx is examined gently because it may be tender on movement. The coccyx is

gently pressed backward to determine if it is movable or fixed. Its tilt is noted as anterior or posterior.

The diagonal conjugate is assessed last because this assessment can be uncomfortable for the client. A moderate amount of constant pressure is needed to depress the perineum adequately. Pressure is better exerted by the examiner's body than by the hand and forearm only. It is recommended that the examiner place the foot (the one on the same side as the examining hand) on a stool and the elbow of the examining arm on the thigh or hip. The needed pressure is then applied and controlled by the trunk of the examiner's body. For this examination, the fingers and wrist should form a straight line with the forearm.

The examiner locates the sacrum with the examining fingers and, with the middle finger, "walks" up the sacrum until the promontory is reached or until the examiner can no longer reach the sacrum. The point where the client's symphysis touches the examiner's hand is marked with the thumb of the opposite hand, and the distance is measured in centimeters by a ruler (Fig. 21-25). In obstetrical examining rooms, a ruler is often fixed to the wall for this measurement.

Often, the examiner will not reach the sacral promontory. The examiner should become familiar with the "reach" of his or her examining fingers and record the findings as greater than (>) the centimeters of this

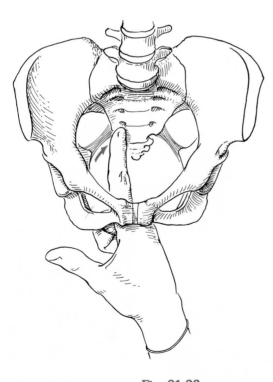 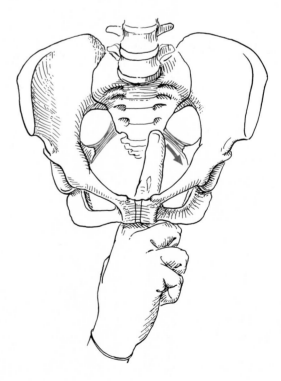

Fig. 21-23
Measurement of the width of the sacrosciatic notch.

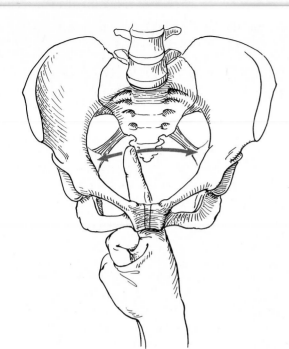

Fig. 21-24
Measurement of the interspinous diameter.

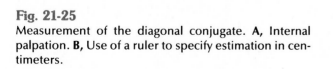

A

B

Fig. 21-25
Measurement of the diagonal conjugate. **A,** Internal palpation. **B,** Use of a ruler to specify estimation in centimeters.

reach. Normally the diagonal conjugate is greater than 12.5 cm.

The examining hand is withdrawn from the vagina, and the intertuberous diameter is measured. Using both thumbs, the examiner externally traces the descending rami down to the tuberosities. The examiner then makes a fist and attempts to insert the fist between the tuberosities to measure the transverse diameter of an outlet (Fig. 21-26). The intertuberous

diameter is usually 10 to 11 cm. Again, the examiner knows the span of his or her own fist and estimates the intertuberous diameter accordingly.

An instrument called the Thom's pelvimeter can be used to measure the intertuberous diameter (Fig. 21-27). This instrument has two arches that are held against the tuberosities by the examiner's thumbs. The precise intertuberous diameter can be determined by calibrations on the instrument's midportion.

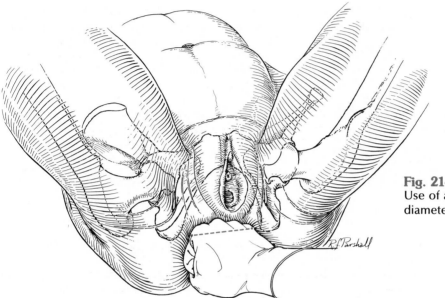

Fig. 21-26
Use of a fist to estimate the intertuberous diameter.

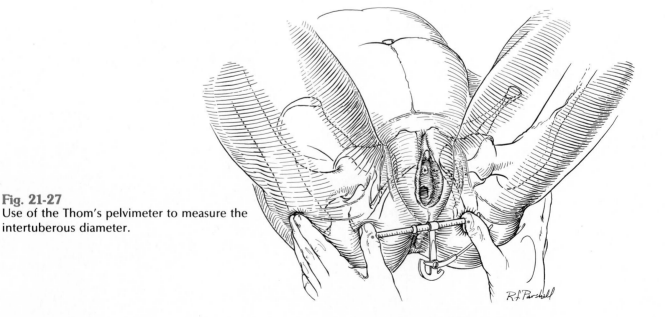

Fig. 21-27
Use of the Thom's pelvimeter to measure the intertuberous diameter.

In summary, the areas of bony pelvic examination and the assessment descriptors for these areas are noted as follows:

Sequence of areas of bony pelvis examination	Assessment descriptors
1. Subpubic arch	Less than 90 degrees; more than 90 degrees
2. Side walls	Parallel; convergent; divergent
3. Ischial spines	Size: small; average; large
	Prominence: blunt; prominent; encroaching
4. Sacrosciatic notch Sacrospinous ligament	Estimated width or length in centimeters or finger breadths (FB)
	Usual length 3 to 4 cm
5. Opposite pelvic side	Symmetrical; asymmetrical
6. Interspinous diameter	Estimated length in centimeters
	Usual length 10.5 cm
7. Sacrum	Concave; straight; convex
8. Coccyx	Position: straight; projects anteriorly; projects posteriorly
	Movability: movable; fixed
9. Diagonal conjugate	Actual length or length greater than the measurement the examiner can reach
	Usual length 12.5 cm
10. Intertuberous diameter	Actual length in centimeters if Thom's pelvimeter is used or an estimated length using a closed fist
	Usual length 10 to 11 cm

SUMMARY

I. First visit
  A. Complete physical examination, including the female genital examination (see Chapter 26, "Integration of the Physical Assessment")
  B. Abdominal assessment (prenatal portion)
    1. Palpation
      a. Fundal height
      b. Fetal position, using Leopold's maneuvers
    2. Auscultation—fetal heart rate
  C. Bony pelvis assessment
    1. Subpubic arch
    2. Side walls
    3. Ischial spine
    4. Sacrospinous ligament
    5. Opposite side
    6. Interspinous diameter
    7. Sacrum
    8. Coccyx
    9. Diagonal conjugate
    10. Intertuberous diameter
II. Repeat visits
  A. Regional examinations as indicated by history and current condition
  B. Weight
  C. Blood pressure
  D. Urine screening for glucose and protein
  E. Abdominal assessment
    1. Palpation
      a. Fundal height
      b. Fetal position, using Leopold's maneuvers
    2. Auscultation—fetal heart rate

BIBLIOGRAPHY

Aladjem, S., editor: Obstetrical practice, St. Louis, 1980, The C.V. Mosby Co.

American College of Obstetricians and Gynecologists: Standards for ambulatory care, Chicago, 1974, The College.

Bailey, R.E.: Mayes' midwifery: a textbook for midwives, ed. 9, London, 1976, Cassell & Collier Macmillan, Ltd.

Caldwell, W.E., Moloy, H.C., and Swenson, P.C.: The use of the roentgen ray in obstetrics: anatomical variations in the female pelvis and their classification according to morphology, Am. J. Roentgenol. **41**:505, 1939.

Fogel, C.I., and Woods, N.F.: Health care of women: a nursing perspective, St. Louis, 1981, The C.V. Mosby Co.

Gant, N.F., and others: A clinical test for predicting the development of acute hypertension in pregnancy, Am. J. Obstet. Gynecol. **120**:1, 1974.

Greenhill, J.P., and Friedman, E.A.: Biological principles and modern practice of obstetrics, Philadelphia, 1974, W.B. Saunders Co.

Hickman, M.A.: An introduction to midwifery, Oxford, 1978, Blackwell Scientific Publications, Ltd.

Humenick, S.S.: Analysis of current assessment strategies in the health care of young children and childbearing families, East Norwalk, Conn., 1982, Appleton-Century-Crofts.

Martin, L.L.: Health care of women, Philadelphia, 1978, J.B. Lippincott Co.

Niswander, K.R.: Obstetrics: essentials of clinical practice, ed. 2, Boston, 1981, Little, Brown & Co.

Page, E.W., Willee, C.A., and Villee, D.B.: Human reproduction: the core content of obstetrics, gynecology and perinatal medicine, ed. 2, Philadelphia, 1976, W.B. Saunders Co.

Oxhorn, H., and Foote, W.: Human labor and birth, New York, 1975, Appleton-Century-Crofts.

Romney, S.L., and others: Gynecology and obstetrics: the health care of women, New York, 1975, McGraw-Hill Book Co.

Spellacy, W.N.: Management of the high risk pregnancy, Baltimore, 1976, University Park Press.

Walker, J., MacGillivray, I., and Macnaughton, M.C.: Combined textbook of obstetrics and gynecology, ed. 9, Edinburgh, 1976, Churchill Livingstone.

Willson, J.R., Carrington, E.R., and Ledger, W.J.: Obstetrics and gynecology, ed. 7, St. Louis, 1983, The C.V. Mosby Co.

CHAPTER 22

MUSCULOSKELETAL ASSESSMENT AND EXAMINATION OF THE JOINTS

The skeletal system is made up of 206 bones and the joints by which they articulate. Bone, cartilage, and connective and hematopoietic (myeloid) tissues make up this system. These structures (1) provide support for the body, (2) allow movement as those muscles attached to the bones shorten in contraction (thereby pulling the bones), and (3) provide for the formation of red blood cells.

The musculoskeletal system is comprised of more than 600 voluntary or striated muscles and constitutes the principal organ of movement, as well as a repository for metabolites. The muscle mass accounts for as much as 40% of the weight of the adult man.

It is the partial contracture of skeletal muscle that makes all the characteristic postures of human beings possible, including the upright position that distinguishes the anthropoid.

Seven types of joint motion have been defined. These movements are flexion, extension, abduction, adduction, internal rotation, external rotation, and circumduction (Figs. 22-1 to 22-4).

Flexion is the bending of the joint to approximate the bones it connects, thereby decreasing the joint angle. *Extension* is the straightening of a limb so that the joint angle is increased, the placement of the distal segment of a limb in such a position that its axis is continuous with that of the proximal segment, or the pulling or dragging force exerted on a limb in a direction away from the body.

Abduction is the movement of a limb away from the midline of the body or one of its parts. *Adduction* is the movement of a limb toward the central axis of the body or beyond it.

Internal rotation is the turning of the body part inward toward the central axis of the body. *External rotation* is the turning of the body part away from the midline.

Circumduction is the movement of a body part in a circular pattern. This is not a singular motion but a combination of the other motions.

Muscles are categorized according to the type of joint movement produced by their contraction. Muscles, thus, are flexors, extensors, adductors, abductors, internal rotators, external rotators, or circumflexors. Muscles shorten on contraction and in so doing exert pull on the bones to which they are attached to move them closer together. Most muscles attach to two bones that articulate at an intervening joint. Generally, one bone moves while the other is held stable. This is caused by simultaneous shortening of other muscles. The body of the muscle that produces movement of an extremity generally lies proximal to the bone that is moved.

Thus, the joint, with its synovial membrane, capsule, ligaments, and the muscles that cross it, is considered to be the functional unit of the musculoskeletal system. This discussion of musculoskeletal assessment assumes that the practitioner has an understanding of the anatomy and physiology of the joints involved.

The examination of neuromuscular coordination begins as the practitioner first meets and observes the client, and it continues as the client advances into the room, sits, rises from a sitting position, climbs onto the examining table, lies down, and rolls over. The practitioner should note the speed, coordination, and strength of motion. He or she should particularly note clumsy, awkward, or involuntary movements, as well as tremor or fasciculation. An estimate of muscle strength may be gained from the handshake of the client. During the interview the flamboyance or paucity of gesture may provide valuable clues to the client's personality and general mobility.

The chief complaint of the client may indicate the direction for emphasis of the physical assessment. The

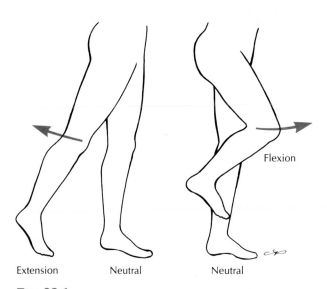

Fig. 22-1
Joint motion. *Left,* Extension of the right knee and hip, increasing the joint angle. *Right,* Flexion of the right knee and hip, decreasing the joint angle.

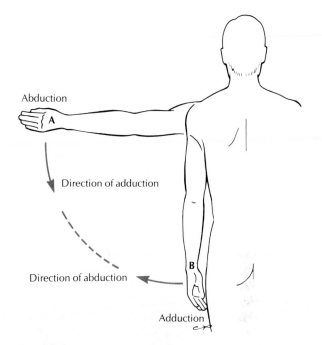

Fig. 22-2
Joint motion. Abduction is the movement of a limb away from the midline of the body, as seen in position *A.* Position *B* illustrates an arm in adduction, the movement of a limb toward the central axis of the body.

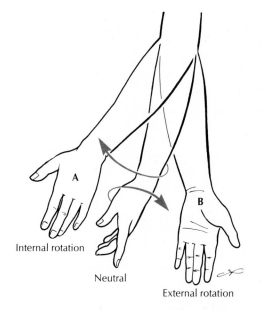

Fig. 22-3
Joint motion. Internal rotation is the turning of a body part inward toward the midline, as seen in position *A.* Position *B* illustrates external rotation, the turning of a body part away from the midline.

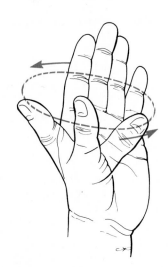

Fig. 22-4
Joint motion. Circumduction is the movement of a body part in a circular pattern.

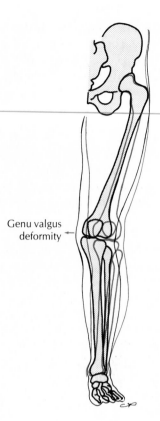

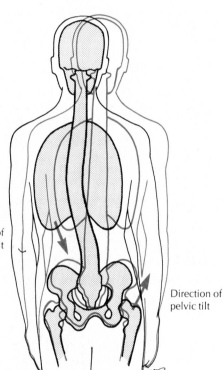

Fig. 22-8
Valgus deformity of the leg: deviation of the leg toward the midline (knock-knee). This condition was called varus deformity in earlier times. Red outline figure shows normal position; black, the deformity.

Genu valgus deformity

Direction of thoracic tilt

Direction of pelvic tilt

Fig. 22-9
Deformity of the spine. Scoliosis is the lateral deviation of the spine. Red outline figure shows the normal position; black, the deformity.

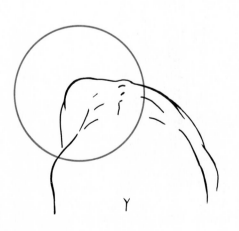

Fig. 22-10
The rotary deformity of scoliosis produces a hump or "razor back" deformity. This deviation is best demonstrated by asking the client to bend at the waist.

be observed. The protrusion may be made more obvious by asking the client to bend over to touch his toes. It is best observed from behind the client (Fig. 22-10).

Kyphosis is a flexion deformity (Fig. 22-11, *B*). When the angle of the defect is sharp, the apex is called a gibbus.

Lordosis (swayback) is an extension deviation of the spine commonly in the lumbar area (Fig. 22-11, *C*).

Measurement of the extremities

The musculoskeletal examination frequently includes the measurement of the extremities for length and circumference. Measurements of length are made when the symmetry of two limbs is questioned or to determine whether limbs are in normal range. The measurements are made with the client lying relaxed on a hard surface (examining table) with the pelvis level and the hips and knees fully extended and with both hips equally adducted. Frequently, apparent discrepancies in limb size are a result of position.

The length of the upper extremity is the distance from the tip of the acromion process to the tip of the middle finger; the shoulder is adducted and the other joints are at neutral zero (anatomical position—limb in extension). The length of the lower extremity is the distance from the lower edge of the anterosuperior iliac spine to the tibial malleolus (Table 22-1).

Table 22-1
Anatomical guideposts for measuring extremities

Area	From	To
Entire upper extremity	Tip of acromion process	Tip of middle finger
Upper arm	Tip of acromion process	Tip of olecranon process
Forearm	Tip of olecranon process	Styloid process of ulna
Entire lower extremity	Lower edge of anterosuperior iliac spine	Tibial malleolus
Thigh	Lower edge of anterosuperior iliac spine	Medial aspect of knee joint
Lower leg	Medial aspect of knee	Tibial malleolus

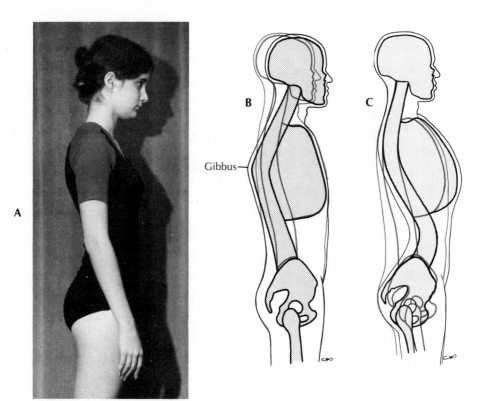

Gibbus

Fig. 22-11
A, Normal curvature of the spine. **B,** Deformity of the spine. Kyphosis is flexion of the spine. When the angle of the defect is sharp, the apex is called a gibbus. **C,** Deformity of the spine. Lordosis (swayback) is extension of the spine. It is most commonly found in the lumbar area. Red outline figure shows the normal position; black, the deformity.

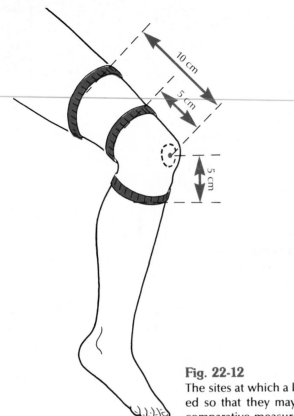

Measurement of muscle mass

The muscles are examined for gross hypertrophy or atrophy. Only in the markedly obese client are changes in muscle mass difficult to assess. The difference in the firm, hypertrophic muscle of the athlete and the limp, atrophic muscle of the paralytic is obvious both on inspection and on palpation with the finger. Although muscle size is largely a function of the use or disuse of the muscle fibers, changes in the size of muscles may be indicative of disease. Malnutrition and lipodystrophy tend to reduce muscle size and markedly weaken the strength of contraction. Lack of neutral input resulting from lesions of the spinal cord or peripheral motor neuron may lead to a reduction in muscle size of as much as 75% of the normal volume; this may occur over as short a time as 3 months. Measurements taken of limbs at their maximum circumference may provide a baseline for comparison when swelling or atrophy are suspected or in subsequent routine examination.

Fig. 22-12
The sites at which a limb is measured are carefully noted so that they may be accurately located for future comparative measurements.

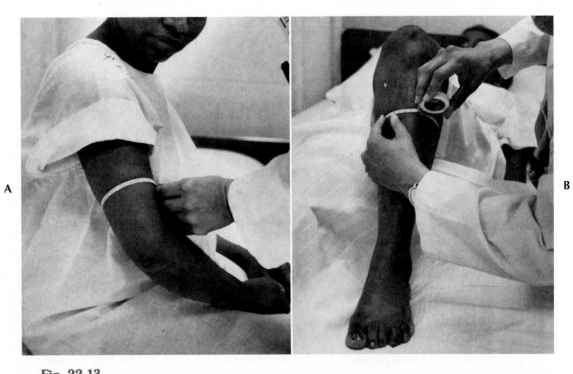

Fig. 22-13
A, Measurement of upper midarm circumference. **B,** Measurement of midgastrocnemius circumference.

The limbs should be in the same position and the muscles in the same state of tension each time measurements are performed. Several corresponding points may be measured above and below the patella and olecranon process. Some clinics routinely measure at 10 cm below and at points 10 and 20 cm above the midpatella to provide uniformity. At any rate, a small diagram showing the points measured (Fig. 22-12) will obviate ambiguity. Differences in symmetry or of limb size at different times of less than 1 cm are not significant (Fig. 22-13).

PALPATION

Palpation is used in the examination of the musculoskeletal system to detect swelling, localized temperature changes, and marked changes in shape.

The consistency of the muscle on palpation is noted.

Muscle tone, or tonus, is the tension that is present in the resting muscle. It is also seen in the slight resistance felt when the relaxed limb is passively moved.

While palpating the muscle, the examiner should be alert to fasciculations, which are involuntary contractions or twitchings of groups of muscle fibers.

The client should be requested to tell the examiner of any sensation he has while the muscles and tendons are being felt. The client's descriptions of pain or tenderness on palpation are recorded.

Tendon stretch reflexes, described in Chapter 23 on neurological assessment, are generally altered in muscle disease, especially if the peripheral nerves are involved. For instance, the tendon reflexes are diminished in muscular dystrophy and polymyositis in proportion to the loss of muscle strength. A lengthened reflex cycle is characteristic of hypothyroidism, whereas a shortened period is indicative of the hypermetabolic state.

TESTING OF MUSCULOSKELETAL FUNCTION
Screening test for muscle strength

Although muscle weakness in adults is generally mild and transitory, it may be the outcome of musculoskeletal, neurological, metabolic, or infectious problems. Therefore, an evaluation is necessary. A simple screening test has been suggested that can be performed in less than 5 minutes and allows the examiner to find nearly any muscle or reflex abnormality.

Muscle strength may be assessed throughout the full range of motion for each muscle or group of muscles.

Table 22-2
Screening test for muscle strength

Muscles tested	Client activity	Examiner activity	Muscles tested	Client activity	Examiner activity
Ocular musculature			Biceps	Flex arm	Pull to extend arm
			Triceps	Extend arm	Push to flex arm
Lids	Close eyes tightly	Attempt to resist closure	Wrist musculature	Extend hand	Push to flex
				Flex hand	Push to extend
Yoke muscles	Track object in six cardinal positions		Finger muscles	Extend fingers	Push dorsal surface of fingers
Facial musculature	Blow out cheeks	Assess pressure in cheeks with fingertips		Flex fingers	Push ventral surface of fingers
				Spread fingers	Hold fingers together
	Place tongue in cheek	Assess pressure in cheek with fingertips	Hip musculature	In supine position raise extended leg	Push down on leg above the knee
	Stick out tongue, move it to right and left	Observe strength and coordination of thrust and extension	Hamstring, gluteal, abductor, and adductor muscles of leg	Sit and perform alternate leg crossing	Push in opposite direction of the crossing limb
Neck muscles	Extend head backward	Push head forward	Quadriceps	Extend leg	Push to flex leg
	Flex head forward	Push head backward	Hamstring	Bend knees to flex leg	Push to extend leg
	Rotate head in full circle	Observe mobility, coordination	Ankle and foot muscle	Bend foot up (dorsiflexion)	Push to plantar flexion
	Touch shoulders with head	Observe range of motion		Bend foot down (plantar flexion)	Push to dorsiflexion
Deltoid	Hold arms upward	Push down on arms	Antigravity muscles	Walk on toes	
				Walk on heels	

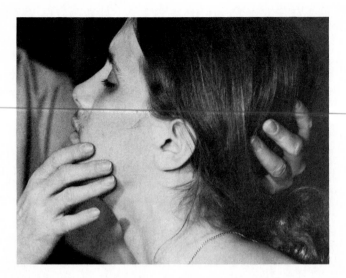

Fig. 22-14
Assessment of the neck musculature. The client flexes his head backward while the examiner attempts to break the extension.

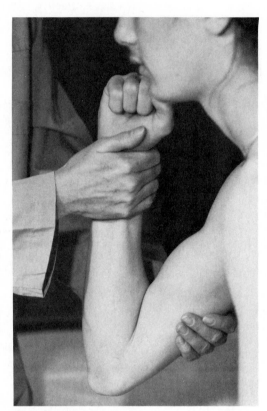

Fig. 22-15
Assessment of biceps strength. The client flexes his arm while the examiner attempts to pull the arm into extension.

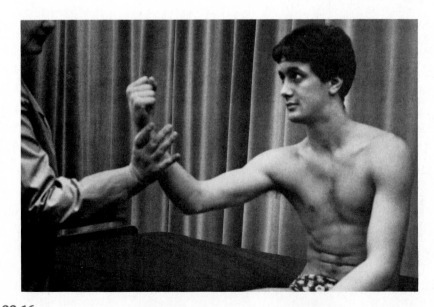

Fig. 22-16
Assessment of triceps strength. The client attempts to extend his arm while the examiner attempts to push the arm into a flexed position.

However, several screening examinations have been designed. One is described in Table 22-2. The usual method of testing is manual and subjective. Resistance is applied to the muscles; the client is placed in the position that best allows movement through the full range. The muscle contractions are graded according to the examiner's judgment of the client's responses. The test allows for a systematic testing of muscle groups from head to toe. As he walks into the examining room and undresses, the client is carefully observed for cues to neurological and motion deficit. He is carefully observed to ascertain that the chief complaint is verifiable by physical evidence. The following procedure may then be used:

1. The examiner assesses the ocular musculature by asking the client to close his eyes tightly as the examiner attempts to open the lids. The client is instructed to look up, down, right, and left as the examiner checks for lid lag and appropriate tracking of the eyes.
2. The examiner assesses the facial musculature by asking the client to blow out his cheeks while the examiner assesses the pressure against the fingers held against the resultant cheek bulge. The client is then asked to put his tongue into the cheek, and the tension created in this bulge is tested. The client is then asked to stick out his tongue and to move it to the right and left.
3. The examiner assesses the neck musculature by asking the client to extend his head backward while standing erect as the examiner attempts

to break the extension (Fig. 22-14). The client is then asked to bend his chin toward his chest forcefully as far as he is able while the examiner attempts to bend the chin upward. The client is asked to touch each shoulder with his head and to rotate the head in a full circle.

4. The examiner tests the deltoid muscles by asking the client to hold his arms upward while the examiner tries to push them down. The client is asked to extend his arms while the examiner attempts to press them down.
5. The examiner tests the biceps by asking the client to fully extend his arms and then to try to flex them while the examiner attempts to pull them into extension (Fig. 22-15).
6. The examiner tests the triceps by asking the client to flex his arms and then to extend them while the examiner attempts to push them into a flexed position (Fig. 22-16).
7. The examiner assesses the wrist and finger musculature by asking the client to extend his hand and then to try to resist the examiner with the hand up, alternately with the fingers out or together, in an attempt to flex the wrist (Fig. 22-17). The handshake provides a measure of the strength of the grasp (Fig. 22-18). Finger strength is assessed by pushing on the dorsal surface of the fingers while the client tries to extend them and on the ventral surface while he tries to further flex the fingers. Finger strength may be assessed by trying to move the

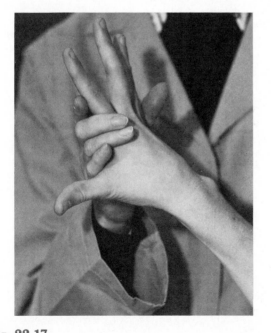

Fig. 22-17
Assessment of wrist strength. The client pushes against the examiner's hand in an attempt to flex the wrist.

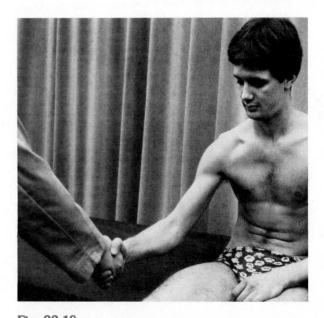

Fig. 22-18
The handshake provides a measure of the strength of the hand grasp.

fingers together as the client attempts to spread them (Fig. 22-19).

8. The examiner assesses hip strength by asking the client to assume the supine position and then to raise the extended leg while the examiner attempts to hold it down.

9. The examiner assesses the hamstring, gluteal, abductor, and adductor muscles of the leg by asking the client to sit and perform alternate leg crossing (Fig. 22-20).

10. The examiner tests quadriceps muscle strength by asking the client to extend a leg stiffly as the examiner tries to bend it (Fig. 22-21).

11. The examiner assesses the hamstring muscles by asking the client to bend his knees as the examiner tries to straighten them (Fig. 22-22).

12. The examiner assesses the ankle and foot musculature by asking the client to exert upward foot pressure and then big toe pressure against the examiner's hands.

13. The client is asked to walk naturally for a short distance to observe gait (if the examiner has not already done so). Then the client is asked to take a few steps on his toes and a few steps on his heels.

The following criteria for recording the grading of muscle strength have been frequently used:

Functional level	Lovett scale	Grade	Percentage of normal
No evidence of contractility	Zero (0)	0	0
Evidence of slight contractility	Trace (T)	1	10
Complete range of motion with gravity eliminated	Poor (P)	2	25
Complete range of motion with gravity	Fair (F)	3	50
Complete range of motion against gravity with some resistance	Good (G)	4	75
Complete range of motion against gravity with full resistance	Normal (N)	5	100

Some examiners prefer simple descriptive words, such as *paralysis, severe weakness, moderate weakness, minimum weakness,* and *normal.* Disability is considered to exist if the muscle strength is less than grade 3; external support may be required to make the involved part functional, and activity of the part cannot be achieved in a gravity field.

There is an expectation that muscle strength will be greater in the dominant arm and leg. Movements should be coordinated and painless.

Muscle fasciculations are checked for in the face, neck, torso, and extremities. A sharp tap to the muscle mass may induce this visible twitching.

Neurological adequacy can be assessed by examining the pupillary reflex and the fundus. Pyramidal tract function is evaluated through the use of deep tendon reflex tests, including Babinski's sign and the client's ability to perform voluntary muscle movements.

Cerebellar tract function may be elicited by asking the client to stand erect with his eyes closed and then checking Romberg's sign. The client is then asked to touch his finger to his nose and to rapidly rotate his hands inward and outward. Sensory perception is assessed by checking for pain, vibration, and temperature responses. (Neural function tests are described in Chapter 23 on neurological assessment.) *The musculoskeletal screening test is the only one performed unless the examiner suspects a musculoskeletal problem.* Another example of the screening examination has been developed by the house staff of Mayo Clinic as described in the boxed material below. A more extensive discussion of range of motion and joint examination, which may be helpful in a more inclusive examination, follows.

Survey of motor function*

	Right	Left
Arise from chair, arms folded		
Walk on toes	_____	_____
Walk on heels	_____	_____
Hop	_____	_____
Squat fully and rise		
Lift foot to step	_____	_____
Step up on step	_____	_____
Abduct arms to horizontal	_____	_____
Reach overhead (full extension)	_____	_____
Wing scapulae	_____	_____

Supine position

Lift head off table
Hands on occiput, rise to a sitting position
Flex thigh, lifting extended leg _____ _____

Prone position

Fully extend neck
Lift head and shoulders off table, hands on buttocks

*The survey has been designed by the house staff of Mayo Clinic and may be used as a substitute for specific tests of muscle strength for very young children and for adults who are unable to cooperate with specific muscle testing. The survey is judged to be of greatest value in conditions defined by muscle weakness.

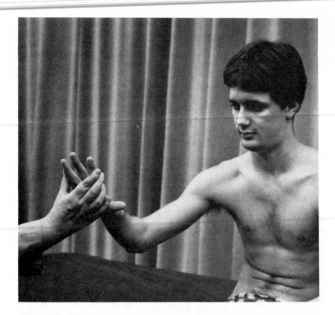

Fig. 22-19
Finger strength is assessed as the examiner resists the client's attempts to spread them.

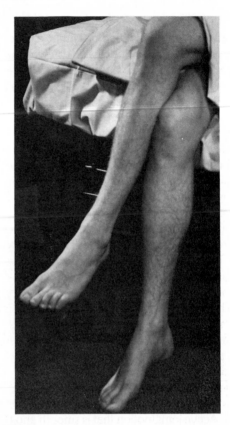

Fig. 22-20
Alternate leg crossing for assessment of hamstring, gluteal, abductor, and adductor muscle strength.

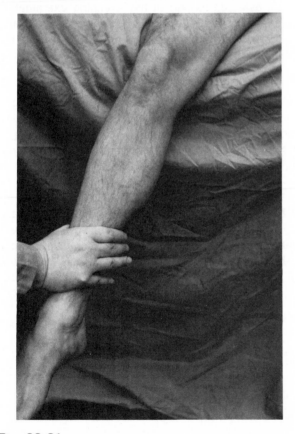

Fig. 22-21
Assessment of quadriceps muscle strength. The client attempts to straighten the leg while the examiner attempts to flex it.

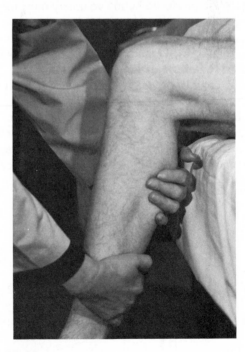

Fig. 22-22
Assessment of hamstring muscle strength. The client flexes his knees while the examiner tries to straighten them.

Table 22-3
Testing for muscle strength and range of joint motion—cont'd

Movement	Muscles	Motor nerves	Positions for testing	Instructions and tests for muscle strength
FINGERS—cont'd				
Abduction	Prime movers (Fig. 73†) Interossei dorsales Abductor digiti minimi	Ulnar nerve (cervical 8, thoracic 1) Ulnar nerve (cervical 8)	Standing, sitting, supine (fingers together)	"Spread your fingers as far apart as possible." Pressure is exerted against the outside surfaces of the fingers being tested to resist spread of the fingers (Fig. 74).
Adduction	Prime movers: interossei palmares (Fig. 75†)	Ulnar nerve (cervical 8, thoracic 1)	Standing, sitting, supine (fingers apart)	"Put your fingers together. Press them hard against each other." An attempt is made to pull them apart (Fig. 76).

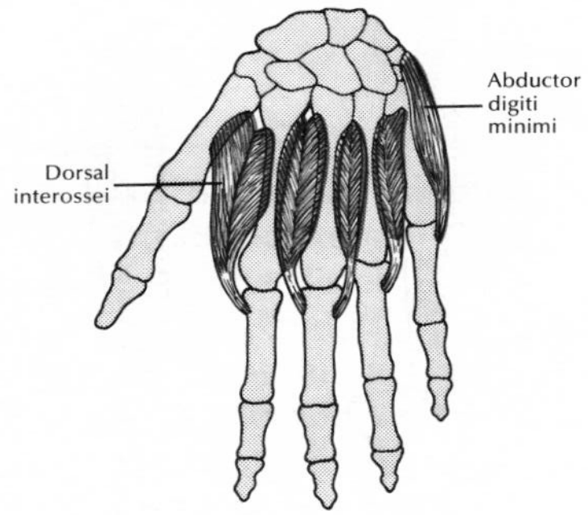

Fig. 74

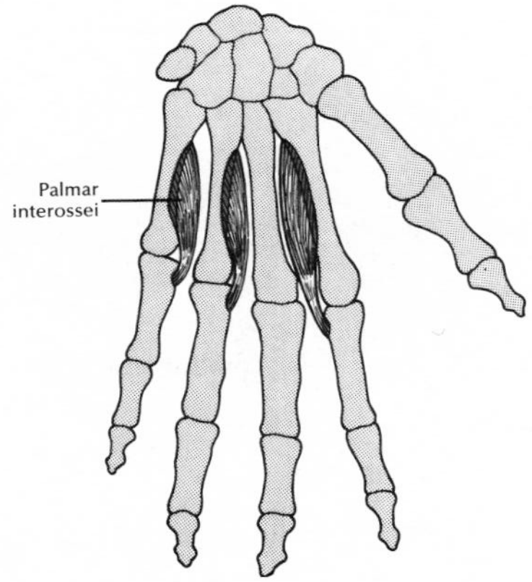

Fig. 76

Fig. 73

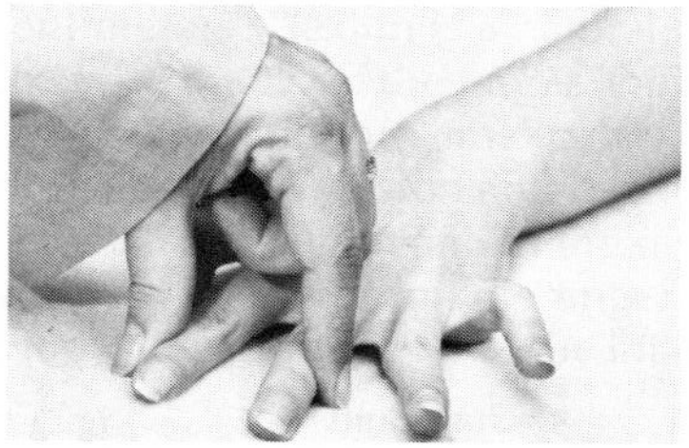

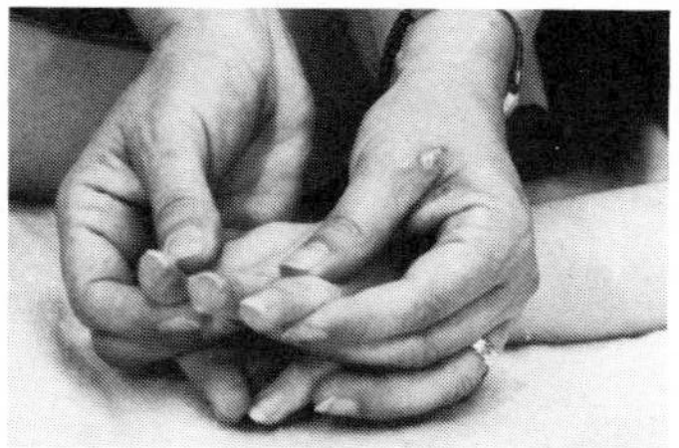

Fig. 75

HIP

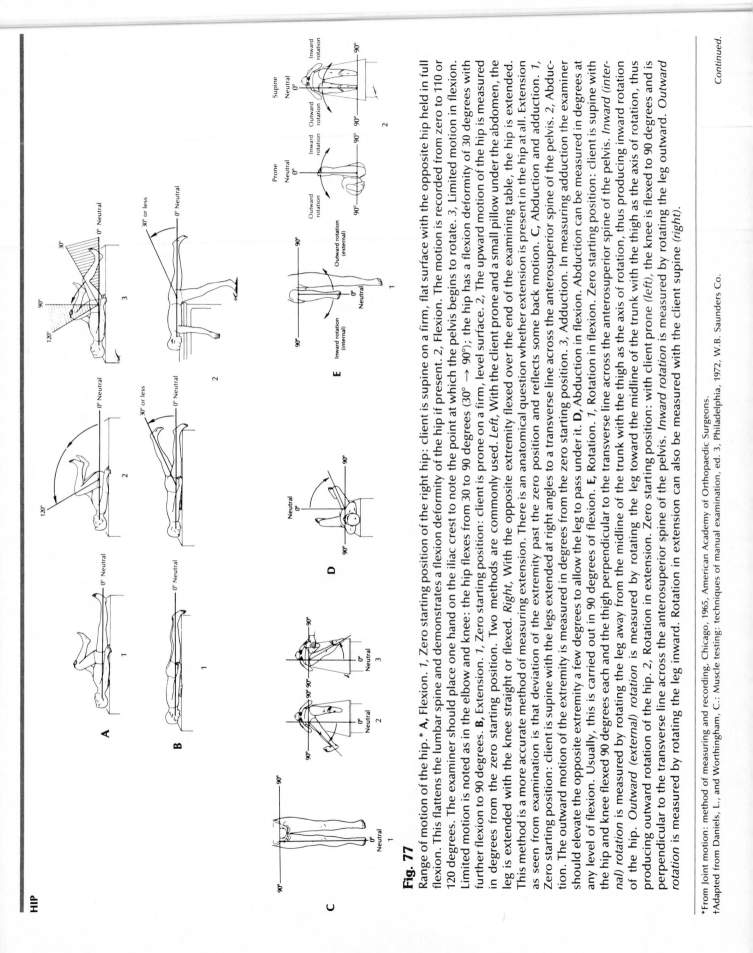

Fig. 77

Range of motion of the hip.* **A,** Flexion. *1,* Zero starting position of the right hip: client is supine on a firm, flat surface with the opposite hip held in full flexion. This flattens the lumbar spine and demonstrates a flexion deformity of the hip if present. *2,* Flexion. The motion is recorded from zero to 110 or 120 degrees. The examiner should place one hand on the iliac crest to note the point at which the pelvis begins to rotate. *3,* Limited motion in flexion. Limited motion is noted as in the elbow and knee: the hip flexes from 30 to 90 degrees (30° → 90°); the hip has a flexion deformity of 30 degrees with further flexion to 90 degrees. **B,** Extension. *1,* Zero starting position: client is prone on a firm, level surface. *2,* The upward motion of the hip is measured in degrees from the zero starting position. Two methods are commonly used. *Left,* With the client prone and a small pillow under the abdomen, the leg is extended with the knee straight or flexed. *Right,* With the opposite extremity flexed over the end of the examining table, the hip is extended. This method is a more accurate method of measuring extension. There is an anatomical question whether extension is present in the hip at all. Extension as seen from examination is that deviation of the extremity past the zero position and reflects some back motion. **C,** Abduction and adduction. *1,* Abduction. The examiner should elevate the opposite extremity a few degrees to allow the leg to pass under it. **D,** Abduction in flexion. Abduction can be measured in degrees at any level of flexion. Usually, this is carried out in 90 degrees of flexion. **E,** Rotation. *1,* Rotation in flexion. Zero starting position: client is supine with the hip and knee flexed 90 degrees each and the thigh perpendicular to the transverse line across the anterosuperior spine of the pelvis. *Inward (internal) rotation* is measured by rotating the leg away from the midline of the trunk with the thigh as the axis of rotation, thus producing inward rotation of the hip. *Outward (external) rotation* is measured by rotating the leg toward the midline of the trunk with the thigh as the axis of rotation, thus producing outward rotation of the hip. *2,* Rotation in extension. Zero starting position: with client prone *(left),* the knee is flexed to 90 degrees and is perpendicular to the transverse line across the anterosuperior spine of the pelvis. *Inward rotation* is measured by rotating the leg outward. *Outward rotation* is measured by rotating the leg inward. Rotation in extension can also be measured with the client supine *(right).*

*From Joint motion: method of measuring and recording, Chicago, 1965, American Academy of Orthopaedic Surgeons.
†Adapted from Daniels, L., and Worthingham, C.: Muscle testing: techniques of manual examination, ed. 3, Philadelphia, 1972, W.B. Saunders Co.

Continued.

Table 22-3
Testing for muscle strength and range of joint motion—cont'd

Movement	Muscles	Motor nerves	Positions for testing	Instructions and tests for muscle strength
HIP—cont'd				
Flexion	Prime movers (Fig. 78†)		Sitting, supine	"Draw your knees up to your chest."
	Psoas major	Femoral nerve (lumbar 2, 3)		"Bend your right [left] knee up to your chest."
	Iliacus	Femoral nerve (lumbar 2, 3)		Resistance is applied to the anterior surface of the leg proximal to the knee (Fig. 79).
	Accessory muscles			
	Sartorius			
	Rectus femoris			
	Tensor fasciae latae			
	Pectineus			
	Adductor brevis			
	Adductor longus			
	Adductor magnus (oblique fibers)			
Extension	Prime movers (Fig. 80§)		Prone	"Lift your right [left] leg toward the ceiling."
	Gluteus maximus	Inferior gluteal nerve (lumbar 5; sacral 1, 2)		Resistance is applied to the dorsal surface of the leg proximal to the knee (Fig. 81).
	Semitendinosus	Sciatic nerve (lumbar 4, 5; sacral 1, 2)		
	Semimembranosus	Sciatic nerve (lumbar 5; sacral 1, 2)		
	Biceps femoris (long head)	Sciatic nerve (sacral 1, 2, 3)		

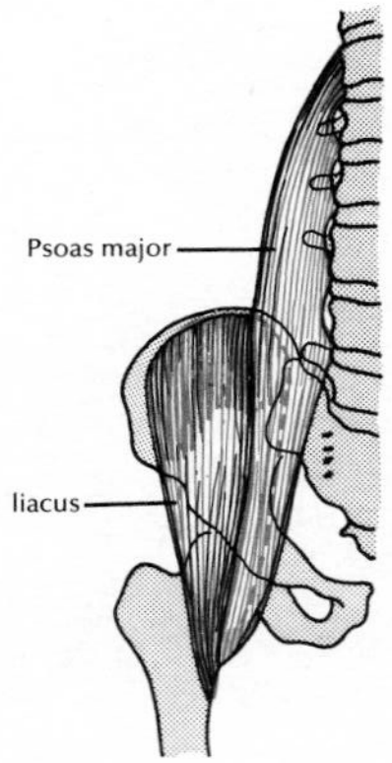

Fig. 78

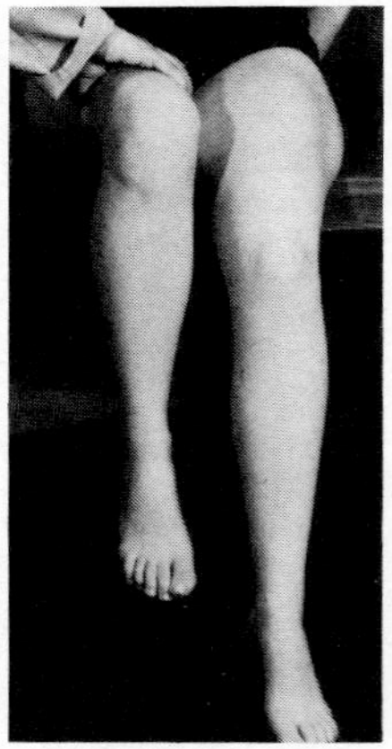

Psoas major

Iliacus

Fig. 79

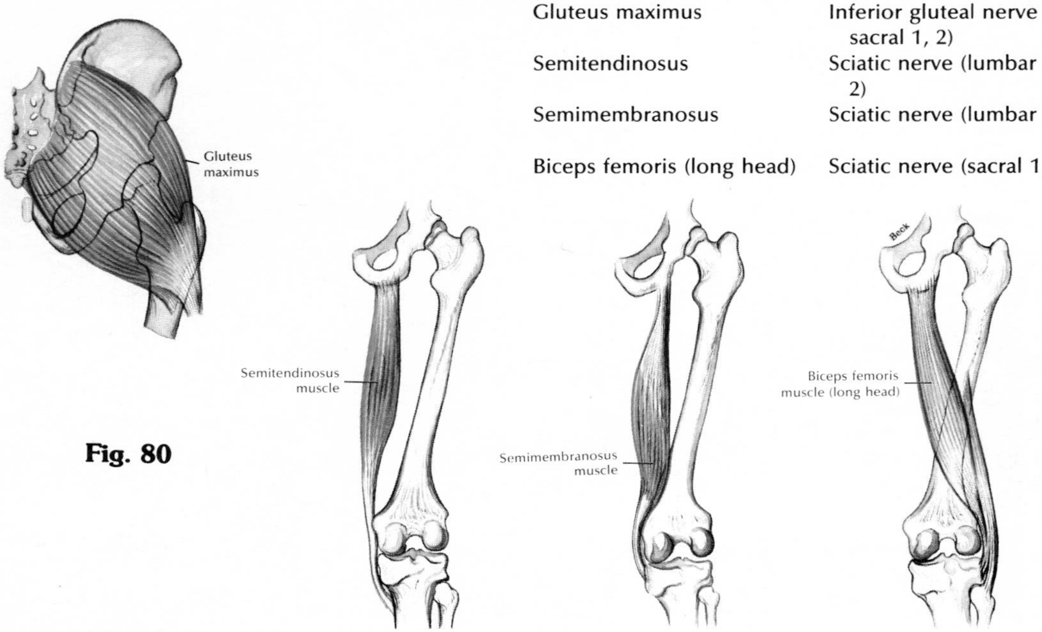

Fig. 80

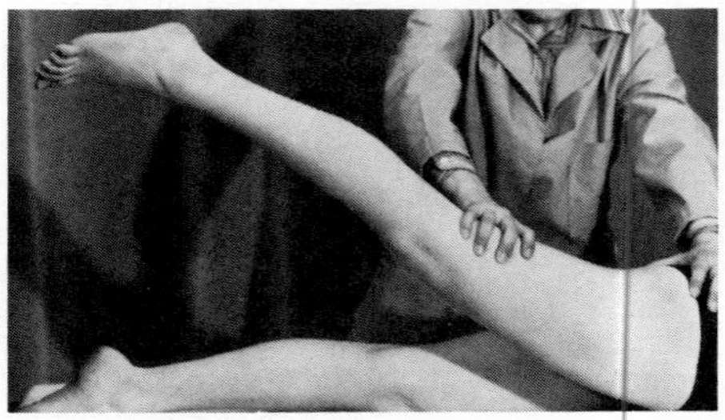

Gluteus maximus

Fig. 81

Semitendinosus muscle

Semimembranosus muscle

Biceps femoris muscle (long head)

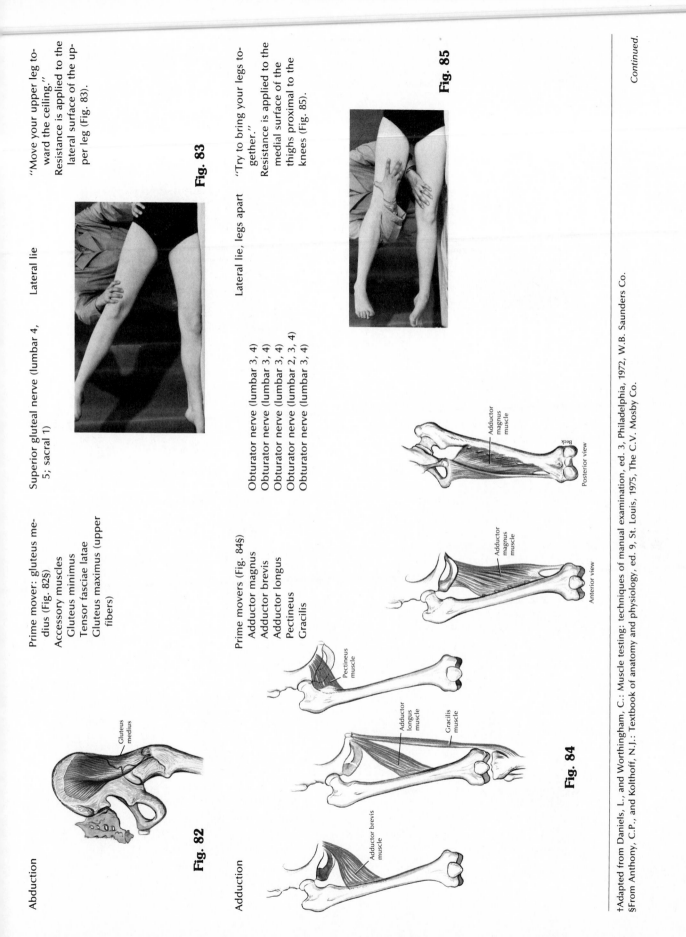

| Abduction | Prime mover: gluteus medius (Fig. 82§) Accessory muscles Gluteus minimus Tensor fasciae latae Gluteus maximus (upper fibers) | Superior gluteal nerve (lumbar 4, 5; sacral 1) | Lateral lie | "Move your upper leg toward the ceiling." Resistance is applied to the lateral surface of the upper leg (Fig. 83). |
| Adduction | Prime movers (Fig. 84§) Adductor magnus Adductor brevis Adductor longus Pectineus Gracilis | Obturator nerve (lumbar 3, 4) Obturator nerve (lumbar 3, 4) Obturator nerve (lumbar 3, 4) Obturator nerve (lumbar 2, 3, 4) Obturator nerve (lumbar 3, 4) | Lateral lie, legs apart | "Try to bring your legs together." Resistance is applied to the medial surface of the thighs proximal to the knees (Fig. 85). |

Fig. 82

Fig. 83

Fig. 84

Fig. 85

†Adapted from Daniels, L., and Worthingham, C.: Muscle testing: techniques of manual examination, ed. 3, Philadelphia, 1972, W.B. Saunders Co.
§From Anthony, C.P., and Kolthoff, N.J.: Textbook of anatomy and physiology, ed. 9, St. Louis, 1975, The C.V. Mosby Co.

Continued.

Table 22-3
Testing for muscle strength and range of joint motion—cont'd

Movement	Muscles	Motor nerves	Positions for testing	Instructions and tests for muscle strength
HIP—cont'd				
Rotation (knees extended) Internal	Prime movers (Fig. 86S) Gluteus minimus	Superior gluteal nerve (lumbar 4, 5; sacral 1)	Sitting (legs about a foot apart at ankle) 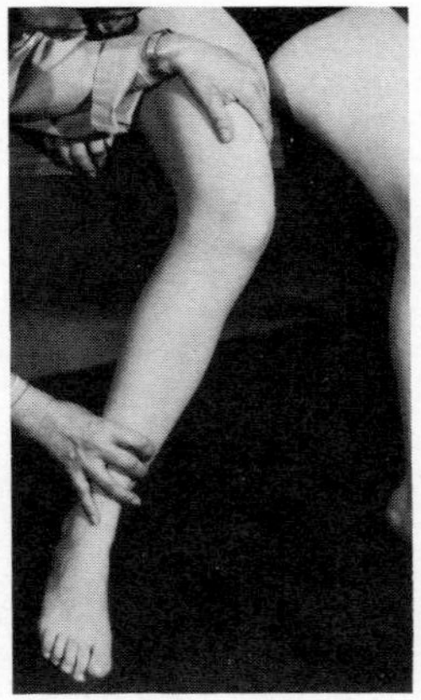	"Pivot your right hip inward—your foot will move away from your body." Resistance is applied toward the midline at the lateral surface of the ankle (Fig. 87).
	Tensor fasciae latae	Superior gluteal nerve (lumbar 4, 5; sacral 1)		
	Accessory muscles Gluteus medius (anterior fibers) Semitendinosus Semimembranosus			
External	Prime movers (Fig. 88†) Obturator externus	Obturator nerve (lumbar 3, 4)	Sitting 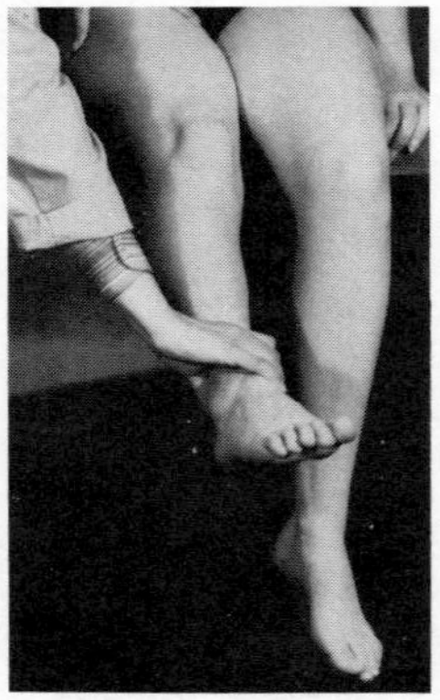	"Rotate your hip outward; your foot will turn in." Resistance is applied to the medial aspect of the ankle (Fig. 89).
	Obturator internus	Obturator nerve (lumbar 5; sacral 2, 3)		
	Quadratus femoris	Obturator nerve (lumbar 5; sacral 1)		
	Piriformis	Obturator nerve (sacral 1, 2)		
	Gemellus superior	Obturator nerve (lumbar 5; sacral 1, 2, 3)		
	Gemellus inferior	Obturator nerve (lumbar 5; sacral 1)		
	Gluteus maximus	Obturator nerve (lumbar 5; sacral 1, 2)		
	Accessory muscles Sartorius Biceps femoris (long head)			
Rotation (knees flexed)	Prime mover: sartorius Accessory muscles External rotators of hip Flexors of hip, knee	Femoral nerve (lumbar 2, 3, 4)	Supine (knees flexed)	"Rotate your knees outward. Bend them toward the table. Bring them as close as you can to the table." Resistance is applied to the lateral aspects of the knees.

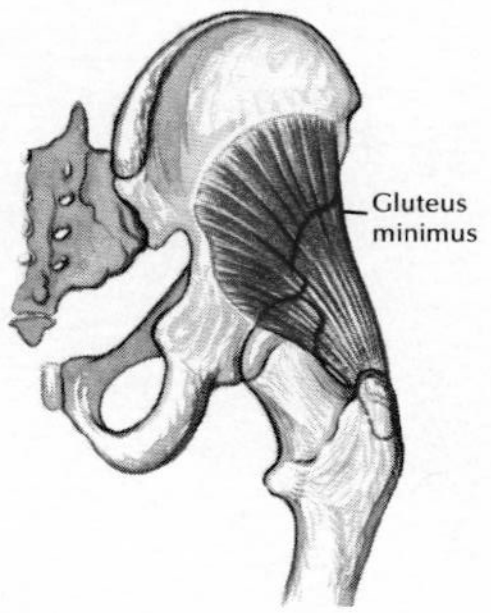

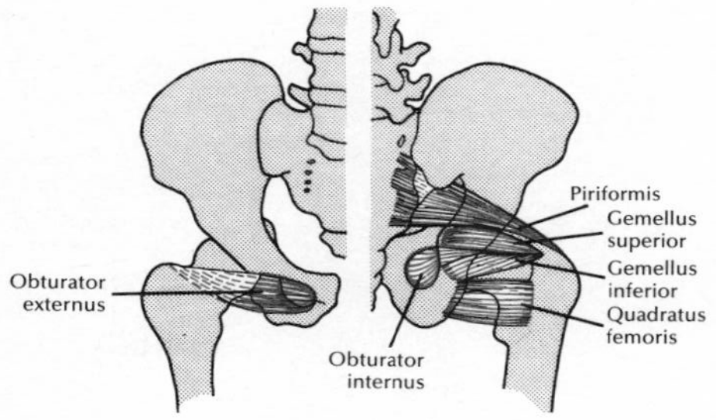

Fig. 86

Gluteus minimus

Fig. 87

Fig. 88

Piriformis
Gemellus superior
Gemellus inferior
Quadratus femoris
Obturator internus
Obturator externus

Fig. 89

Movement	Muscles	Motor nerves	Positions for testing	Instructions and tests for muscle strength
Abduction	Prime mover: tensor fasciae latae Accessory muscles Gluteus medius Gluteus minimus	Superior gluteal nerve (lumbar 4, 5; sacral 1)	Supine	"Bend your knees out." Resistance is applied to the upper outer aspect of each leg.

KNEE

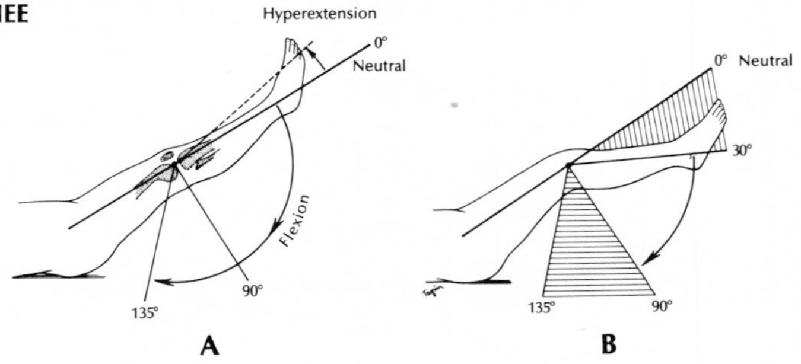

Fig. 90
Range of motion of the knee.* **A,** Flexion. Zero starting position: the extended straight knee with client either supine or prone. *Flexion* is measured in degrees from the zero starting point. *Hyperextension* is measured in degrees opposite to flexion at the zero starting point. **B,** Measurement of limited motion of the knee. The terminology for recording limited motion of the knee is similar to that of the elbow and hip: (1) the knee flexes from 30 to 90 degrees (30° → 90°); (2) the knee has a flexion deformity of 30 degrees with further

Movement	Muscles	Motor nerves	Positions for testing	Instructions and tests for muscle strength
Flexion	Prime movers (Fig. 91§) Biceps femoris (long head) Biceps femoris (short head) Semitendinosus Semimembranosus Accessory muscles Popliteus Sartorius Gracilis Gastrocnemius	Sciatic nerve (sacral 1, 2, 3) Sciatic nerve (lumbar 4, 5; sacral 1, 2) Sciatic nerve (lumbar 4, 5; sacral 1, 2, 3) Sciatic nerve (lumbar 4, 5; sacral 1, 2, 3)	Prone	"Bend your right [left] leg. Try to touch your heel to the back of your leg." Resistance is applied to the dorsal aspect of the ankle (Fig. 92).

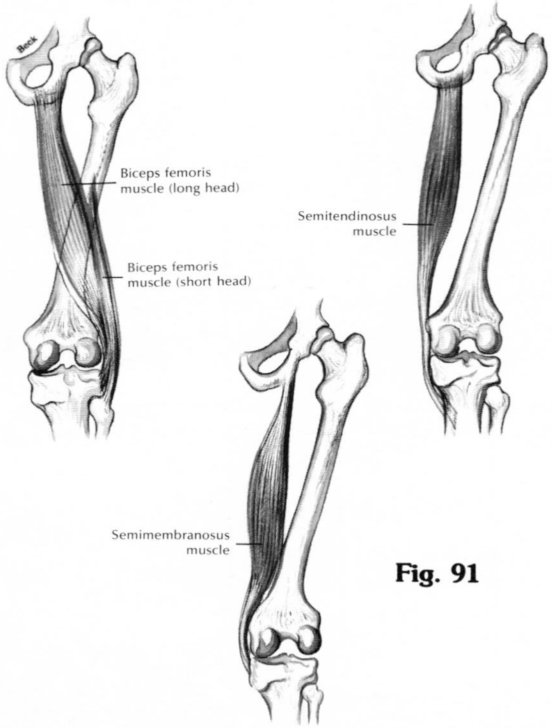

Fig. 91

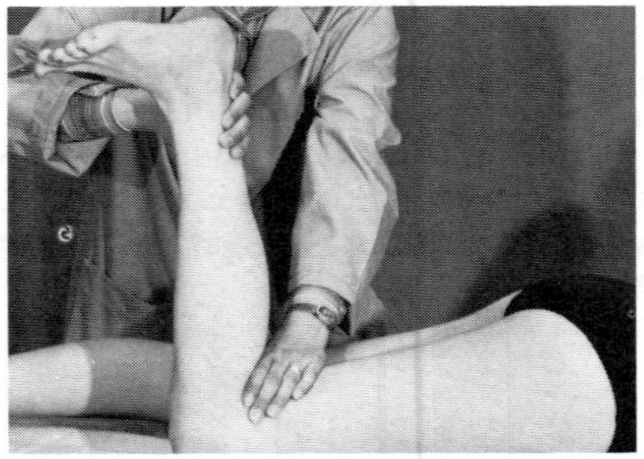

Fig. 92

*From Joint motion: method of measuring and recording, Chicago, 1965, American Academy of Orthopaedic Surgeons.
†Adapted from Daniels, L., and Worthingham, C.: Muscle testing: techniques of manual examination, ed. 3, Philadelphia, 1972, W.B. Saunders Co.
§From Anthony, C.P., and Kolthoff, N.J.: Textbook of anatomy and physiology, ed. 9, St. Louis, 1975, The C.V. Mosby Co.

Continued.

response to stretch of the fibers. In the case of the gastrocnemius muscle, the stretch can be achieved by dorsiflexion of the foot. Occasionally massage is helpful in relaxing the spasm. Fasciculations may frequently be observed before and after the cramp and are further evidence of the hyperexcitability of the neuromuscular unit. Electromyogram recordings show high-frequency action potentials during the cramp. These muscle spasms have greater frequency when the client is dehydrated or sweating and in the pregnant client.

The cause of the pain associated with muscle cramp has not been determined but is thought by some to be caused by the increased metabolic needs of the hyperactive muscles and to the collection of the metabolic waste products such as lactic acid within the muscle.

MUSCLE ENZYME LEVELS

Destructive diseases of striated muscle fibers result in the loss of enzymes from the intracellular compartment of the muscle. The enzymes enter the blood and can be measured. The usual laboratory analysis of serum enzymes includes alkaline phosphatase, lactic dehydrogenase (LDH), serum glutamic oxaloacetic transaminase (SGOT), and creatine phosphokinase (CPK). Enzymes are found in all tissues. Since high concentrations of these enzymes are found in the heart and liver, elevated serum level values may result from myocardial infarction or hepatitis. However, CPK, although present in the heart and brain, is most concentrated in the striated muscle. The level may rise from a normal level of 0 to 65 international units (IU) to more than 1,000 IU in clients with destructive lesions of the striated muscles.

MYALGIA

"I hurt all over" is frequently the chief complaint for the diffuse muscle pain that accompanies many types of systemic infection, for example, influenza, measles, rheumatic fever, brucellosis, dengue fever, or salmonellosis. Soreness and aching are other descriptive terms for this type of involvement. Little is known of the cause. *Fibromyositis* (myogelosis) is the term used to describe the inflammation of the fibrous tissue in muscle, fascia, and nerves. The client may complain of pain and tenderness in a muscle after exposure to cold, dampness, or minor trauma.

Firm, tender zones occasionally several centimeters in diameter are found on palpation. Palpation, active contraction, or passive stretching increases the pain. Intense pain localized to a smaller group of muscles may be a result of epidemic myalgia, also called pleurodynia, "painful neck," or "devil's grip." Intense pain at the beginning of neurological involvement has been seen in poliomyelitis and herpes zoster.

The pain of poliomyelitis is described as marked during the initial involvement of the nerve, whereas the later sensation of the paralyzed muscle is said to be one of aching. The segmental pattern of the intense pain of herpes zoster is caused by the inflammation of spinal nerves and dorsal root ganglia that occurs 3 to 4 days before the skin eruption.

The initial symptoms of rheumatoid arthritis may be diffuse muscular soreness and aching, which may antedate the joint involvement by weeks or months. The muscles are tender, and the client describes the pain as occurring not at the time of activity but hours later. An increased sedimentation rate or a positive latex fixation test may support the conclusion of rheumatoid involvement.

ELECTROMYOGRAPHY

The electromyogram is the graph generated from the electrical potential of individual muscles. The test is accomplished by inserting needles directly into the muscle being studied and recording the potential with the muscle at rest, with slight voluntary contractions, and at maximum flexion. Whereas the heart can be sampled from a number of surface electrode positions, the skeletal muscles are variable in size, widely separated, and numerous. Therefore, no small number of leads can give an adequate picture of their activity. Furthermore, surface electrodes yield only a summation of the underlying activity. To ascertain the bursts of individual muscle units, sterile needle electrodes must be used to register the activity.

Thus, the electromyogram must be done for one muscle at a time. Information obtained from the tracing is useful in determining neural adequacy of the muscle and the presence of intrinsic muscle disease.

MUSCLE BIOPSY

Muscle biopsy was first used by Cachenne in 1868. Currently the use of muscle biopsy is believed to be indicated for five clinical problems: (1) atrophy of the muscle that is progressive (when doubt exists to whether the disease is myogenic or neurogenic); (2) localized inflammatory disease of the muscle wherein biopsy may contribute to isolating the causative agent, thus allowing institution of the appropriate therapeutic regimen; (3) certain metabolic diseases wherein the histological or biological data, or both, thus provided may help to identify the disease; (4) fever associated with many visceral and cutaneous lesions wherein biopsy of the muscle may reveal further connective tissue and vascular involvement to support the conclusions of a generalized involvement; and (5) trauma wherein the biopsy may further define the degree of nerve and muscle injury.

ASSESSMENT OF GAIT

Gait is evaluated in both phases—the stance and the swing—for rhythm and smoothness. *Stance* is considered to consist of three processes: (1) heel strike—the heel contacts the floor or ground; (2) midstance—body weight is transferred from the heel to the ball of the foot; and (3) push-off—the heel leaves the ground (see Chapter 7, General assessment).

The *swing* phase also consists of three processes: (1) acceleration; (2) swing through—the lifted foot travels ahead of the weight-bearing foot; and (3) deceleration—the foot slows in preparation for the heel strike.

The description of the observation of the client's gait should include: *phase* (conformity); *cadence* (symmetry, regular rhythm); *stride length* (symmetry, length of swing); *trunk posture* (related to phases); *pelvic posture* (related to phases); and *arm swing* (symmetry, length of swing).

If pain is present, it should be described in relationship to the phases of gait.

EXAMINATION OF BONES AND JOINTS
Bones

Bones are examined for deformity or tumors. Bones are also examined for integrity by testing resistance to a deforming force. Palpation of the bone is performed to assess the presence of pain or tenderness. Tenderness of a bone may indicate tumor, inflammation, or the aftermath of a trauma. Frequently, traumatic injuries are associated with damage to both bone and nerve. Paralysis of the ulnar and median nerves in the hand is frequently the result of a hand injury and may result in a clawlike posture of the hand.

Joints
Signs and symptoms of disorders

Pain, swelling, partial or complete loss of mobility, stiffness, weakness, and fatigue are the signs and symptoms most frequently associated with disorders of the joints. Joint disease may be indicated by skin that feels warm, is red, has lesions, or is ulcerated. In the condition of psoriatic arthritis the lesions and the nails have been shown to be involved in about 50% of cases. Pitting is the most commonly recognized change. There may be isolated pitting of a single nail or the pitting may be *uniformly* distributed across the nails.

Pain. *Pain* is the symptom that most frequently causes the client to seek help, and understanding the character of the pain may be helpful in determining its cause in the physical assessment of the involved joints. The client should be encouraged to try to recall those events occurring before the onset of pain because most individuals tend to forget minor injuries or unusual physical activity in the weeks before the pain began. The client is unlikely to correlate symptoms and signs of infection in the months before with his current joint pain. The nature of the onset of pain is also important because rheumatoid symptoms are known to begin gradually, whereas gouty attacks are characterized by sudden onset that frequently wakes the client from sleep.

The client frequently has difficulty in localizing the pain associated with joint disease. His description may involve large areas of the body, that is, "my neck" (while moving his hand from his head to the thoracic vertebra), "my back," or "all down my arm." This difficulty in localizing the pain may be related to whether the pain is deep or superficial and whether a nerve is involved.

The locations or distribution of the pain may also provide valuable information. Rheumatoid involvement is known to be migratory, that is, involving first one joint, which improves, than another. On the other hand most infectious arthritis is confined to one joint. The joint involvement in rheumatoid arthritis tends to be symmetrical, whereas that of gout, psoriatic arthritis, and Reiter's syndrome tends to occur initially in one or two joints but becomes polyarticular in later stages. Spondylitis is first detected in the spine and then spreads to peripheral joints (centrifugal spread), whereas rheumatoid arthritis starts peripherally in the hands and feet and then involves the large joints of the hips, shoulders, and spine in the later stages of the disease (centripetal spread).

The time that pain occurs may also be diagnostic. The individual with osteoarthritis generally reports that the pain is made worse by increased use of the affected joint and, thus, frequently has pain later in the day or when tired. The individual with rheumatoid arthritis generally reports stiffness and pain that occurs early in the morning and some improvement when he forces himself to exercise the part.

Questions directed to a description of referred pain may prove helpful. Spinal nerve root involvement is frequently felt in peripheral tissues. For instance, lumbosacral nerve root irritation (sciatica) may be experienced as pain in the thigh or the knee on the involved side. The area of referred pain corresponds with the segmental innervation of the structures. The description of this type of pain may include words associated with paresthesias, that is "prickling," "like an electric shock," "pins and needles," and "numbing." Pain of muscle origin may be described by such words as "pulled" or "charley horse." Joint pain descriptions may be noted along a spectrum from dull, aching, or stiff to excruciating and intolerable.

A knowledge of those measures known to alleviate the pain may also be valuable diagnostically. Some of these have already been discussed, for example, exercise for rheumatoid arthritis and rest for osteoarthritis.

Limitation of range of motion. The client may voluntarily limit the motion of a joint in response to pain. Spasm of the muscles involved in the movement of a joint may limit its motion. Mechanical obstruction to movement may accompany bony overgrowth and scar tissue. Limitation of motion in a joint is accompanied by weakness and atrophy of the muscles that are involved.

Decreased range of motion is observed in joints in which there is inflammation of surrounding tissues, arthritis, fibrosis, or bony fixation (ankylosis).

Deformity. Deformities of the joint include absorption of tissues, flexion contracture, and bony overgrowth. Absorption may produce a flail joint such that the bones making the joint move erratically. Deformities result from scarring phenomena following inflammation and infection.

Swelling. The amount of swelling of the joint may range from difficult to detect to visually evident fluid within the joint, that is, visible or palpable as a bulging of the joint capsule. Pressure on the sac at one point causes the fluid within to shift and may lead to bulging at another site. The sac may feel from soft to tense, and the involvement may be symmetrical or unilateral. Frequently, the swelling is fusiform. Redness, warmth, swelling, and pain in a joint are the classical descriptors of an inflammantory process. The inflammation may be within the joint itself or in the soft tissue surrounding

it. Swelling may also result from intraarticular effusion, synovial thickening, or bony overgrowth. The swelling may also result from the deposition of fat in the region adjacent to the joint.

The synovial membrane is not palpable in normal joints. The palpation of a "boggy" or "doughy" consistency generally indicates a thickened or otherwise abnormal synovial membrane.

Heberden's or Bouchard's nodes of the fingers or bony spurs, particularly in the knees, are typical of osteoarthritis.

Tenderness. Inflammatory processes cause joints to be tender. Arthritis, tendonitis, bursitis, and osteomyelitis are associated with tenderness in and around a joint. An attempt should be made to determine the anatomical structure that is tender.

Increased temperature. Heat over a joint is indicative of inflammation and suggests rheumatoid arthritis. Symmetrical comparison of joints for temperature is indicated when one joint is hot. The backs of the fingers are used when comparing temperature.

Redness. Vasodilation or inflammation is noted in the skin overlying a tender joint affected by septic arthritis and gouty arthritis.

Crepitation. Crepitation (crackling or grating sounds) produced by motion of the joint is caused by irregularities of the articulating surfaces. The coarseness of surface may involve the cartilage or the bony capsule.

A systematic assessment of individual joints may be made during the performance of the head to toe physical examination, or all the joints may be examined at a preselected time during the examination. As with all

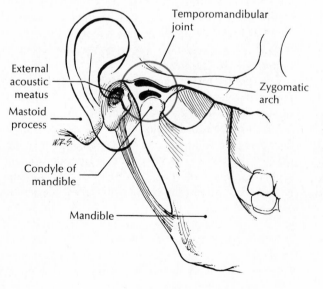

Fig. 22-23
The temporomandibular joint. A fibrocartilaginous disk divides the articulation point into two synovial cavities. Note the proximity to external acoustic meatus.

bilateral structures, the paired joints should be compared.

The joints that are given special consideration are the temporomandibular, sternoclavicular, manubriosternal, shoulder, elbow, wrist, hip, knee, and ankle.

Temporomandibular joint

The temporomandibular joint is the articulation between the mandible and the temporal bone (Fig. 22-23). The joint is divided into two cavities as a fibrocartilaginous disk. Swelling is observed as a tumescence over the joint but must be considerable to be visible. Palpation is accomplished by placing the fingertips anterior to the external meatus of the ear. In the normal joint, there is a depression over the joint. Swelling may make this indentation difficult to feel. The jaw is palpated while it is moved through its range of motion: opening and closure of the mouth, protrusion (jutting of the jaw), retrusion (tucking in of chin), and side-to-side sliding of the mandible. The normal range of distance between the upper and lower incisors is 3 to 6 cm. Lateral motion of the jaw may be measured by asking the client to protrude the jaw and move it from side to side. The distance is measured by the distance that the midline of the lower lip deviates in each direction. The normal range of motion is 1 to 2 cm (Fig. 22-24). "Clicks" may be heard on movement and may be regarded as normal.

Sternoclavicular joint

The sternoclavicular joint is located at the juncture of the clavicle and the manubrium of the sternum. The joint is divided into two synovial cavities by a disk of cartilage and fibrous material. The joint is reinforced by a fibrous capsule and ligaments (Fig. 22-25). The obtuse angle formed by the junction of the manubrium and body of the sternum is called the angle of Louis and has been used as a landmark for counting the ribs. Observation of this joint is readily accomplished because there is little tissue overlying it. Swelling, redness, bony overgrowth, and dislocation are not difficult to see. Swelling of the joint appears as a smooth, round bulge. Although this joint is often overlooked, it is often involved following surgery of the neck. Palpation is done with the fingertips. Movements of the shoulder are dependent on the normal function of this joint. Inflammation of the sternoclavicular joint may result in pain on movement of the shoulder girdle.

Manubriosternal joint

The hyaline cartilage–lined joint covers the articular surface of the second rib and those of the manubrium and body of the sternum (see Fig. 22-25)). Little tissue overlies this joint. Observation is thus a more accurate method of examination. Observation is the only technique of examination because movement of the joint is minimal.

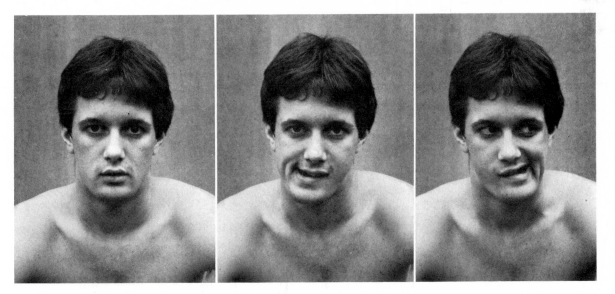

Fig. 22-24
Lateral motion is determined by asking the client to move the lower jaw from side to side. The distance measured is the distance the midline of the lower lip deviates in each direction. The midline of the stationary upper lip may be used as the baseline.

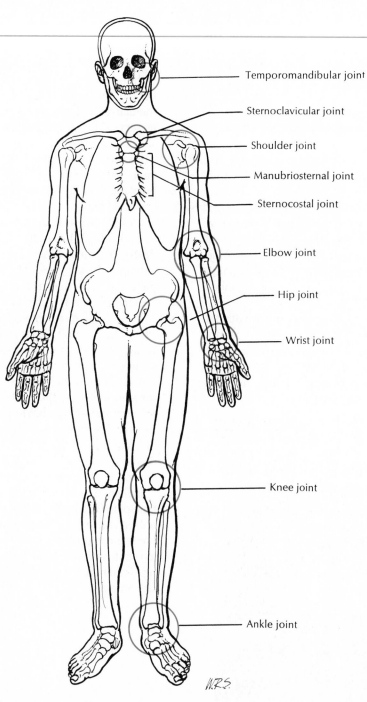

Fig. 22-43
Results of the examination of joints may be summarized by circling the joint involved and briefly noting the pathological condition.

Fig. 22-44
Straight leg-raising test.

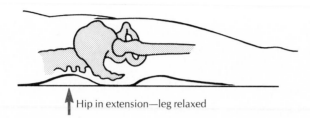

Hip in extension—leg relaxed

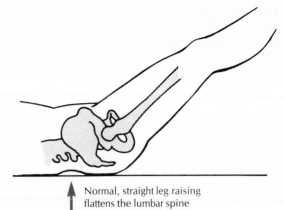

Normal, straight leg raising
flattens the lumbar spine

SUMMARY

I. Muscle
  A. Inspection
    1. Size—swelling
    2. Shape, contour, symmetry
    3. Strength
    4. Involuntary movement
  B. Palpation
    1. Tenderness
    2. Masses
    3. Heat
  C. Range of motion against resistance—screening examination
    1. Position
      a. Head extension and flexion
      b. Arm extension and flexion
      c. Wrist extension and flexion
      d. Finger extension and flexion
      e. Leg extension and flexion
      f. Ankle extension and flexion
    2. Standing
      a. Back posture—flexion and rotation
    3. Walk on toes, heels, hop
II. Joints
  A. Inspection
    1. Size—swelling
    2. Shape—contractures
    3. Redness
  B. Palpation
    1. Effusion
    2. Heat
    3. Masses
  C. Auscultation—crepitation
  D. Range of motion

BIBLIOGRAPHY

Adams, R.: Diseases of the muscle, New York, 1975, Harper & Row, Publishers.

Beetham, W., and others: Physical examination of the joints, Philadelphia, 1965, W.B. Saunders Co.

Daniels, L., and Worthingham, C.: Muscle testing: techniques of manual examination, ed. 3, Philadelphia, 1972, W.B. Saunders Co.

Enneking, W.F., and Sherrard, M.G.: Physical diagnosis of the musculoskeletal system, Gainesville, Fla., 1969, Storter Printing Co., Inc.

Goodgold, J., and Eberstein, A.: Electrodiagnosis of neuromuscular diseases, Baltimore, 1972, Williams & Wilkins.

Hoppenfield, S.: Physical examination of the spine and extremities, New York, 1976, Appleton-Century-Crofts.

Joint motion: method of measuring and recording, Chicago, 1965, American Academy of Orthopaedic Surgeons.

Knapp, M.E.: Electromyography, Postgrad. Med. **47:**213, 1970.

Layzer, R.B., and Rowland, L.P.: Cramps, N. Engl. J. Med. **285:**31, 1971.

Mann, R.A., editor: DuVries, surgery of the foot, ed. 5, St. Louis, 1984, The C.V. Mosby Co.

McCarty, D.J., editor: Arthritis, ed. 9, Philadelphia, 1979, Lea & Febiger.

Moosa, A.: Paediatric electrodiagnosis, Arch. Dis. Child. **46**(6):149, 1972.

Polley, H.F., and Hunder, G.G.: Physical examination of the joints, Philadelphia, 1978, W.B. Saunders Co.

Rosse, C., and Clawson, D.: Introduction to the musculoskeletal system, New York, 1970, Harper & Row, Publishers.

Walton, J.N.: Disorders of voluntary muscle, ed. 3, Baltimore, 1974, Williams & Wilkins.

Yates, D.A.: The electrodiagnosis of muscle disorders, Proc. R. Soc. Med. **65:**617, 1972.

CHAPTER 23

NEUROLOGICAL ASSESSMENT

The neural system provides integration for all the functions of the body, but the system also derives its homeostatic balance from the appropriate functioning of the peripheral organs. The cells of the central nervous system, for example, depend on an adequate supply of glucose for their metabolic processes, and this supply can be maintained only when those tissues that play a role in intermediary metabolism function well. This balance makes neurological assessment a part of all the components of the history and the physical examination.

The neurological system controls cognitive and voluntary behavioral processes and the subconscious and involuntary bodily functions of the organism (see boxed material below). The major functions of the nervous system are reception (sensory), integration, and adaptation. That is, the normal nervous system receives stimuli from the environment, compares the adaptive processes necessary to adjustment to the environment with the functions the body is currently employing, and effects changes as necessary to assure homeokinesis or survival.

Equipment needed for neurological assessment includes vials of coffee, vanilla, tobacco, and oil of cloves for olfactory assessment and vials of glucose solution (sweet), salt solution, vinegar or lemon juice (sour), and quinine (bitter) for taste assessment. Test tubes of water are used for assessment of hot and cold temperature perception. Also necessary are an ophthalmoscope, a Snellen's chart for visual acuity, a Rosenbaum pocket-vision screener, a tuning fork, a reflex hammer, a tongue blade, an applicator, and a wisp of cotton.

The *mental status examination* is an integral part of the neurological examination. In the context of the total assessment of health, however, this appraisal occurs much earlier in the examination. Most examiners make assessments of mental status while obtaining the client's history and do special tests immediately afterward (see the boxed material on p. 533).

CRANIAL NERVE FUNCTION
CN I: olfactory nerve

The olfactory nerve is sensory in function and makes possible the sense of smell, or olfaction.

The peripheral neurons of the olfactory nerve are bipolar neurons. The ciliated, distal neurons penetrate the nasal mucosa in the roof of the nose, the upper septum, and the medial wall of the superior nasal concha. Unless the individual sniffs or inspires deeply, most of the inspired air does not contact the olfactory epithelium; during normal respiration, inspired air does not rise this high in the nares. Deep inspiration or sniffing causes a sudden rush of air into the upper nose and initiates swirling or turbulence of air around the olfactory mucosa. The central, unmyelinated axons are grouped in 15 to 20 bundles that pass through the cribriform plate of the ethmoid bone to synapse within the olfactory bulb. The second-order neurons course posteriorly from the bulb to the olfactory trigone, where they divide into medial and lateral striae. The medial striae terminate in the cortex of the medial subcallosal gyrus and the inferior portion of the cingulate

---

Neurological physical examination

The remainder of the neurological physical examination may be performed as five areas of investigation:
1. Assessment of cranial nerve function
2. Assessment of proprioception and cerebellar function
3. Musculoskeletal assessment (see Chapter 22)
4. Assessment of sensory function
5. Assessment of reflexes

---

gyrus. The lateral striae terminate in the uncus, the anterior portion of the hippocampal gyrus, and amygdaloid nucleus. Testing the sense of smell is an examination of the integrity of the entire system. When the same odor is smelled continuously, the olfactory cells are thought to be fatigued because a decreased awareness of odor is reported on long exposures.

Clinical examination

The client is asked to close his eyes (if the substance can be identified visually), occlude one nostril, and attempt to identify familiar substances with the open one, sniffing or inhaling deeply. The substances should be mildly aromatic (volatile oils and liquids) and unambiguous, such as coffee, cigarettes, soap, peanut butter, toothpaste, oranges, vanilla, chocolate, and oils of wintergreen, lemon, lime, almond, and cloves. It has been shown that the most easily identified substances are coffee, oil of almond, chocolate, and oil of lime. Strongly aromatic compounds should be avoided in determining olfactory function because the vapors may prevent the perception of weaker substances. Substances that stimulate either gustatory receptors or trigeminal branches of the nasal mucosa should also be avoided, including chloroform, oil of peppermint, camphor, ammonia, alcohol, and formaldehyde.

The substances are housed in test tubes that are kept closed until the examiner is prepared to present them to the client.

The client is asked whether he smells anything; then he attempts to identify the substance. The process is repeated for each nostril to determine symmetry (Fig. 23-1).

Both the number of substances used as stimuli and the number of correct responses should be recorded, along with differences in sensitivity from one nostril to the other.

If the client has difficulty identifying substances, he should be asked whether he is able to smell anything at all. In addition, the examiner should determine whether the nasal passages are patent.

Anosmia is the loss of the sense of smell or the inability to discriminate vapors. Diminution of the ability to smell is termed hyposmia. The client is not always aware of a deficit in olfaction. A pathophysiological condition of the nasal mucosa or olfactory bulb or tract can interfere with the sensation of smell.

The individual with an impaired sense of smell also has difficulty in identifying flavors. Since the tongue has receptors for only sweet, salt, sour, and bitter, these must be regarded as the true tastes and will be retained in hyposmia and anosmia. However, flavor perception is a synthesis of odor, taste, and perceptions from stimulation of end organs in the mouth and pharynx. The individual with CN I involvement may complain only of loss of the sense of taste. The examiner should note that olfactory acuity is thought to be more acute before eating than after a meal.

The mucosal surfaces are examined when the client has difficulty in smelling, since an inflammation of the mucous membranes (viral, bacterial) decreases the sense of smell. Allergic rhinitis and excessive cigarette smoking commonly cause anosmia or hyposmia.

Lesions of the sinuses may result in distortion or hallucinations of smell but do not result in a loss of olfactory sensation. Unilateral loss of smell may be an early indication of a neoplasm involving the olfactory bulb or tract. Total anosmia may follow head trauma, especially fractures involving the cribriform plate. Parosmia is a perversion of the sense of smell that sometimes accompanies trauma or tumors of the uncus. Olfactory hallucinations that are offensive are known as cacosmia.

CN II: optic nerve

The optic nerve is described in Chapter 11 on eye assessment (note the sections on examination of visual acuity, visual fields, the pupils—tests of pupillary constriction, retinal fields, and the optic disc). Fig. 23-2 illustrates an examination for unilateral protrusion of an eye.

Cranial nerves and their functions

I	Olfactory	Sense of smell
II	Optic	Visual acuity
III	Oculomotor	Movement of eye muscles
		Upper lid opening
		Pupillary reflexes
IV	Trochlear	Movement: superior oblique eye muscles
V	Trigeminal	Sensory for face
		Motor to muscles of mastication
VI	Abducens	Movement of lateral rectus eye muscle
VII	Facial	Motor to muscles of facial expression
		Sensory: taste, anterior two thirds of tongue
VIII	Acoustic	Auditory acuity
		Position in space: balance
IX	Glossopharyngeal	Sensory position in space
		Motor to uvula
		Soft tissue of palate
		Sensory: taste in posterior one third of tongue
X	Vagus	Motor to muscles of pharynx, larynx
XI	Hypoglossal	Motor to tongue
XII	Spinal accessory	Motor to sternocleidomastoid muscles and trapezius muscles

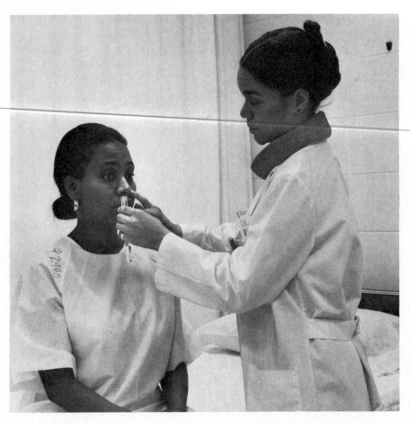

Fig. 23-1
Testing for ability to smell. The client is asked to sniff as the test tube containing the test substance is placed beneath the nostril. The examiner holds the other nostril closed.

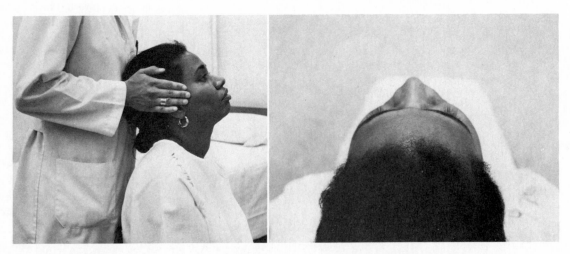

Fig. 23-2
An examination for unilateral protrusion of an eye. The examiner stands behind the client and slowly extends the neck. The eyelashes should be sighted simultaneously for both eyes if they are similar in size and position.

CN III: oculomotor nerve, CN IV: trochlear nerve, CN VI: abducens nerve

The oculomotor, trochlear, and abducens nerves are also described in Chapter 11 (note the sections on neuromuscular and extraocular muscle function—tests of eye movement).

Doll's head maneuver (vestibular oculogyric reflex)

Rapid turning of the head to one side results in ocular deviation to the contralateral side. In deep coma or other conditions resulting in paralysis of the oculomotor nerves or muscles, conjugate gaze to the contralateral side may be diminished or lost.

CN V: trigeminal nerve

The trigeminal nerve is motor to the muscles of mastication and sensory to the face and to the mucosa of the nose and mouth in perceiving touch, temperature, and pain.

The nuclei of the trigeminal nerve are located in the midportion of the pons. The bulk of the cell bodies of the sensory portion of the trigeminal nerve lies in the gasserian ganglion, with the remainder in the mesen-

cephalic nucleus. The sensory fibers to the gasserian ganglion are contained in one of the three proximal divisions of the nerve: ophthalmic, maxillary, or mandibular (Fig. 23-3). Peripheral nerve endings of the ophthalmic branch are sensory to the cornea, conjunctiva, upper lid, forehead, bridge of the nose, and scalp as far posteriorly as the vertex. The maxillary division of CN V conducts sensation from the skin of the lateral aspect of the nose, cheek, upper teeth, and jaw and from the mucosa of the lower nasal cavity, nasopharynx, hard palate, and uvula. The mandibular division contains the motor fibers that innervate the masseter, temporal, pterygoid, and digastric muscles. This division is also sensory to the skin of the lower jaw, pinna of the ear, anterior portion of the external auditory canal, side of the tongue, lower gums, lower teeth, floor of the mouth, and buccal surface of the cheek.

Afferent fibers from the gasserian ganglion enter the lateral portion of the pons and bifurcate into ascending and descending branches. The ascending branches pass to the main sensory nucleus responsible for the sensation of touch and to the mesencephalic nucleus that serves proprioception from the muscles of masti-

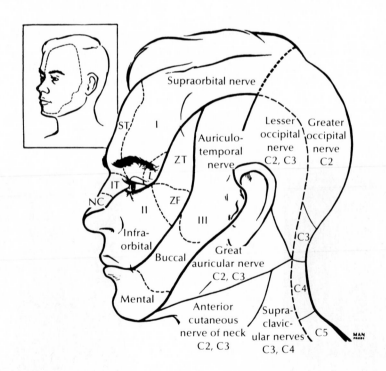

Fig. 23-3
Cutaneous fields of the head and upper part of the neck. Inset shows the area of sensory loss in the face following resection of the trigeminal nerve. The cutaneous fields of the three branches of the trigeminal nerve are identified as *I*, ophthalmic; *II*, maxillary; and *III*, mandibular. (From Haymaker, W., and Woodhall, B.: Peripheral nerve injuries, ed. 2, Philadelphia, 1959, W.B. Saunders Co.)

of first one hand and then the other with the eyes closed (Fig. 23-19). The client is then asked to repeat this activity several times while gradually increasing the speed of performance.

The client may be asked to touch his nose and then the examiner's finger at a distance of about 18 inches (Figs. 23-20 and 23-21). This maneuver is also repeated with increasing speed. The finger-to-finger test involves asking the client to spread the arms broadly and then to bring them together in the midline. It is done slowly and then rapidly with the eyes open and then closed. The client is asked to pat and then use a polishing motion on the examiner's hand, progressively increasing the speed (Figs. 23-22 and 23-23).

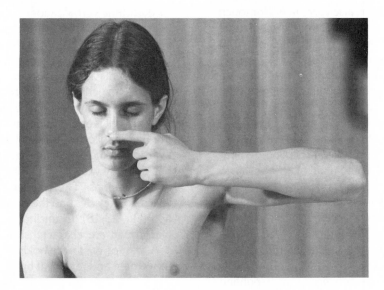

Fig. 23-19
Test of cerebellar function. The client is asked to alternately touch his nose with the tip of the index finger of each hand, repeating the motion with increasing speed.

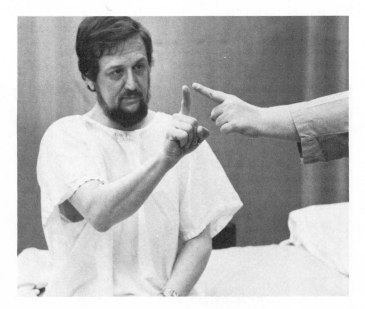

Fig. 23-20
Test of cerebellar function. The client is asked to touch the examiner's finger, which is placed about 18 inches from the client's eye.

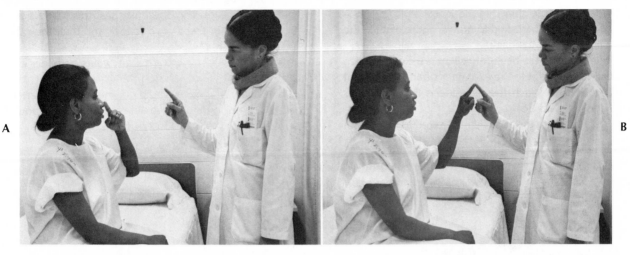

Fig. 23-21
Test of cerebellar function. **A,** The client is asked to touch her nose with an index finger and then, **B,** to touch the examiner's index finger at a distance of about 18 inches, repeating the motion with increasing speed.

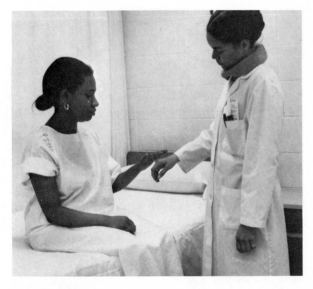

Fig. 23-22
Test of cerebellar function. The client is asked to pat the examiner's hand, progessively increasing the speed of motion.

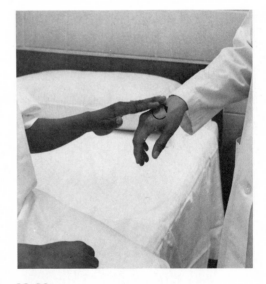

Fig. 23-23
Test of cerebellar function. The client is asked to make a polishing (circular) motion on the volar surface of the examiner's hand, progressively increasing the speed of motion.

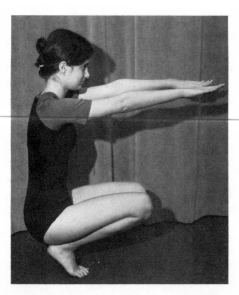

Fig. 23-30
Test of the proprioceptive system. The client is asked to do a knee bend without support.

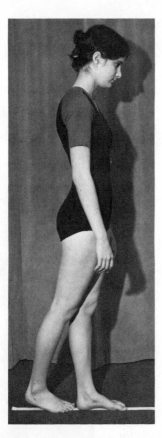

Fig. 23-31
Test of the proprioceptive system. The client is asked to walk a straight line placing heel to toe.

The client who is reasonably steady may be asked to do a knee bend from a standing position without support (Fig. 23-30).

The client is asked to walk a straight line, placing the heel of the leading foot against the toe of the other foot (Fig. 23-31).

The client is asked to pull against the resistance of the examiner's hands, and the client's hands are released without warning. The client with cerebellar disease may have difficulty in starting and stopping movement. Thus, there may be excessive after-movement or rebound, so that the client hits himself.

DEFINITIONS

decomposition of movement Movements smoothly coordinated in the normal individual are performed in several parts.

dysdiadochokinesia Disturbance in the ability to stop one movement and follow it by the opposite action, such as supination and pronation of hands.

dysmetria Disturbance in the ability to stop a movement

These definitions may be helpful in recording signs observed in cerebellar or proprioceptive dysfunction (see the boxed material below).

Comparison of disorders of the cerebellum, posterior columns, and vestibular neurons

Cerebellar dysfunction

Ataxia not made worse in darkness or with eyes closed	Dysmetria
	Dysdiadochokinesia
	Scanning speech
Clumsiness	Hypotonia
Poor coordination	Asthenia
Decomposition of movement	Tremor
	Nystagmus

Posterior column dysfunction

Ataxia made worse in darkness or with eyes closed	Astereognosis
	Loss of two-point discrimination
Positive Romberg's sign	
Inability to recognize limb position	Loss of vibratory sensation

Vestibular dysfunction

Nystagmus	
	Nausea
	Vomiting
	Ataxia

SENSORY FUNCTION

The equipment needed for sensory testing includes a cotton wisp or soft brush, a safety pin, test tubes for cold and warm water, a tuning fork, and calipers or a compass with dull points.

Although it is not necessary to evaluate sensation over the entire skin surface, stimuli should be applied strategically so that the dermatomes and major peripheral nerves are tested. A minimum number of test sites would include areas on the forehead, cheek, hand, lower arm, abdomen, foot, and lower leg.

As a general rule, the more distal area of the limb is checked first. In the screening examination the nerve may be assumed to be intact if sensation is normal at its most peripheral extent. If evidence of dysfunction is found, the site of the dysfunction must be localized and mapped. This means determining the boundaries of the loss of sensation. A lucid method of recording would include a sketch of the region involved and a description of the sensory change.

The intensity of the stimulus is kept to a minimum level on initial application. Gradual increases in magnitude may be made until the client is aware of the stimulus.

Variation in sensitivity of skin areas is seen in the normal client, so that a stronger stimulus is required over the back, the buttocks, and areas where the skin is heavily cornified. Symmetry of sensation is established by checking first one spot and then its mirror image area.

The client's eyes should be closed during evaluation of sensory modalities. The visual cuing that occurs when the client is able to see the examiner apply the stimulus may lead to false positive responses in the client who is highly sensitive to suggestion.

Spurious results to sensory testing are risked when either the client or the examiner is fatigued. Inattention to instruction or lack of motivation may lead to an impression of sensory loss.

The examiner should avoid predictable patterns in applying the stimulus. That is, the examiner should vary testing sites and timing so that the client cannot predict the response he is expected to give.

DEFINITIONS

anesthesia Absence of touch sensation.
hyperesthesia Greater than normal sensation to touch stimuli.
hypoesthesia Less than normal sensation to touch stimuli.
paresthesia Abnormal or perverted sensation; may include burning, itching, pain, or the feel of an electrical shock.

The preceding definitions may be helpful in recording sensory dysfunction.

Light touch sensation

Light touch and deep touch are mediated by different nerve endings. Sensory fibers for simple touch enter the spinal cord and travel upward before crossing to enter the anterior spinothalamic tract to the thalamus. Light touch is the sensory system that is least often obtunded. Both anterior spinothalamic tracts must suffer destruction before transmission of light touch is lost.

Light touch is tested by touching the skin with a wisp of cotton (Fig. 23-32) or a soft brush (Fig. 23-33). Pressure is applied in such a way that sensation is stimulated but not enough to perceptibly depress the skin. The client is instructed to say, "Yes," or "Now," when he feels his skin being touched. The hair of the skin should be avoided when testing for touch sensation in

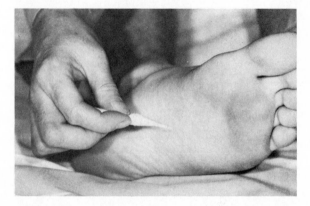

Fig. 23-32
Test of sensation of light touch using a wisp of cotton applied firmly enough to stimulate the sensory nerve endings but not so much that the skin is indented.

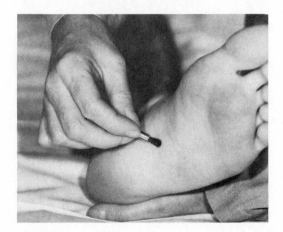

Fig. 23-33
Test of light touch sensation using a soft brush.

the skin. The follicles are innervated with sensory fibers that are stimulated by movement of the hair. Instances of distortion of sensation or anesthesia are recorded.

Tactile localization (point localization). The client is asked to point to the spot where he was touched.

Pain sensation

Pain and temperature fibers both travel in the dorsolateral fasciculus for a short distance, after which they cross and continue to the thalamus in the lateral spinothalamic tract.

Superficial pain. The evaluation of the sensory perception of superficial pain and pressure may be conducted through the use of the sharp and dull points of a safety pin (Figs. 23-34 and 23-35); however, recent studies have indicated a risk of infection with safety pins and some examiners use the hub (dull) and point (sharp) of a hypodermic needle. The client is asked to say, "Sharp," "Dull," or "Can't tell," when he feels the pin touch his skin. At least 2 seconds should be allowed between successive tests to avoid summation effects (several successive stimuli perceived as one). Pain sensation may be lost in the presence of lesions of the tegmentum of the brainstem.

Deep pressure. Deep pressure is tested over the eyeball, Achilles tendon, forearm, and calf muscles.

Temperature sensation

In the screening examination, temperature assessment need not be done when pain sensation is found to be within normal limits. When it is performed, the stimuli are tubes filled with warm and cold water that are rolled against the skin sites to be tested. The examiner tests the stimuli on his own skin to avoid burning the client and to provide a comparison. The client is asked to say, "Hot," "Cold," or "Can't tell." The tubes are applied to a sufficient number of areas to ascertain that all dermatomes are included.

Vibration sensation

The normal client is able to distinguish vibration when the base of a vibrating tuning fork is applied to a bony prominence such as the sternum, elbow, or ankle. The client perceives the vibration as a buzzing or tingling sensation.

The greatest sensitivity to vibration is seen when the tuning fork is vibrating between 200 and 400 cycles per second. A large tuning fork is suggested, since the decay of vibration occurs more slowly in the larger instrument.

After the client closes his eyes, the vibrating tuning fork may be applied to the clavicles, spinous processes, elbows, finger joints, knees, ankles, and toes (Fig. 23-36). The client is asked to say, "Yes," or "Now," (1) when he first feels the vibrations and (2) when the vibrations stop. The examiner must emphasize to the client the importance of signifying the cessation of the feeling of vibration. The examiner may damp the vibrations of the tuning fork to move along more rapidly.

Vibratory sensation is diminished in the older client (after 65 years of age), particularly in the extremities.

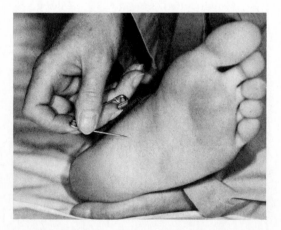

Fig. 23-34
Evaluation for superficial pain using the sharp point of a safety pin.

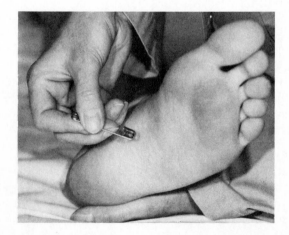

Fig. 23-35
Alternate use of the dull end of the pin for evaluation of pain.

Tactile discrimination

Tactile discrimination requires cortical integration. Three types of tactile discrimination that are tested clinically include (1) stereognosis, (2) two-point discrimination, and (3) extinction. Afferent fibers for vibration, proprioception, and stereognosis are found to take one of three courses after entering the spinal cord: they (1)

synapse immediately with motor cells to form a reflex arc, (2) run superiorly in the dorsal column to the cerebellum, or (3) travel in dorsal columns to the medulla and cross-run to the thalamus.

Stereognosis. Stereognosis is the act of recognizing objects on the basis of touching and manipulating them. This is a function of the parietal lobes of the cerebral cortex. Objects used to test stereognosis should be universally familiar items, such as a key or coin (Fig. 23-37).

Two-point discrimination. Two-point discrimination is defined as the ability to sense whether one or two areas of the skin are being stimulated by pressure. This may be done with pins. One pin is held in each hand and both are applied to the skin simultaneously. The client is asked if he feels one or two pinpricks. This determination may also be accomplished using calipers or a compass with dull points (Fig. 23-38).

In the adult client there is considerable variability of perceptual ability over the different parts of the body. The following are minimum distances between the two points of the calipers at which the normal adult is capable of sensing simultaneous stimulation:

Tongue: 1 mm
Fingertips: 2.8 mm
Toes: 3 to 8 mm
Palms of hands: 8 to 12 mm
Chest, forearms: 40 mm
Back: 40 to 70 mm
Upper arms, thighs: 75 mm

Extinction. The normal client, when touched in corresponding areas on both sides of the body, perceives touch in both areas. The failure to perceive touch on one side is called the extinction phenomenon. Impairment of the extinction phenomenon is frequently noted in lesions of the sensory cortex.

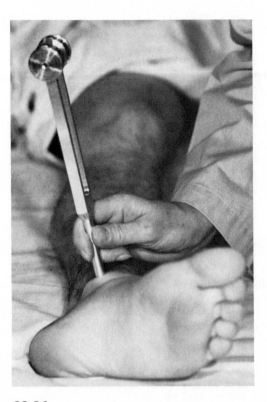

Fig. 23-36
Test of sensitivity to vibration. The base of the vibrating tuning fork is applied to bony prominences such as the sternum, elbow, or ankle.

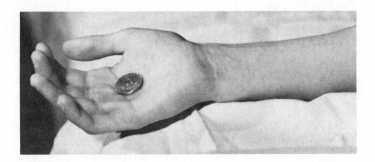

Fig. 23-37
Test for stereognosis. The normal client can discriminate a familiar object (coin, key) by touching and manipulating it.

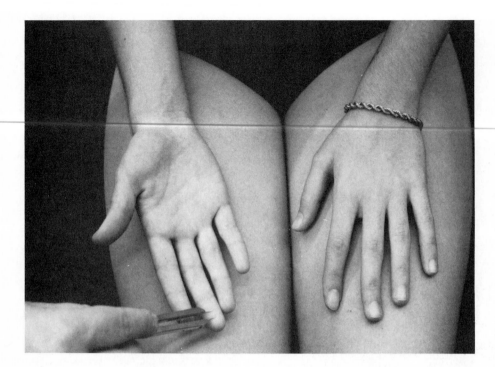

Fig. 23-38
Test for two-point discrimination.

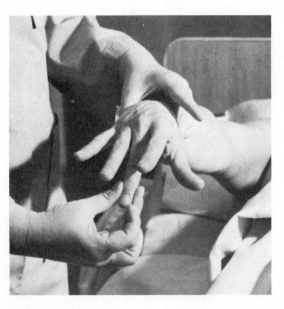

Fig. 23-39
Test of kinesthetic sensation. The normal client can discriminate the position of his body parts. With the client's eyes closed, the examiner changes the position of a finger. The client describes how the position was changed.

Kinesthetic sensation (position awareness)

Kinesthetic sensation is that facilitated by proprioceptive receptors in the muscles, tendons, and joints. Perception of the position, orientation, and motion of limbs and body parts is obtained from kinesthetic sensations.

With the client's eyes closed and the joint in a neutral position, the examiner changes the position of one finger of the client's hand. It is important that the joint be held at the lateral aspect. The client is asked to describe how the position of the finger was changed. The finger is always moved to a neutral position before it is moved again (Fig. 23-39). This procedure may be done for any joint.

Graphesthesia

The normal client can discern the identity of letters or numbers inscribed on the palm of the hand, back, or other areas with a blunt object.

Patterns of sensory loss

Loss of discriminatory sensation may indicate a lesion of the posterior columns or sensory cortex. Bilateral sensory loss in both lower extremities suggests a peripheral neuropathy, such as diabetic neuropathy. Often the pattern of sensory loss is useful in establishing a diagnosis. Some common patterns of sensory deficit are described in Table 23-2.

Sensory loss resulting from disease in a single peripheral nerve may be mapped over the skin surface distribution of that nerve. The nerves most commonly

Table 23-2

Patterns of sensory loss

Pathological involvement	Common cause	Characteristics
Peripheral nerve	Metabolic disorders, such as diabetes or nutritional deficiencies	Peripheral structures more frequently involved—"glove and stocking" involvement—may involve all sensory modalities
Specific peripheral nerve or root	Trauma Vascular occlusion	May map area of sensory loss specific to area innervated by the nerve and distal to the pathological lesion
Dorsal root		Loss of sensation in the segmented distribution (dermatome)
Spinal cord—hemisection (Brown-Séquard's syndrome)	Trauma Medullary lesion Extramedullary lesion	Loss of pain and temperature perception on contralateral side, one or two segments below the lesion Loss of position sense, two-point discrimination, and vibratory sensation on ipsilateral side below the lesion
Brainstem	Trauma Neoplasm Vascular occlusion	Loss of pain and temperature sensation on contralateral side of body, ipsilateral side of face
Thalamus	Trauma Neoplasm Vascular occlusion	Loss of sensory modalities on contralateral side of body
Cortex—lesions of post-cortical cortex	Trauma Neoplasm Vascular occlusion	Loss of discriminatory sensation on contralateral side of body Loss of position sense, two-point discrimination, or stereognosis

involved in disease include the medial, radial, ulnar, sciatic, femoral, and peroneal nerves. The examiner should be knowledgeable of the sensory, motor, and reflex distribution of these and other major nerves (Fig. 23-40). Body surface projections of the major nerves are seen in Fig. 23-41.

Pathophysiological conditions involving the dorsal root may result in sensory loss distributed over the dermatome for that root (Fig. 23-42). Clear description of sensory loss for a given segment may be difficult to obtain, since a good deal of sensory overlap occurs between the distribution of one root and another.

Both nerve and root sensory loss may result from disease involving a plexus. This phenomenon is frequently observed for the brachial plexus. Superior brachial plexus lesions involve C5 and C6, resulting in sensory loss in the shoulder and in the lateral arm and forearm. In addition, there may be weakness of the shoulder muscles. Inferior brachial plexus lesions involve C8 and T1, resulting in sensory loss of the medial surface of the arm and in weakness of the arm muscles.

Text continued on p. 562.

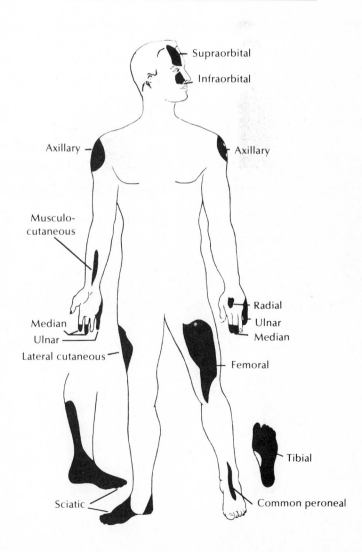

Fig. 23-40

Areas of sensory loss from peripheral nerve lesions. (From Prior, J.A., and Silberstein, J.S.: Physical diagnosis: the history and examination of the patient, ed. 4, St. Louis, 1973, The C.V. Mosby Co.)

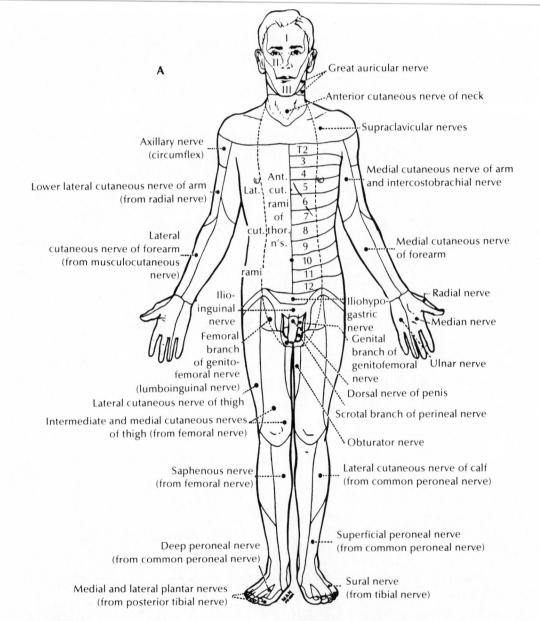

Fig. 23-41
Cutaneous fields of peripheral nerves from the anterior (**A**) and posterior (**B**) aspects. (From Haymaker, W., and Woodhall, B.: Peripheral nerve injuries, ed. 2, Philadelphia, 1959, W.B. Saunders Co.)

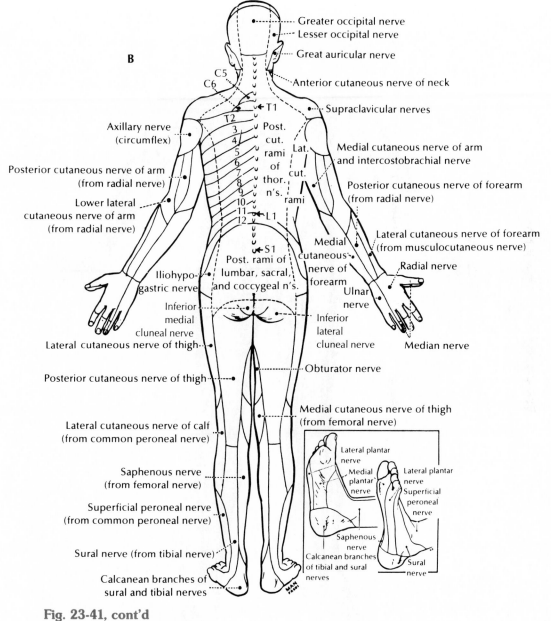

B

Greater occipital nerve
Lesser occipital nerve
Great auricular nerve
C5
C6
Anterior cutaneous nerve of neck
T1
Supraclavicular nerves
Axillary nerve
(circumflex)
T2
3
4
5
6
7
8
9
10
11
12
Post. cut. rami of thor. n's.
Lat. cut. rami
Medial cutaneous nerve of arm
and intercostobrachial nerve
Posterior cutaneous nerve of arm
(from radial nerve)
Posterior cutaneous nerve of forearm
(from radial nerve)
Lower lateral
cutaneous nerve of arm
(from radial nerve)
L1
Lateral cutaneous nerve of forearm
(from musculocutaneous nerve)
S1
Medial
cutaneous
nerve of
forearm
Radial nerve
Post. rami of
lumbar, sacral,
and coccygeal n's.
Iliohypo-
gastric nerve
Ulnar
nerve
Inferior
medial
cluneal nerve
Inferior
lateral
cluneal nerve
Median nerve
Lateral cutaneous nerve of thigh
Posterior cutaneous nerve of thigh
Obturator nerve
Medial cutaneous nerve of thigh
(from femoral nerve)
Lateral cutaneous nerve of calf
(from common peroneal nerve)
Lateral plantar
nerve
Medial
plantar
nerve
Lateral plantar
nerve
Superficial
peroneal
nerve
Saphenous nerve
(from femoral nerve)
Superficial peroneal nerve
(from common peroneal nerve)
Saphenous
nerve
Sural
nerve
Sural nerve (from tibial nerve)
Calcanean branches
of tibial and sural
nerves
Calcanean branches of
sural and tibial nerves

Fig. 23-41, cont'd
For legend see opposite page.

Pathophysiological conditions of the thalamocortical fibers on the cortex result in a loss of those cortical integrating functions (kinesthesia, two-point discrimination, stereognosis). Cortical mapping of the brain is seen in Fig. 23-43; the cortical integrating center for peripheral sensory phenomena is in the postcentral gyrus. Gross perceptions of vibration, pain, temperature, and crude touch may be retained.

The degree of awareness of the client is often recorded in relation to the manner in which he reacts to external stimuli according to the following: alert, cooperative, orientation intact, responds to spoken

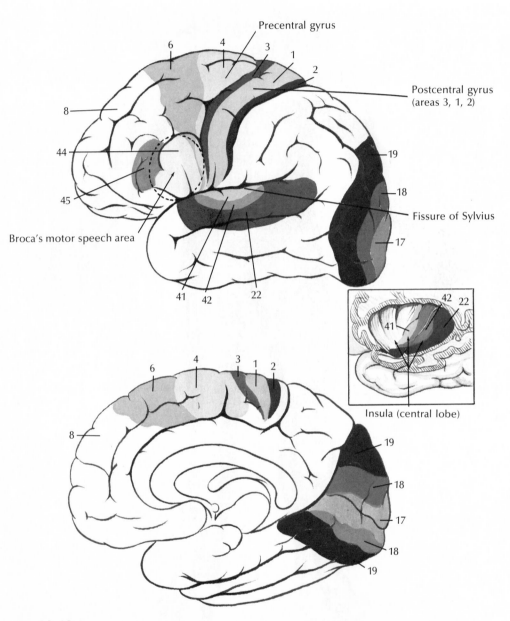

Fig. 23-43

Map of the human cortex. Identity of each numbered area is determined by structural differences in the neurons that compose it. Some areas whose functions are best understood are the following: areas *3, 1,* and *2,* somatic sensory areas; area *4,* primary motor area; area *6,* secondary motor area; area *17,* primary visual area; areas *18* and *19,* secondary visual areas; areas *41* and *42,* primary auditory areas; area *22,* secondary auditory area. Area *44* and the posterior part of area *45* constitute the approximate location of Broca's motor speech area. (From Anthony, C.P., and Kolthoff, N.J.: Textbook of anatomy and physiology, ed. 9, St. Louis, 1975, The C.V. Mosby Co. Modified from Brodmann, K.: Feinere Anatomie des Grosshirns. In Handbuch der Neurologie, Berlin, 1910, Springer-Verlag.)

words and commands, responds to tactile stimuli, responds to painful stimuli, does not respond to stimuli.

REFLEXES
Deep tendon reflex

The skeletal muscles contract when they are stretched by contraction of the antagonistic muscle, by the pull of gravity, or by external manipulation. The muscles will also contract when their tendons are stretched. These principles form the basis for an understanding of the deep tendon reflex (DTR). Afferent fibers for the reflex arise from both the muscle itself and the tendon.

Muscle spindles or fusiform capsules have been identified in abundance in skeletal muscles, particularly in antigravity muscles. The spindles are capsules surrounding two to ten specialized muscle cells known as intrafusal fibers; these spindles are parallel with surrounding muscles and are attached to them by connective tissue. Both ends of the intrafusal fiber consist of striated contractile tissue, whereas the central portion, the nuclear bag, is expanded and nucleated. These bags are innervated, but primary afferent fibers are stimulated to carry impulses when the bag is stretched or otherwise deformed. On reaching the spinal cord, these action potentials activate the alpha motor neurons. The alpha motor neurons terminate at the endplates of the skeletal muscle and stimulate their contraction (Fig. 23-44).

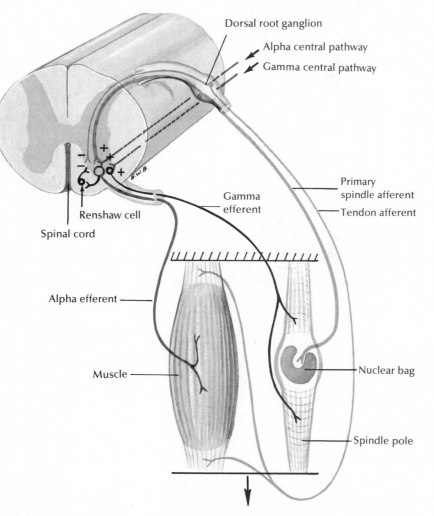

Fig. 23-44

Neural basis for the stretch reflex. Afferent fibers from muscle spindle and tendon organs and efferent fibers to muscle and spindle (gamma fibers) are shown. Excitation is indicated by plus signs, inhibition by minus signs. The Renshaw cell is an interneuron that provides recurrent inhibition to the active motoneuron pool. Muscle is rigidly fixed at the upper end and subject to stretch in the direction of the arrow at the lower end. (From Schottelius, B.A., and Schottelius, D.D.: Textbook of physiology, ed. 18, St. Louis, 1978, The C.V. Mosby Co.)

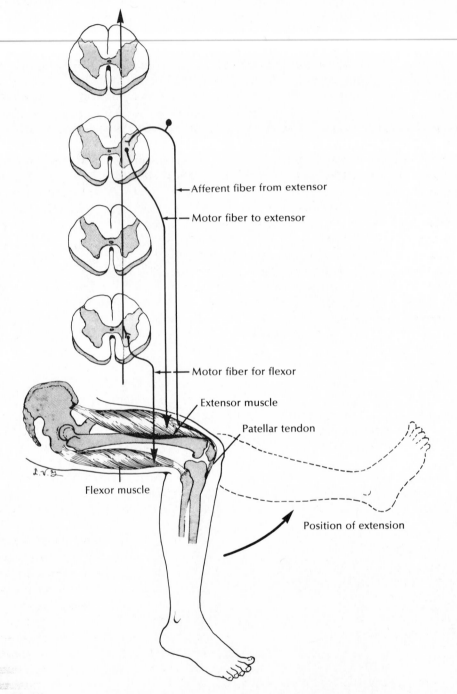

Afferent fiber from extensor

Motor fiber to extensor

Motor fiber for flexor

Extensor muscle

Patellar tendon

Flexor muscle

Position of extension

Fig. 23-45
Tendon reflex (knee jerk or patellar tendon reflex). Note that the patellar tendon of the extensor muscle is attached to the tibia below the knee. (From Schottelius, B.A., and Schottelius, D.D.: Textbook of physiology, ed. 18, St. Louis, 1978, The C.V. Mosby Co.)

Afferent nerve fibers (gamma afferent fibers) encased in a fibrous capsule are called Golgi tendon organs or tendon end organs and are found in the tendons of skeletal muscles. Stretching of the muscle deforms and activates these afferent nerves, which end on and inhibit the alpha motor neurons. The threshold for activation of the Golgi organs is significantly greater than that of the muscle spindles, and these organs are thought to modulate excessive stretching through inhibition of the muscle spindle (autoinhibition).

Another cell that may inhibit reflex contraction of a muscle is the Renshaw cell, an interneuron between axons of motor nerves. The full nature of this inhibition is not understood.

Golgi efferent nerves terminate in the muscle spindles and may regulate their sensitivity.

Fig. 23-45 illustrates the tendon reflex, using patellar tendon reflex as an example. The patellar tendon of the quadriceps muscle, an extensor muscle of the upper leg, is attached to the tibia. Deforming this tendon with a reflex hammer causes the muscle to be stretched, activating the muscle spindles, and thereby the primary afferent nerve, in terminating on the alpha motor nerve in the cord segment (L3 and L4). The action potential thus stimulates the alpha efferent fibers, resulting in shortening of the quadriceps muscle,

which pulls up the tibia to extend the leg. Dysfunction of the tendon reflex, then, could be attributed to lesions of the afferent or efferent arc of the nerve or to lesions of the muscle, tendon, or spinal segment involved.

Assessment of the DTRs allows the examiner to obtain information about the function of the reflex arcs and spinal cord segments without implicating other cord segments or higher neural structures.

Reflexes may be altered in pathophysiological changes involving the sensory pathways from the tendons and muscles or the motor component, that is, the corticospinal or corticobulbar pathways (upper motor neuron), or the anterior horn cells or their axons (lower motor neuron).

The best muscle contraction is obtained in testing deep muscle tendons when the muscle is slightly stretched before the tendon is stretched (tapped with the reflex hammer).

Augmentation of the reflex may be obtained by isometrically tensing muscles not directly involved in the reflex arc being tested. For example, the client may be asked to clench the fists or to lock the fingers together and pull one hand against the other (Jendrassik's maneuver) (Fig. 23-46) as the examiner attempts to elicit reflexes in the lower extremity. To reinforce the reflex arcs of the upper extremities, the client may be asked to clench the jaws or to set the quadriceps.

Elicitation of reflexes

Three categories of reflexes are described: (1) DTRs, elicited by deforming (tapping) a tendon (synonyms are muscle stretch reflexes, muscle jerks, and tendon jerks); (2) superficial or cutaneous reflexes, obtained by stimulating the skin; and (3) pathological reflexes, which are usually present only in disease.

Reflexes may be graded for the record as follows:

4^+ or $++++$	Brisk, hyperactive, clonus of tendon associated with disease
3^+ or $+++$	More brisk than normal, not necessarily indicative of disease
2^+ or $++$	Normal
1^+ or $+$	Low normal, slightly diminished response
0	No response

The symmetry of the reflex from one side of the body to the other is also recorded. Differences in response on one side of the body may be helpful in locating the site of the lesions.

A succinct method of recording the reflex findings is the stick figure representation (Fig. 23-47). This expresses both amplitude and symmetry well.

Jaw closure reflex. The maxillary reflex, or jaw jerk, is elicited by tapping; the examiner's thumb is placed on the midline of the client's chin but below the lip,

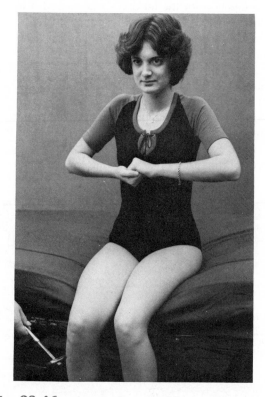

Fig. 23-46
Augmentation maneuver for deep tendon reflexes.

8. Medications taken regularly
   a. By practitioner's prescription
   b. By self-prescription

Developmental data

The assessment of the development of the child is discussed in Chapter 4, "Developmental Assessment." The history of the child's development is a component of that assessment and should provide clues that indicate when a more formal assessment is indicated. The initial history should include the following:

1. The age at which the child attained specific developmental achievements
   a. Held head erect
   b. Rolled over
   c. Sat alone
   d. Walked alone
   e. Said first words
   f. Used sentences
   g. Controlled feces
   h. Learned urinary continence
2. A comparison of this child's development with siblings or other children his age
3. Any periods of decreased or increased growth
4. Questions regarding school achievement are included in the review of systems but may be appropriate to incorporate into the developmental assessment if early delays have been noted.

Table 24-3
Recommended immunization schedules for infants and children not initially immunized at usual recommended times in early infancy

Timing	Preferred schedule	Recommended schedules			Comments
		Alternatives			
		#1	#2	#3	
First visit	DTP #1, OPV #1, Tuberculin test (PPD)	MMR, PPD	DTP #1, OPV #1, PPD	DTP #1, OPV #1, MMR, PPD	MMR should be given no younger than 15 mo old.
1 mo after first visit	MMR	DTP #1, OPV #1	MMR, DTP #2	DTP #2	
2 mo after first visit	DTP #2, OPV #2	—	DTP #3, OPV #2	DTP #3, OPV #2	—
3 mo after first visit	(DTP #3)	DTP #2, OPV #2	—	—	In preferred schedule, DTP #3 can be given if OPV #3 is not to be given until 10-16 mo.
4 mo after first visit	DTP #3 (OPV #3)	—	(OPV #3)	(OPV #3)	OPV #3 optional for areas for likely importation of polio (e.g., some southwestern states).
5 mo after first visit	—	DTP #3, (OPV #3)	—	—	
10-16 mo after last dose	DTP #4, OPV #3, or OPV #4	DTP #4, OPV #3, or OPV #4	DTP #4, OPV #3, or OPV #4	DTP #4, OPV #3, or OPV #4	—
Preschool	DTP #5, OPV #4, or OPV #5	DTP #5, OPV #4, or OPV #5	DTP #5, OPV #4, or OPV #5	DTP #5, OPV #4, or OPV #5	Preschool dose not necessary if DTP #4 or #5 given after fourth birthday.
14-16 yr old	Td	Td	Td	Td	Repeat every 10 yr.

From American Academy of Pediatrics: Report of the Committee on Infectious Diseases, ed. 19, Evanston, Ill., 1982.
Alternative #1 can be used in those more than 15 months old if measles is occurring in the community.
Alternative #2 allows for more rapid DTP immunization.
Alternative #3 should be reserved for those whose access to medical care is compromised by poor compliance.
DTP, Diphtheria and tetanus toxoids with pertussis vaccine.
OPV, Oral, attenuated poliovirus vaccine contains types 1, 2, and 3.
Tuberculin test, Mantoux (intradermal PPD) preferred. Frequency of tests depends on local epidemiology. The Committee recommends annual or biennial testing unless local circumstances dictate less frequent or no testing.
MMR, Live measles, mumps, and rubella viruses in a combined vaccine.
Td, Adult tetanus toxoid (full dose) and diphtheria toxoid (reduced dose) in combination.
For all products used, consult manufacturer's brochure for instructions for storage, handling, and administration. Biologics prepared by different manufacturers may vary, and those of the same manufacturer may change from time to time. The package insert should be followed for a specific product.

Nutritional data

The questions regarding nutrition will vary depending on the age of the child. The information obtained for the infant, who is growing rapidly, is usually more detailed and specific than the history obtained for the older child.

I. Early infancy
  A. The type of feeding (breastfeeding, commercial formula, or home-prepared formula)
  B. Frequency of feedings
  C. Amount consumed with each feeding and during a 24-hour period
  D. Any changes in feeding (such as from breastfeeding to bottle feeding and time of change)
  E. Any problems observed with feeding (such as colic or spitting)
  F. How long does mother plan to continue breastfeeding or bottle feeding
  G. Vitamin, iron, or fluoride supplements (including the name of the preparation, when it was started, the amount given, and the method of administration)
  H. Solid foods (including the type—commercially prepared or home prepared, the amount given, how they are given—by spoon or in bottle, and the frequency)
  I. Water (including the amount given, frequency offered, given plain or with a sweetener)
  J. Infant's appetite and his reaction to eating

  If the infant is breastfeeding additional questions about the mother need to be asked:
  1. How the mother cares for her breasts
  2. Her program of daily exercise, rest, and diet
  3. Medications being taken (specify name, frequency, purpose, and effectiveness) (The boxed material below provides a list of drugs that are known to be excreted in human milk and to have side effects in breastfed infants.)
  4. The mother's feelings about breastfeeding
  5. The support she receives from family members

  If the infant is receiving bottle feedings, it is important to learn if he is held for all feedings. The baby who receives a bottle of milk

---

Examples of medicants, foods, and sundries that are excreted in breast milk and may affect infants

Analgesics
  Codeine in habituated doses
  Heroin in habituated doses
  Meperidine in habituated doses
  Morphine in habituated doses
  Propoxyphene in IV
  Sodium salicylate in high doses
Antihistamines
Antimicrobials
  Ampicillin
  Chloramphenicol
  Penicillin
  Sulfonamides
  Tetracyclines
Depressants
  Barbiturates
    Long-acting, hypnotic doses
    Short-acting, hypnotic doses
  Others
    Alcohol
    Bromides, hypnotic doses
    Chloral hydrate
    Diazepam
    Reserpine

Diuretics
  Hydrochlorothiazide, chlorothiazide
Hormonal compounds
  Iodides
  Oral contraceptives
  Pregnane beta-diol
  Propylthiouracil
  Thyroid
Anthraquinone derivatives
  Cascara
  Danthron
Social drugs (legal)
  Caffeine
  Tobacco
Social drugs (illegal)
  Abuse drugs: stimulants, depressants, narcotics, psychedelics in high doses
Miscellaneous
  Anticoagulants, oral
  DDT
  Ergotrate maleate
  Fluorides
  Foods: white navy beans, corn, egg white, chocolate, unripe fruit, pickles, peanuts, cottonseed, and wheat

Data from Levin, R.: In Herfindal, E.T., and Hirschman, J., editors: Clinical pharmacy and therapeutics, Baltimore, 1975, Williams & Wilkins.

Table 24-4
Average heart rate for infants and children at rest

Age	Average rate
Birth	140
1st mo	130
1-6 mo	130
6-12 mo	115
1-2 yr	110
2-4 yr	105
6-10 yr	95
10-14 yr	85
14-18 yr	82

Table 24-5
Amplitude, quality of the heart rate, and site, as they relate to differential diagnosis of heart dysfunction in young infants and children

Amplitude, quality, site	Cardiac dysfunction
Narrow, thready	Congestive heart failure Severe aortic stenosis
Bounding	Patent ductus arteriosus Aortic regurgitation
Pulsation in suprasternal notch	Aortic insufficiency Patent ductus arteriosus Coarctation of the aorta
Palpable thrill in suprasternal notch	Aortic stenosis Valvular pulmonary stenosis Coarctation of the aorta, occasionally patent ductus arteriosus

Data from Kempe, C.H., and others: Current pediatric diagnosis and treatment, ed. 5, Los Altos, Calif., 1978, Lange Medical Publications.

Table 24-6
Variations in respiration with age

Age	Rate/minute
Premature	40-90
Newborn	30-80
1 yr	20-40
2 yr	20-30
3 yr	20-30
5 yr	20-25
10 yr	17-22
15 yr	15-20
20 yr	15-20

Data from Lowrey, G.H.: Growth and development of children, Chicago, 1978, Year Book Medical Publications, Inc.

include noting that the column of mercury is rising steadily, inserting no more than ½ inch, and observing a decrease in the child's effort to push against the thermometer. It is normal for the child to push against the thermometer as the rectal sphincter muscles contract in response to the stimulus. The practitioner waits until the sphincter relaxes before continuing to insert. The thermometer is held firmly enough to keep the child from pushing it out. Care must be taken to hold the thermometer firmly but not to push it in further. Also, the child must be held securely to prevent jerking and pushing the thermometer further into the rectum.

Obtaining an oral temperature reading is usually reserved for children who are 5 to 6 years of age and older. The child must be able to understand not to bite on the glass thermometer and to keep his mouth closed during the procedure. Sometimes, the child's health condition interferes with being able to use this method, for example, mouth breathing or limited intellectual functioning.

An axillary temperature can be obtained on any child and reduces the risk of injury and is less intrusive. It can be done when the child objects to the rectal temperature and the oral temperature is not appropriate. The thermometer is placed in the axilla and the arm held close to the body. The child can be restrained by using the "hug" if necessary.

Temperature regulation is less exact in children than adults. The rectal temperature is normally higher in infants and young children, and the average temperature is above 99° F (37.2° C) until the age of 3 years. The increase in temperature with even a minor infection is usually greater in infants and young children than in adults. However, young infants with a severe infection may have a normal or subnormal temperature.

Pulse and respiration. Apprehension, crying, and physical activity, as well as the examination procedure itself, can alter a child's heart and respiratory rates. Thus, it is desirable to take these measurements while the child is at rest, either sleeping or lying quietly. If the child has been active, the measurement is delayed until the child has relaxed about 5 to 10 minutes.

The child's pulse is to be examined for rate, rhythm, quality, and amplitude, just as in an adult. Auscultation of the heart—measuring the apical pulse—is the most easily obtained pulse in a young infant. The average heart rate of the infant at birth is 140 beats per minute. At 2 years of age the child's heart has adjusted downward to 110. At 10 years the rate is 85, and by the time the child reaches age 18, his pulse may be observed to have lowered to 82. A child, usually an adolescent, who engages in exercise regularly, such as swimming laps, may exhibit a much slower rate, that is, in the 60s.

Table 24-4 lists the average heart rates for children from birth to 18 years. Heart rhythm in children is not always regular. Often it reflects the phasic action of the heart in relation to the respiratory cycle. This is called sinus arrhythmia, and it is considered normal in children.

Palpation of the brachial and the femoral pulses is an essential step in the examination of the young infant. Irregularities often are the first signs of serious heart dysfunction. The amplitude and time of appearance of the femoral pulse are expected to equal those of the brachial pulse. Absence or weakness of the femoral pulse alerts the examiner to the possibility of coarctation of the aorta in the young infant. Table 24-5 compares some differences in amplitude, quality, and site and how they may relate to the differential diagnosis of heart disorders in children.

The respiratory rate may be obtained by inspection and/or auscultation. The average range of normal respirations is 30 to 80 per minute in the newborn period as compared with 20 to 30 in the 2-year-old. By 10 years of age the rate has adjusted to 17 to 22, and by age 20 it averages 15 to 20 respirations per minute. Table 24-6 exhibits variations in respiration with age.

Blood pressure. The levels of systolic and diastolic blood pressure gradually increase during childhood, and there is normally a considerable variation in a child's pressure. The systolic pressure of the child may be raised by crying, vigorous exercise, or anxiety. It is therefore appropriate to choose a time when the child is quiet and comfortable to obtain this measurement.

The National Task Force on Blood Pressure Control in Children has recommended that children 3 years of age or older should have their blood pressure measured annually as part of their regular health care. The child of this age is usually able to cooperate when the procedure for obtaining a blood pressure measurement is explained to him. The blood pressure of the child under 3 years of age is not routinely measured unless there are indications of underlying problems such as renal or cardiac disease.

The most common method of measuring the blood pressure of the child is still auscultation using a mercury or aneroid sphygmomanometer. The selection of the cuff size and the method of measuring the blood pressure are described in Chapter 7, "General Assessment, Including Vital Signs." Pediatric cuffs can be obtained in several sizes for newborns, infants, and children. A pediatric stethoscope with a small diaphragm is also essential when measuring the blood pressure of a young child. The systolic pressure is recorded as that point at which the Korotkoff sounds are initially heard. The diastolic pressure is recorded for the point at which the fourth phase Korotkoff sound is heard, when the

sound first becomes muffled. In young children the fourth and fifth sounds frequently occur simultaneously, and sometimes the Korotkoff sounds are heard all the way to zero.

The Doppler instrument, although relatively expensive, is useful with young infants and children. Infants are often intrigued by the audible sounds that the Doppler emits and become happily excited. The Doppler measures systolic blood pressure, which is the first sound heard. The reliability for accurate diastolic pressure measurement has not yet been documented.

The flush method is used with the young infant or child when a Doppler is not available and provides only a measure of mean pressure. This method is described in Chapter 7, "General Assessment, Including Vital Signs."

The blood pressure measurements obtained should be recorded on appropriate blood pressure charts such as those developed by the National Task Force on Blood Pressure Control in Children (Figs. 24-6 and 24-7) that were based on studies supported by the National Heart, Lung and Blood Institute. They allow the examiner to record the blood pressure measurements in serial fashion, determine how this child compares with other children his age, and observe a trend or pattern for this child over a period of time.

Growth measurements

The routine measurement of growth is a screening procedure rather than a diagnostic procedure. Growth is a continuous process that needs to be evaluated over time. Successive, serial measurements plotted on a standardized growth chart provide objective information about the individual child's rate and pattern of growth as compared with the general population. The information obtained is useful in providing reassurance to parents and professionals regarding the child who is growing normally, assessing the nutritional status of the child, and identifying the child who may have abnormalities affecting the various growth parameters.

The three parameters of growth routinely measured during each examination of the child under 3 years of age are recumbent length, body weight, and head circumference. For the child over 3 years of age it is sufficient to obtain standing height and weight measurements only. Assessment of body segments, skinfold thickness, bone age, and dentition may be used for further study of body growth but are not usually included in the routine physical examination.

The growth charts published by the National Center for Health Statistics (NCHS) in 1976 should be used to record growth measurements (see Fig. 24-29). They

Areas of assessment
General inspection

The survey or general inspection is discussed in Chapter 7, "General Assessment, Including Vital Signs." The general inspection of the child includes the many observations described in Chapter 7. The examiner also needs to keep in mind those physical and behavioral characteristics that are expected for the individual child at his present chronological age. Chapter 4, "Developmental assessment," describes normal physical and behavioral changes that occur during the development of the child.

Some of the physical changes to be observed are the normal changes in facies, posture, and body contour (Fig. 24-12); changes in gait; and the development of secondary sex characteristics. The criteria for assessing pubertal status developed by Tanner are useful in describing the child's stage of pubertal development and are outlined as follows*:

Boys: genital (penis) development

Stage 1 Preadolescent: testes, scrotum, and penis are of about the same size and proportion as in early childhood

Stage 2 Enlargement of scrotum and testes; skin of scrotum reddens and changes in texture; little or no enlargement of penis at this stage

Stage 3 Enlargement of penis, which occurs at first mainly in length; further growth of testes and scrotum

Stage 4 Increased size of penis with growth in breadth and development of glans; testes and scrotum larger; scrotal skin darkened

Stage 5 Genitalia adult in size and shape

Girls: breast development

Stage 1 Preadolescent: elevation of papilla only

Stage 2 Breast bud stage: elevation of breast and papilla as small mound; enlargement of areolar diameter

Stage 3 Further enlargement and elevation of breast and areola, with no separation of their contours

Stage 4 Projection of areola and papilla to form a secondary mound above the level of the breast

Stage 5 Mature stage: projection of papilla only, due to recession of the areola to the general contour of the breast

Both sexes: pubic hair

Stage 1 Preadolescent: the vellus over the pubes is not further developed than that over the abdominal wall, i.e., no pubic hair

Stage 2 Sparse growth of long, slightly pigmented, downy hair, straight or slightly curled, chiefly at the base of the penis or along the labia.

Stage 3 Considerably darker, coarser, and more curled; The hair spread sparsely over the junction of the pubes

Stage 4 Hair now adult in type, but area covered is still considerably smaller than in the adult; no spread to the medial surface of thighs

---

*From Tanner, J.M.: Growth at adolescence, ed. 2, Oxford, 1962, Blackwell Scientific Publications, Inc.

Stage 5 Adult in quantity and type with distribution of the horizontal (or classically feminine pattern); spread to medial surface of thighs but not up linea alba or elsewhere above the base of the inverse triangle (Spread up linea alba occurs later and is rated Stage 6.)

Both sexes: axillary hair

Stage 1 Preadolescent: no axillary hair

Stage 2 Scanty growth of slightly pigmented hair

Stage 3 Hair adult in quality and quantity

Observations are made regarding the child's development during the examination, and the findings may indicate that a more formal assessment is indicated.

The child's behavior is also observed and described. Is this a quiet, shy child or an active, restless child? Is this child comfortable during the visit or anxious and afraid? Does the child respond to the parent or other adults in an appropriate way? Each child is uniquely himself, and it is a challenge to observe and record a description of any child's behavior. It is also necessary to keep in mind that the behavior seen during a visit for health care may not be typical for that child.

Skin

The examination of the skin provides valuable information about the general health of the child and evidence of specific skin problems. The skin of the entire body should be noted at each examination. The normal condition of the skin changes with age, and it is helpful to become familiar with those changes seen in children.

The skin of the newborn is soft, smooth, and appears almost transparent. The superficial vessels are prominent, giving the skin its red color. A mild degree of jaundice is present after the second or third day in normal infants; if the jaundice is severe or occurs in the first 24 hours, however, the examiner should consider the presence of a serious problem. Small papular patches, called nevus flammeus, may be present over the occiput, forehead, and upper eyelids in the newborn period and usually disappear by the end of the first year of life. The nose and cheeks are frequently covered by small white papules caused by plugging of the sebaceous glands during the neonatal period. Both sweat and sebaceous glands are present in the newborn but do not function until the second month of life. Some desquamation is common during the first weeks and varies in individual babies. Mongolian spots, which are blue, irregularly shaped flat areas, are found in the sacral and buttocks area of some infants, usually those who have more darkly pigmented skin. These usually disappear by the end of the first or second year but occasionally persist for a longer time. There is a considerable amount of fine hair, called lanugo, over the body of the newborn, which is lost during the first weeks of life. The nails of the full-term newborn are

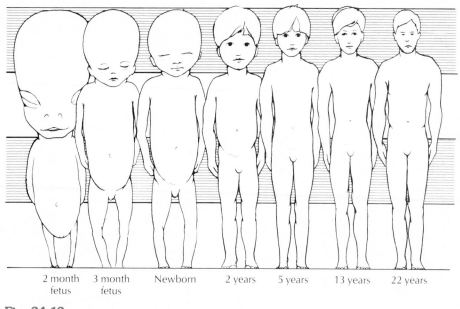

| 2 month fetus | 3 month fetus | Newborn | 2 years | 5 years | 13 years | 22 years |

Fig. 24-12
Changes in body proportions from before birth to adulthood.

well formed and firm in contrast to those of the premature infant, which are imperfectly formed.

During the first year of life there is a continuing increase in the proportion of subcutaneous fat, and raw areas resulting from skin rubbing against skin are more prevalent in young obese infants. This is called intertrigo. During the second year of life there is a decrease in the proportion of subcutaneous fat, and intertrigo is less common.

After the first year of life the normal child shows little changes in the skin until the onset of puberty, when there is considerable development of both sweat and sebaceous glands. Associated with the development of the sebaceous glands is acne vulgaris, which is so common in its mildest forms that it is sometimes considered a normal physiological change. Early evidence of acne is the occasional comedo, or blackhead, on the nose and chin. At age 13 or 14, papules and small pustules may begin to appear, and by age 16 many children will have recovered completely. There are also changes in the amount and distribution of hair. Hair growth becomes heavier; the appearance of pubic, axillary, and most of the more prominent body hair is influenced by sexual development during adolescence.

Lymph nodes

Lymph nodes in children have the same distribution as that found in adults, but the nodes are usually more prominent until the time of puberty. The amount of lymphoid tissue is considerable at birth and increases steadily until after puberty. It is common to find shotty,

discrete, movable, small, nontender nodes in the occipital, postauricular, anterior and posterior cervical, parotid, submaxillary, sublingual, axillary, epitrochlear, and inguinal areas in the normal healthy child. Lymph nodes are examined during the examination of each part of the body.

Head and neck

The shape of the newborn infant's head is often asymmetrical as a result of the molding that occurs during the passage through the birth canal, and it may be a few days or weeks before the normal shape is restored. The newborn has a skull that molds easily because the bones of the cranium are not fused, which allows some overlapping of the bones. Trauma may result in caput succedaneum or cephalohematoma. *Caput succedaneum* is an edematous swelling of the superficial tissues of the scalp that is manifested by a generalized soft swelling not bounded by suture lines. This is temporary and is usually resolved within the first few days of life. *Cephalohematoma* occurs as a result of bleeding into the periosteum and results in swelling that does not cross the suture line. Most cephalohematomas are absorbed within 2 weeks to 3 months. Flattening of the head is often seen in normal children but can also be indicative of problems such as mental retardation or rickets.

The sutures of the skull are palpated and can usually be felt as ridges until the age of 6 months. The fontanels are palpated during each examination of the infant and young child to determine the size, shape, and presence of any tenseness or bulging. Normally, the posterior fontanel closes by 2 months of age and the anterior fontanel closes by the end of the second year (Fig. 24-13). Tenseness or bulging of the fontanels is most easily detected when the child is in a sitting position and should be assessed when the child is quiet. Bulging of the fontanels is evidence of intracranial pressure. The fontanels may be depressed when the infant is dehydrated or malnourished. Early closure or delayed closure of the fontanels should be noted. Early closure may result from microcephaly and delayed closure from prolonged intracranial pressure.

The importance of measuring the head circumference of the child up to 3 years of age has already been discussed.

Transillumination of the skull is a useful procedure in the initial examination of the infant and for any infant with an abnormal head size. Transillumination is carried out in a completely darkened room with an ordinary flashlight equipped with a rubber adaptor. The light is placed against the infant's head. If the cerebrum is absent or greatly thinned, as from increased intracranial pressure, the entire cranium lights up. Often, defects transilluminate in a more limited way. Auscultation of the skull may reveal bruits, which are commonly found in normal children up to 4 years of age. After the age of 4, bruits are evidence of problems such as aneurysms or increased intracranial pressure.

The young infant's scalp is inspected for evidence of crusting, which often results from a seborrheic dermatitis.

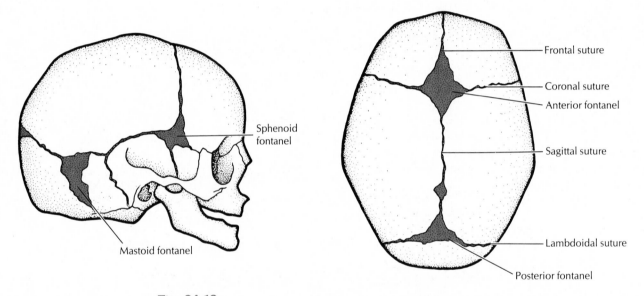

Fig. 24-13
Skull bones of the infant, showing fontanels and sutures.

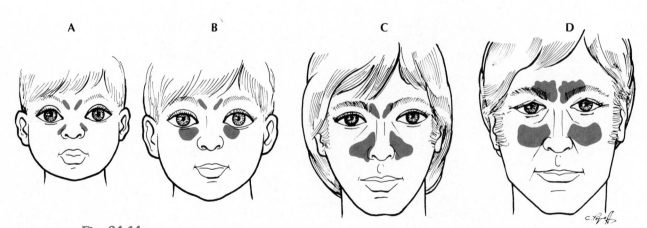

Fig. 24-14
Development of the frontal and maxillary sinuses. **A,** Early infancy. **B,** Early childhood. **C,** Adolescence. **D,** Adulthood.

The shape of the face is inspected. A facial paralysis is most easily observed when the child cries or smiles and the asymmetry is increased. An abnormal or unusual facies may indicate a chromosomal abnormality such as Down's syndrome.

The frontal and maxillary sinuses should be percussed by the direct method and palpated in the child over 2 or 3 years of age. Until that age the sinuses are too small and poorly developed for percussion or palpation (Fig. 24-14).

The submaxillary and sublingual glands are palpated in the same way as in the adult examination. Local swelling of the parotid gland is most easily determined by observing the child in the sitting position with the head raised and the neck extended and by noting any swelling below the angle of the jaw. The swollen parotid gland may be felt by palpating downward from the zygomatic arch. Unilateral or bilateral swelling of the parotid gland is usually indicative of mumps.

The neck is examined with the child lying flat on his back. The size of the neck is noted. The neck of the infant normally is short; it lengthens at about 3 or 4 years of age. The lymph nodes are palpated, as are the thyroid gland and trachea. The sternocleidomastoid muscle is carefully palpated. A mass on the lower third of the muscle may indicate a congenital torticollis. Finally, the mobility of the neck is determined by lifting the child's head and turning it from side to side. Any resistance to flexion may be indicative of meningeal irritation.

Eyes

The examination of the eyes is most easily accomplished when the child is able to cooperate. The school age child is able to participate, and the examination is carried out as described in Chapter 11 on assessment of the eyes. The infant and young child are much more of a challenge to the examiner.

Visual function at birth is limited but improves as the structures develop. Vision may be grossly tested in the very young infant by noting the pupillary response to light; this is one of the most primitive visual functions and is normally found in the newborn infant. The blink reflex is also present in normal newborns and young infants. The infant will blink his eyes when a bright light is introduced. At 5 or 6 weeks of age the child should be able to fixate and give some evidence of following a bright toy or light. At 3 or 4 months of age the infant begins to reach for objects at different distances. At 6 to 7 months of age, the infant can have a funduscopic examination performed. For children 3 to 6 years of age Snellen's E chart can be used. The child is asked to hold his fingers in the same direction as the fingers of the E (Fig. 24-15). The young child is normally farsighted and does not achieve visual acuity of 20/20 until the age of 7 years.

Tests for strabismus (squint, cross-eye), which is an imbalance of the extraocular muscles, are of importance because strabismus can lead to amblyopia exanopsia (lazy eye), a functional loss of vision in one eye that occurs when there is a disconjugate fixation. Early

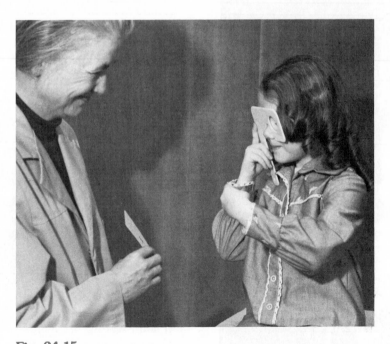

Fig. 24-15
Preparing the child for participation in testing of visual acuity.

substantial bilateral hearing loss. This loss is often associated with personality changes that may further complicate the history-taking process. Hearing loss has been shown to be associated with suspiciousness and irritability. Communication techniques that are used with the partially deaf client should include a commonly accepted vocabulary and simple, direct questions. The examiner should face the client so that the client can clearly see the lips and eyes. In cases of extreme hearing loss, electronic amplifying equipment or even an old-fashioned speaking tube may be used. Since shouting obscures the consonants and only amplifies vowels, this process should be avoided with the client who has a hearing loss. In instances where the client is totally deaf, it may be necessary to communicate entirely in writing. When the interview has to be conducted in writing, only the most pertinent questions should be asked, since this process is quite exhausting for the majority of such clients. It may be wiser to identify only that a symptom exists at the first interview and to establish other clues, such as how long and how much, at a subsequent interview.

Vision perception diminishes from the middle years onward. One of the changes that can be seen during the interview is a change in pupil size. The reduction in pupil size limits the amount of light that reaches the retina. The client may appear to have slow adaptation and a degree of blindness. These changes may be compensated by increasing the illumination without glare and by using color contrast. The client's ability to follow directions may be markedly increased by using color contrast in the furniture and walls of the room. "Sit in the yellow chair" may be an easier task than "Sit in the middle chair." If written interview forms are used, a high-wattage lamp, placed so that the light is reflected onto the page and not the client's eyes, may improve the responses that the client can make. Since light-dark adaptation occurs more slowly, the level of general illumination in examining rooms should be the same level of brightness. Differences in intensity of lighting should be avoided. Floor and table lamps should not be used; these frequently appear as spots of bright light surrounded by dark or dim spaces and are confusing to the individual with slow visual adaptation.

As previously mentioned, a sensory loss that makes the history taking of the elderly client difficult is the apparent decrease in the perception of pain. In the laboratory the aging client perceives and responds to cutaneous and visual pain-producing stimuli to a lesser degree than the healthy young adult. A more intense stimulus is required to evoke a response in the older client. Further evidence of sensory loss with aging is the lessening of hypersensitivity reactions. Thus, the aging client may not report symptoms attested to by younger individuals in the early stages of some illnesses.

Laboratory testing has shown that there is a loss of tactile perception that accompanies aging. Thus, "I don't know why I fell" may mean that the client did not feel the object under the sole of his foot that caused him to trip. Furthermore, his loss of visual acuity may have made the object difficult to see.

One of the common fallacies of thinking that must be avoided by the examiner of aging clients is that general intelligence declines as a function of advancing years. Although some of the older correlation studies would seem to support this conclusion, more recent, controlled studies deny this phenomenon. Studies performed on individuals at various time intervals in their lives (using them as their own controls) have shown an increase in intelligence test scores that continued to 55 or 60 years of age. Furthermore, there is little evidence to support the fact that a decline of intelligence occurs even after age 60 unless systemic or neurological disorders are superimposed. Impaired oxygen delivery to central nervous system structures, such as that which accompanies decreased cerebral blood perfusion, is cited as the major cause of intellectual deterioration. Thus, the examiner should interact with the aging client with respect for both the intelligence and the experience the client's years have granted him.

Although the general intelligence has been shown to remain intact, there may be an uneven decline in some of those intellectual skills thought to comprise intelligence. Problem-solving skills involving numerical manipulation, analogies, block design, and number series suffer loss starting in early adult years. However, this may be a disuse phenomenon; if so, it should be less likely to be found in individuals using these skills in their careers, such as engineers, who constantly challenge their mathematical skills. Vocabulary skills and inventories of available information show little change from early adulthood through the aging years. For some aged clients memory appears to be less efficient for recent events than for those of the distant past. This failure to relate events in the immediate past has also been correlated with the physical health of the client (particularly the temporal lobe); the older person in good health has much less of an orodeficit.

As with any individual, learning that involves the unlearning of previously held information is the most difficult type of learning for the older client. By virtue of his greater number of learning years, the client may have a good deal to unlearn during the acquisition of most new information. Thus, difficulties for the aging person in learning new tasks may be understood.

When disorders of memory or learning ability are

Plate 6

Skin changes in the elderly client.

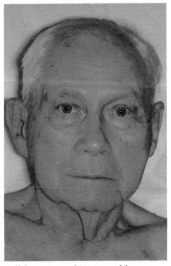

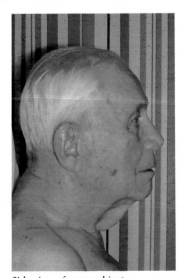

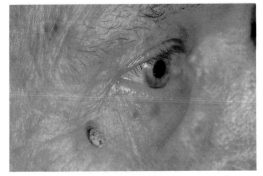

Close-up to emphasize skin wrinkling, sagging, and a prominent seborrheic keratosis.

Full face view of 84-year-old man.

Side view of same subject.

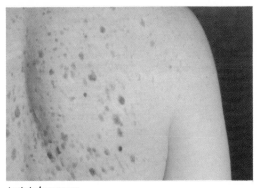

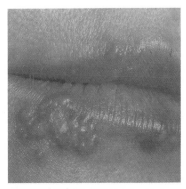

Actinic keratoses.

Herpes simplex.

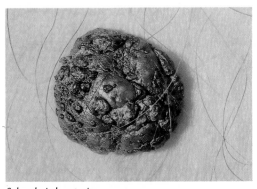

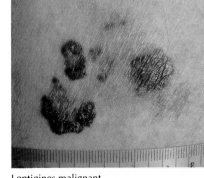

Seborrheic keratosis.

Lentigines malignant.

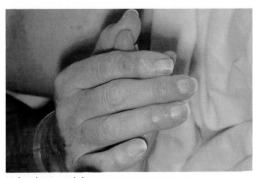

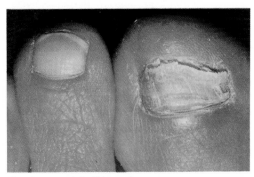

Heberdon's nodules.

Onychomycosis (nail fungus).

Pharmaceutical history

It is particularly important to assess the medicines prescribed for the older client and those nonprescription medicines he is ingesting at his own discretion. In addition to a careful drug history taken at the initial interview, a periodic review of drug intake is important to the care of the elderly client.

Many of the drugs frequently prescribed for common medical problems pose a greater danger to the aged client than to the younger adult. Mucosal irritation and bleeding of the gastrointestinal tract caused by aspirin, digitalis intoxication, bizarre or hypersensitive reactions to barbiturates, bleeding phenomena as a result of heparin, potassium depletion resulting from diuretics, and extrapyramidal symptoms resulting from phenothiazine and phenylbutazone toxicity are known to have a higher incidence in older adults. The changes in reaction to drugs may be caused by diminished central nervous system function, altered metabolism, and a reduction in elimination of drugs as a result of the functional decline of both the liver and the kidney.

Frequently, iatrogenic illness is not identified, because practitioners do not recognize symptoms as drug induced, since they are part of the stereotype of old age: slowed reaction time, confusion, disorientation, loss of memory, tremors, loss of appetite, noncompliant behavior, or anxiety.

Chronic laxative abuse is frequently seen in the elderly and may explain symptoms of potassium deficiency or general malnourishment. Tranquilizers and sleeping medications are also recognized as being frequently used by the elderly.

Just as important as the drugs that are being used are those that have been ordered by a physician and not taken. Some clients do not fill prescriptions. Other stop taking medicine because they feel better. The examiner may ask to see the containers of all drugs that are currently being taken and advise the client to bring all of his medicine with him on future visits so that the examiner may see them firsthand. This will allow the practitioner to count the pills remaining and to calculate whether they are being taken as prescribed. This may also obviate confusion from descriptions such as, "It is a little yellow one with a mark in the middle."

PHYSICAL APPRAISAL

The approach to the physical examination in the elderly is essentially identical to that performed on a client of any age. However, special techniques may be used to assure comfort and avoid rushing the elderly client. Time is invested in gaining trust. A pace is selected that is relaxed and invites the client to be comfortable. The client should feel free to establish his own pace. The examiner may need to allow more time for response to requests such as a change of position. The

examiner should note evidence of muscle weakness or lack of coordination so that assistance may be given to the client when he needs help in moving or turning.

Patience is the most helpful asset in dealing with the elderly. Valuable information may be lost because the practitioner did not wait to see the full range of response to a test. A hurried and annoyed manner of dealing with the elderly client may cause tension such that the client retreats or makes minimum attempts to comply with procedures.

The following review of examinations includes only those parameters that may differ in the aged client as compared to the younger adult.

General inspection

There is an average lifetime height loss of 2.9 cm for men and 4.9 cm for women. This change is attributed to the thinning of cartilages between bones. The decline in height begins at age 50. The 1983 Metropolitan Insurance Weights (see Appendix B) are based on data from persons 25 to 59 years old. Comparison with data from ages 70 to 90 years of age reveals that the average weights are similar to 1983 Metropolitan Insurance reference weights. However, those persons older than 90 years of age were 7% below the Metropolitan Insurance reference weights.

With loss of connective tissue, contours appear sharper and hollows are deeper, especially the orbits and axillae. Muscles appear more prominent.

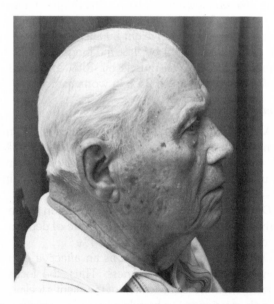

Fig. 25-2
Signs that aging changes are occurring in the individual may be observed in the skin. Please note the white, thinning, and coarse hair; sagging skin folds; wrinkling; and lentigines in this 84-year-old white man.

Because cartilage continues to be laid down in old age, the ears and nose of the elderly client may be larger and appear more prominent in relation to the face. The earlobes elongate as does the nose.

Wrinkling and relaxation (sagging) of the skin are recognized as signs of the aging process, as are the loss of pigmentation and thinning of the hair. The skin may be the source of external clues that aging changes are occurring: gray hair, sagging skin folds, wrinkling, and lentigines (Figs. 25-2 and 25-3).

The age at which graying of the hair is observed is largely influenced by genetic factors. In whites graying is observed at age 34 ±10 years. By the age of 50 one half of the population has hair that is 50% gray. Japanese men start to gray at about 30 to 34 years of age, whereas Japanese women follow about 5 years later. Blacks are observed to have the onset of graying at 44 ±10 years.

Some skin changes are known to be associated with aging. There is a flattening of the dermal-epidermal rete pegs. There is a loss of Langerhans' cells, mast cells, and blood vessels. The melanophores are fewer in number and less active. The rate of cell turnover is decreased as well. Immune function declines as androgen production declines, and the sebaceous glands decline in function. The eccrine sweat gland cells flatten and become atrophic and accumulate lipofuscin. Furthermore, the rate, volume, and sodium content of sweat are diminished.

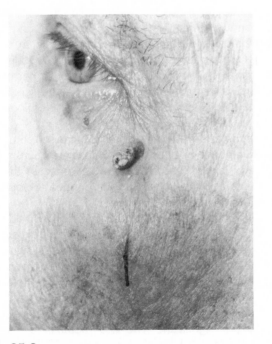

Fig. 25-3
Close-up demonstrating lentigines, hyperkeratosis, sagging of upper eyelid, and wrinkling of the skin.

Connective tissues

Connective tissue consists of two major components: ground substance made up of mucopolysaccharides in the form of a hydrated gel and fibrous proteins, collagen, elastin, and reticular fibers. These substances are synthesized by fibroblasts. Age-related changes in ground substance are seen in the increase in density of the gel and a loss of water. The volume occupied by the ground space is reduced as fiber density increases. Diffusion is impaired and cell mobility is reduced.

As tissues age, collagen fibers increase in number and in size and cross-linkage develops between fibers. The solubility of collagen is decreased, the collagen is stiffer, and the elastic property is reduced. Fibers of elastin also develop cross-linkage as they age and undergo dehydration. The fibers become more rigid and are under continued stress to fray and fragment. Reticular fibers are known to decrease with age.

As a result of these changes, the skin loses its elasticity and wrinkles. Joints become stiffened by an increase in fibrous tissue around them. Lungs lose elastic recoil. The costal cartilages become stiff. Loss of hydration from intervertebral disks results in shrinking of stature. The chambers of the heart are less distensible. The arteries become rigid, valves stiffen, and pacemaker cells may be replaced by collagen.

Skin

The skin of elderly people appears thin and translucent. Atrophy of the epidermal structures results from the degeneration of collagen and elastin. In addition there is a loss of subcutaneous fat and increased vascular fragility. The skin is dry and thick. There is a loss of skin turgor over the extremities, and, therefore, the skin of the forehead is recommended for the pinch-fold test for dehydration. The elderly have less scalp, axillary, and pubic hair, and the hair of the eyebrows and other facial hair in women becomes coarse.

Eccrine sweat gland and sebaceous gland production is diminished, and the skin is dry and flaky. As a result of the decline in melanophore activity, the skin appears pale.

Nail growth slows. Normal findings also include cherry angiomas, small red papular lessions.

For further discussion, the reader is referred to pp. 639-641.

Muscle

Muscle mass is subject to a 30% loss between the ages of 30 and 80. Muscle cells show signs of aging: an increase in lipid content and the accumulation of the insoluble pigment, lipofuscin. Muscles are hypotonic and atrophic. Muscle contours are less evident and add to a sagging appearance of the soft tissue.

A stooped posture and reduction in arm swing to

Biochemical assessment of deficient nutrients in the elderly is needed for the following nutrients:

1. Vitamin A
2. Thiamin
3. Riboflavin
4. Iron
5. Calcium
6. Pyridoxine

Mean protein intake was adequate in most dietary studies of the elderly. However, in some studies (Ten-State Nutrition Study and Hanes Survey), the mean protein intake was below the comparison standard for low income black men, black and white women, and high income women.

The elderly are at high risk for deficient dietary intake of essential nutrients and for body stores of the nutrients. The elderly are more likely than young adults to have low or deficient blood levels of serum albumin, protein, hemoglobin, as well as hematocrit.

Mucous membranes, skin, and nails. The mucous membranes, skin, and nails may provide many clues to nutritional status in the elderly. Vitamin B_6 and riboflavin deficiency may be evident in examination of the mouth. Glossitis, cheilosis, angular stomatitis, and bleeding gums may be caused by lack of vitamin B.

Vitamin C deficiency. Indicators that the client has vitamin C deficiency include irregular hairs with broken ends, poor wound healing, and ecchymoses and petechiae of the skin. Gingival tissues become edematous and erythematous and ulcerate and bleed spontaneously as a result of defective collagen formation.

Vitamin A deficiency. Dermatitis or dry, "toadlike" and follicular hyperkeratoses are associated with vitamin A deficiency. The mucous membrane of the mouth is hyperplastic and hyperkeratotic.

Iron deficiency. Koilonychia (spoon nails) are associated with iron deficiency. Generalized pallor of the oral mucosa is a prominent sign. Localized papillary atrophy of the tongue can progress to total denudation. White spots on the nail may be related to zinc deficiency. Bands across the nails may reflect protein deficiency.

Table 25-3
Drug-vitamin relationships

Drug	Nutrient absorption interference
Aspirin	Vitamin C, folate
Tetracycline	Vitamin C
Cardiac glycosides	Riboflavin
Hydralazine	Vitamin B_6
Colchicine	Vitamin B_{12}
Biguanidines	Vitamin B_{12}

Tissue maintenance and repair. The synthesis of structural proteins and enzymes by cells is dependent on protein availability. In addition, immune competence is related to protein status.

• • •

Certain drugs interfere with vitamin utilization. The drug-vitamin relationships are explained in Table 25-3.

Head and neck

Eyes. The loss of fat from the orbit causes a sunken appearance of the eyes and senile ptosis. Loss of neuromuscular stimulation and cells and loss of control of the muscles of accommodation and the iris may cause contracted, unequal pupils, and the pupillary response to light may be sluggish.

The lacrimal glands decrease in tear production with aging, so that the eyes may appear dry and lusterless. However, the lacrimal ducts may stenose and the lower lid sag so that tears flow onto the cheeks giving the impression of increased tears. Other eye changes may include arcus senilis, scleral discolorations, and diminution of pupil size. Arcus senilis is the accumulation of a lipid substance on the cornea. It characteristically appears as a grayish arc or complete circle almost at the edge of the cornea. It may be seen as a dotlike accumulation even in those individuals in their 20s or 30s. As more of the lipid is deposited, the cornea may be completely infiltrated, thickened, and even raised in appearance. The iris may frequently have pale brown discolorations. This condition occurs earlier in persons with hyperlipidemia. The cornea tends to cloud with age.

Table 25-4
Visual changes in the elderly

Visual function	Changes with aging
Lens transparency	Decreased
Acuity	Decreased
Accommodation to far object	Improved
Accommodation to near object	Decreased
Astigmatism	Corneal shape more spherical
Adaptation (light to dark)	Reduced
Color vision	Decreased; pastels discriminated less readily; color blindness worse
Flicker adaptation	Decreased
Peripheral vision	Decreased
Pupillary response	Decreased response to light changes; pupil smaller
Intraocular fluid reabsorption	Decreased; glaucoma more likely

Presbyopia. The amount the eye can alter its refractive power in focusing on a far object and a near object is called the amplitude of accommodation. When the ciliary muscle is relaxed (in viewing objects at a distance), the tension on the zonules is decreased and the lens is flattened. Contraction of the ciliary muscle (in viewing near objects) causes the muscle to shorten, the zonules are relaxed, and the tension on the capsule is relieved, allowing a near object to come into focus on the retina. The shape of the accommodated lens is determined by the lens capsule, which is thinner at the central anterior and posterior surfaces. Thus, both center lens surfaces bulge during accommodation. Added to the bulging lens with accommodation to near objects, the eyes converge and pupils constrict.

The amplitude of accommodation decreases progressively with age, a condition known as presbyopia. The reduction in near vision results from loss of elastic properties of the capsule, hardening or sclerosis of the lens substance, and weakening of the ciliary muscle. A subjective blur criterion is used for measuring the amplitude of accommodation.

At age 10 the dioptric power of the lens may be increased by about 14 diopters; by age 20 this is reduced to 11 diopters; at 40 it is about 6 diopters; and at 50 years or greater, it is less than 2 diopters (Table 25-4).

Loss of elasticity and transparency of the lens causes vision changes, requiring many aging individuals to wear corrective lenses. Normal changes in the eye may predicate changes in the eyeglasses every 3 to 5 years. The examiner should assess visual acuity with the client wearing his glasses and determine how long the client has had them (Figs. 25-4 and 25-5).

Peripheral vision is diminished in the aged. In addition, there is a decrease in the rate of dark adaptation. Sclerotic changes in the iris result in a small (miotic) and somewhat fixed pupil. Light reflexes are sluggish and accommodation is poor. Restriction of upward movement occurs with age. The aged person may have to tip the head back further and further to look up. Smooth pursuit eye movements are impaired and slowed. An elevation in the threshold for visible light perception has been noted, along with a loss of visual acuity in dim lighting. The elderly are also less able to perceive purple colors.

The number of vitreous floaters increases with age. Glaucoma ad cataracts are other problems frequently associated with aging. Surgical removal of the cataract and ocular correction will obviate the loss of vision.

The ophthalmoscopic examination reveals mildly narrowed vessels, granular pigment in the macula, drusen in the posterior pole, and a loss of bright macular and foveal reflexes. The fundus itself lacks luster and may be more yellow in appearance.

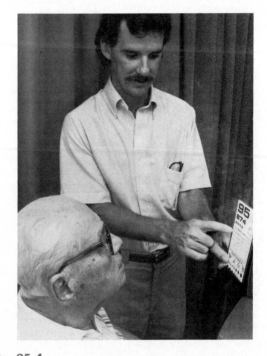

Fig. 25-4
Visual acuity testing with the Rosenbaum pocket (handheld) chart.

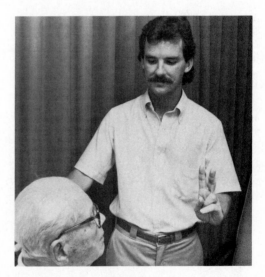

Fig. 25-5
Visual acuity testing by asking the client to identify the number of fingers extended by the examiner. The test is used only when the client is unable to identify shapes from printed materials.

Ears

Outer ear. Aging changes begin to appear in the outer ear between 30 and 50 years of age. The skin becomes dry and less resilient, and connective tissue is lost.

Hair growth may be noted along the periphery of the helix, anthelix, and tragus of the pinna. The hairs are coarse and wirelike.

The pinna increases in both length and width during the process of aging (Fig. 25-6). The skin of the ears may be dry and earlobes elongated.

The ear wax is drier among older persons, and there is a decrease in the wax-producing ceruminous glands.

Middle ear. The eardrum is more translucent and rigid. Elasticity and atrophy of muscle tissue are reduced. Calcification of ligaments and ossification and fixation of the middle ear bones have been described.

Inner ear. A degeneration of hair cells beginning in the basal part of the cochlea and extending to the apex is associated with old age deafness. The damage is associated with the organ of Corti. Typically the lesion

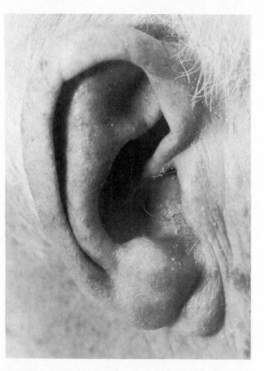

Fig. 25-6
Close-up of ear. Notice the lengthening of the earlobe, dryness of the skin, and seborrheic scaling.

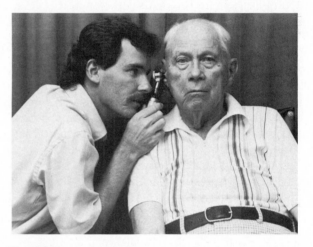

Fig. 25-7
Otoscopic examination of the ear in the elderly client.

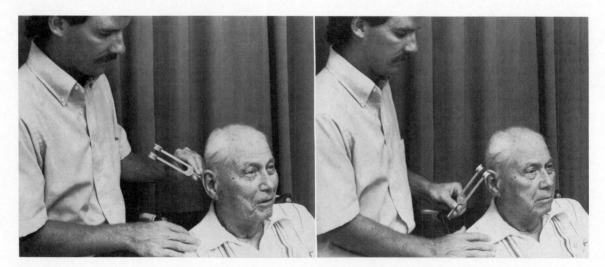

Fig. 25-8
Rinne test in the elderly client.

is confined to a few millimeters of the basal position. The reason for the loss of sensory cells is not clear (Fig. 25-7).

Lipofuscin is found in the neuronal cytoplasm of aging subjects. There are no data to support the idea that lipofuscin interferes with function. The stria vascularis is a network of capillaries that secretes endolymph and is important to the generation of the direct current potential that sensitizes the hair cells of the cochlea. Atrophy of the stria vascularis has been associated with presbycusis when no change was identified in the organ of Corti.

Atrophic changes in the spiral ligament, alterations in mass and stiffness of the basilar membrane, and modifications in middle ear mechanics may also account for aging changes in hearing.

Central mechanism of presbycusis. The inner ear transduces the mechanical vibrations of the middle ear into the electrical impulses of the auditory nerve. The characteristic of the aging central auditory system is that the brain of the older person receives the impulse (hears) but does not understand the words.

Most elderly persons have more hearing difficulties than younger adults. Over half the persons in the United States with bilateral hearing losses are 65 years or older. Hearing loss in the elderly is most frequently the result of presbycusis or otosclerosis. *Presbycusis* is the loss in perception of auditory stimuli that accompanies degenerative changes of the neural structures of the inner ear or the auditory nerve, or both. It is the most common auditory disorder in the entire population. The first symptom is the loss of high-frequency tones. Threshold increases for auditory perception at all frequencies for pure tone. The rate of impaired hearing loss (defined as elevated thresholds in the traditional

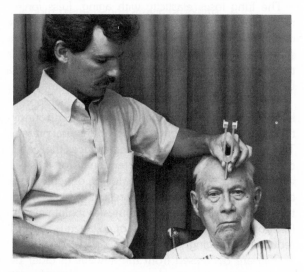

Fig. 25-9
Weber test in the elderly client.

"speech" frequencies—500, 1,000, and 2,000 Hz) increases sharply after age 65 to include 25% of the population at age 75. The average pure tone response in the speech frequencies is a relatively valid prediction of intellegibility of normal speech. This definition of impairment ignores the test tones most likely to be depressed in aging ears, notably frequencies above 2,000 Hz where speech energies of the voiceless consonants (sing, *th*in) and higher pitched environmental sounds predominate.

A mild loss of speech frequency noises may pose little problem for the older person when listening to normal, well-articulated conversation spoken in a quiet room. However, when speech is masked by environmental noise or when the talker delivers the message at a rate greater than 160 words per minute, the higher frequencies have a more important role.

Otosclerosis is a common condition of the otic capsule in which abnormally excessive bone cells are deposited. This generally results in fixation of the footplate of the stapes in the oval window; occasionally, however, the otosclerotic process may affect the cochlea, resulting in a neural deafness (Figs. 25-8 and 25-9).

Hearing loss, which affects almost all elderly people, may have severe psychological effects resulting from social isolation.

Nose. The sense of smell is markedly diminished in the older adult because of a decrease of olfactory nerve fibers and atrophy of the remaining fibers.

Mouth. Atrophy of the papillae of the lateral edges of the tongue is common in persons past age 45. There is a decline in the number of papilla and in the number of taste buds per papilla. One of the indications of loss of taste perception is that the elderly need to be exposed to eleven times the concentration of sugar required by younger clients to sense sweetness. All taste modalities (sweet, salty, sour, bitter) decline with age. However, sweet and salty tastes are lost first.

Examination of the mouth. Oral changes that accompany normal aging include tooth loss, a decrease in secretion of saliva, atrophy of the oral mucosa, atrophy of the muscles of mastication, and loss of acuity of taste.

Referral to dentist. Elderly persons have more unmet dental needs and make fewer visits to the dentist than any other age group in the United States. Tooth loss increases with age. Approximately 20% of the individuals in the 45 to 64 age group are edentulous; by age 65, 50% have no teeth, and the value reaches 60% for those older than 75 years. Tooth loss is not a normal aging process; older persons lose teeth because they have dental disease. The condition that most frequently leads to tooth loss is periodontal disease. There are several conditions that, when recog-

have been measured and may explain the elderly client's complaints of anorexia and difficulty in digesting meals.

The elderly have a higher incidence of gastrointestinal disorders. Older individuals have increased esophageal spasms and contractions and weaker activity of the lower esophageal sphincter. Dysphagia (difficulty in swallowing) is a common complaint of the elderly. Gastric acid secretion is impaired. Atrophic gastritis is more common. A decline in motility of the gastrointestinal system has been noted. The reduction in colonic motility may result in a number of dysfunctions including constipation.

Constipation is a frequent complaint. However, although a decline in the motility of the gastrointestinal tract has been proved to occur with advancing years, it has been shown that 90% of individuals over 60 years of age have at least one bowel movement a day.

Gastrointestinal bleeding in the older client. The percentage of clients with upper gastrointestinal bleeding was 48% in 1970. The mortality for persons with upper gastrointestinal bleeding is 7% to 10%.

Biliary disease in the aging client. Biliary disease affects 15% to 20% of all adults, and the incidence rises steadily with age. It is estimated that 35% to 80% of elderly persons have gallstones by age 75 with a 2:1 ratio of women to men. Some 40% of clients with gallstones have no symptoms.

Colorectal cancer. The incidence of colon cancer begins to rise significantly at the ages of 40 to 45. Some 116,000 cases of colorectal cancer are detected in the United States each year. Colon cancer discovered before symptoms develop is usually localized in the bowel wall, and the 5-year survival is greater than 85%. Most colon cancer originates from neoplastic polyps.

Liver. Liver weight is known to decrease with advancing age. A decrease in the number of liver cells has been documented, and the number of mitochondria is decreased. A reduction of liver blood flow, particularly the portal fraction, has been shown. No alteration in liver function tests has been noted. Impaired metabolism of some drugs occurs with aging.

Impaired biliary secretion has been noted. Protein synthesis is reduced.

Medications. In the management of older persons taking oral drugs, the following changes in gastrointestinal function must be considered: (1) decreased absorption; (2) decreased protein binding of the drug, since liver proteins such as albumin are decreased; (3) altered metabolism of the drug, which may be related to diminished enzyme production; (4) decreased renal excretion; (5) change in distribution; and (6) variation

in target sensitivity. The presence of side effects are carefully monitored to observe the client's response to therapy.

Endocrine system

Pituitary gland. The human pituitary gland decreases minimally in size (not more than 20%) with aging. The pituitary cells respond less to hypothalamic increasing hormones.

Antidiuretic hormone (ADH). Neurohypophyseal function has been shown to be impaired in aged rats. In the human the maximum achievable urine osmolality decreases with increasing age. The decrease in maximum urine-concentrating ability is also related to diminished ability of the kidney cells of the distal convoluted tubules and collecting ducts to respond to ADH and the decreased glomerular filtration rate that occurs with age. The development of dilutional hyponatremia following the stress of surgery in the elderly led to the theory that there is a disturbance in the release of ADH.

Prolactin. Until about age 45, prolactin levels in men are about 60% those found in women. One study has indicated that serum levels fall in women and increase in men as a result of aging.

Growth hormone. Women of normal weight and ages 20 to 30 years have greater plasma growth hormone levels than those ages 40 to 59 years. Obese women have no decline in growth hormone with age. In men no change in growth hormone levels has been noted with age. Production of growth hormone is known to be increased in hypoglycemia; some 20% of the elderly do not have this response. Surges of growth hormone known to occur during sleep in young individuals do not occur in the elderly.

Thyroid gland. Recent studies indicate a modest (not exceeding 15%) decrease of T_4 but not T_3 occurs with advancing age in healthy individuals, as well as an increase in thryroid stimulating hormone (TSH). The basal metabolic rate is known to decrease with age, but this is related to a reduction in muscle mass. The prevalence of thyroid nodules may increase with age.

The diagnosis of hyperthyroidism and hypothyroidism is more difficult in the elderly. The older person is more likely to have signs and symptoms indicating involvement of only one system, such as heart disease with congestive failure.

Some investigation has been done to examine the effect of thyroid hormones on the aging processes. Aging changes could not be attributed to the hypothyroid state, but accelerated aging of collagen has been observed in hyperthyroid states.

In normal persons the serum level of parathyroid hormone (PTH) and osteoclastic activity increases after age 40 in both sexes. However, the serum level in women may be almost twice that found in men of the same age. It has been suggested that the increase in PTH may be secondary to a decrease in calcium absorption from the gastrointestinal tract.

It has been shown that the renal production of biologically active 1,25 $(OH)_2$ vitamin D is important in the absorption of calcium and is decreased with aging. It has been shown that estrogen administration, provision for a calcium intake of 1,000 mg per day, and weight bearing exercises improve the condition.

Adrenal gland

Glucocorticoid (cortisol). Plasma cortisol and secretion rates are stable with healthy aging, but the secretion rate is known to decrease by 30% over the life span.

Adrenal androgens. A decrease in urinary excretion of 17-ketosteroids to about half the value seen in young adults has been documented.

Aldosterone. The aldosterone secretory rate, plasma concentration and metabolic clearance rate, and urinary excretion decline with age. The secretion of renin by the juxtaglomerular cells is decreased in the elderly, and in many individuals no renin increase is seen with sodium secretion.

Pancreas

Insulin. Basal levels of insulin have not been observed to change with age, nor is there clear evidence of a change in sensitivity to insulin.

Glucagon. Glucagon release is not changed with aging.

Diabetic hyperosmolar coma is a condition that is confined almost entirely to the elderly. The main sign of the problem is a markedly elevated blood sugar level (750 to 2,000 mg/dl). Adult onset diabetes mellitus is observed to have a high incidence among the elderly. Most are managed successfully with diet and oral hypoglycemics, and few require insulin.

There is some evidence that accelerated aging accompanies the diabetic state. Decreased replication of both the B and A cells of the pancreatic sites has been documented. A more rapid rate of cell death of the endothelial cells in capillaries results in microangiopathy. The thickening of the capillary basement membrane observed in most aged subjects occurs more rapidly in diabetics.

Muscle cells and fibroblasts of diabetic persons have decreased replications in cell culture.

The altered characteristics of collagen formation are also indicative of accelerated aging. Juvenile diabetics have been noted to have collagen resembling that of much older persons. Bone mass is decreased.

Glucose tolerance in the older individual. The ability to metabolize a glucose load is influenced by a client's age, activity, and diet. Aging is known as one of the most important factors influencing performance on glucose tolerance testing. The 1- and 2-hour glucose values progressively rise at the rate of 10 mg/dl for each decade beyond age 50. A decrease in tissue sensitivity to insulin is the major factor responsible for the diminution in glucose tolerance. Failure to correct the glucose tolerance test for age would result in as many as 70% of the clients above the age of 70 being labeled diabetic.

A further compromise of ability of older persons to metabolize glucose is related to inactivity. The effect of inactivity is to diminish tissue sensitivity to insulin. The glucose tolerance test results may also be affected by drugs such as thiazides, furosemide, chlorthalidone, and high doses of phenytoin (Dilantin).

Genitourinary system

Because of the decreased cardiac output, blood flow to the kidneys and glomerular filtration rate are markedly diminished in the aged, leading to a loss of kidney function.

Structural changes in the kidneys result in aging changes in renal function. There is a gradual decline in renal plasma flow (RPF), in glomerular filtration rate (GFR), and in renal tubular resorptive capacity.

There is reduced renal excretion of many substances. In day-to-day activities the changes produce no signs or symptoms. The danger to the elderly client is that the aging kidneys fail to respond effectively to rapid or massive changes in fluid and electrolyte balance.

Renal plasma flow is thought to decline at the rate of 10% per decade as a result of a decline in cardiac output and changes in renal arterioles. The decline in RPF affects the cortex of the kidneys, whereas normally medullary blood flow persists.

The glomerular filtration rate decreases from 120 ml per 1.73 m^2 (body surface) in young adults to 80 ml per 1.73 m^2 in the elderly person. A more precise study of creatinine clearance indicates the values are normal to the midforties and then decline at the rate of 8 ml per minute per 1.73 m^2 per decade. The resorptive capacity of the renal tubules progressively diminish with aging.

The two most common signs of genitourinary dysfunction in the elderly are nocturnal frequency of micturition and incontinence of urine.

In addition to the frequency of urination, the volume passed during each episode should be investigated. Small amounts of urine passed frequently may be the result of a mucosal irritation caused by inflammation or trauma. Large volumes of urine passed frequently may be the result of chronic renal failure or poorly regulated

reflexes may be elicited in the healthy elderly adult. As a rule of progression, reflexes are preserved in the arms but lost in the lower legs at first. Muscle strength deteriorates less rapidly than coordination.

Achilles reflexes (ankle jerks) may diminish and disappear in some cases. The plantar reflex may be difficult to elicit. The superficial reflexes such as the abdominal reflexes may disappear (Fig. 25-18).

Immune response and aging

The thymus gland undergoes a process of involution that begins at sexual maturity and is complete by 45 to 50 years of age. The cellular mass at age 50 is only 5% to 10% of the maximum size. The thymus serves both as a site for cellular differentiation and as an endocrine gland. Thymic hormones play a role in the differentiation of lymphocytes. The hormones follow a similar

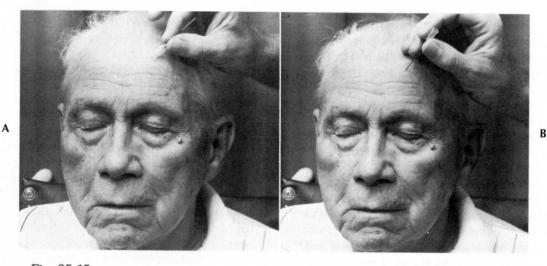

Fig. 25-15
Sensory examination of cranial nerve V, ophthalmic branch. **A,** The client is asked to identify the pressure stimulus that he has been taught to identify as "dull." The tool used is a no. 23 needle, which is disposable and helps to prevent cross-contamination between clients. **B,** The client is asked to identify the pain stimulus that he has been taught to identify as "sharp."

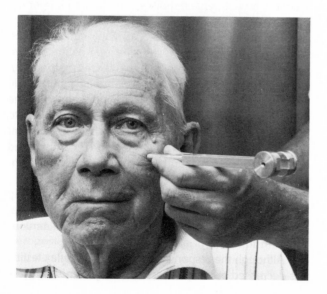

Fig. 25-16
Sensory examination of cranial nerve V—maxillary branch. The client is asked to identify the presence or absence of vibration in a tuning fork placed over a bony prominence.

decline to the number of thymic cells; thymic hormone can no longer be detected in humans more than 60 years of age.

Immature lymphocytes from the bone marrow enter the cortex of the thymus gland. This transit of lymphocytes decreases with age as does the capacity to differentiate immature lymphocytes.

Lymphocytes from elderly persons are more suscep-

tible to damage by ionizing radiation, ultraviolet light, and mutagenic drugs. Furthermore, recovery from radiation damage is impaired in the elderly.

The total number of lymphocytes does not appear to change with aging, nor does the total concentration of immunoglobulins. However, the concentration of IgA and IgG is increased in the elderly, whereas IgM is decreased.

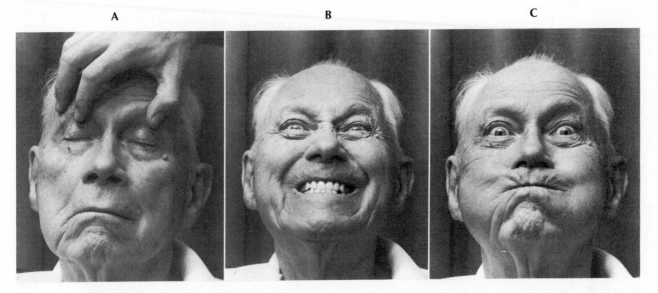

A **B** **C**

Fig. 25-17
Motor examination of cranial nerve VII. **A,** The client is asked to close his eyes against the resistance of the examiner. **B,** The client is asked to smile as wide as possible (to grimace). **C,** The client is asked to blow out his cheeks as much as possible.

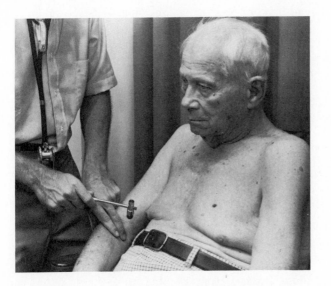

Fig. 25-18
Reflex assessment. Elicitation of biceps reflex.

Autoantibodies to nucleic acids, smooth muscle, mitochondria, lymphocytes, gastric parietal cells, immunoglobulin, and thyroglobulin have been found with increased frequency in older humans. In one study of healthy blood donors over 60 years of age, approximately two thirds had one or more autoantibodies. It has been suggested that autoantibodies and circulating immune complexes contribute to the pathological changes that occur with aging.

The response of elderly persons to foreign antigens decreases with age. Furthermore, the antibody response is maintained for a shorter time. There is no difference in the number of macrophages or lymphocytes in older animals. But there is a decrease in the activity of helper T cells coupled with increased suppressor T cell activity and defects in the B lymphocytic function.

Infections in the elderly

Some bacterial pathogens such as gram-negative bacilli are more likely to occur in older clients than in young adults. On the other hand, some pathogens are less likely to affect the elderly.

The elderly person may have altered signs and symptoms to a given pathogen from the young adult. Older clients with pneumonia are less likely to complain of cough, and elderly clients with meningitis often deny stiff neck. Sometimes the symptoms of infection are ignored by the client who feels his pains are signs of other conditions of aging. For instance the stiff neck of meningitis might be confused with cervical osteoarthritis. A heart murmur might lead the clinician to suppose the more common condition of arteriosclerosis in the elderly, whereas bacterial endocarditis might be suspected in the younger adult.

Both the incidence and mortality from many bacterial infections are higher in the elderly. The effectiveness of the immune system declines with age, and the older person is more likely to have predisposing illnesses.

Bacterial pneumonia has become a major cause of morbidity and mortality in the older client. The elderly client with pneumonia is more likely to develop bacteremia and complications such as emphysema and meningitis. The pneumonia of the elderly has been described as latent, without chills or cough. Lethargy may be the first sign of pneumonia. Pneumococcal infection is more likely to result in high fever, pleuritic chest pain, and chills. Most elderly will be tachypneic and have decreased breath sounds, basilar rales, "e" to "a" sounds, and bronchial breath sounds.

The incidence of *bacterial meningitis* is increasing in the aged, as is the mortality. Bacterial infection may spread from the urinary tract, the lung, the ear in otitis media, or the infected sinus.

The inflammatory reaction in the pia and arachnoid causes complaints of neck stiffness and pain and may be seen in the protective reflexes (Kernig's and Brudzinski's signs). Cerebral edema and inflammation may result in headache, confusion, or lethargy. Papilledema and other cranial nerve involvement may be evident.

Delay in making a diagnosis has resulted from attributing changes in mental status to senility or psychosis, stroke, and cerebral anoxia.

Bacterial endocarditis is caused by streptococci and staphylococci in 25% to 80% of cases of endocarditis in the elderly. About 50% of these clients had a prior history of rheumatic fever. Bacterial endocarditis has become more common in the elderly population. The signs and symptoms of malaise, anorexia, weight loss, and neurological findings are often attributed to other diseases.

The elderly have a higher incidence of urinary tract infections than the younger adult population. The incidence is 3% in men aged 65 to 70 but rises to 20% after the age 70. In women, the urinary infection rate is 20% after 65 and 23% to 50% after the age of 80. The incidence for both sexes increases markedly among the institutionalized elderly.

Most older persons with urinary tract infections are asymptomatic. Urinary tract infection symptoms such as dysuria, frequency, hesitancy, and incontinence may occur but may be difficult to interpret.

Viral infections. Influenza is common among the elderly. Some 70% of the deaths caused by pneumonia and influenza occurred in persons older than 65, and 95% of those persons had underlying chronic disease. Clients with pneumonia and cardiovascular disease were at greatest risk.

The symptoms of influenza are usually more prolonged and severe in the elderly but are of the typical respiratory and generalized nature. Some arrive for medical treatment with confusion, stupor, and coma.

Herpes zoster is a disease that occurs primarily in the older adult. Both the severity of the infection and neuralgia that follows the eruption of vesicles increase with age.

Respiratory syncytial virus causes an influenza-like disease in the elderly. Symptoms observed in clients infected with this virus include rhinorrhea, sore throat, anorexia, malaise, headache, and sore throat. Although pneumonia may occur, rhinorrhea is more common.

Viral gastroenteritis may result from rotavirus and calicirvirus, as has been demonstrated in outbreaks of gastroenteritis in nursing homes for the elderly. The rotavirus infection is typified by initial symptoms of nausea and vomiting for 1 to 2 days, followed by profuse, watery diarrhea of 1 to 5 days. Calicivirus produces milder symptoms. Vomiting occurs in about 40% of infected persons, whereas diarrhea occurs universally.

Temperature regulation

An absent or diminished febrile response is frequently observed in elderly clients. The assessment of a low body temperature (36° C [96.9° F] or lower) occurs more frequently among the elderly than other age groups.

Changes in laboratory tests observed in the elderly

It is important to keep in mind that the ranges of normal published in textbooks and many laboratory handbooks are derived from studies of persons aged 20 to 40. A number of serum and blood components have been shown to change with aging.

A gradual increase in fasting blood sugar and decline in glucose tolerance have been demonstrated in aging persons. Blood cholesterol concentrations have been shown to increase with aging. A decline in the concen-

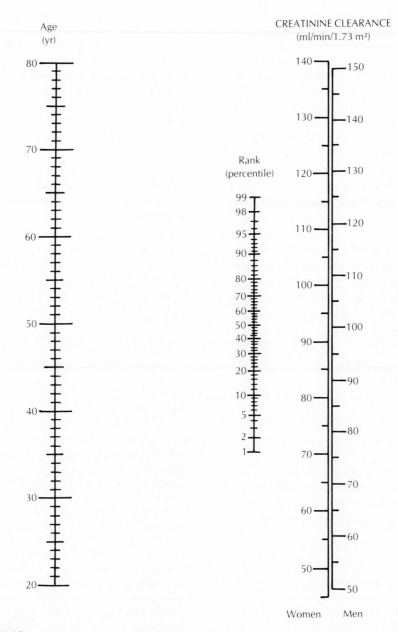

Fig. 25-19
Nomogram for ascertaining percentile rank in creatinine clearance. Nomogram is constructed for use with creatinine determinations done by automated "total chromogen" method. A line through the subject's age and creatinine clearance intersects the percentile rank line at a point indicating the subject's age-adjusted percentile rank. (From Rowe, J.W., and others: Ann. Intern. Med. **84**:567, 1976.)

tration of circulating thyroid hormone, triiodothyronine, may be responsible for some alterations in homeostasis.

Although the total serum protein concentration is not changed, with age, albumin concentration declines. Blood urea nitrogen concentration is known to increase significantly with age.

The most significant change in serum enzymes is a marked increase in the concentration of alkaline phosphatase.

The hemoglobin and red blood cell counts are known to decline with advancing age as the testosterone effect is withdrawn. White blood cell counts are lower in the elderly as well.

Variability in aging

There is considerable support for the idea that the rate of aging, like the rate of growth, may vary between individuals and that a person may age more rapidly in some parts of the body than others. The variations in child growth have been widely investigated. Much less effort has been devoted to determining biological age in the elderly. The most common approach has been to combine a large number of age-related parameters to a multiple regression equation to predict the biological age. Factor analysis of a test battery has also been used. Little clinical application of the data to predict longitudinal changes or mortality has been made. One study showed the biological age of unhealthy persons to be higher. Borkan and Norris used the following variables in determination of biological age:

1. Forced expiratory volume at 1 second.
2. Vital capacity
3. Maximum breathing capacity
4. Systolic blood pressure
5. Diastolic blood pressure
6. Hemoglobin
7. Serum albumin
8. Serum globulin
9. Creatinine clearance (Fig. 25-19)
10. Auditory threshold
11. Visual acuity
12. Visual depth perception
13. Basal metabolic rate
14. Cortical bone percentage
15. Creatinine excretion
16. Hand grip strength
17. Maximum work rate
18. Tapping time (medium targets)
19. Tapping time (close targets)
20. Reaction time—simple
21. Reaction time—choice
22. Foot reaction time
23. Plasma glucose tolerance test

This is a cross-sectional analysis, and the data cannot determine that an individual is aging faster than his chronological age mates or whether the changes are the result of the aging processes alone or of disease. The values allow an assessment of the individual at a particular point in time. One of the findings of the study was that men who appeared to be older than their chronological age were biologically older as well. Furthermore, the study followed subjects to their demise, and those who were biologically older at the time they were measured were noted to die sooner.

Elderly abuse

There is an estimated nationwide occurrence of 500,000 to 1,000,000 cases of abuse of elderly persons in the United States each year. The types of abuse may include actual assault but could encompass neglect such as failure to change an immobile person's position or arrange for toileting. Abuse could also occur from improper administration of medication, such as oversedation.

The examiner should bear these facts in mind when working with the older client.

BIBLIOGRAPHY

Agate, J.N.: The practice of geriatric medicine, ed. 2, London, 1970, William Heinemann Medical Books, Ltd.

Berman, N.: Geriatric cardiology, Lexington, Mass., 1982, D.C. Heath & Co.

Borkan, G.A., and Norris, A.H.: Assessment of biological age using a profile of physical parameters, Gerontology **35**:177, 1980.

Brocklehurst, J.C.: Textbook of geriatric medicine and gerontology, Edinburgh, 1973, Churchill Livingstone, Inc.

Buckley, E.C. III, and Dorsey, F.C.: The effect of aging on serum immunoglobulin concentrations, J. Immunol. **105**:964, 1970.

Busse, E.W., and Pfeiffer, E., editors: Behavior and adaptation in late life, Boston, 1969, Little, Brown & Co.

Butler, R.N., and Lewis, M.I.: Aging and mental health, ed. 3, St. Louis, 1982, The C.V. Mosby Co.

Caird, F.I., and Judge, T.G.: Assessment of the elderly patient, London, 1974, Pitman Publishing, Ltd.

Dybkkar, R., Lauritzen, M., and Krakauer, R.: Relative preference values for clinical chemical and haematological quantities in "healthy" elderly people, Acta Med. Scand. **209**:1, 1981.

Elkowitz, E.B.: Geriatric medicine for the primary care practitioner, New York, 1981, Springer Publishing Co., Inc.

Food and Nutrition Board, National Academy of Sciences: Recommended dietary allowances, Washington, D.C., 1980, National Academy of Sciences.

Gregerman, R., and Bierman, E.L.: Aging and hormones. In Williams, R.H., editor: Textbook of endocrinology, Philadelphia, 1981, W.B. Saunders Co.

Harper, A.E.: Recommended dietary allowances for the elderly, Geriatrics **33**:73, 1978.

Hershey, D.: Life span and factors affecting it, Springfield, Ill., 1974, Charles C Thomas, Publisher.

Jones, H.E.: Trends in mental abilities, 1958, Institute of Child Welfare, University of California.

Kenney, R.A.: Physiology of aging: a synopsis, Chicago, 1982, Year Book Medical Publishers, Inc.

McCue, J.D., editor: Medical care of the elderly, Lexington, Mass., 1983, D.C. Heath & Co.

Maurer, J.F., Rupp, R.R.: Hearing and aging, New York, 1979, Grune & Stratton, Inc.

National High Blood Pressure Coordinating Committee, Washington, D.C., September, 1979, U.S. Government Printing Office.

Owens, W.J.: Age and mental abilities: a second adult follow-up, J. Educ. Psychol. **67**:311, 1966.

Pitt, B.: Psychogeriatrics: an introduction to the psychiatry of old age, New York, 1982, Churchill Livingston, Inc.

Post, F.: The clinical psychiatry of late life, Oxford, 1965, Pergamon Press, Ltd.

Reichel, W., editor: Clinical aspects of aging, Baltimore, 1978, Williams & Wilkins.

Roe, D.: Geriatric nutrition, Englewood Cliffs, N.J., 1983, Prentice-Hall, Inc.

Rossman, I.: Clinical geriatrics, ed. 2, Philadelphia, 1979, J.B. Lippincott Co.

Russell, R., McGandy, R., and Jelliffe, D.: Reference weights: practical considerations, Am. J. Med. **75**(5):767, 1984.

Shanas, E.: Health status of older people, Am. J. Public Health **64**:261, 1974.

Steinberg, F.U.: Care of the geriatric patient, ed. 6, St. Louis, 1983, The C.V. Mosby Co.

Samiy, A.H., editor: Clinical geriatric medicine, Med. Clin. North Am. **67**(2):263, 1983.

Schrier, R.W.: Clinical internal medicine in the aged, Philadelphia, 1982, W.B. Saunders Co.

Texter, E.C., Jr.: The aging gut: pathophysiology, diagnosis and management, New York, 1983, Masson Publishing USA, Inc.

4. Determine auditory acuity (CN VIII).
5. Perform Weber and Rinne tests.

I. Examine nose.
  1. Determine patency of each nostril.
  2. Test for olfaction (CN I).
  3. Determine position of septum.
  4. Inspect mucosa, septum, and turbinates with nasal speculum.

J. Examine mouth and pharynx.
  1. Inspect lips, total buccal mucosa, teeth, gums, tongue, sublingual area, roof of mouth, tonsillar area, and pharynx.
  2. Test glossopharyngeal nerve (CN IX) and vagus nerve (CN X) ("ah" and gag reflex).
  3. Test hypoglossal nerve (CN XII) (tongue movement).
  4. Test taste (CN VII).

K. Complete examination of cranial nerves.
  1. Test trigeminal nerve (CN V) (jaw clenching, lateral jaw movements, corneal reflex, pain, and light touch to face).
  2. Test facial nerve (CN VII). (Client raises eyebrows, shows teeth, puffs cheeks, keeps eyes closed against resistance.)
  3. Test spinal accessory nerve (CN XI) (trapezius and sternocleidomastoid muscles).

L. Palpate temporomandibular joint.

M. Observe range of motion of the head and neck.

N. Palpate nodes (preauricular, posterior auricular, occipital, tonsillar, submaxillary, submental, anterior cervical, posterior cervical, supraclavicular, and infraclavicular nodes).

O. Palpate carotid arteries.

P. Palpate thyroid gland.

Q. Palpate for position of trachea.

R. Auscultate carotid arteries and thyroid gland.

IV. *Client is sitting on the bed or examining table, total chest uncovered if male, breasts covered if female (Fig. 26-2). Examiner is standing behind client.*

A. Examine back.
  1. Inspect spine.
  2. Palpate spine.
  3. Inspect skin and thoracic configuration.
  4. Palpate muscles and bones.
  5. Palpate costovertebral area, asking client about tenderness.

B. Examine lungs (apices and lateral and posterior areas). NOTE: Apical, posterior, and lateral lung regions can usually be examined from a position behind client.

  1. Observe respiration and total thorax.
  2. Palpate for thoracic expansion and tactile fremitus.
  3. Percuss systematically.
  4. Determine diaphragmatic excursion.
  5. Auscultate systematically.
  6. Auscultate for vocal fremitus.

V. *Client is sitting on the bed or examining table, uncovered to the waist. Examiner is facing client (Fig. 26-3).*

A. Examine breasts.
  1. Observe breasts with client's arms and hands at the side; above the head; and pressed into the hips, eliciting pectoral contraction.
  2. Observe breasts with client leaning forward.
  3. Ask client about lesions; if present, palpate them.
  4. If large breasts, perform a bimanual examination.

B. Palpate axillary nodes.

C. Examine lungs (anterior areas).
  1. Inspect configuration and skin.
  2. Palpate for tactile fremitus.
  3. Percuss lungs systematically.
  4. Auscultate lungs systematically.

D. Examine heart.
  1. Inspect precordium.
  2. Palpate precordium.
  3. Auscultate precordium.
  4. Observe external jugular vein and internal jugular pulsations.

VI. *Client is supine. Examiner is at the right side of client (Fig. 26-4).*

A. Examine breasts.
  1. Palpate breasts systematically.
  2. Attempt to express secretion from the nipples.

B. Examine heart.
  1. Inspect precordium.
  2. Palpate precordium.
  3. Auscultate precordium.
  4. Observe jugular venous pulses and pressures.

C. Measure blood pressure (both arms).

D. Examine abdomen.
  1. Inspect abdomen.
  2. Auscultate bowel sounds, aorta, renal arteries, and femoral arteries.
  3. Percuss and measure liver.
  4. Percuss spleen.
  5. Palpate liver, spleen, inguinal and femoral node and hernia areas, general abdomen, and femoral pulses systematically.
  6. Test abdominal reflexes.

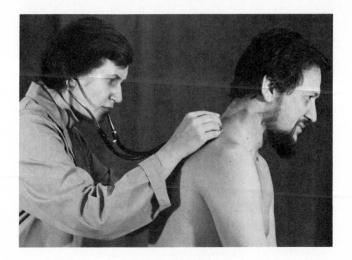

Fig. 26-2
Client seated, examiner behind client.

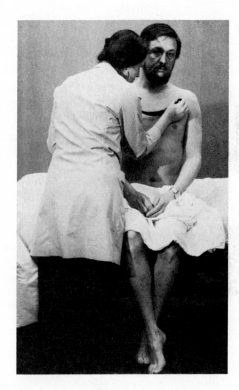

Fig. 26-3
Client seated (uncovered to waist), examiner facing client.

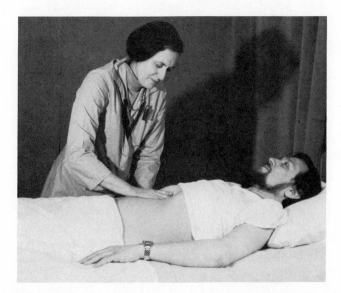

Fig. 26-4
Client lying on back, examiner at client's right side.

E. Examine genitals of male client.
   1. Inspect penis, uretheral opening, and scrotum.
   2. Palpate scrotal contents.
F. Examine lower extremities.
   1. Inspect skin, hair distribution, muscle mass, and skeletal configuration.
   2. Palpate for temperature, texture, edema, popliteal pulses, posterior tibial pulses, and dorsal pedal pulses.
   3. Test range of motion.
   4. Test strength.
   5. Test sensation (pain, light touch, and vibration).
   6. Test position sense.
VII. *Client* is sitting on the bed or examining table. *Examiner* is standing in front of client (Fig. 26-5).
   A. Assess neural system.
      1. Elicit deep tendon reflexes (biceps, triceps, brachioradialis, patellar, and Achilles reflexes).
      2. Test for Babinski's reflex.
      3. Test for coordination of upper and lower extremities.
   B. Test upper extremities for strength, range of motion sensation, vibration, and position.

VIII. *Female client* is in lithotomy position, genital area uncovered. *Examiner* is sitting, facing the genital area.
   A. Examine genitalia.
      1. Inspect genitalia.
      2. Palpate external genital area.
      3. Perform speculum examination.
      4. Take smears and cultures.
      5. Perform bimanual vaginal examination.
   B. Examine rectum: perform bimanual recto-vaginal examination.
IX. *Client* is standing. *Examiner* is standing next to client (Fig. 26-6).
   A. Examine spine.
      1. Observe with client bending over.
      2. Test for range of motion.
   B. Assess neural system.
      1. Observe gait.
      2. Perform Romberg test.
      3. Observe heel and toe walks.
   C. Test for inguinal and femoral hernias.
X. *Male client* is standing and leaning over examination table.
   A. Examine rectum.
   B. Palpate rectum.
   C. Palpate prostrate.
   D. Palpate seminal vesicles.

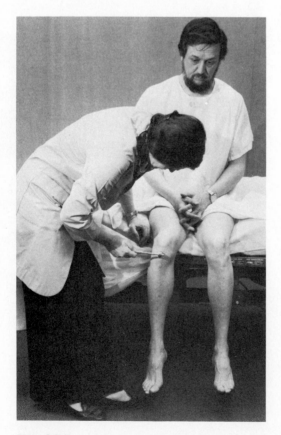

Fig. 26-5
Client seated, examiner facing client.

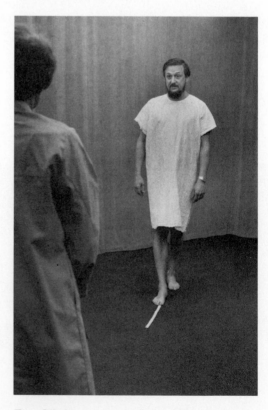

Fig. 26-6
Client standing, examiner standing.

RECORDING OF THE PHYSICAL EXAMINATION

In recording the physical examination, the practitioner is continuously attempting to achieve a balance between conciseness and comprehensiveness. The record should describe what was seen, heard, palpated, and percussed. Whenever appropriate, the exact description is written; evaluations such as "normal," "good," or "poor" are avoided or used judiciously. Too frequently, a major system, such as the cardiovascular system, is described in one word, "normal." This description does not indicate what components of that system were assessed or the examiner's parameters of normal.

Conciseness is achieved through the use of outlines, phrases, and abbreviations. Grammar is sacrificed, and only essential words are written. Often it is helpful to use a form for recording the physical examination. A form provides an outline into which data can be entered. Forms serve as reminders for completeness. They also save time. And, if they are systematically used by all the members of a health system, they are extremely useful as indices for rapid information identification.

As recommended in the recording of the history (see Chapter 3 on the health history), the beginning practitioner should overrecord. The beginner should record all findings from the examination. With increased skill and discrimination regarding the significance of findings, the practitioner will be able to weed out the irrelevant information and consolidate the significant data.

Table 26-1 is a guideline that is designed to be of assistance to the beginning recorder. The first column indicates the body systems or regions that are examined. The second column contains a list of the areas of recording. These areas should be described for all clients. The third column is a partial list of areas to be recorded if abnormalities are identified in the examination of that system. The fourth column contains examples of recording for each body system or area. The examples of recording do not relate to one client; column four should not be read as an example of the composite physical examination of one client.

Table 26-1
Areas and examples of recording for the physical examination

Area of examination	Descriptions usually recorded	Descriptions recorded in detail if abnormalities are present (partial listing only)	Examples of recording

Vital signs	Temperature: oral or rectal
	Pulse
	Respiration
	Blood pressure: both arms in at least two positions (lying and sitting recommended)
	Weight: indicate if client is clothed or unclothed
	Height: without shoes
		Blood pressure in standing position and in both thighs	T: 98.6° F (oral)
			P: 76/min—strong and regular: R: 16/min
			BP:
			  Lying: R, 110/70/60; L, 112/68/60
			  Sitting: R, 116/74/67; L, 120/76/65
			Wt: 130 lb, unclothed
			Ht: 5 ft 3 in

General health	Appearance as relative to chronological age Apparent state of health Awareness Personal appearance Emotional status Nutritional status Affect Response Cooperation	Handshake Speech Respiratory difficulties Gross deformity Movements Unusual behavior	Slightly obese, alert, white male who looks younger than his stated age of 45. Moves without difficulty; no gross abnormalities apparent. Appears healthy and in no acute distress; is neatly dressed, responsive, and cooperative. Responds appropriately; smiles frequently.
Skin and mucous membranes	Color Edema Moisture Temperature Texture Turgor	Discharge Drainage Lesions: distribution, type, configuration Superficial vascularity Mobility Thickness	*Skin:* Uniformly brown in color; soft, warm, moist, elastic, of normal thickness. No edema or lesions. *Mucous membranes:* Pink, moist, slightly pale.
Nails	Color of beds Texture	Lesions Abnormalities in size or shape Presence of clubbing	Nail beds pink, texture hard, no clubbing.

Continued.

Table 26-1

Areas and examples of recording for the physical examination—cont'd

Area of examination	Descriptions usually recorded	Descriptions recorded in detail if abnormalities are present (partial listing only)	Examples of recording
Hair and scalp	Quantity Distribution Color Texture	Lesions Parasites	*Hair:* Normal male distribution; thick, curly; black color with graying at temples. *Scalp:* Clean, no lesions.
Cranium	Contour Tenderness	Lesions	Normocephalic, no tenderness.
Face	Symmetry Movements Sinuses CN V CN VII	Tenderness Edema Lesions Parotid gland	Symmetrical at rest and with movement. Jaw muscles strong, no crepitations or limitation in movement of temporomandibular joint. Sinus areas not tender. Sensory: pain and light touch intact.
Eyes	Visual acuity Visual fields Alignment of eyes Alignment of eyelids Movement of eyelids Conjunctiva Sclera Cornea Anterior chamber Iris Pupils: size, shape, symmetry, reflexes (PERRLA may be used for "Pupils, equally round, react to light and accommodation") Lens Lacrimal apparatus Ophthalmological examination (disc, vessels, retina, macular areas)	Eyebrows Tonometry Lesions Exophthalmia	Vision (distant with glasses): R, 20/40; L, 20/30; can read newspaper at 18 in. Visual fields full. Alignment: no deviation with cover test; light reflex equal; palpebral fissure normal. Extraocular movements: bilaterally intact; no nystagmus, ptosis, lid lag. Conjunctiva: clear, slightly injected around area of R inner canthus. Sclera: white. Cornea: clear, arcus senilis, R eye. Anterior chamber: not narrowed. Iris: blue, round. Pupils: PERRLA. Lens: clear. Funduscopic examination: normal veins and arteries; disc round, margins well defined, color yellowish pink; macular areas normal; no arteriolovenous (A-V) nicking, hemorrhages, or exudates. Lacrimal system: no swelling or discharge. Corneal reflex: present.
Ears	Auricle Canal Otoscopic examination (color, presence of landmarks) Rinne and Weber tests	Position Discharge Pathological alterations, present on otoscopic examination Lesions Mastoid tenderness General tenderness	Auricle: no lesions, canal clean. Otoscopic examination: drum intact, color gray, landmarks present. Hearing: finger rub heard in both ears at 3 ft. Rinne and Weber tests: normal, AC 2× > BC.
Nose	Patency of each nostril Olfaction Turbinates and mucous membranes	External nose Vestibule Transillumination of sinuses	Nostrils patent, odors identified. Septum: slightly deviated to R. Turbinates and membranes: pink, moist, no discharge.
Oral cavity	Buccal mucosa Gums Teeth (decayed, missing, filled) Floor of mouth Hard and soft palate Tonsillar areas Posterior pharyngeal wall	Breath odor Lips Lesions Laryngoscopic examination Palpation of mouth Parotid duct	Membranes: pink and moist, no lesions. Gums: no edema or inflammation. Teeth: 3D, 1M, 10F (approximately). Palate: intact, moves symmetrically with phonation, gag reflex present. Tonsils: present, not enlarged. Pharynx: pink and clean. Tongue: strong, midline, moves symmetrically.

Table 26-1
Areas and examples of recording for the physical examination—cont'd

Area of examination	Descriptions usually recorded	Descriptions recorded in detail if abnormalities are present (partial listing only)	Examples of recording
	Taste Tongue position and movement		Taste: able to differentiate sweet and sour.
Neck	Movements: rotation and lateral bend Symmetry Thyroid gland Tracheal position Glands and nodes	Postural alignment Tenderness Tone of muscles Lesions Masses	Full ROM, strong symmetrically, thyroid not palpable, trachea midline, no enlargement of head and neck regional nodes.
Breasts	Axillary nodes Supraclavicular nodes Infraclavicular nodes Breasts: observation and palpation Nipples and areolar areas Discharge Masses	Retraction Dimpling	No nodes palpable—axillary, infraclavicular, or supraclavicular; no masses, retraction, or discharge; L breast slightly larger than R breast, otherwise symmetrical at rest and with movement. Nipples symmetrically positioned.
Chest and respiratory system	Shape of thorax Symmetry of thorax Respiratory movements Respiratory excursion Palpation: tactile fremitus, tenderness, masses Percussion notes Diaphragmatic excursion and level Auscultation: breath sounds, adventitious sounds	Adventitious sounds Deformity Use of accessory muscles of respiration Vocal fremitus Egophony, bronchophony, whispered pectoriloquy	Thorax oval, AP diameter < lateral diameter; symmetrical at rest and with movements; excursion normal; tactile fremitus equal bilaterally; no masses or tenderness; percussion tones resonant, diaphragmatic excursion 5 cm bilaterally between T10 and T12; vesicular breath sounds bilaterally; no adventitious sounds.
Central cardiovascular system	Position in which the heart was examined; lying, sitting, left lateral, recumbent Inspection: bulging depression, pulsation (precordial and juxtaprecordial) Palpation: thrusts, heaves, thrills, friction rubs Point of PMI Auscultation: rate and rhythm, character of S_1, character of S_2, comparison of S_1 in aortic and pulmonic areas, comparison of S_1 and S_2 in major auscultatory areas, presence or absence of extra sounds—if present, description	Murmur or extra sound: whether systolic or diastolic; intensity; pitch; quality; site of maximum transmission; effect of position, respiration, and exercise; radiation	Examined in sitting and lying positions; no abnormal pulsations or lifts observed; PMI in the 5th ICS, slightly medial to the LMCL; no abnormal pulsations palpated. Apical pulse: 72, regular; S_1 single sound; S_2 splits with inspiration; A_2 is louder than P_2, S_1 heard loudest at apex, S_2 heard loudest at base; no murmurs or other sounds.
Arterial pulses	Radial pulse: rate, rhythm; consistency and tenderness of arterial wall Amplitude and character of peripheral pulses: superficial temporal, brachial, femoral, popliteal, posterior tibial, dorsal pedal Carotid pulses: equality, amplitude, thrills, bruits	Any abnormality: analysis of type	Radial pulse: bilaterally equal, regular, strong; no tenderness or thickening of vessels; 76/min. Peripheral pulses:

	Right	*Left*
Temporal	As above	As above
Brachial	As above	As above
Femoral	As above	As above
Popliteal	Not felt	Not felt
Posterior tibial	As above	As above
Dorsal pedal	As above	As above

Carotid pulses: equal, strong, no bruits.

Continued.

WORKSHEET FOR RECORDING A PHYSICAL EXAMINATION

Vital signs

Temperature _____ Respiration _____ BP (L) Arm (R)

_____ Supine _____

_____ Sitting _____

_____ Standing _____

Height _____ Weight _____ (Stripped or clothed)

General

Skin, hair, nails, mucous membranes

Head

Scalp _____

Face _____

(CNs, V, VII) _____

_____

Sinus areas _____

Nodes _____

Cranium _____

Eyes

Visual acuity _____

Visual fields _____

Ocular movements (CNs, III, IV, VI) _____

Corneal light reflex _____

Lids, lacrimal organs _____

Conjunctiva, sclera _____

Cornea (CN V) _____

Lens and media _____

Pupils: Pupillary reflexes (CN III) _____

Light, direct and consensual _____

Near point _____

Fundi (CN II) _____

Intraocular pressure _____

Ears

External structures _____

Canal _____

Tympanic membranes _____

Hearing (CN VIII) _____

Nose

Septum _____

Mucous membranes _____

Patency _____

Olfactory sense (CN I) _____

Oral cavity
Lips _____
Mucous membranes _____
Gums _____
Teeth _____
Palates and uvula (CNs IX and X) _____
Tonsillar areas _____
Tongue (CN XII) _____
Floor _____
Voice _____
Breath _____

Neck
General structure _____
Trachea _____
Thyroid _____
Nodes _____
Muscles (CN XI) _____

Breasts and area nodes

_____
_____
_____

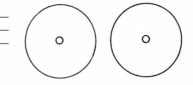

Chest, respiratory system
Chest shape _____
Type of respiration _____
Expansion _____
Fremitus _____
General palpation _____
Percussion _____
_____ Diaphragmatic excursion: (R) _____ cm (L) _____ cm
Breath sounds _____
_____
_____
_____
_____
Adventitious sounds _____
_____

Cardiovascular system
Rate and rhythm: Radial (palpation) _____
                Apical (auscultation) _____
Precordium: Inspection _____
           Palpation _____
           Auscultation _____
             S_1 _____
             S_2 _____
             S_3 _____
             S_4 _____
            Extra sounds _____
            Murmur(s): Systolic _____
                  Diastolic _____
Carotid arteries _____
Jugular venus pulse and pressure _____

Description of peripheral pulses

	Brachial	Radial	Femoral	Popliteal	Dorsal pedal	Post. tibial
R						
L						

WORKSHEET FOR RECORDING A PHYSICAL EXAMINATION—cont'd

Abdomen and inguinal areas

Contour, tone _____

Scars, marks _____

Auscultation _____

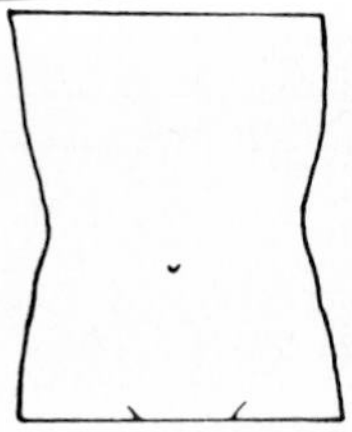

Liver _____ Span _____ cm at RMCL

Spleen _____

Kidneys _____ CVA tenderness _____

Bladder _____

Hernias _____

Masses _____

Palpation _____

Percussion _____

Genitalia and area nodes

_____

_____

_____

_____

Rectal examination

Musculoskeletal system

Gait _____

Deformities _____

Joint evaluation _____

Muscle strength _____

Muscle mass _____

Range of motion _____

Spine

Contour _____

Position _____

Motion _____

Nervous system

Mental status _____

Language _____

Cranial nerves (summarize) _____

Motor: Coordination: Upper extremities _____

Lower extremities _____

Involuntary movements _____

Deep tendon reflexes:

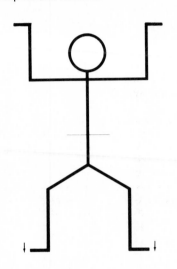

Note: +s denote finger jerks, brachioradialis, biceps, triceps, reflexes, 4-quadrant abdominal scratch reflexes, patellar Achilles reflexes, and plantar reflexes. Abdominal reflexes are recorded as 0 or +. Scale: 0-4 (++++); normal = 2 (++).

Sensory

Light touch _____

Pain (pinprick) _____

Vibration _____

Position _____

CHAPTER 27

CLINICAL LABORATORY PROCEDURES

The information obtained through the physical examination is augmented and in many cases verified through the judicious use of laboratory diagnostic procedures to provide a biochemical data base for use in the analysis of the client's state of health.

The tests most frequently included in a screening workup are a blood chemistry profile, hematology, a serological test for syphilis, urinalysis, a chest roentgenogram, the Papanicolaou (Pap) cytological examination for cancer diagnosis, hormonal evaluation of ovarian function in women from puberty onward, a proctoscopic examination, and an electrocardiogram (ECG) for all persons older than 40 years of age.

Blood chemistry profiles characteristically include determinations of sodium, potassium, chloride, calcium, phosphorus, glucose, bilirubin, blood urea nitrogen (BUN), uric acid, total proteins, albumin, cholesterol, serum glutamic-oxaloacetic transaminase (SGOT), lactic dehydrogenase (LDH), and alkaline phosphatase.

The hematology screening examination includes a study of the red blood cell (RBC) count, hematocrit, hemoglobin, mean corpuscular volume, and mean corpuscular hemoglobin concentration. The total white blood cell (WBC) count and a differential count based on morphological types are also included.

Urinalysis is performed for analysis of specific gravity, pH, and the presence of glucose, protein, acetone, blood, and microscopic formed elements.

The procedure for the Pap smear is described in Chapter 20 on assessment of the female genitalia and procedures for smears and cultures.

The tables of normal ranges found in textbooks of clinical pathology are to be considered as relative guidelines. The values are often those of medical or nursing student volunteers and laboratory technicians and thus are not specific as to sex and age.

Furthermore, values vary from one clinical laboratory to another even though the same procedure may be used in each laboratory.

There may be real differences in values observed in geographically separated population groups; for example, generally higher cholesterol values are observed in sample populations in San Francisco. Seasonal changes may also play a role; for example, uric acid levels are observed to be greater in winter than in other seasons.

When abnormal values are observed in test results, the examiner should review the interview data to determine if any circumstances in the client's life-style, environment, drug use, or state of nutrition or hydration may have influenced the value. For instance, an elevated protein-bound iodine (PBI) level and low resin-uptake value (triiodothyronine [T_3]) may indicate that the client has been taking oral contraceptives.

Posture is known to affect laboratory values. Blood albumin, total protein, hemoglobin, cholesterol, and calcium values are known to be higher in the client who has been standing for a long time.

Diet and alcohol may also alter laboratory values. Bilirubin and SGOT values have been shown to be elevated during fasting. High fat content in the diet will produce hyperlipemia. High-protein meals may produce an increased BUN level. Most professionals are aware of the possibility of increased blood glucose values incurred as a result of a "carbohydrate binge." Alcohol consumption or alcoholic liver damage has been shown to result in increased levels of uric acid, glucose, calcium, phosphorus, LDH, SGOT, creatine phosphokinase (CPK), alkaline phosphatase, and triglycerides, accompanied by a low PBI level and albumin-globulin (A/G) ratio.

The blood specimens collected from a dehydrated individual will show the values to be consistent with the more concentrated fluid. These include increased levels of sodium, potassium, chloride, calcium, phosporus, glucose, BUN, uric acid, cholesterol, total protein, globulin, LDH, SGOT, and creatinine.

The overhydrated client might be expected to have decreased concentrations of sodium, potassium, chloride, calcium, phosphorus, BUN, uric acid, albumin, total proteins, and cholesterol in the blood.

Improper handling of specimens may also result in erroneous test results. Test tubes that have been washed with detergent and poorly rinsed may cause spuriously elevated calcium, sodium, and potassium levels.

Possible applications of results of laboratory procedures include the following:

1. Provision of health assessment parameters of both a morphological and biochemical nature that are unavailable through the health history and physical examination.
2. Confirmation of a biochemical state of health when physical examination findings are negative.
3. Provision of further information in the differential diagnosis of disease. For example, the client with easy fatigability, shortness of breath on exertion, dizziness on exercise, and pale buccal mucosa may have a diagnosis of anemia confirmed through the results of screening hematological studies.
4. Provision of a gauge of the severity of disease. The degree of anemia that is disclosed may determine the therapeutic regimen for the client. The milder form of iron deficiency anemia may well be ameliorated in time through diet and rest, allowing the client's blood-forming organs to make up the deficit. Medication may be necessary for more severe involvement, and blood replacement by transfusion may be necessary for marked reduction in hemoglobin and RBCs.
5. Provision of biochemical clues that will indicate appropriate dosages of medication. A serum iron determination may be made for the client who is suspected of having iron deficiency anemia to substantiate the physical examination findings. The serum iron levels may be used to monitor the efficiency of the treatment regimen.

BLOOD CHEMISTRY PROFILE

Automated machines are available in many pathology laboratories for the purpose of performing chemistry tests. These machines commonly perform six to twenty-four determinations, using a single small sample of blood. Two types of machines are used. The first type is a discrete sample analyzer (DSA), which separates the sample into as many chambers as there are tests to be performed. Translated into the language of technician-performed testing, this means the sample is separated into an individual test tube for each ordered test. The second type is a continuous flow analyzer (CFA), which separates the sample within a single tubing into discrete sections through the use of bubbles. These sections pass through the tubing, stopping at specific sites for analysis. Some caution must be used with these machines to be certain that the tubing is thoroughly cleaned between samples.

Most of these machines provide a printout sheet that records the client's data against a range of normal for the particular instrument.

Blood chemistry tests are performed on venous samples that are obtained following a period of fasting (usually at least 6 hours).

Some of these machines provide test results at a rate of greater than 3,000 per minute and thus provide significantly more data at less cost to the consumer.

In general, the machines are carefully self-calibrated and are more accurate than the results produced when humans do the testing.

One disadvantage to the practitioner and the client is more data may be generated than is actually necessary to assess the client's health status.

Electrolytes

Some electrolytes that are routinely analyzed in a screening examination include sodium (Na^+), potassium (K^+), chloride (Cl^-), and carbon dioxide (CO_2) combining power.

Plasma is an aqueous solution (90% water) that contains approximately 1% electrolytes.

The distribution of electrolytes in the normal individual is represented by the following values:

Na^+ 136 to 142 mEq/L	Cl^- 95 to 103 mEq/L
K^+ 3.8 to 5 mEq/L	PO_4^{3-} 1.8 to 2.6 mEq/L
Ca^{2+} 4.5 to 5.3 mEq/L	SO_4^{2-} 0.2 to 1.3 mEq/L
Mg^{2+} 1.5 to 2.5 mEq/L	HCO_3^- 21 to 28 mEq/L
	Protein $\cong$ 17 mEq/L

The distribution of these ions in the plasma is compared with those of the interstitial and cellular fluids in Fig. 27-1.

Electrolytes are carefully controlled through a variety of physical and chemical mechanisms, so that the range of normal for each of these compartments is quite narrow.

Sodium

Sodium is the major cation of the body. It is the most abundant extracellular ion and as such plays a prominent role in the osmolality of the extracellular fluid. The ion is necessary to the resting potential of excitable cells. The intake of sodium in the average adult diet is 10 to 12 g, but the amount is variable.

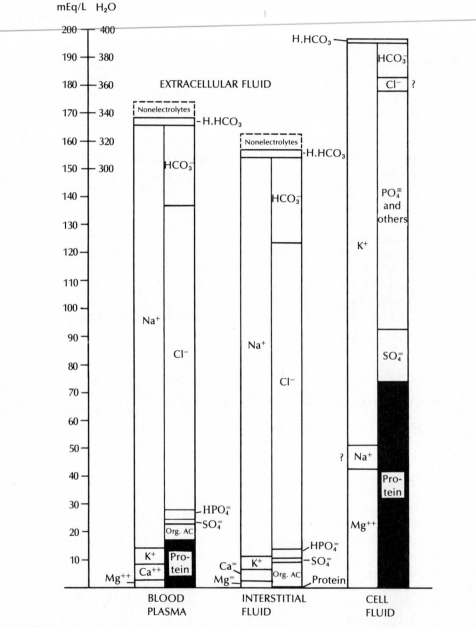

Fig. 27-1

Electrolyte distribution in the fluid compartment of the body. The column of figures on the left (200, 190, 180, and so on) indicates amounts of cations or anions; the figures on the right (400, 380, 360, and so on) indicate the sum of cations and anions. Note that chloride and sodium values in cell fluid are questioned. It is probable that at least muscle intracellular fluid contains some sodium but no chloride. (From Anthony, C.P., and Thibodeau, G.A.: Textbook of anatomy and physiology, ed. 11, St. Louis, 1983, The C.V. Mosby Co. Adapted from Mountcastle, V.B., editor: Medical physiology, vol. 2, ed. 14, St. Louis, 1980, The C.V. Mosby Co.; after Gamble, J.L.: Harvey Lect. **42:**247, 1946-1947.)

The kidney plays the principal role in homeostasis of sodium in the body fluids. Aldosterone is secreted by the adrenal cortex as a result of the activation of the renin angiotensin system when the whole blood sodium concentration or blood volume is decreased or when the potassium concentration is increased. ACTH directly stimulates the cells of the adrenal cortex. Thus, aldosterone is also secreted in times of stress. Aldosterone facilitates the reabsorption of sodium in the distal tubule of the kidney.

The concentration of the ions is necessarily dependent on the water content of the blood. Although the whole blood sodium content might stay constant, the concentration of the sodium ions will be greater when water stores are less in quantity.

Osmotic diuretic agents, such as mannitol and glucose, are known to carry out sodium with them. In some cases of acidemia, the concentration of SO_4^{2-}, Cl^-, PO_4^{3-}, and organic acids overwhelms the kidneys' capacity to secrete H^+ and NH_3 while exchanging Na^+. Thus, the ions are excreted in the urine with a fixed base, which is sodium for the most part. In conditions where potassium is lost from the cellular compartment, sodium replaces the ion. This situation may occur in acidosis or when the sodium-potassium pump is malfunctioning.

SERUM SODIUM: NORMAL VALUES AND DEVIATIONS

Normal values: 136 to 142 mEq/L
Normal osmolality of the blood: 280 to 295 mOsm/L

Deviations	Cause
Hyponatremia	Dehydration with loss of electrolytes
	Sweating
	Diarrhea
	Burns
	Nasogastric tube
	Addison's disease
	Diuretics
	Mercurial
	Chlorothiazide
	Chronic renal insufficiency
	Chronic glomerulonephritis
	Pyelonephritis
	Starvation
	Diabetic acidosis
	Water retention or dilution
	Cirrhosis
	Congestive heart failure
	Renal insufficiency
	Excessive ingestion of water
	Overhydration with intravenous therapy
Hypernatremia (uncommon)	Deficient water intake
	Excessive water loss—lack of antidiuretic hormone (ADH)
	Cushing's disease
	Primary hyperaldosteronism

Potassium

Potassium is the most abundant intracellular cation; since the majority of potassium is found within the cells, the total body content of the ion cannot be measured readily. Furthermore, the relationship between intracellular potassium and serum potassium is a highly dynamic one. For instance, intracellular potassium readily leaves the cell in the event of serum potassium deficiency. Potassium ions compete with hydrogen ions for excretion by the kidney; potassium is excreted largely by this mechanism, although some may be lost in sweat and gastrointestinal secretions.

The importance of homeokinetic control of extracellular potassium ions relate to the function of potassium in neuromuscular excitability. The resting membrane potential of the cells of these tissues is directly related to the ratio of intracellular potassium concentrations.

SERUM POTASSIUM: NORMAL VALUES AND DEVIATIONS

Normal values: 3.8 to 5 mEq/L

Deviations	Cause	Possible effects
Hyperkalemia	$\downarrow$ Excretion of K^+	Changes in ECG; >8 mEq/L
	Kidney disease	Widened P wave
	Intestinal obstruction	Symmetrical peaking of T wave
	Addison's disease	Widened QRS complex
	Hypoaldosteronism	Depressed S-T segment; >11 mEq/L
	Iatrogenic K^+ replacement therapy	Ventricular fibrillation
	Trauma	Heart block in diastole
	Burns	Neuromuscular changes
	Diuretics such as spironolactone that cause $\downarrow$ K^+ excretion	Flaccidity
	K^+ shift from tissues	Muscle paralysis
	Muscle crush	Numbness
	Acidosis	Tingling
Hypokalemia	$\downarrow$ Ingestion of K^+	Changes in ECG
	$\uparrow$ Excretion of K^+	Flattening and inversion of T wave
	Prolonged gastrointestinal suctioning	Prominent U wave
	Vomiting	Sagging of S-T segment
	K^+ depleting diuretics	Muscle weakness
	Excessive administration of bicarbonate (K^+ enters the cells)	Malaise
	Cirrhosis	Apathy
	Cushing's disease	Nausea and vomiting
	Treatment with steroids	$\downarrow$ Reflexes
	Aldosteronism	$\downarrow$ Smooth muscle tone
	Excessive licorice intake	Distention
	Intravenous infusion of K^+ free fluids	Paralytic ileus
	Fasting, starvation	$\downarrow$ Diastolic blood pressure
		Impairment of renal tubular function
		Polyuria

Chloride

Chloride is the major anion of the body and in general is found to behave in concert with sodium. More precisely, the chloride passively follows sodium in its transport through membranes. Chloride plays a prominent role in acid-base balance. In acidemia, Cl^- concentration is increased, and thus more Cl^- is associated with sodium. In alkalemia, more bicarbonate (HCO_3^-) is associated with sodium. Chloride deficit leads to increased reabsorption of bicarbonate in the distal tubules of the kidney and thereby leads to alkalemia. Since chloride is necessary to the synthesis of hydrochloric acid in the stomach, excessive loss of gastric secretions leads to alkalemia. Chloride is also lost from the intestinal tract in diarrhea or as a result of intestinal fistula. Chloride is excreted in the urine with cations in diuresis.

SERUM CHLORIDE: NORMAL VALUES AND DEVIATIONS

Normal values: 95 to 103 mEq/L

Deviations	Cause	Possible effects
Hypochloremia	Hypokalemic alkalosis Ingestion of potassium compounds that do not contain chloride Potassium-sparing diuretics Excessive loss of gastric secretions Vomiting Nasogastric tube	Associated with ↓ K^+ and ↑ CO_2 combining power
Hyperchloremia (rare)	Diarrhea Iatrogenic Ammonium chloride ingestion	Fistulas

Calcium

Plasma calcium (Ca^{2+}) occurs in three forms. About half of the calcium is bound to protein. Calcium in this form does not diffuse through the capillary wall. A second, nonionized, nondiffusable group of calcium compounds makes up approximately 5% of the plasma calcium. Somewhat less than half (45%) of the plasma calcium is ionized. This third form of calcium diffuses through the capillary membrane and is physiologically active.

The effects of calcium on skeletal and cardiac muscle, nerve tissue, and bone are due to the ionized calcium. The ionized calcium of the plasma is maintained within a fairly narrow range ($\pm 5\%$) as a result of the influence of parathyroid hormone (PTH) and thyrocalcitonin (TCT). PTH increases plasma ionized calcium by increasing absorption of calcium from the intestinal tract and reabsorption of calcium from the renal tubules of the kidney and by absorbing calcium salts from the bones through its action of osteoclasts. TCT lowers serum ionized calcium by increasing depositions of calcium in the bones through its influence on the osteoblasts.

A metabolite of vitamin D increases the absorption of calcium from the intestine through the stimulation of a calcium-binding protein.

SERUM CALCIUM: NORMAL VALUES AND DEVIATIONS

Normal values
Adults:
  Ionized: 4.2 to 5.2 mg/dl
          2.1 to 2.6 mEq/L
  Total: 9 to 10.6 mg/dl
          4.5 to 5.3 mEq/L
Infants: 11 to 13 mg/dl

Deviations	Cause	Possible effects
Hypercalcemia	↑ PTH ↓ TCT } Hyperparathyroidism associated with alkaline phosphatase) ↑ Vitamin D intake ↑ Absorption of Ca^{2+} in intestine ↑ Reabsorption of Ca^{2+} in renal tubules Acidosis Paget's disease Destructive bone lesions Osteoporosis Immobilization Hypothyroidism Malignancy (associated with hypergammaglobulinemia) ↓ Urinary excretion Na^+ depletion Thiazide diuretics	Polyuria; polydipsia ↓ Neuromuscular excitability Skeletal muscle (↓ tone, weakness, atrophy) Smooth muscle (↓ tone, observed in such signs as nausea, vomiting, and constipation) Heart muscle Shortening of Q-T interval of the ECG Arteriovenous block ↓ Plasma phosphate Renal calculi caused by precipitation of calcium phosphate ($Ca_3[PO_4]_2$) Alkalosis Ataxia Hyperreflexia
Hypocalcemia	↑ TCT ↓ PTH } Hypoparathyroidism ↓ Absorption of Ca^{2+} from the gastrointestinal tract Steatorrhea Sprue Celiac disease Acute pancreatitis ↓ Vitamin D (hypovitaminosis) Hypoalbuminemia Pregnancy Diuretic ingestion Starvation ↓ Magnesium	↓ Neuromuscular excitability (tetany) Prolongation of the S-T segment of the ECG Osteomalacia in adults Rickets in children

Phosphorus

The serum level of phosphate (PO_4^{3-}) generally bears a combination relationship with serum calcium concentration. Parathyroid hormone increases the amount of phosphate absorbed in the intestinal tract, since phosphate is absorbed when calcium is absorbed. The excretion of phosphate is accomplished largely by the kidney and is determined by the fact that phosphate is a threshold substance. Thus, the kidney regulates the serum phosphate level by secreting phosphate when the serum level exceeds 1 mMol/L and retaining phosphate when the serum concentration is less.

SERUM PHOSPHORUS: NORMAL VALUES AND DEVIATIONS

Normal values
Adults: 3 to 4.5 mg/dl
           1.8 to 2.6 mEq/L
Children: 4 to 7 mg/dl
           2.3 to 4.1 mEq/L

Deviations	Cause	Possible effects
Hyperphos-phatemia	↑ TCT ↑ Growth hormone ↑ Ingestion of PO_4^{3-} Chronic glomerulo-nephritis Sarcoidosis	Associated with ↓ BUN, creatinine Symptoms of hypocalce-mia Associated with ↓ gamma globulin
Hypophos-phatemia	↑ PTH ↓ Ingestion of PO_4^{3-} Hyperinsulinism	↓ ATP Symptoms of hypercalce-mia Associated with indications of hypoglycemia

Magnesium

Magnesium (Mg^{2+}) influences muscular activity in much the same direction as does calcium. The ion appears to be necessary for the coenzyme activity in the metabolism of carbohydrate and protein.

SERUM MAGNESIUM: NORMAL VALUES AND DEVIATIONS

Normal values: 1.5 to 2.5 mEq/L
                   1.8 to 3 mg/dl

Deviations	Cause	Possible effects
Hypermag-nesemia	↑ Ingestion of Mg^{2+} (milk of magnesia)	↓ Neuromuscular excitation ↓ Muscle tone
Hypomag-nesemia	Malabsorption syndrome Acute pancreatitis	↑ Neuromuscular excitation (tetany) Peripheral vasodilatation Arrhythmias

Gases and pH

The blood gases are not usually tested in the screening examination but may be indicated as necessary tests by clinical signs such as cyanosis or hyperventilation.

Oxygen

Tests for blood oxygen analysis are generally performed on arterial blood. The blood may be tested for oxygen content, hemoglobin saturation, and the gas tension (PaO_2, arterial blood; PvO_2, venous blood). The oxygen content of the blood reflects the hemoglobin concentration. At standard temperature and pressure 1.34 ml of oxygen combines with 1 g of hemoglobin at full saturation. The oxygen saturation of hemoglobin is a comparison of the percentage of oxygen that is bound to hemoglobin with the total amount that it is possible for the hemoglobin to carry. The erythrocyte carries 98.5% of the oxygen in the blood bound to hemoglobin. Since the normal hemoglobin content of the adult male is 15 g/dl, the oxygen-carrying capacity is approximately 20 ml/dl of blood, or 20 vol%.

BLOOD OXYGEN: NORMAL VALUES AND DEVIATIONS

Normal values

	Arterial blood	Mixed venous blood
Content:	15 to 23 vol%	
Saturation:	94% to 100%	70% to 75%
Tension:	95 to 100 mm Hg	35 to 40 mm Hg

Deviations	Cause	Possible effects
Anoxic hypoxia	Inadequate environmental O_2 supply, such as occurs in high altitude (acute) Impaired respiratory exchange	Low Pa_{O_2} Inadequate saturation of the arterial blood with oxygen Cyanosis ↑ Respiratory rate
Chronic hypoxia	Living at high altitude	↑ O_2 carrying capacity as RBCs increase
Anemic hypoxia	↓ Hemoglobin Competition for hemoglobin-binding sites (carbon monoxide poisoning)	↓ Saturation of hemoglobin possible
Stagnant hypoxia	↓ Circulatory function (failure to deliver O_2 to tissues) Cardiac failure Shock Peripheral impairment of flow (embolism)	Blood O_2 values may be normal
Histotoxic hypoxia	↓ Ability of cells to take up or use O_2, such as in poisoning	
Hyperoxia	Pure O_2 delivered at 1 atmosphere (766 mm Hg)	Bronchitis in 12 to 24 hours Fall in vital capacity in 60 hours Retrolental fibroplasia

At standard conditions arterial blood contains 0.3 ml of oxygen dissolved in 100 ml of plasma; this exerts a pressure of 100 mm Hg. The amount of oxygen combined with hemoglobin is decreased with an increase in temperature, acidity, and carbon dioxide tension ($PaCO_2$, arterial blood; $PvCO_2$, venous blood).

Carbon dioxide

Carbon dioxide in the blood occurs in three forms: as bicarbonate, combined with protein (carbamino), and in simple solution. Carbon dioxide in an aqueous solution is in potential equilibrium with carbonic acid. The enzyme carbonic anhydrase is necessary to the catalysis of the equilibrium:

$$CO_2 + H_2O \rightleftharpoons H_2CO_3$$

The only test for carbon dioxide that is generally performed as part of the screening battery is the carbon dioxide–combining power, which measures the buffering capacity of the blood. The sample is collected, and the serum is removed after clotting and centrifugation. The carbon dioxide tension of the serum is equilibrated to normal alveolar tensions of 40 mm Hg. The bicarbonate is converted to carbon dioxide by hydrolysis, and the gas that is given up is measured. Subtraction of the known amount of dissolved carbon dioxide in the blood gives a value that is essentially that of bicarbonate alone.

Normal $PaCO_2$: 35 to 45 mm Hg
Normal $PvCO_2$: 41 to 55 mm Hg
Normal arterial whole blood HCO_3^-: 22 to 26 mEq/L
Normal venous whole blood HCO_3^-: 22 to 26 mEq/L

The base excess (BE) is a measure of alkaline substances in the blood. This includes bicarbonate and other bases in the blood.

Normal arterial BE: −2 to +2
Normal venous BE: −2 to +2

pH

Hydrogen ion concentration of the blood is reflected in the pH value. The degree of alkalinity or acidity of the body is important in that many enzymes are active only within narrow pH ranges. Furthermore, many other physiological processes are pH dependent, notably respiration. Acidosis is the process whereby an individual develops acidemia, the accumulation of excess hydrogen ions in the blood—or decreased pH. The affected person is described as acidotic.

Alkalosis, on the other hand, is the process whereby alkalemia is incurred. Alkalemia may be defined as decreased hydrogen ion concentration in the blood—or increased pH—and the individual may be described as alkalotic.

The Henderson-Hasselbalch equation describes pH relationships:

$$pH = pK + \log \frac{base}{acid}$$

pK is the dissociation constant (the ability to release hydrogen ions of the acid described). In the human being the bicarbonate ion is the most important buffering system, since the ion is present in large quantities. Thus, the equation may be written:

$$pH = 6.1 + \log \frac{HCO_3^-}{H_2CO_3}$$

The ratio $\dfrac{HCO_3^-}{H_2CO_3} = \dfrac{20}{1}$ in the normal person.

The bicarbonate ion is controlled by the lungs through the expiration of carbon dioxide and the kidneys, which control excretion of bicarbonate and hydrogen ions.

WHOLE BLOOD pH: NORMAL VALUES AND DEVIATIONS

Normal values
Arterial: 7.38 to 7.44 (7.40)
Venous: 7.30 to 7.41 (7.36)

Deviations
Acidemia (acidosis): <pH 7.35
Alkalemia (alkalosis): >pH 7.45

Glucose

Sucrose, lactose, and starches make up the majority of the carbohydrates ingested by humans. Slight amounts of alcohol, lactic acid, pyruvic acid, pectins, and dextrins are also consumed. These carbohydrates are hydrolyzed in the intestinal tract and broken down to the monosaccharides: glucose (80%), fructose (10%), and galactose (10%), in which form they are absorbed into the bloodstream.

Glucose is the principal form of fuel for cellular function; the liver can convert fructose and galactose to glucose, so that all the absorbed sugars can be used. Fats and proteins may also be converted to glucose during fasting states or in times of increased glucose use, as in exercise. Glucose in excess of energy needs is converted to storage forms. The body is capable of storing about 100 g of glucose as glycogen. The majority of the remainder of glucose is converted to fat, but some is converted to amino acids.

The pancreatic hormones, insulin and glucagon, play a prominent role in glucose metabolism, as well as in the metabolism of protein and lipid. Insulin is produced by the beta cells of the pancreas, and its secretion is primarily determined by the concentration of blood glucose. The secretion of insulin is increased by an increase from basal of blood glucose; it is decreased as the concentration of blood glucose becomes less than normal. Blood insulin values in excess of normal produce the following major changes in glucose metabolism: (1) the rate of glucose metabolism is increased by facilitating the transport of glucose into the cells via facilitated diffusion, (2) the process of glycogen storage is enhanced, (3) the process of glucose entry into fat cells is enhanced and fat storage increased, and (4) the process of glucose entry into muscle cells is enhanced.

On the other hand, a decrease of blood insulin is accompanied by (1) glycogenolysis, a breakdown of glycogen to glucose, and (2) glyconeogenesis, the manufacture of glucose by the liver from amino acids derived from protein stores and from glycerol derived from fat stores. These two processes are functions of glucagon.

Thus, blood glucose concentration in the fasting state is maintained within reasonably narrow limits. Blood glucose determination at any one time will provide data concerning the state of the body's metabolism for that specific point in the individual's daily cycle. However, the practitioner must bear in mind that the metabolic processes are determined by the state of nutrition and the energy expenditure. The normal individual, in dynamic equilibrium, will show remarkable variation throughout the day; the picture is even more complex in disease.

Care of specimens for blood glucose determination deserves special attention; glucose values for whole blood decrease 10 mg/dl per hour (at room temperature) unless a satisfactory preservative is employed. Fluoride is currently recognized as the most effective preservative.

Glucose analysis is accomplished by reducing and enzymatic methods. In both cases, a protein-free filtrate of the blood sample is tested. The reducing methods include the Folin-Wu and Somogyi-Nelson tests, both of which consist of color changes that occur in copper solutions. The enzymatic (glucose oxidase) tests measure hydrogen peroxide that is released during the enzymatic conversion of glucose to gluconic acid.

Blood glucose values are 120 to 130 mg/dl in mild hyperglycemia, and greater than 500 mg/dl in marked hyperglycemia.

BLOOD GLUCOSE: NORMAL VALUES AND DEVIATIONS

Normal values

Serum or plasma: 70 to 110 mg/dl (Folin-Wu)
                 65 to 90 mg/dl (Somogyi-Nelson)
                 65 to 90 mg/dl (glucose oxidase)

Deviations	Cause	Possible effects
Hyperglycemia	Diabetes mellitus (most common cause)	Ketoacidosis
	Pancreatic insufficiency	Diuresis if >160 to 180 mg/1 bond
	Cushing's disease	$\downarrow$ CO_2 combining
	Treatment with steroids	power >500 mg/dl
	$\uparrow$ Catecholamines	
	Pheochromocytoma	
	Pancreatic neoplasm	
	Hyperthyroidism (look for hydrocholesterolemia)	
	Thiazide diuretics	
Hypoglycemia	Beta cell neoplasm (hyperinsulinism)	
	Addison's disease	
	Hypothyroidism	
	Hepatocellular disease	
	Starvation (late)	
	Glycogen storage diseases	

A rising blood glucose concentration stimulates excessive insulin secretion in some individuals. Some amino acids (leucine) may also stimulate excessive beta cell secretion. Thus, glucose levels may be depleted as the insulin effects are manifested.

Two-hour postprandial glucose test. The 2-hour postprandial glucose test consists of the serial collection of samples of blood glucose determination following a 100 g carbohydrate meal given to a client who has fasted for 12 hours. The following represent hyperglycemia results:

Time	Blood glucose determination
1 hour after meal	>170 mg/dl
2 hours after meal	>120 mg/dl

Glucose tolerance test. The glucose tolerance test is performed in the fasting individual following the ingestion of 100 g of glucose; the blood glucose level rises 30 to 60 mg/dl above the fasting level by 30 minutes. By the end of an hour the blood glucose level begins to decline (20 to 50 mg/dl), and after 2 to 3 hours returns to the fasting level. Urine specimens are collected. Glucose does not appear in the urine of the normal individual during the course of the glucose tolerance test. The glucose tolerance test shows elevated values in the period following myocardial infarction.

Bilirubin

Bilirubin is a pigment that is mainly derived from the breakdown of heme in the hemoglobin of RBCs in Kupffer's cells of the reticuloendothelial system. The pigment has a golden hue and is the major pigment found in bile. Plasma containing the pigment enters the hepatic parenchymal cells and is enzymatically conjugated with glucuronic acid in preparation for excretion. The conjugated bilirubin is soluble in an aqueous medium and is actively excreted into the bile. A small amount of the conjugated bilirubin is returned to the blood and accounts for the direct-reacting bilirubin found in the plasma of normal subjects. Because it passes through membranes, it may be detected in the urine.

Intestinal bacteria act on bilirubin to form urobilinogen. Since urobilinogen is highly soluble, it is readily reabsorbed through the intestinal mucosa into the blood and is for the most part recycled in the liver back to the intestine; some, however, is excreted in the urine.

Bilirubin is analyzed through its reaction (color change) with diazo reagents; this is the basis of van den Bergh's test. The conjugated form reacts expediently with the diazo reagents in aqueous solution and is called direct reacting. The unconjugated form must be treated with methyl alcohol for the reaction to occur and is called indirect reacting.

Bilirubin is called unconjugated, free, or indirect reacting before it is combined with glucuronic acid in the liver cell. It does not cross the membranes of the capillary or of the glomerular capsule. After combination with glucuronic acid in the hepatic cells, bilirubin is referred to as conjugated, glucuronide, or direct reacting. But the routine test gives only the total value.

The occurrence of jaundice (yellowish tint of the skin) represents the failure to remove or excrete the bilirubin. The skin may appear jaundiced when serum bilirubin levels are about three times the normal value. In most individuals pigmentation of the tissues is visible when serum bilirubin levels exceed 1.5 mg/dl.

SERUM BILIRUBIN: NORMAL VALUES AND DEVIATIONS

Normal values
Total: 0.1 to 1.2 mg/dl
Newborn total: 1 to 12 mg/dl

Deviations	Cause	Possible effects
Hyperbilirubinemia	Destruction of red cells Hemolytic diseases (↓ hemoglobin) Hemorrhage Hematoma Hepatic dysfunction	Jaundice
↑ Unconjugated bilirubin	Autoimmune disease Transfusion-initiated hemolysis Hemolytic diseases Sickle cell anemia Pernicious anemia Glucuronyl transferase deficiency (hemolytic disease of the newborn) Hemorrhage (bleeding into body cavities) Hematoma Impaired hepatic uptake of bile (infectious or toxic hepatitis)	Brain damage (22 mg/dl or more)
↑ Conjugated bilirubin	Impaired glucuronide excretion Hepatocellular disease (infectious, toxic, or autoimmune hepatitis) Cirrhosis Obstruction of biliary ducts Calculi Tumor Extrinsic pressure Cholangiolitis	"Regurgitation" of conjugated bilirubin back into the blood

Blood urea nitrogen

Urea is the end product of protein metabolism and is formed through deamination of amino acids in the liver. Urea is excreted by the kidneys.

Ingestion of protein does not cause a significant change in the BUN level. However, in the interest of accuracy this test is done in the fasting individual.

The severity of uremia is an indicator of the seriousness of renal involvement.

BUN: NORMAL VALUES AND DEVIATIONS

Normal values
8 to 18 mg/dl
Normal values tend to be higher in men than in women.

Deviations	Cause
Increased BUN level of uremia	High protein intake Dehydration Protein catabolism Burns Intestinal obstruction Gastrointestinal hemorrhage Renal disease Glomerulonephritis Pyelonephritis Prostatic hypertrophy
Decreased BUN level	↓ Protein ingestion Starvation Liver dysfunction Cirrhosis (loss of 80% to 85% hepatic function)

Creatinine

The metabolism of creatinine phosphate, a high-energy compound produced in skeletal muscle, results in the production of creatinine. The serum creatinine level does not vary markedly with diet or exercise and may be regarded as an indicator of total muscle mass.

Creatinine clearance by the kidney has been used as a measure of renal function. In addition to the serum creatinine level being fairly constant, creatinine clearance as a measure offers another advantage to the client in that an intravenous injection of the substance used in the clearance study is not needed. Renal plasma clearance of creatinine (C) is equal to the rate of creatinine excretion (UV) divided by the plasma concentration of creatinine (P):

$$C = \frac{UV}{P}$$

Since endogenous creatinine is fully filtered in the glomerulus and not reabsorbed by the tubules, its clearance is a useful clinical tool for estimation of the glomerular filtration rate (GFR). Thus, the removal of creatinine from the blood is a measure of renal efficiency. As renal function declines, the creatinine level rises.

SERUM CREATININE: NORMAL VALUES AND DEVIATION

Normal values

0.6 to 1.2 mg/dl
Normal values for men are slightly higher than for women.

Deviation	Cause	Possible effects
Hypercreatinemia	Renal disease (75% of nephrons are nonfunctional)	Signs of renal failure
	Chronic glomerulonephritis	
	Nephrosis	
	Pyelonephritis	
	Hyperthyroidism	

Uric acid

Uric acid production is the final step in purine metabolism. Uric acid is not in stable solution at a normal human blood pH of 7.4. Uric acid is continuously produced in the human being and is excreted by the kidney. The quantity of uric acid found in the urine is about 10% of that which is filtered. Thus, it is obvious that uric acid is reabsorbed in the proximal tubules. It has been further shown that uric acid is secreted in the proximal tubules.

However, reabsorption overrides this process, and the plasma uric acid represents the balance of uric acid production and excretion.

SERUM URIC ACID: NORMAL VALUES AND DEVIATION

Normal values

Women: 2 to 6.4 mg/dl
Men: 2.1 to 7.8 mg/dl

Deviation	Cause	Possible effects
Hyperuricemia (gout)	↑ Destruction of nucleic acid and purine products	Monosodium urate precipitate in joints (tophi)
	Chronic lymphocytic and granulocytic leukemia	Often associated with hyperlipidemia, atheromatosis
	Multiple myeloma	
	Chronic renal failure	
	Fasting	
	↑ Ingestion of protein	
	↓ Excretion of uric acid	Impaired clearance of uric acid
	Gout	

Deviation	Cause	Possible effects
	Fasting	
	Toxemia of pregnancy	
	Glomerulonephritis	
	Thiazide diuretics	
	Alpha-lipoprotein deficiency (Tangier disease)	
	Hypoparathyroidism	
	↑ Salicylate ingestion	
	Ethanol ingestion	

Monosodium urate deposits may occur in the presence of a normal serum uric acid value.

Hypouricemia is seldom observed unless the client is being treated with allopurinol, which depresses uric acid production.

Total proteins

Plasma proteins make up approximately 7% of the plasma volume. Albumin and globulin in the free state, as well as in combination with lipid and carbohydrate substances, are the major plasma proteins. Through the application of zone electrophoresis and ultracentrifugation, the plasma proteins have been defined as albumin, the globulins (alpha-1, alpha-2, beta-1, beta-2, and gamma), lipoproteins, and fibrinogen. Separation through centrifugation is possible because the sedimentation rate at high speeds is determined by molecular size and shape. Electrophoresis is the process of migration of charged particles in an electrolyte solution through which an electrical current is passed. The proteins move at various rates, depending on size, shape, and electrical charge. Immunoelectrophoresis separates the immune globulin fractions through a combination of electrophoresis and immunodiffusion.

The plasma proteins are large molecules that do not readily diffuse through the capillary membrane. The small amount of protein that does pass through the capillary wall is taken up by the lymphatic system and returned to the blood. It has been demonstrated that the plasma protein concentration exceeds that of the interstitial space nearly four times. Since the plasma proteins are the only dissolved substances in the plasma that do not pass through the capillary membrane, they are responsible for plasma oncotic pressure. Thus, proteins help to regulate intravascular volume. The plasma proteins also serve as buffers in acid-base balance and as binding and transporting agents for lipids, triglycerides, hormones, vitamins, calcium, and copper. In addition, they participate in blood coagulation. Furthermore, in the event that body tissues become depleted of protein, plasma proteins may be used for replenishment. The liver synthesizes nearly all of the plasma albumin and fibrinogen and about one half of the globulins.

Familial lipoprotein lipase deficiency and familial hypertriglyceridemia have not been shown to be related to coronary artery disease. Monogenic hypercholesterolemia is the result of a defect in LDL uptake by peripheral cells. Affected individuals may have cutaneous xanthomas, xanthelasma, and retinal lipemia.

Laboratory tests of plasma lipids and lipoproteins include total cholesterol, total triglyceride, HDL, LDL, cholesterol/HDL ratio, phenotype determination, and centrifugation and separation.

Clinically significant hyperlipoproteinemia is said to exist with the following values:

Age of subject	Total plasma cholesterol	Plasma triglyceride
20 years	200 mg/dl	140 mg/dl
20 years	240 mg/dl	200 mg/dl

Phospholipids

Lecithin and sphingomyelin are the major serum phospholipids. Phospholipids are constituents of both HDLs and LDLs.

Normal serum phospholipid values: 150 to 375 mg/dl

TOTAL SERUM LIPIDS: NORMAL VALUES AND DEVIATIONS

Normal values: 350 to 800 mg/dl (adult)

Deviations	Cause	Predominant lipoprotein
Cholesterol: marked elevation; triglyceride: no change or elevation	↑ Ingestion of cholesterol	LDL (Type IIa)
Cholesterol: elevation; triglyceride: no change or elevation	↑ Cholesterol manufacture by liver Obesity Hereditary ↓ LDL catabolism Hypothyroidism Hereditary	LDL (Type IIa) or LDL and VLDL (Type IIb)
	↓ Remnant removal Hypothyroidism Hereditary	Remnants (Type III) or VLDL and chylomicrons (Type V)

Cholesterol: no change or elevation; triglyceride; elevation	↑ Triglyceride synthesis
	Dietary intake (caloric)
	Alcohol
	Hyperinsulinism
	  Obesity
	  Corticosteroids
	Estrogen
	Hereditary
		VLDL (Type IV) or VLDL and chylomicrons (Type V)

	↓ Triglyceride clearance Insulin (diabetes) Hypothyroidism Renal failure Hereditary	VLDL (Type IV) or VLDL and chylomicrons (Type V)

Cholesterol

Exogenous cholesterol is absorbed from the small intestine into the lymph. Endogenous cholesterol is formed by all the cells of the body. Most of the endogenous cholesterol in the plasma is formed by the liver from acetate. It is the endogenous cholesterol that is measured in blood chemistry profiles. A control mechanism exists for these two processes, since endogenous cholesterol production is inhibited when cholesterol ingestion is increased. Cholesterol is present in the plasma primarily as LDLs. The LDL cholesterol is taken up by most peripheral tissues. This is a modified receptor process. In addition, most tissues are capable of cholesterol synthesis. Increased uptake of LDL inhibits cellular cholesterol production and decreased uptake results in increased cholesterol synthesis in the peripheral cells.

Cholesterol testing was the forerunner of serum lipid analysis and has served as a valuable but debatable tool for prediction of coronary artery disease caused by atheromatous or arteriosclerotic artery disease.

Because the liver esterifies cholesterol, the ratio of esterified to unesterified cholesterol may be considered an indication of liver function. The normal serum esterified cholesterol value ranges from 20% to 30%.

Obstruction of the biliary ducts is typified by an increased cholesterol level with a decrease in the amount of esterified cholesterol.

SERUM CHOLESTEROL: NORMAL VALUES AND DEVIATIONS

Normal values: 150 to 250 mg/dl

Deviations	Cause	Possible effects
Hypercholesterolemia (marked: >400 mg/dl)	Liver disease Nephrotic stage of glomerulonephritis Familial hypercholesterolemia Hypothyroidism Pancreatic dysfunction Diabetes mellitus	Associated with ↑ alkaline phosphatase, ↑ bilirubin, ↑ BUN, ↑ creatinine

Hypocholesterolemia (significant: <150 mg/dl)	↓ Ingestion of cholesterol
	Malnutrition
	Fasting
	Liver disease
	Megaloblastic or hypochromic anemia
	↑ Estrogen
	↑ Thyroid hormone
	Hypermetabolic states
	  Fever
	  Exercise	

Enzymes

Enzymes are individual molecules or aggregates of protein molecules occurring in globular form. Enzymes act as catalysts to biochemical reactions. In the event of cellular destruction of an organ or tissue, the cytoplasmic enzymes are released into the plasma from the diseased cells. Enzymes are categorized by their functional effect. These groupings are called isoenzymes. Isoenzymes are enzymes with the same functional effect but with variations in configuration and physical characteristics. The isoenzyme content of many tissues and structures has been determined. There is sufficient variation in the enzyme content of the various organs that changes in the enzyme concentration in the blood may serve as an indicator of the site of disease. Electrophoresis may be used to separate these proteins. Serum enzyme determination results are also used to assess tissue rejection following transplantation procedures.

SGOT, serum LDH, and serum alkaline phosphatase determinations are included in most screening laboratory examinations. Enzyme determinations currently and commonly encountered in clinical practice are described in this section.

Serum glutamic-oxaloacetic transaminase (SGOT)

SGOT is found in many tissues. The transaminase enzymes catalyze the conversion of an amino acid to a keto acid; another keto acid is converted to an amino acid in the glycolytic cycle. This enzyme catalyzes conversions of glutamic and oxaloacetic acids. High tissue concentrations of SGOT have been demonstrated for the heart and liver, but appreciable amounts are found in RBCs, muscle, and kidney.

Colorimetric and spectrophotometric techniques are used in determining the serum concentration of these enzymes. Elevated levels of the enzyme may be identified 8 hours after tissue damage occurs. In the case of a single injury (such as myocardial infarction) that is not followed by further damage, the enzyme reaches a peak level in 24 to 36 hours and declines to basal levels in about 4 to 6 days.

The SGOT concentration is directly related to the degree of cellular damage.

SGOT: NORMAL VALUES AND DEVIATION

Normal values: 8 to 33 U/dl (Reitman-Frankel)
10 to 40 mU/ml (SMA 12/60)

Deviation	Cause
Elevation of SGOT values	Myocardial infarction
Elevation greater than 1,000	Hepatocellular disease
U/ml (or more than 10	Infectious or toxic hepatitis
times normal)	Liver necrosis
Elevation to 40 to 100 U/ml	Tachyarrhythmias
	Congestive heart failure
	Myocarditis
	Pericarditis
	Pulmonary infarction
	Cirrhosis
	Cholangitis
	Pancreatitis
	Metastatic liver disease

Deviation	Cause
	Generalized infection (infectious mononucleosis)
	Trauma
	Shock
	Muscle disease
	Muscular dystrophy
	Dermatomyositis
	Skeletal muscle damage
	Generalized infection

Serum glutamic-pyruvic transaminase (SGPT)

SGPT catalyzes conversions between glutamic and pyruvic acid in the glycolytic pathway. The liver contains the highest concentration of SGPT, but the enzyme is prominent in kidney, heart, and skeletal muscle. The pattern of release of SGPT is similar to SGOT in the face of cellular damage, although more damage than that necessary to produce an elevation of SGOT is generally present when SGPT levels are increased.

SERUM SGPT: NORMAL VALUES AND DEVIATION

Normal values: 5 to 35 U/ml (Reitman-Frankel)

Deviation	Cause
Elevation of SGPT values	
Marked elevation	Infectious or toxic hepatitis
	Infectious mononucleosis
Moderate elevation	Obstructive jaundice
	Postnecrotic cirrhosis
Slight elevation	Cirrhosis
	Myocardial infarction

Lactic dehydrogenase (LDH)

The tissue concentrations of LDH mimic those of SGOT. Furthermore, elevations in serum LDH levels correlate with the same conditions underlying increases in SGOT concentrations. LDH catalyzes the conversions between pyruvate and lactate in the glycolytic cycle. Following myocardial infarction, serum LDH levels increase five to six times in the first 48 hours and may remain elevated for 6 to 10 days. LDH has been separated into five isoenzymes, making it a sharper diagnostic tool. These isoenzymes may be separated by electrophoresis.

A variety of colorimetric tests are available for assessment of this serum enzyme concentration.

A hemolyzed blood specimen may give spuriously high values for LDH concentration in the serum, since the damaged RBCs give up LDH; this will be reflected in the concentration of the enzyme in the sample.

Since the 1970s, particular emphasis has been placed on the use of the isoenzymes of LDH. There are five isoenzymes of LDH, designated LDH_1 to LDH_5. Normally LDH_2 is greater than LDH_1 in the serum. However, the myocardium has an abundant LDH_1 content, and following myocardial infarction, the serum value of LDH_1 may exceed LDH_2. Thus, the LDH_1/LDH_2 ratio becomes greater; this is referred to as a reversed or flipped ratio. Increases in LDH_1 also occur in hemolytic states, hyperthyroidism, megaloblastic anemia, renal disease, and gastric malignancy.

SERUM LDH: NORMAL VALUES AND DEVIATION

Normal values: 200 to 400 U/ml (Wroblewski)
100 to 225 mU/ml (SMA 12/60)

Deviation	Cause
Evaluation of LDH values	
Elevation greater than 1,400 Wroblewski units	Hemolytic disorders (marked hemolysis)
	Pernicious anemia
	Myocardial infarction
Elevation of 500 to 700 Wroblewski units	Chronic viral hepatitis
	Malignant neoplasms
	Liver
	Kidney
	Brain
	Skeletal muscle
	Heart
	Destruction of lung tissue
	Pulmonary emboli
	Pneumonia
	Destruction of renal tissue
	Infarction
	Infection
	Generalized viral infection

Alkaline phosphatase

Determinations of serum alkaline phosphatase levels are frequently used to determine the presence of liver and bone cell disease, since the enzyme has its greatest content in these two tissues. However, it is also found in significant concentrations in intestine, kidney, and placenta. The enzyme is thought to catalyze reactions in the process of bone matrix formation, because increased serum alkaline phosphatase levels correlate with osteoblastic activity. The isoenzymes from the liver, bone, intestine, kidney, and placenta can be separated by electrophoresis; thus, the source of the enzyme can be determined. Synthesis of alkaline phosphatase is thought to be small in the normal hepatic cell. The serum alkaline phosphatase level reflects placental function and may be used to monitor the progress of pregnancy.

A low alkaline phosphatase level may be associated with hypophosphatemia, hypothyroidism, or vitamin C deficiency.

SERUM ALKALINE PHOSPHATASE: NORMAL VALUES AND DEVIATION

Normal values

Adults: 1.5 to 4.5 U/dl (Bodansky)
4 to 13 U/dl (King-Armstrong)
0.8 to 2.3 U/ml (Bessey-Lowry)
30 to 100 mU/ml (SMA 12/60)

Children: 5 to 14 U/dl (Bodansky)
3.4 to 9 U/ml (Bessey-Lowry)
15 to 30 U/dl (King-Armstrong)
(The level in children is about three times that of the adult.)

Deviation	Cause
Elevation of alkaline phosphatase values	
Marked elevation (15 U/dl or more—Bodansky)	Liver disease
	Obstructive disease
	Neoplasm
	Bone disease
	Paget's disease
	Sarcoma
	Metastatic carcinoma
Slight to moderate elevation (8 to 10 U/dl—Bodansky)	Liver disease
	Cholangitis
	Cirrhosis
	Hyperparathyroidism
	Osteomalacia
	Renal infarction, tissue rejection

Acid phosphatase

Acid phosphatase occurs in greatest amount in prostatic tissue. In the normal individual the enzyme is excreted in prostatic fluids. However, in prostatic metastatic carcinoma, the serum acid phosphatase level rises and thus becomes a tool in differential diagnosis.

Normal serum acid phosphatase values: 1 to 4 U/dl (King-Armstrong)

Creatine phosphokinase (CPK)

CPK catalyzes the phosphorylation of creatine by adenosine triphosphate (ATP). The greatest tissue content of CPK is found in skeletal and cardiac muscle, although significant amounts occur in the brain. The serum CPK level may be elevated as a result of intramuscular injection or following surgery and returns to basal levels in 24 to 48 hours. Since CPK is not produced by the liver, elevated serum values of this enzyme may help eliminate liver disease in differential diagnosis.

Recent investigations have shown the usefulness of measuring the three isoenzymes of CPK, designated as M, B, and MB. The M isoenzyme is present in skeletal and cardiac muscle, the B isoenzyme is found in the brain, and the MB isoenzyme is found in relatively high concentrations in the cardiac muscle but is also present in the skeletal muscle. The MB fraction has specific predictability in relation to myocardial infarction; it is typically the first enzyme detectable in abnormal concentration in serum following myocardial damage. The isoenzyme is first detectable 3 to 5 hours after infarction and reaches its peak in 12 to 24 hours, with a rapid decline to normal values in 24 to 48 hours.

CPK–MB is also elevated in individuals with muscle trauma, polymyositis, muscular dystrophy, neuromuscular disease, pulmonary embolism, tachyarrhythmias, and unstable angina.

SERUM CPK: NORMAL VALUES AND DEVIATION

Normal values: 0 to 200 units (Sigma)
Men: 5 to 50 mU/ml (Oliver-Rosalki)
Women: 5 to 30 mU/ml (Oliver-Rosalki)

Deviation	Cause
Elevation of serum CPK values	Muscle disease
	Duchenne's muscular dystrophy (early)
	Dermatomyositis
	Polymyositis
	Trauma
	Myocardial infarction
	Encephalitis
	Bacterial meningitis
	Cerebrovascular accident
	Hepatic coma
	Uremic coma
	Strenuous exercise
	Ingestion of salicylates

Aldolase

Aldolase catalyzes the splitting of fructose 1,6-diphosphate into glyceraldehyde phosphate and dihydroxyacetone phosphate. Aldolase occurs in greatest concentration in skeletal and heart muscle, but the liver contains a moderate amount, and all tissues contain some of the enzyme.

SERUM ALDOLASE: NORMAL VALUES AND DEVIATION

Normal values: 3 to 8 U/dl (Sibley-Lehninger)

Deviation	Cause
Elevation of serum aldolase values	Muscle disease
	Progressive muscular dystrophy
	Dermatomyositis
	Trichinosis
	Myocardial infarction
	Viral hepatitis
	Hepatic cellular necrosis
	Granulocytic leukemia
	Carcinomatosis

Amylase

Pancreatic amylase is synthesized in the pancreatic cells and secreted into the pancreatic ducts for transport to the duodenum, where it catalyzes the hydrolysis of starch and glycogen. Elevated serum amylase levels may be used to monitor damage to pancreatic cells. Although the salivary glands produce amylase, diseases of these cells do not affect the serum lipase level.

SERUM AMYLASE: NORMAL VALUES AND DEVIATION

Normal values: 60 to 150 U/dl (Somogyi)

Deviation	Cause
Elevation of serum amylase values	Acute pancreatitis

Lipase

Lipase is synthesized by the pancreatic cells and secreted into the pancreatic ducts for transport to the duodenum, where it catalyzes the hydrolysis of triglycerides to fatty acids. Elevation of serum lipase concentrations indicates damage to pancreatic cells. Serum lipase levels remain elevated longer following acute pancreatitis than do amylase levels.

SERUM LIPASE: NORMAL VALUES AND DEVIATION

Normal values: 0 to 1.5 U/ml (Cherry-Crandall)

Deviation	Cause
Elevation of serum lipase values (lipasemia)	Acute pancreatitis

Cholinesterase

Cholinesterase (ChE) catalyzes the hydrolysis of acetylcholine and other cholinesters and has been classified as "true" cholinesterase or as pseudocholinesterase. True cholinesterase, or acetylcholinesterase, is more rapid in its action on acetylcholine and is found in greatest concentration in the brain and in RBCs. Pseudocholinesterase is found in plasma but not in the erythrocytes and is thought to be manufactured by the liver. Both of these enzymes are inactivated by organophosphates. Testing of acetylcholinesterase provides an indication of toxicity from insecticides containing these compounds.

Normal ChE (RBC) values: 0.65 to 1.00 pH units
Pseudocholinesterase (plasma): 0.5 to 1.3 pH units

SCREENING HEMATOLOGICAL EXAMINATIONS

The hemogram, or complete blood cell count (CBC), includes the following determinations: RBC count, hematocrit (HCT), hemoglobin (Hgb), white blood cell (WBC) count, and differential WBC count. Other commonly performed hematological examinations are determinations of the mean corpuscular volume (MCV), mean corpuscular hemoglobin (MCH), and mean corpuscular hemoglobin concentration (MCHC).

Red blood cells
RBC count

Erythropoiesis, the manufacture of RBCs, occurs in the bone marrow. Erythropoietin, a hormone produced by the kidney exposed to hypoxia, plays a prominent role in the control of erythropoiesis.

Electronic counting devices (such as the Coulter device) are faster and produce more accurate blood cell determinations than those of a technician counting the smear under a microscope.

Both anemias and polycythemias are classified as relative if they result from changes in plasma volume.

RED BLOOD CELLS: NORMAL COUNTS AND DEVIATIONS

Normal counts
Men: 4.6 to $6.2 \times 10^6/\mu l$
Women: 4.2 to $5.4 \times 10^6/\mu l$

Deviations	Cause	Possible effects
Elevated RBC count (polycythemia)	Bone marrow hyperplasia (polycythemia vera)	Hyperviscosity of blood Tendency toward thrombosis Sluggish blood flow to tissues (tissue hypoxia) Hypervolemia Headache Tinnitus Dizzines Ruddy cyanosis
Decreased RBC count (anemia)	RBC production deficiency states Protein Iron Vitamin B$_{12}$ Folic acid Toxicity (depressed bone marrow) Metabolites (urea, creatinine) Drugs (chloramphenicol) Ionizing radiation Hypothyroidism Hereditary (thalassemia)	Pallor Fatigue Rapid pulse Irritability Headache Dizziness Postural hypotension Menstrual irregularities Angina Shortness of breath

Hematocrit

The hematocrit examination is used to determine the volume-packed (centrifuged) RBCs in 100 ml of blood.

Normal hematocrit values
Men: 40% to 54%
Women: 38% to 47%

Hemoglobin

Hemoglobin consists of heme, a pigmented compound containing iron, and globin, a colorless protein. Hemoglobin binds with oxygen and carbon dioxide. The hemoglobin molecule binds oxygen and transports it to the periphery; it binds carbon dioxide as it is transported to the lung.

Normal hemoglobin values
Men: 13.5 to 18 g/dl
Women: 12.0 to 16 g/dl

Mean corpuscular volume

The MCV test measures RBCs in terms of individual cell size. The value can be calculated through the use of the following formula:

$$MCV = \frac{HCT}{RBC}$$

The result is expressed in microcubic millimeters per blood cell.

Normal MCV: 80 to 94 μmm^3

This test is used to classify anemias as microcytic (RBC size smaller than normal), normocytic, or macrocytic (larger than normal).

Deviations	Cause
Microcytic anemia	Hypochromic Iron deficiency Thalassemia Chronic infections Chronic renal disease Malignancy
Normocytic anemia	Hypochromic Lead poisoning Chronic infection Chronic renal disease Malignancy Normochromic Hemorrhage Hemolytic anemia Bone marrow hypoplasia Splenomegaly
Macrocytic anemia	Normochromic Pernicious anemia Folic acid deficiency Hypothyroidism Hepatocellular disease

Mean corpuscular hemoglobin

The MCH examination measures the hemoglobin concentration of the individual RBCs. Expressed in picograms (micromicrograms), it can be calculated by dividing the hemoglobin in grams by the RBCs:

$$MCH = \frac{Hgb}{RBC}$$

The test allows the classification of anemia as hypochromic or normochromic.

Normal MCH values: 27 to 31 pg

Mean corpuscular hemoglobin concentration

The MCHC test measures the concentration of hemoglobin in grams per dl of RBCs. Expressed in percentages, it can be calculated using the following formula:

$$MCHC = \frac{Hgb\ (g)}{HCT}$$

Normal mean cell hemoglobin concentration: 32% to 36%

An elevation of MCHC is seen only in hereditary spherocytosis.

Sedimentation rate

The erythrocyte sedimentation rate (ESR) is the speed with which RBCs settle in unclotted blood. The speed with which the RBCs settle is dependent on the concentration of the various plasma protein fractions and on the concentration of the RBCs. The cells settle out more rapidly when the plasma concentration is high and the RBC count is low. Increased concentration of fibrinogen or of the globulins speeds up the rate of sedimentation. The rate of settling is accelerated in many inflammatory conditions, in pregnancy, and in multiple myeloma. The sedimentation rate is decreased is sickle cell anemia; this may be caused by the abnormal shape and stickiness of the RBCs.

Normal ESR rate (Westergren)

Men under 50:   <15 mm/hr
Men over 50:   <20 mm/hr
Women under 50: <20 mm/hr
Women over 50:   <30 mm/hr

Microscopic RBC examination

A stained smear of whole blood is examined microscopically to assess the morphological characteristics of the RBCs.

Normal RBC: nonnucleated, biconcave disk, 7 μ to 8 μ in diameter; contains 95% hemoglobin

Nucleated RBCs may be observed in periods of marked erythropoiesis as a result of marrow stimulation. These immature cells are released from the marrow and are found in the circulating blood.

Reticulocytes. A reticulocyte is a precursor to the RBC, is larger than the normal RBC, and stains more with basic dye. The center does not appear pale, as does the normal RBC. In the normal individual 0.5% to 1.5% reticulocytes are present in the circulating blood. During periods of accelerated erythropoiesis the number of reticulocytes in the general circulation increases. The reticulocyte count is generally elevated as a result of hemorrhage or hemolysis.

Nuclear fragments. Structures that represent the degenerated nucleus of the erythroblast are seen as coarse dots, blue lines, and imperfect rings in the smear.

Basophilic stippling. The term basophilic stippling refers to the presence of hemogenous blue dots observed in RBCs treated with Wright's stain. This stippling may indicate thalassemia or toxic manifestations, resulting in abnormal hemoglobin production.

Siderotic granules. Granules of iron-containing substances in addition to hemoglobin may be seen in some cells of smears of RBCs treated with Prussian blue dye. The cells are termed siderocytes and are increased in number following splenectomy and during the course of hemolytic anemias.

Heinz bodies. The RBCs of the individual with glucose-6-phosphate dehydrogenase deficiency may contain inclusion bodies containing denatured hemoglobin called Heinz bodies, for example, in thalassemias.

Poikilocytosis. A poikilocyte is an RBC of abnormal shape. Poikilocytosis refers to the presence of abnormally shaped RBCs in the blood. Leptocytes (target, or "Mexican hat," erythrocytes) are characterized by a central pigment bulls-eye area surrounded by a clear area, which is ringed by a hemoglobinated peripheral border. This type of erythrocyte is seen in the blood of individuals with hemoglobin C or A, or a combination of C and S. They are frequently seen in thalassemia. Liver disease has been shown to be present in some individuals with demonstrated poikilocytosis. The sickle cell disease is characterized by long, crescent-shaped cells.

Anisocytosis. Anisocytosis is the term used for blood that contains erythrocytes with excessive variations in size.

Platelets (thrombocytes). Platelets may be seen in the microscopic examination of whole blood smears. The platelets are granular fragments of cytoplasm of megakaryocytes in the bone marrow. The platelets are largely phospholipids and polysaccharides. They are carriers for a variety of enzymes for clotting factors and serotonin. Thus, platelets play a major role in blood coagulation.

Thrombocytopathy refers to platelet cells of unusual size or shape.

PLATELETS: NORMAL COUNT AND DEVIATIONS

Normal count: 300,000/μl

Deviations	Cause
Thrombocytopenia	Bone marrow depression
Thrombocytosis	Polycythemia
	Splenectomy

WHITE BLOOD CELLS: NORMAL COUNTS AND DEVIATIONS

Normal counts: 4,500 to 11,000/μl whole blood

Deviations	Cause
Elevated WBC count (leukocytosis)	Leukemia
	Bacterial infection
	Polycythemia (resulting from bone marrow stimulation)
Decreased WBC count (leukopenia)	Bone marrow depression
	Ionizing radiation
	Chloramphenicol

Deviations	Cause
	Phenothiazines
	Sulfonamides
	Phenylbutazone
	Agranulocytosis
	Acute viral infection
	Acute alcohol ingestion

White blood cells
WBC count

The WBC count is the assessment of the number of WBCs (leukocytes) in 1 µl of whole blood. The WBCs function to protect the body against infectious disease. Neutrophils and monocytes destroy microorganisms by phagocytosis. Lymphocytes and plasma cells are thought to produce antibodies. Eosinophils play a role in allergy. Granulocytes, monocytes, and some lymphocytes are produced in the bone marrow; lymphocytes are produced in the lymph nodes and thymic tissue. Disease processes may result in changes within individual leukocyte groups, which may include morphological and functional changes and variations in total numbers. These alterations may provide valuable clues that can be used in differential diagnosis.

Differential WBC count

Six different types of WBCs have been identified in the blood: polymorphonuclear neutrophils (PMNs), polymorphonuclear eosinophils (PMEs), polymorphonuclear basophils (PMBs), monocytes, lymphocytes, and plasma cells. Platelets (thrombocytes) are particles of megakaryocytes.

Increased granulation of leukocytes may indicate toxicity reactions.

A shift to the left means that increased numbers of immature neutrophils are present in the specimen and that they are band forms rather than lobulations. Acute stress to the bone marrow and severe bacterial infection may cause the release of early granulocytes. Increased lobulation (3 to 6) or segmentation of neutrophils is often observed in association with vitamin B_{12} deficiency.

Mild to moderate leukocytosis associated with mild to moderate lymphocytosis is characteristic of chronic infections such as tuberculosis. In relative lymphosytosis, the total number of circulating lymphocytes remains constant, but the WBC count is low because of neutropenia. Relative lymphocytosis is normal between 4 months and 4 years of age.

Monocytosis may occur even with no increase in WBCs.

Abnormal white blood cells of diagnostic importance

Plasma cells. Plasma cells are not normally found in the circulating blood. The presence of plasma cells in the blood predicates the necessity to differentiate multiple myeloma, infectious mononucleosis, serum sickness, and rubella.

Downey cells. Downey cells are abnormal lymphocytes that differ from the normal cells in size, cytoplasmic structures (vacuolated, foamy), and immature chromatin pattern. These cells are observed in individuals with infectious mononucleosis, viral disease (hepatitis), and allergic states.

LE cell. The LE cell is a polymorphonuclear leukocyte, generally a neutrophil that contains an inclusion body. The inclusion body has been shown to be denatured nuclear protein that is being phagocytosed by the neutrophil. The LE cell, which can be induced in the laboratory in the presence of LE factor, is present in the blood of many individuals who have lupus erythematosus.

DIFFERENTIAL WBC COUNT: NORMAL PERCENTAGES AND DEVIATIONS

Normal differential count

Type of cell	Percentage of total WBC count	Range
Neutrophils (PMNs)	56%	50% to 70%
Eosinophils (PMEs)	2.7%	5% to 6%
Basophils (PMBs)	0.3%	0 to 1%
Lymphocytes	34%	20% to 40%
Monocytes		0 to 7%

Deviations	Cause
Neutrophilic leukocytosis	Bacterial infections
	Pneumonia
	Systemic infections
	Inflammatory disease
	Rheumatic fever
	Rheumatoid arthritis
	Pancreatitis
	Thyroiditis
	Carcinoma
	Trauma (tissue destruction)
	Burns
	Crush injury
	Stress
	Cold
	Heat
	Exercise
	Electroshock therapy
	Panic, fear, anxiety
	Increased catecholamines
	Increased corticosteroids
	Cushing's disease
	Acute gout
	Diabetes mellitus
	Lead poisoning
	Acute hemorrhage
	Hemolytic anemia

Deviations	Cause
Neutrophilopenia	Acute viral infections
	Bone marrow disease
	Nutritional deficiency
	Vitamin B_{12}
	Folic acid
Basophilic leukocytosis	Myeloproliferative diseases
	Myelofibrosis
	Polycythemia vera
Basophilopenia	Anaphylactic reaction
Eosinophilic leukocytosis	Allergic manifestations
	Asthma
	Hay fever
	Parasitic infestations
	Roundworm
	Flukes
	Malignancy (Hodgkin's disease)
	Colitis
	Eosinophilic granulomatosis
	Eosinophilic leukemia
Lymphocytosis	Leukemia (80% to 90% of total
	WBCs)
	Infectious diseases
	Infectious mononucleosis
	Pertussis
	Viral infections with exanthema
	Measles
	Rubella
	Roseola
	Chickenpox
	Thyrotoxicosis
	Cushing's disease
Monocytosis	Typhoid fever
	Tuberculosis
	Subacute bacterial endocarditis
	Malaria

DETECTION OF SYPHILIS (LUES)

Syphilis is the disease caused by the spirochete *Treponema pallidum*. The disease is described in terms of its early or late manifestations or in terms of primary, secondary, and tertiary stages. It is transmitted by intimate mucous membrane contact or in utero. The destructiveness of the organism is attributed to its invasiveness and the elaboration of a weak endotoxin. Immunity is established by a single infection. One to 4 months after contraction of syphilis, two distinct antibodies appear in the serum. The complement fixation and flocculation diagnostic tests are based on one of these, syphilitic reagin, which combines with certain tissue lipids. *T. pallidum* is sensitive to penicillin. Thus, detection provides an opportunity for curative intervention.

Immunological tests for syphilis

The first serological test for syphilis (STS) was devised by Wassermann and, along with Kolmer's modification that superseded it, was a complement fixation test. Wassermann used extract from a syphilitic liver that had as its reactive ingredient cardiolipin, which is found in many tissues and is not actually specific for syphilis. Thus, it was fortuitous that the syphilitic reagin reacted with it. A lipoidal substance is found in spirochetes that is thought to be similar to the cardiolipin lipoprotein complex, which would explain the reaction.

The procedure for the complement fixation test involves first mixing the sample serum with cardiolipin reagent. The antigen-antibody reaction serves to bind the complement, removing it from the reaction. Sheep blood indicator is then added to the mixture. Hemolysis of the blood cells indicates the presence of free complement. If the cells do not hemolyze, complement is absent because of an earlier antigen-antibody reaction. False positive results may occur if the serum contains anticomplement activity.

The flocculation tests include the Venereal Disease Research Laboratory (VDRL), rapid plasma reagin (RPR), Kahn, Hinton, Kline, and Mazzini tests. These tests are performed by adding a suspension of cardiolipin antigen particles to the sample serum. If the syphilitic reagin (antibody) is present, it produces clumping, or flocculation. The reaction is quantitated by the degree of flocculation.

T. pallidum immobilization (TPI) test

Nichols strain of pathogenic spirochetes can be cultured in rabbits. These spirochetes are incubated with the suspected serum for the TPI test. If the specific antibody is present, the spirochetes are immobilized. This reaction can be observed under the microscope. Other treponema spirochetes are known to give positive reactions to this test.

Reiter protein complement fixation (RPCF) test

The nonpathological Reiter strain of spirochetes can be cultured in artificial media for the RPCF test. Antigen has been prepared from this strain and used in a complement fixation technique.

Fluorescent treponemal antibody absorption (FTA-ABS) test

In the FTA-ABS test, nonspecific cross-reacting antibodies are absorbed from the suspected serum through the use of the Reiter treponema antigen. The remaining serum is incubated on a smear of killed Nichols spirochetes. Following this, a solution containing fluorescent antibodies produced against human globulins is exposed to the sample.

Accuracy of test results

The STS tests are reported to produce as many as 25% to 45% biological false positive (BFP) results. That is, many positive tests have been reported for individuals who definitely have not been exposed to or do not have syphilis. Further investigation has shown these individuals to have acute viral or bacterial infections, hypersensitivity reactions, or a recent vaccination; in some cases such individuals have been found to have chronic systemic illness, such as collagen disease, malaria, or tuberculosis.

Positive test results obtained from nonspecific methods may be confirmed with the FTA-ABS test, which yields positive results midway through or at the end of the primary stage. Thus, in screening procedures a flocculation STS test is done initially and is followed up with the more specific FTA-ABS test.

All tests for syphilis give positive results in the secondary stage.

Antibiotic therapy may cause tests for syphilis to be negative.

Darkfield examination

Serous fluid exudate may be removed from a syphilitic lesion by pipet. *T. pallidum,* if present, may then be identified by darkfield microscopy. This provides positive identification of the spirochete and may be the earliest method of identification, since antibodies are not apparent until late in the primary stage.

URINALYSIS

The urine examined for screening purposes is generally a voided specimen collected without regard to circadian variation of the components; that is, it is voided at any time during the 24-hour period. More accuracy can be expected in electrolyte determination and less likelihood of bacterial contamination can be expected if a midstream or clean-catch specimen is employed. Ideally, the urine is collected on the client's arising, following a period of 12 hours in which no fluids were taken. The urine should be tested within 2 hours following its collection; spurious results may be obtained if urine is allowed to stand for long periods at room temperature; the urine pH is greater, bacteria multiply, and leukocytes and casts are known to deteriorate.

The standard urinalysis includes description of appearance, determination of specific gravity, pH, glucose, protein ketones, and microscopic examination of urinary sediment.

Appearance

The normal color of urine is pale golden yellow. Diluted urine is even more pale in hue. The color is only reported in the event of abnormality. Orange, red, and brown hues of the urine may be associated with porphyria, hemoglobinuria, urobilinuria, or bilirubinemia. Porphyria may be indicated by urine that becomes burgundy red on exposure to light.

Deviations	Cause
Orange hue	Bile
	Ingestion of phenazopyridine (Pyridium)
Red hue	Blood
	Porphyria
	Urates
	Ingestion of dihydroxyanthraquinone (Dorbane)
Brown hue	Blood (melanin may turn black on standing)

Specific gravity

The specific gravity of the urine provides an indicator of the ability of the kidney to concentrate urine. The test is reported as the ratio of the weight of the urine tested to the weight of water.

Normal specific gravity of the urine
1.016 to 1.022 (in states of euhydration)
1.001 to 1.035 (range of normal without reference to hydration)

Low values suggest renal tubular dysfunction. Concentrated urine is observed in ADH deficiency.

pH

pH OF URINE: NORMAL pH AND DEVIATION

Normal pH: freshly voided urine is generally acidic, with a pH of 4.6 to 8

Deviation	Cause
Alkaline urine	Metabolic alkalemia (except hypokalemic chloremia)
	Proteus infections
	Aged specimen

Glucose

The presence of glucose is not a normal finding for urine. Although glucose is freely filtered by the renal glomerulus, it is fully reabsorbed by the tubules. Only when the blood glucose levels reach the tubular maximum (T_m) of glucose (320 mg/min) or plasma threshold of 160 to 190 mg/dl is the kidney unable to completely reabsorb it. Glycosuria may indicate that the individual has a low renal threshold for glucose. The most common cause, however, is the presence of diabetes mellitus. Occasionally after high carbohydrate intake, the blood glucose level may be high enough to allow spilling of glucose into the urine. Both reducing and enzymatic tests may be used to identify urinary glucose.

The practitioner may measure both blood and urinary glucose concentrations through the means of dipsticks, chemically treated papers that change color on exposure to glucose. Color charts provided with the testing materials allow standard comparison and subsequent identification of the degree of glucose concentration of the tested body fluid.

Deviation	Cause
Glucosuria	Diabetes mellitus
	Increased intracranial pressure
	Cushing's disease
	Pheochromocytoma
	Pregnancy

Protein

Tests for the protein content in urine depend on the principle that protein precipitates in the presence of heat in acidic urine. Sulfosalicylic acid is the acid most frequently used for this purpose. An estimate of the protein content is made from the density of the precipitate as follows:

Precipitate description	Value	Percent protein
Faintly cloudy	1+	
Cloudy but transparent	2+	0.1
Opaque with clumping	3+	0.2 to 0.3
Dense, solid gel	4+	0.5

Normally, very small amounts of protein appear in urine that are not detectable by routine methods. Even trace quantities are an indication that follow-up should be done. A 24-hour quantitation of the protein excreted by the kidneys may be done. In addition, an electrophoretic determination of the type of protein in the urine may be done. Albumin is the most frequently encountered protein, since its molecular size is smaller than that of the globulins or fibrinogen.

The urine specimen of women may be contaminated with vaginal secretions. In many agencies it has become routine to use a clean-catch urine collection technique to obviate this protein contamination.

Bence Jones protein is an abnormal protein that appears in the urine of individuals with multiple myeloma.

URINARY PROTEIN: NORMAL EXCRETION AND DEVIATION

Normal excretion: 0.1 g/24 hr

Deviation	Cause
Proteinuria	Pregnancy
	Strenuous physical exercise
	Orthostatism
	Fever
	Kidney disease
	Glomerulonephritis
	Nephrotic syndrome
	Neoplasm
	Infarction
	Postrenal infection

Acetone and diacetic acid (ketone bodies)

Ketones are products of fat metabolism and are increased in the blood during periods when increased fats are being used as fuel, such as in starvation, after glycogen stores have been depleted. In diabetes mellitus, the lack of insulin makes glucose relatively unavailable to the cells, so that fats are again metabolized in greater quantity. The blood ketones are increased more rapidly than they can be metabolized and are excreted in the urine. Acetone determinations are indicated whenever the urinary glucose test is positive or blood glucose is elevated.

The acetone level of urine may be tested with a chemically treated dipstick that changes color in the presence of ketone bodies. This is read against a standard scale provided with the test papers.

Microscopic examination of urinary sediment

The normal urinary sediment may contain one or two RBCs as well as WBCs and an occasional cast. All other substances are considered pathological.

Red blood cells. Since RBCs are too large to filter through the glomerulus, the presence of blood in the urine indicates bleeding within the genitourinary tract. Common causes are calculi, cystitis, neoplasm, tuberculosis, and glomerulonephritis.

White blood cells. WBCs may indicate infection in any part of the genitourinary tract. Glomerulonephritis is typified by the presence of WBCs, casts, and bacteria. As a rule, pyuria from the kidney is associated with proteinuria, whereas only very small amounts of protein are present in the urine of the individual with an infection of the lower urinary tract.

Casts. Gelled protein and cellular debris precipitated in the renal tubules and molded to the tubular lumen are called casts. Portions of these casts may break off and are found in the urine. The casts are hyaline, granular, or cellular in nature. Epithelial casts are made up of columnar renal epithelium or round cells. The hyaline casts are almost transparent and consist of homogeneous protein. The granular casts are dark colored and a degenerated form of the hyaline casts. The tubular shape of the casts has led to the use of the term *cylindruria.*

Casts consisting of WBCs are typical of pyelonephritis and the exudative stage of acute glomerulonephritis. Casts containing RBCs may appear clear or yellow.

The deposition of amyloid substance in urinary casts gives them a waxy appearance.

Urine that contains hyaline casts and protein may indicate a nephrotic syndrome.

Crystals. The acidity or alkalinity of the urine determines the type of crystals that may be identified in it. A urine with low pH is characterized by calcium oxalate, cystine, uric acid, and urate crystals. Alkaline urine is most frequently associated with carbonate crystals and amorphous phosphates.

EXAMINATION OF THE STOOL

In most cases a stool specimen is obtained by asking the individual to defecate, but digital removal of feces from the rectum can be done to facilitate collection when time constraints so dictate. Frequently a laxative is recommended to soften the stool, particularly if the individual has given a history of constipation. Because chemical analyses are calculated on the basis of daily output, the entire stool is sent to the laboratory. The feces are analyzed for size, shape, consistency, and color.

The normal individual excretes 100 to 200 g of feces daily. The volume depends on the fluid content of the bowel. About 500 to 1,000 ml of chyme (liquid stool) are delivered to the colon each day, but most of the water and electrolytes are reabsorbed, primarily in the proximal colon. Sodium is absorbed, and chloride follows passively. The gradient established results in absorption of water. In addition, bicarbonate ions are secreted by the colon, and an equal amount of chloride is absorbed. About one fourth of the stool is solid material, which consists of the undigested residue of food, intestinal mucus and epithelium, bacteria, fat, and waste materials from the blood.

The rapid passage of stool through the colon in diarrhea results in larger stools (by volume) containing more liquid. Diarrhea is generally caused by inflammation of the colon but may also result from malabsorption syndromes.

A fecalith or stercolith is a dried, hardened fecal mass.

Color

The normal color of the stool is brown as a result of food pigments as well as the breakdown products of bilirubin. Bilirubin is converted to biliverdin (green bile) by intestinal bacteria and then to stercobilin (a brown substance). Increased motility of the stool in diarrhea may result in green stools because of the presence of biliverdin that was allowed insufficient time for bacterial conversion in the colon.

Melena is a black stool caused by gastrointestinal bleeding (more than 100 ml) high enough in the tract that it is partially digested. Bleeding of the lower gastrointestinal tract is observed as bright- to dark-red blood in the stool. The guiac test for occult blood is described in Chapters 17 and 18 on assessing the abdomen and rectosigmoid region.

Deviation	Cause
Melena	Esophagitis
	Esophageal varices
	Hiatus hernia
	Gastritis
	Peptic ulcer
	Carcinoma
Presence of bright- to dark-red blood	Polyps of the colon
	Carcinoma of the colon
	Diverticulitis
	Colitis
	Hemorrhoids

Ingestion of iron or bismuth compounds may cause the stool to be green to black. Green vegetables ingested in excessive amounts may also turn the stool green. A dietary intake that contains a good deal of milk but is low in protein may result in a light-colored stool.

Odor

The odor of feces and flatus is the result of bacterial action and depends on the colonic bacterial flora and the type of food ingested.

The normal stool is 10% to 20% fat. An excessive amount of fat in the stool is termed *steatorrhea*. The stool may appear grossly oily. Steatorrhea may be the result of pancreatic or small bowel malabsorption problems or liver disease. Sudan stain is an iodine compound that colors fat droplets, rendering them visible under the microscope. Excessive fat loss in the stool may also be associated with deficiency of the fat-soluble vitamin D.

Quantitative evaluation of fecal fat content is sometimes performed. In the performance of this test, the amount of dietary fat is usually controlled at 100 g of fat per day. A 3-day stool collection containing more than 5 g of fat for each day is considered pathological.

Microscopic examination

The stool may be examined under the microscope to identify ova and parasites. At least three separate specimens are examined, since one negative examination is not sufficient to rule out the infestation.

The presence of WBCs in the stool is indicative of an inflammation in the gastrointestinal tract.

BIBLIOGRAPHY

Bauer, J.D.: Clincial laboratory methods, ed. 9, St. Louis, 1982, The C.V. Mosby Co.

Cromwell, L., and others: Medical instrumentation for health care, Englewood Cliffs, N.J., 1976, Prentice-Hall, Inc.

Eastham, R.D.: Clinical hematology, ed. 4, Baltimore, 1974, Williams & Wilkins.

French, R.M.: Guide to diagnostic procedures, ed. 4, New York, 1975, McGraw-Hill Book Co.

Henry, J.B.: Todd-Sanford-Davidsohn Clinical diagnosis and management by laboratory methods, Philadelphia, 1979, W.B. Saunders Co.

Ravel, R.: Clinical laboratory medicine, ed. 2, Chicago, 1973, Year Book Medical Publishers, Inc.

Skydell, B., and Crowder, A.S.: Diagnostic procedures: a reference for health practitioners and a guide to patient counseling, Boston, 1975, Little, Brown and Co.

Tilkian, S.M., and Conover, M.B.: Clinical implications of laboratory tests, ed 3, St. Louis, 1983, The C.V. Mosby Co.

Wallach, J.: Interpretation of diagnostic tests: a handbook synopsis of laboratory medicine, ed. 2, Boston, 1974, Little, Brown & Co.

Widmann, F.K.: Goodale's clinical interpretation of laboratory tests, ed. 7, Philadelphia, 1973, F.A. Davis Co.

TABLES OF NORMAL VALUES

Abbreviations used in tables

<	= less than	mg	= milligram	ng	= nanogram
>	= greater than	ml	= milliliter	pg	= picogram
dl	= 100 ml	mM	= millimole	μEq	= microequivalent
gm	= gram	mm Hg	= millimeters of mercury	μg	= microgram
IU	= International Unit	mIU	= milliInternational Unit	μIU	= microInternational Unit
kg	= kilogram	mOsm	= milliosmole	μl	= microliter
mEq	= milliequivalent	mμ	= millimicron	μU	= microunit

Table A-1
Whole blood, serum, and plasma chemistry

Component	System	Typical reference intervals		
		Conventional units	Factor*	Recommended SI units†
Acetoacetic acid				
Qualitative	Serum	Negative	—	Negative
Quantitative	Serum	0.2-1.0 mg/dl	98	19.6-98.0 μmol/L
Acetone				
Qualitative	Serum	Negative	—	Negative
Quantitative	Serum	0.3-2.0 mg/dl	172	51.6-344.0 μmol/L
Albumin				
Quantitative	Serum	3.2-4.5 g/dl (salt fractionation)	10	32-45 g/L
		3.2-5.6 g/dl (electrophoresis)		32-56 g/L
		3.8-5.0 g/dl (dye binding)		38-50 g/L
Alcohol, ethyl	Serum or whole blood	Negative—but presented as mg/dl	0.22	Negative—but presented as mmol/L
Aldolase	Serum			
	Adults	3-8 Sibley-Lehninger U/dl at 37° C.	7.4	22-59 mU/L at 37° C
	Children	Approximately 2 times adult levels		Approximately 2 times adult levels
	Newborn	Approximately 4 times adult levels		Approximately 4 times adult levels

*Factor, Number factor (note that units are not presented).
†Value in SI units, Value in conventional units × factor.
‡Usually not measured in blood (preferred specimen in urine, hair, or nails except in acute cases where gastric contents are used).

☐ From Henry, J.B.: Todd-Sanford-Davidsohn clinical diagnosis and management by laboratory methods, ed. 17, Philadelphia, 1984, W.B. Saunders Co.

Table A-1
Whole blood, serum, and plasma chemistry—cont'd

Component	System	Typical reference intervals		
		Conventional units	**Factor**	**Recommended SI units**
Alpha-amino acid nitrogen	Serum	3.6-7.0 mg/dl	0.714	2.6-5.0 mmol/L
δ-Aminolevulinic acid	Serum	0.01-0.03 mg/dl	76.3	0.76-2.29 μmol/L
Ammonia	Plasma	20-120 μg/dl (diffusion)	0.554	11.1-67.0 μmol/L
		40-80 μg/dl (enzymatic method)		22.2-44.3 μmol/L
		12-48 μg/dl (resin method)		6.7-26.6 μmol/L
Amylase	Serum	60-160 Somogyi units/dl	1.85	111-296 U/L
Argininosuccinic lyase	Serum	0-4 U/dl	10	0-40 U/L
Arsenic‡	Whole blood	<7 μg/dl	0.13	<0.91 μmol/L
Ascorbic acid (vitamin C)	Plasma	0.6-1.6 mg/dl	56.8	34-91 μmol/L
	Whole blood	0.7-2.0 mg/dl		40-114 μmol/L
Barbiturates	Serum, plasma, or Whole blood	Negative	—	Negative
Base excess	Whole blood			
Male		−3.3 to +1.2 mEq/l	1	−3.3 to +1.2 mmol/L
Female		−2.4 to +2.3 mEq/l		−2.4 to +2.3 mmol/L
Base, total	Serum	145-160 mEq/l	1	145-160 mmol/L
Bicarbonate	Plasma	21-28 mM	1	21-28 mmol/L
Bile acids	Serum	0.3-3.0 mg/dl	10	3.0-30.0 mg/L
Bilirubin	Serum			
Direct (conjugated)		Up to 0.3 mg/dl	17.1	Up to 5.1 μmol/L
Indirect (unconjugated)		0.1-1.0 mg/dl		1.7-17.1 μmol/L
Total		0.1-1.2 mg/dl		1.7-20.5 μmol/L
Newborns total		1-12 mg/dl		17.1-205.0 μmol/L
Blood gases				
pH	Whole blood	7.38-7.44 (arterial)	1	7.38-7.44
		7.36-7.41 (venous)		7.36-7.41
P_{CO_2}	Whole blood	35-40 mm Hg (arterial)	0.133	4.66-5.32 kPa
		40-45 mm Hg (venous)		5.32-5.99 kPa
P_{O_2}	Whole blood	95-100 mm Hg (arterial)	0.133	12.64-13.30 kPa
Bromide	Serum	0-5 mg/dl	0.125	0-0.63 mmol/L
BSP (Bromsulphalein) (5mg/kg)	Serum	Less than 6% retention 45 min after injection	0.01	Fraction retention <0.06 at 45 min after dye injection
Calcium				
Ionized	Serum	4-4.8 mg/dl	0.25	1.0-1.2 mmol/L
		2.0-2.4 mEq/l	0.5	
		30-58% of total	0.01	0.30-0.58 of total
Total	Serum	9.2-11.0 mg/dl	0.25	2.3-2.8 mmol/L
		4.6-5.5 mEq/l	0.5	23-28 mmol/L
Carbon dioxide (CO_2 content)	Whole blood (arterial)	19-24 mM	1	19-24 mmol/L
	Plasma or serum (arterial)	21-28 mM		21-28 mmol/L
Carbon dioxide	Whole blood (venous)	22-26 mM	1	22-26 mmol/L
	Plasma or serum (venous)	24-30 mM		24-30 mmol/L
CO_2 combining power	Plasma or serum (venous)	24-30 mM	1	24-30 mmol/L
CO_2 partial pressure (P_{CO_2})	Whole blood (arterial)	35-40 mm Hg	0.133	4.66-5.32 kPa
	Whole blood (venous)	40-45 mm Hg		5.32-5.99 kPa
Carbonic acid (H_2CO_3)	Whole blood (arterial)	1.05-1.45 mM	1	1.05-1.45 mmol/L
	Whole blood (venous)	1.15-1.50 mM		1.15-1.50 mmol/L
	Plasma (venous)	1.02-1.38 mM		1.02-1.38 mmol/L

Continued.

Table A-1

Whole blood, serum, and plasma chemistry—cont'd

Component	System	Conventional units	Factor	Recommended SI units
		Typical reference intervals		
Component	**System**	**Conventional units**	**Factor**	**Recommended SI units**
Carboxyhemoglobin (carbon monoxide hemoglobin)	Whole blood			Fraction hemoglobin saturated
	Suburban nonsmokers	<1.5% saturation of hemoglobin	0.01	<0.015
	Smokers	1.5-5.0% saturation		0.015-0.050
	Heavy smokers	5.0-9.0% saturation		0.050-0.090
Carotene, beta	Serum	40-200 μ/dl	0.0186	0.74-3.72 μmol/L
Ceruloplasmin	Serum	23-50 mg/dl	10	230-500 mg/L
Chloride	Serum	95-103 mEq/l	1	95-103 mmol/L
Cholesterol				
Total	Serum	150-250 mg/dl (varies with diet, sex, and age)	0.026	3.90-6.50 mmol/L
Esters	Serum	65-75% of total cholesterol	0.01	Fraction of total cholesterol: 0.65-0.75
Cholinesterase (Pseudocholinesterase)	Erythrocytes	0.65-1.3 pH units	1	0.65-1.3 units
	Plasma	0.5-1.3 pH units		0.5-1.3 units
		8-18 IU/l at 37° C	1	8-18 U/L at 37° C
Citrate	Serum or plasma	1.7-3.0 mg/dl	52	88-156 μmol/L
Copper	Serum, plasma			
Male		70-140 μg/dl	0.157	11.0-22.0 μmol/L
Female		80-155 μg/dl		12.6-24.3 μmol/L
Cortisol	Plasma			
8 AM–10 AM		5-23 μg/dl	27.6	138-635 nmol/L
4 PM–6 PM		3-13 μg/dl		83-359 nmol/L
Creatine as creatinine	Serum or plasma			
Male		0.1-0.4 mg/dl	76.3	7.6-30.5 μmol/L
Female		0.2-0.7 mg/dl	76.3	15.3-53.4 μmol/L
Creatine kinase (CK)	Serum			
Male		55-170 U/l at 37° C	1	55-170 U/L at 37° C
Female		30-135 U/l at 37° C	1	30-135 U/L at 37° C
Creatinine	Serum or plasma	0.6-1.2 mg/dl (adult)	88.4	53-106 μmol/L
		0.3-0.6 mg/dl (children <2 yr)		27-54 μmol/L
Creatinine clearance (endogenous)	Serum or plasma and urine			
Male		107-139 ml/min	0.0167	1.78-2.32 ml/s
Female		87-107 ml/min		1.45-1.79 ml/s
Cryoglobulins	Serum	Negative	—	Negative
Electrophoresis, protein	Serum	Percent		Fraction of total protein
Albumin		52-65% of total protein	0.01	0.52-0.65
Alpha-1		2.5-5.0% of total protein	0.01	0.025-0.05
Alpha-2		7.0-13.0% of total protein	0.01	0.07-0.13
Beta		8.0-14.0% of total protein	0.01	0.08-0.14
Gamma		12.0-22.0% of total protein	0.01	0.12-0.22
		Concentration		
Albumin		3.2-5.6 gm/dl	10	32-56 g/L
Alpha-1		0.1-0.4 gm/dl		1-4 g/L
Alpha-2		0.4-1.2 gm/dl		4-12 g/L
Beta		0.5-1.1 gm/dl		5-11 g/L
Gamma		0.5-1.6 gm/dl		5-16 g/L
Fats, neutral (see Triglycerides)				
Fatty acids				
Total (free and esterified)	Serum	9-15 mM	1	9-15 mmol/L
Free (non-esterified)	Plasma	300-480 μEq/l	1	300-480 μmol/L
Ferritin	Serum			
Male		15-200 ng/ml		15-200 μg/L
Female		12-150 ng/ml		15-150 μg/L
Fibrinogen	Plasma	200-400 mg/dl	0.01	2.00-4.00 g/L
Fluoride	Whole blood	<0.05 mg/dl	0.53	<0.027 mmol/L

Table A-1

Whole blood, serum, and plasma chemistry—cont'd

Component	System	Typical reference intervals		
		Conventional units	**Factor**	**Recommended SI units**
Folate	Serum	5-25 ng/ml (bioassay)	2.27	11-56 nmol/L
		>2.3 ng/ml (radioassay)		>5.2 nmol/L
	Erythrocytes	166-640 ng/ml (bioassay)		376-1452 nmol/L
		>140 ng/ml (radioassay)		>318 nmol/L
Galactose	Whole blood			
Adults		None	—	None
Children		<20 mg/dl	0.055	<1.1 mmol/L
Gamma globulin	Serum	0.5-1.6 gm/dl	10	5-16 g/L
Globulins, total	Serum	2.3-3.5 gm/dl	10	23-35 g/L
Glucose, fasting	Serum or plasma	70-110 mg/dl	0.055	3.85-6.05 mmol/L
	Whole blood	60-100 mg/dl		3.30-5.50 mmol/L
Glucose tolerance				
Oral	Serum or plasma			
Fasting		70-110 mg/dl	0.055	3.85-6.05 mmol/L
30 min		30-60 mg/dl above fasting		1.65-3.30 mmol/L above fasting
60 min		20-50 mg/dl above fasting		1.10-2.75 mmol/L above fasting
120 min		5-15 mg/dl above fasting		0.28-0.83 mmol/L above fasting
180 min		Fasting level or below		Fasting level or below
Intravenous	Serum or plasma			
Fasting		70-110 mg/dl		3.85-6.05 mmol/L
5 min		Maximum of 250 mg/dl		Maximum of 13.75 mmol/L
60 min		Significant decrease		Significant decrease
120 min		Below 120 mg/dl		Below 6.60 mmol/L
180 min		Fasting level		Fasting level
Glucose 6-phosphate dehydrogenase (G6PD)	Erythrocytes	250-500 units/10⁶ cells	1	250-500 μunits/cells
		1200-2000 mIU/ml packed erythrocytes	1	1200-2000 U/L packed erythrocytes
γ-Glutamyl transferase	Serum	5-40 IU/l	1	5-40 U/L at 37° C
Glutathione	Whole blood	24-37 mg/dl	0.032	0.77-1.18 mmol/L
Growth hormone	Serum	<10 ng/ml	1	<10 μg/L
Guanase	Serum	<3 nM/ml/min	1	<3 U/L at 37° C
Haptoglobin	Serum	60-270 mg/dl	0.01	0.6-2.7 g/L
Hemoglobin	Serum or plasma			
Qualitative		Negative	—	Negative
Quantitative		0.5-5.0 mg/dl	10	5-50 mg/L
	Whole blood			
Female		12.0-16.0 g/dl	10	1.86-2.48 mmol/L
Male		13.5-18.0 g/dl		2.09-2.79 mmol/L
α-Hydroxybutyrate dehydrogenase	Serum	140-350 U/ml	1	140-350 kU/L
17-Hydroxycorticosteroids	Plasma			
Male		7-19 μg/dl	10	70-190 μg/L
Female		9-21 μg/dl		9-21 μg/L
After 24 USP Units of ACTH				
IM		35-55 μg/dl		350-550 μg/L
Immunoglobulins	Serum			
IgG		800-1801 mg/dl	0.01	8.0-18.0 g/L
IgA		113-563 mg/dl		1.1-5.6 g/L
IgM		54-222 mg/dl		0.54-2.2 g/L
IgD		0.5-3.0 mg/dl	10	5.0-30 mg/L
IgE		0.01-0.04 mg/dl		0.1-0.4 mg/L
Insulin	Plasma			
Bioassay		11-240 μIU/ml	0.0417	0.46-10.00 μg/L
Radioimmunoassay		4-24 μIU/ml		0.17-1.00 μg/L
Insulin tolerance (0.1 unit/kg)	Serum			
Fasting		Glucose of 70-110 mg/dl	0.055	Glucose of 3.85-6.05 mmol/L
30 min		Fall to 50% of fasting level	0.01	Fall to 0.5 of fasting level
90 min		Fasting level		Fasting level

Continued.

Table A-1
Whole blood, serum, and plasma chemistry—cont'd

Component	System	Conventional units	Factor	Recommended SI units
		Typical reference intervals		
Iodine				
Butanol-extraction (BEI)	Serum	3.5-6.5 μg/dl	0.079	0.28-0.51 μmol/L
Protein bound (PBI)	Serum	4.0-8.0 μg/dl		0.32-0.63 μmol/L
Iron, total	Serum	60-150 μg/dl	0.179	11-27 μmol/L
Iron binding capacity	Serum	250-400 μg/dl	0.179	54-64 μmol/L
Iron saturation	Serum	20-55%	0.01	Fraction of total iron binding capacity: 0.20-0.55
Isocitric dehydrogenase	Serum	50-240 units/ml at 25° C (Wolfson-Williams Ashman units)	0.0167	0.83-4.18 U/L at 25° C
Ketone bodies	Serum	Negative	—	Negative
17-Ketosteroids	Plasma	25-125 μg/dl	0.01	0.25-1.25 mg/L
Lactic acid (as lactate)	Whole blood			
Venous		5-20 mg/dl	0.111	0.6-2.2 mmol/L
Arterial		3-7 mg/dl		0.3-0.8 mmol/L
Lactate dehydrogenase (LDH)	Serum	(lactate → pyruvate) 80-120 units at 30° C	0.48	38-62 U/L at 30° C
		(pyruvate → lactate) 185-640 units at 30° C	0.48	90-310 U/L at 30° C
		(lactate → pyruvate) 100-190 U/l at 37° C	1	100-190 U/L at 37° C
Lactate dehydrogenase isoenzymes	Serum			Fraction of total LDH
LDH$_1$ (anode)		17-27%	0.01	0.17-0.27
LDH$_2$		27-37%		0.27-0.37
LDH$_3$		18-25%		0.18-0.25
LDH$_4$		3-8%		0.03-0.08
LDH$_5$ (cathode		0-5%		0.00-0.05
Lactate dehydrogenase (heat stable)	Serum	30-60% of total	0.01	Fraction of total LDH: 0.30-0.60
Lactose tolerance	Serum	Serum glucose changes similar to glucose tolerance test	—	Serum glucose changes similar to glucose tolerance test
Lead	Whole blood	0-50 μg/dl	0.048	0-2.4 μmol/L
Leucine aminopeptidase (LAP)	Serum			
Male		80-200 U/ml (Goldbarg-Rutenberg)	0.24	19.2-48.0 U/L
Female		75-185 U/ml (Goldbarg-Rutenberg)		18.0-44.4 U/L
Lipase	Serum	0-1.5 U/ml (Cherry-Crandall)	278	0-417 U/L
		14-280 mIU/ml	1	14-280 U/L
Lipids, total	Serum	400-800 mg/dl	0.01	4.00-8.00 g/L
Cholesterol		150-250 mg/dl	0.026	3.9-6.5 mmol/L
Triglycerides		10-190 mg/dl	0.109	1.09-20.71 mmol/L
Phospholipids		150-380 mg/dl	0.01	1.50-380 g/L
Fatty acids (free)		9.0-15.0 mM/l	1	9.0-15.0 mmol/L
		300-480 μEq/l	0.01	300-480 μmol/L
Phospholipid phosphorus		8.0-11.0 mg/dl	0.323	2.58-3.55 mmol/L
Lithium	Serum	Negative	—	Negative
Therapeutic interval		0.5-1.4 mEq/l	1	0.5-1.4 mmol/L
Long-acting thyroid-stimulating hormone (LATS)	Serum	None	—	None
Luteinizing hormone (LH)	Serum			
Male		6-30 mIU/ml	0.23	1.4-6.9 mg/L
Female		Midcycle peak: 3 times baseline value		Midcycle peak: 3 times baseline value
		Premenopausal <30 mIU/ml		Premenopausal <5 times baseline value
		Postmenopausal >35 mIU/ml		Postmenopausal >5 times baseline value

Table A-1

Whole blood, serum, and plasma chemistry—cont'd

Component	System	Typical reference intervals		
		Conventional units	**Factor**	**Recommended SI units**
Macroglobulins, total	Serum	70-430 mg/dl	0.01	0.7-4.3 g/L
Magnesium	Serum	1.3-2.1 mEq/l	0.5	0.7-1.1 mmol/L
		1.8-3.0 mg/dl	0.41	0.7-1.1 mmol/L
Methemoglobin	Whole blood	0-0.24 g/dl	10	0.0-2.4 g/L
		<1% of total hemoglobin	0.01	Fraction of total hemoglobin: <0.01
Mucoprotein	Serum	80-200 mg/dl	0.01	0.8-2.0 g/L
Muramidase	Serum	4-13 mg/l		4-13 mg/L
Non-protein nitrogen (NPN)	Serum or plasma	20-35 mg/dl	0.714	14.3-25.0 mmol/L
	Whole blood	25-50 mg/dl		17.9-35.7 mmol/L
5'Nucleotidase	Serum	0-1.6 units at 37° C	1	0-1.6 units at 37° C
Ornithine carbamyl transferase	Serum	8-20 mIU/ml at 37° C	1	8-20 U/L at 37° C
Osmolality	Serum	280-295 mOsm/kg	1	280-295 mmol/L
Oxygen				
Pressure (Po_2)	Whole blood (arterial)	95-100 mm Hg	0.133	12.64-13.30 kPa
Content	Whole blood (arterial)	15-23 volume %	0.01	Volume fraction: 0.15-0.23
Saturation	Whole blood (arterial)	94-100%		0.94-1.00
pH	Whole blood (arterial)	7.38-7.44	1	7.38-7.44
	Whole blood (venous)	7.36-7.41		7.36-7.41
	Serum or plasma (venous)	7.35-7.45		7.35-7.45
Phenylalanine	Serum			
Adults		<3.0 mg/dl	0.061	<0.18 mmol/L
Newborns (term)		1.2-3.5 mg/dl		0.07-0.21 mmol/L
Phosphatase				
Acid phosphatase	Serum	0.13-0.63 U/l at 37° C (paranitrophenylphosphate)	16.67	2.2-10.5 U/L at 37° C
Alkaline phosphatase	Serum	20-90 IU/l at 30° C (paranitrophenylphosphate in AMP buffer)	1	20-90 U/L at 30° C
Phospholipid phosphorus	Serum	8-11 mg/dl	0.323	2.6-3.6 mmol/L
Phospholipids	Serum	150-380 mg/dl	0.01	1.50-3.80 g/L
Phosphorus, inorganic	Serum			
Adults		2.3-4.7 mg/dl	0.323	0.78-1.52 mmol/L
Children		4.0-7.0 mg/dl		1.29-2.26 mmol/L
Potassium	Plasma	3.8-5.0 mEq/l	1	3.8-5.0 mmol/L
Prolactin	Serum			
Female		1-25 ng/ml	1	1-25 µg/L
Male		1-20 ng/ml		1-20 µg/L
Proteins	Serum			
Total		6.0-7.8 g/dl	10	60-78 g/L
Albumin		3.2-4.5 g/dl		32-45 g/L
Globulin		2.3-3.5 g/dl		23-35 g/L
Protein fractionation		See electrophoresis		See electrophoresis
Protoporphyrin	Erythrocytes	15-50 µg/dl	0.018	0.27-0.90 µmol/L
Pyruvate	Whole blood	0.3-0.9 mg/dl	114	34-103 µmol/L
Salicylates	Serum	Negative	—	Negative
Therapeutic interval		15-30 mg/dl	0.072	1.44-1.80 mmol/L
		150-300 µg/ml	0.0072	1.08-2.16 mmol/L
Sodium	Plasma	136-142 mEq/l	1	136-142 mmol/L
Sulfate, inorganic	Serum	0.2-1.3 mEq/l	0.5	0.10-0.65 mmol/L
		0.9-6.0 mg/dl as SO_4^{--}	0.104	0.09-0.62 mmol/L as SO_4^{--}
Sulfhemoglobin	Whole blood	Negative	—	Negative

Continued.

Table A-1

Whole blood, serum, and plasma chemistry—cont'd

Component	System	Typical reference intervals		
		Conventional units	Factor	Recommended SI units
Sulfonamides	Serum or whole blood	Negative	—	Negative
Testosterone	Serum or plasma			
Male		300-1200 ng/dl	0.035	10.0-42.0 nmol/L
Female		30-95 ng/dl		1.1-3.3 nmol/L
Thiocyanate	Serum	Negative	—	Negative
Thyroid hormone tests	Serum			
a) Expressed as thyroxine				
T_4 by column		5.0-11.0 μg/dl	13.0	65-143 nmol/L
T_4 by competitive binding—Murphy-Pattee		6.0-11.8 μg/dl		78-153 nmol/L
T_4 RIA		5.5-12.5 μg/dl	13.0	72-163 nmol/L
Free T_4		0.9-2.3 ng/dl		12-30 pmol/L
b) Expressed as iodine				
T_4 by column		3.2-7.2 μg/dl	79.0	253-569 nmol/L
T_4 by competitive binding—Murphy-Pattee		3.9-7.7 μg/dl		308-608 nmol/L
Free T_4		0.6-1.5 ng/dl	79.0	47-119 pmol/L
T_3 resin uptake		25-38 relative % uptake	0.01	Relative uptake fraction: 0.25-0.38
Thyroxine-binding globulin (TBG)	Serum	10-26 μg/dl	10	100-260 μg/L
TSH	Serum	<10μU/ml	1	<10^{-3}IU/L
Transferases				
Aspartate amino transferase (AST or SGOT)	Serum	10-40 U/ml (Karmen) at 25° C 16-60 U/ml (Karmen) at 30° C	0.48	8-29 U/L at 30° C 8-33 U/L at 37° C
Alanine amino transferase (ALT or SGPT)	Serum	10-30 U/ml (Karmen) at 25° C 8-50 U/ml (Karmen) at 30° C	0.48	4-24 U/L at 30° C 4-36 U/L at 37° C
Gamma glutamyl transferase (GGT)		5-40 IU/l at 37° C	1	5.40 U/L at 37° C
Triglycerides	Serum	10-190 mg/dl	0.011	0.11-2.09 mmol/L
Urea nitrogen	Serum	8-23 mg/dl	0.357	2.9-8.2 mmol/L
Urea clearance	Serum and urine			
Maximum clearance		64-99 ml/min	0.0167	1.07-1.65 ml/s
Standard clearance		41-65 ml/min, or more than 75% of normal clearance		0.68-1.09 ml/s or more than 0.75 of normal clearance
Uric acid	Serum			
Male		4.0-8.5 mg/dl	0.059	0.24-0.5 mmol/L
Female		2.7-7.3 mg/dl		0.16-0.43 mmol/L
Vitamin A	Serum	15-60 μg/dl	0.035	0.53-2.10 μmol/L
Vitamin A tolerance	Serum			
Fasting 3 hr or 6 hr after 5000 units		15-60 μg/dl	0.035	0.53-2.10 μmol/L
Vitamin A/kg		200-600 μg/dl		7.00-21.00 μmol/L
24 hrs		Fasting values or slightly above	—	Fasting values or slightly above
Vitamin B_{12}	Serum	160-950 pg/ml	0.74	118-703 pmol/L
Unsaturated vitamin B_{12} binding capacity	Serum	1000-2000 pg/ml	0.74	740-1480 pmol/L
Vitamin C	Plasma	0.6-1.6 mg/dl	56.8	34-91 μmol/L
Xylose absorption	Serum			
Normal		25-40 mg/dl between 1 and 2 hr	0.067	1.68-2.68 mmol/L between 1 and 2 h
In malabsorption		Maximum approximately 10 mg/dl		Maximum approximately 0.67 mmol/L
Dose: Adult		25 g D-xylose	0.067	0.167 mol D-xylose
Children		0.5 g/kg D-xylose		3.33 mmol/kg D-xylose
Zinc	Serum	50-150 μg/dl	0.153	7.65-22.95 μmol/L

Table A-2
Urine

Component	Type of urine specimen	Typical reference intervals		
		Conventional units	Factor	Recommended SI units
Acetoacetic acid	Random	Negative	—	Negative
Acetone	Random	Negative	—	Negative
Addis count	12 hr collection	WBC and epithelial cells		
		1,800,000/12 hr	1	1.8×10^6/12 h
		RBC 500,000/12 hr	1	0.5×10^6/12 h
		Hyaline casts: 0-5000/12 hr	1	5.0×10^3/12 h
Albumin				
Qualitative	Random	Negative	—	Negative
Quantitative	24 hr	15-150 mg/24 hr	1	0.015-0.150 g/24 h
Aldosterone	24 hr	2-26 µg/24 hr	2.77	5.5-72.0 nmol/24 h
Alkapton bodies	Random	Negative	—	Negative
Alpha-amino acid nitrogen	24 hr	100-290 mg/24 hr	0.0714	7.14-20.71 mmol/24 h
δ-Aminolevulinic acid	Random			
	Adult	0.1-0.6 mg/dl	76.3	7.6-45.8 µmol/L
	Children	<0.5 mg/dl		<38.1 µmol/L
	24 hr	1.5-7.5 mg/24 hr	7.63	11.15-57.2 µmol/24 h
Ammonia nitrogen	24 hr	20-70 mEq/24 hr		
		500-1200 mg/24 hr	0.071	35.5-85.2 mmol/24 h
Amylase	2 hr	35-260 Somogyi units/hr	0.185	6.5-48.1 U/h
Arsenic	24 hr	<50 mg/l	0.013	<0.65 µmol/L
Ascorbic acid	Random	1-7 mg/dl	0.057	0.06-0.40 mmol/L
	24 hr	>50 mg/24 hr	0.0057	>0.29 mmol/24 h
Bence Jones protein	Random	Negative	—	Negative
Beryllium	24 hr	<0.05 µg/24 hr	111	<5.55 nmol/24 h
Bilirubin, qualitative	Random	Negative	—	Negative
Blood, occult	Random	Negative	—	Negative
Borate	24 hr	<2 mg/l	16	<32 µmol/L
Calcium				
Qualitative (Sulkowitch)	Random	1+ turbidity	1	1+ turbidity
Quantitative	24 hr			
	Average diet	100-240 mg/24 hr	0.025	2.50-6.25 mmol/24 h
	Low calcium diet	<150 mg/24 hr		<3.75 mmol/24 h
	High calcium diet	240-300 mg/24 hr		6.25-7.50 mmol/24 h
Catecholamines	Random	0-14 µg/dl	10	0-140 µg/L
	24 hr	<100 µg/24 hr (varies with activity)	1	<100 µg/24 h
Epinephrine		<10 ng/24 hr	5.46	<55 nmol/24 h
Norepinephrine		<100 ng/24 hr	5.91	<590 nmol/24 h
Total free catecholamines		4-126 µg/24 hr	1	4-126 µg/24 h
Total metanephrines		0.1-1.6 mg/24 hr	1	0.1-1.6 mg/24 h
Chloride	24 hr	140-250 mEq/24 hr	1	140-250 mmol/24 h
Concentration test (Fishberg)	Random—after fluid restriction			
Specific gravity		>1.025	1	>1.025
Osmolality		>850 mOsm/l	1	>850 mmol/L
Copper	24 hr	0-50 µg/24 hr	0.016	0-0.48 µmol/24 h
Coproporphyrin	Random			
	Adult	3-20 µg/dl	0.015	0.045-0.30 µmol/L
	24 hr			
	Adult	50-160 µg/24 hr	0.0015	0.075-0.24 µmol/24 h
	Children	0-80 µg/24 hr	0.0015	0.00-0.12 µmol/24 hr
Creatine	24 hr			
	Male	0-40 mg/24 hr	0.0076	0-0.30 mmol/24 h
	Female	0-100 mg/24 hr		0-0.76 mmol/24 h
		Higher in children and during pregnancy	—	Higher in children and during pregnancy

Continued.

Table A-2

Urine—cont'd

Component	Type of urine specimen	Typical reference intervals		
		Conventional units	Factor	Recommended SI units
Creatinine	24 hr			
	Male	20-26 mg/kg/24 hr	0.0088	0.18-0.23 mmol/kg/24 h
		1.0-2.0 g/24 hr	8.8	8.8-17.6 mmol/24 h
	Female	14-22 mg/kg/24 hr	0.0088	0.12-0.19 mmol/kg/24 h
		0.8-1.8 g/24 hr	8.8	7.0-15.8 mmol/24 h
Cystine, qualitative	Random	Negative	—	Negative
Cystine and cysteine	24 hr	10-100 mg/24 hr	0.0083	0.08-0.83 mmol/24 h
Diacetic acid	Random	Negative	—	Negative
Epinephrine	24 hr	0-20 μg/24 hr	0.0055	0.00-0.11 μmol/24 h
Estrogens				
Total	24 hr			
	Male	5-18 μg/24 hr	1	5-18 μg/24 h
	Female			
	Ovulation	28-100 μg/24 hr		28-80 μg/24 h
	Luteal peak	22-80 μg/24 hr		22-105 μg/24 h
	At menses	4-25 μg/24 hr		4-25 μg/24 h
	Pregnancy	Up to 45,000 μg/24 hr		Up to 45,000 μg/24 h
	Postmenopausal	Up to 10 μg/24 hr		Up to 10 μg/24 h
Fractionated	24 hr, non-pregnant, midcycle			
Estrone (E^1)	—	2-25 μg/24 hr	3.7	7-93 nmol/24 h
Estradiol (E^2)	—	0-10 μg/24 hr	3.7	0-37 nmol/24 h
Estriol (E^3)	—	2-30 μg/24 hr	3.5	7-105 nmol/24 h
Fat, qualitative	Random	Negative	—	Negative
FIGLU (N-formiminoglutamic acid)	24 hr	<3 mg/24 hr	5.7	<17.0 μmol/24 h
	After 15 g of L-histidine	4 mg/8 hr	5.7	23.0 μmol/8 h
Fluoride	24 hr	<1 mg/24 hr	0.053	0.053 mmol/24 h
Follicle-stimulating hormone (FSH)	24 hr			
	Adult	6-50 Mouse uterine units (MUU)/24 hr	1	4-25 mIU/ml
	Prepubertal	<10 MUU/24 hr	1	4-30 mIU/ml
	Postmenopausal	>50 MUU/24 hr	1	40-50 mIU/ml
	Midcycle	2× baseline		
Fructose	24 hr	30-65 mg/24 hr	0.0056	0.17-0.36 mmol/24 h
Glucose				
Qualitative	Random	Negative	—	Negative
Quantitative	24 hr			
Copper-reducing substances		0.5-1.5 g/24 hr	1	0.5-1.5 g/24 h
Total sugars		Average 250 mg/24 hr	1	Average 250 mg/24 h
Glucose		Average 130 mg/24 hr	0.0056	Average 0.73 mmol/24 h
Gonadotropins, pituitary (FSH and LH)	24 hr	10-50 MUU/24 hr	1	10-50 IU/24 h
Etiocholanolone	24 hr			
	Male	1.4-5.0 mg/24 hr	3.44	4.8-17.2 μmol/24 h
	Female	0.8-4.0 mg/24 hr		2.8-13.8 μmol/24 h
Dehydroepiandrosterone	24 hr			
	Male	0.2-2.0 mg/24 hr	3.46	0.7-6.9 μmol/24 h
	Female	0.2-1.8 mg/24 hr		0.7-6.2 μmol/24 h
11-Ketoandrosterone	24 hr			
	Male	0.2-1.0 mg/24 hr	3.28	0.7-3.3 μmol/24 h
	Female	0.2-0.8 mg/24 hr		0.7-2.6 μmol/24 h
11-Ketoetiocholanolone	24 hr			
	Male	0.2-1.0 mg/24 hr	3.28	0.7-3.3 μmol/24 h
	Female	0.2-0.8 mg/24 hr		0.7-2.6 μmol/24 h
11-Hydroxyandrosterone	24 hr			
	Male	0.1-0.8 mg/24 hr	3.26	0.3-2.6 μmol/24 h
	Female	0.0-0.5 mg/24 hr		0.0-1.6 μmol/24 h

Table A-2
Urine—cont'd

Component	Type of urine specimen	Typical reference intervals		
		Conventional units	Factor	Recommended SI units
11-Hydroxyetiocholanolone	24 hr			
Male		0.2-0.6 mg/24 hr	3.26	0.7-2.0 μmol/24 h
Female		0.1-1.1 mg/24 hr		0.3-3.6 μmol/24 h
Lactose	24 hr	14-40 mg/24 hr	2.9	41-116 μmol/24 h
Lead	24 hr	<100 μg/24 hr	0.0048	<0.48 μmol/24 h
Magnesium	24 hr	6.0-8.5 mEq/24 hr	0.5	3.0-4.3 mmol/24 h
Melanin, qualitative	Random	Negative	—	Negative
3-Methoxy-4-hydroxymandelic	24 hr			
acid (VMA)				
Adults		1.5-7.5 mg/24 hr	5.05	7.6-37.9 μmol/24 h
Infants		83 μg/kg/24 hr	0.0051	0.4 μmol/kg/24 h
Mucin	24 hr	100-150 mg/24 hr	1	100-150 mg/24 h
Muramidase (lysozyme)	24 hr	1.3-36 mg/24 hr		1.3-36 mg/24 h
Myoglobin				
Qualitative	Random	Negative	—	Negative
Quantitative	24 hr	<4 mg/l	1	<4 mg/L
Osmolality	Random	500-800 mOsm/kg water	1	500-800 mmol/kg
Pentoses	24 hr	2-5 mg/kg/24 hr	1	2-5 mg/kg/24 h
pH	Random	4.6-8.0	1	4.6-8.0
Phenosulfonphthalein (PSP)	Urine timed after 6 mg PSP IV			Fraction dye excreted
15 min		20-50% dye excreted	0.01	0.2-0.5
30 min		16-24% dye excreted		0.16-0.24
60 min		9-17% dye excreted		0.09-0.17
120 min		3-10% dye excreted		0.03-0.10
Phenylpyruvic acid, qualitative	Random	Negative	—	Negative
Phosphorus	Random	0.9-1.3 g/24 hr	32	29-42 mmol/24 h
Porphobilinogen				
Qualitative	Random	Negative	—	Negative
Quantitative	24 hr	0-1.0 mg/24 hr	4.42	0-4.4 μmol/24 h
Potassium	24 hr	40-80 mEq/24 hr	1	40-80 mmol/24 h
Pregnancy tests	Concentrated morning specimen	Positive in normal pregnancies or with tumors producing chorionic gonadotropin	—	Positive in normal pregnancies or with tumors producing chorionic gonadotropin
Pregnanediol	24 hr			
Male		0-1.5 mg/24 hr	3.12	0-4.7 μmol/24 h
Female		1-8 mg/24 hr		3-25 μmol/24 h
Peak		1 week after ovulation	—	1 week after ovulation
Pregnancy		<50 mg/24 hr		156 μol/24 h
Children		Negative	—	Negative
Pregnanetriol	24 hr			
Male		0.4-2.4 mg/24 hr	2.97	1.2-7.1 μmol/24 h
Female		0.5-2.0 mg/24 hr		1.5-5.9 μmol/24 h
Children		Up to 1 mg/24 hr		Up to 3 μmol/24 h
Protein, qualitative	Random	Negative	—	Negative
	24 hr	40-150 mg/24 hr	1	40-150 mg/24 h
Reducing substances, total	24 hr	0.5-1.5 mg/24 hr	1	0.5-1.5 mg/24 h
Sodium	24 hr	75-200 mEq/24 hr	1	75-200 mmol/24 h
Solids, total	24 hr	55-70 g/24 hr	1	55-70 g/24 h
		Decreases with age to 30 g/24 hr	—	Decreases with age to 30 g/24 h
Specific gravity	Random			Relative Density (U 20° C/water 20° C)
		1.016-1.022 (normal fluid intake)	1	1.016-1.022 (normal fluid intake)
		1.001-1.035 (range)		1.001-1.034 (range)
Sugars (excluding glucose)	Random	Negative	—	Negative
Titratable acidity	24 hr	20-50 mEq/24 hr	1	20-50 mmol/24 h

Continued.

Table A-2
Urine—cont'd

Component	Type of urine specimen	Typical reference intervals		
		Conventional units	Factor	Recommended SI units
Urea nitrogen	24 hr	6-17 g/24 hr	0.0357	0.21-0.60 mol/24 h
Uric acid	24 hr	250-750 mg/24 hr	0.0059	1.48-4.43 mmol/24 h
Urobilinogen	2 hr	0.3-1.0 Ehrlich Units	—	
	24 hr	0.05-2.5 mg/24 hr or	1.69	0.09-4.23 µmol/24 h
		0.5-4.0 Ehrlich units/24 hr	—	
Uropepsin	Random	15-45 units/hr (Anson)	7.37	111-332 U/h
	24 hr	1500-5000 units/24 hr (Anson)		11-37 kU/h
Uroporphyrins				
Qualitative	Random	Negative	—	Negative
Quantitative	24 hr	10-30 µg/24 hr	0.0012	0.012-0.37 µmol/24 h
Vanillylmandelic acid (VMA)	24 hr	1.5-7.5 mg/24 hr	5.05	7.6-37.9 µmol/24 h
Volume, total	24 hr	600-1600 ml/24 hr	0.001	0.6-1.6 L/24 h
Zinc	24 hr	0.15-1.2 mg/24 hr	15.3	2.3-18.4 µmol/24 h

Table A-3
Synovial fluid

Component	Typical reference intervals		
	Conventional units	Factor	Recommended SI units
Blood-serum-synovial fluid glucose difference	<10 mg/dl	0.055	<0.55 mmol/L
Differential cell count	Granulocytes <25% of nucleated cells	0.01	Granulocyte number fraction: <25% of nucleated cells
Fibrin clot	Absent	—	Absent
Mucin clot	Abundant	—	Abundant
Nucleated cell count	<200 cells/µl	10^6	<2 × 10^8 cells/L
Viscosity	High	—	High
Volume	<3.5 ml	0.001	<0.0035L

Table A-4
Seminal fluid

Component	Typical reference intervals		
	Conventional units	Factor	Recommended SI units
Liquefaction	Within 20 min	1	Within 20 min
Sperm morphology	>70% normal mature spermatozoa	0.01	Number fraction: >0.7 normal, mature spermatozoa
Sperm motility	>60%	0.01	Number fraction: >0.6
pH	>7.0 (average 7.7)	1	>7.0 (average 7.7)
Sperm count	60-150 million/ml	10^3	60-150 × 10^9/L
Volume	1.5-5.0 ml	0.001	0.0015-0.005L

Table A-5
Gastric fluid

Component	Typical reference intervals		
	Conventional units	Factor	Recommended SI units
Fasting residual volume	20-100 ml	0.001	0.02-0.10L
pH	<2.0	1	<2.0
Basal acid output (BAO)	0-6 mEq/hr	1	0-6 mmol/h
Maximum acid output (MAO) (after histamine stimulation)	5-40 mEq/hr	1	5-40 mmol/h
BAO/MAO ratio	<0.4	1	<0.4

Table A-6
Hematology

Component	Typical reference intervals		
	Conventional units	Factor	Recommended SI units
Red cell volume			
Male	20-36 ml/kg body weight	0.001	0.020-0.036 L/kg body weight
Female	19-31 ml/kg body weight	—	0.019-0.031 L/kg body weight
Plasma volume			
Male	25-42 ml/kg body weight	0.001	0.040-0.050 L/kg body weight
Female	28-45 ml/kg body weight	—	0.040-0.050 L/kg body weight
Coagulation and hemostatic tests			
Bleeding time			
Mielke template	2-8 minutes		2-8 min
Simplate	3-8 minutes		3-8 min
Antithrombin III			
Immunologic	21-30 mg/dL		210-310 mg/L
Functional	80-120%		0.8-1.2
Clot retraction	40-94% of serum extruded in 1 hour at 37° C		
Euglobulin clot lysis time	Clot lyses between 2 and 4 hours at 37° C		
Factor assays (procoagulant)	0.5-1.5 U/mL		0.5-1.5
Factor VIII antigen (Factor VIIIR:Ag; Laurell)	0.5-1.5 U/mL		0.5-1.5
Ristocetin cofactor (Factor VIIIR:RCoF)	0.5-1.5 U/mL		0.5-1.5
Factor XIII (screening test)	Clot insoluble in 5M urea at 24 hours		
Fibrinogen	200-400 mg/dL		2-4 g/dL
Fibrinogen split products	10 ug/mL		10 mg/L
Partial thromboplastin time (PTT)	Depends upon phospholipid reagent used, typically 60-85 seconds		
Activated PTT	Depends upon activator and phospholipid reagents used, typically 20-35 seconds		
Plasminogen			
Immunologic	10-20 mg/dL		100-200 mg/L
Functional	2.2-4.2 CTA U/mL*		
Prothrombin time	Depends upon thromboplastin reagent used, typically 9.5-12 seconds		
Thrombin time	Depends upon concentration of thrombin reagent used, typically 20-29 seconds		
Whole blood clot lysis time	None in 24 hours		
Complete blood count (CBC)			
Hematocrit			
Male	40-54%	0.01	Volume fraction: 0.40-0.54
Female	38-47%		0.38-0.47%
Hemoglobin			
Male	13.5-18.0 g/dl	0.155	2.09-2.79 mmol/L
Female	12.0-16.0 g/dl		1.86-2.48 mmol/L

*CTA, Committe on Thrombotic Agents

Continued.

Table A-6
Hematology—cont'd

Component	Typical reference intervals		
	Conventional units	Factor	Recommended SI units
Red cell count			
Male	$4.6\text{-}6.2 \times 10^6/\mu l$	10^6	$4.6\text{-}6.2 \times 10^{12}/L$
Female	$4.2\text{-}5.4 \times 10^6/\mu l$		$4.2\text{-}5.4 \times 10^{12}/L$
White cell count	$4.5\text{-}11.0 \times 10^3/\mu l$	10^6	$4.5\text{-}11.0 \times 10^9/L$
Erythrocyte indices			
Mean corpuscular volume (MCV)	80-96 cu microns	1	80-96 fl
Mean corpuscular hemoglobin (MCH)	27-31 pg	1	27-31 pg
Mean corpuscular hemoglobin concentration (MCHC)	32-36%	0.01	Concentration fraction: 0.32-0.36

White blood cell differential (adult)	Mean percent	Range of absolute counts		Mean number fraction†	Range of absolute count
Segmented neutrophils	56%	1800-7000/μl	10^6	0.56	$1.8\text{-}7.8 \times 10^9/L$
Bands	3%	0-700/μl	10^6	0.03	$0\text{-}0.70 \times 10^9/L$
Eosinophils	2.7%	0-450/μl	10^6	0.027	$0\text{-}0.45 \times 10^9/L$
Basophils	0.3%	0-200/μl	10^6	0.003	$0\text{-}0.20 \times 10^9/L$
Lymphocytes	34%	1000-4800/μl	10^6	0.34	$1.0\text{-}4.8 \times 10^9/L$
Monocytes	4%	0-800/μl	10^6	0.04	$0\text{-}0.80 \times 10^9/L$

Component	Conventional units	Factor	Recommended SI units
Hemoglobin A_2	1.5-3.5% of total hemoglobin	0.01	Mass fraction: 0.015-0.035 of total hemoglobin
Hemoglobin F	<2%	0.01	Mass fraction: <0.02

Osmotic fragility

% NaCl	% Lysis Fresh	% Lysis 24 hr at 37° C	Factor	NaCl mmol/L	Lysed fraction Fresh	Lysed fraction 24 h at 37° C
0.2	—	95-100	%NaCl—171	34.2	—	0.95-1.00
0.3	97-100	85-100	% Lysis—0.01	51.3	0.97-1.00	0.85-1.00
0.35	90-99	75-100		59.8	9.90-0.99	0.75-1.00
0.4	50-95	65-100		68.4	0.50-0.95	0.65-1.00
0.45	5-45	55-95		77.0	0.05-0.45	0.55-0.95
0.5	0-6	40-85		85.5	0-0.06	0.40-0.85
0.55	0	15-70		94.1	0	0.15-0.70
0.6	—	0-40		102.6	—	0-0.40
0.65	—	0-10		111.2	—	0-0.10
0.7	—	0-5		119.7	—	0-0.05
0.75	—	0		128.3	—	0

Component	Conventional units	Factor	Recommended SI units
Platelet count	150,000-400,000/μl	10^6	$0.15\text{-}0.4 \times 10^{12}/L$
Reticulocyte count	0.5-1.5%	0.01	Number fraction: 0.005-0.015
	25,000-75,000 cells/μl	10^6	$25\text{-}75 \times 10^9/L$
Sedimentation rate (ESR) (Westergren)			
Men under 50 yrs	<50 mm/hr	1	<15 mm/h
Men over 50 yrs	<20 mm/hr		<20 mm/h
Women under 50 yrs	<20 mm/hr		<20 mm/h
Women over 50 yrs	<30 mm/hr		<30 mm/h
Viscosity	1.4-1.8 times water	1	1.4-1.8 times water
Zeta sedimentation ratio	41-54%	0.01	Fraction: 0.41-0.54

†All percentages are multiplied by 0.01 to give fraction.

Table A-7
Amniotic fluid

	Typical reference intervals		
Component	**Conventional units**	**Factor**	**Recommended SI units**
Appearance			
Early gestation	Clear	—	Clear
Term	Clear or slightly opalescent	—	Clear or slightly opalescent
Albumin			
Early gestation	0.39 g/dl	10	3.9 g/L
Term	0.19 g/dl		1.9 g/L
Bilirubin			
Early gestation	<0.075 mg/dl	17.1	<1.28 μmol/L
Term	<0.025 mg/dl		<0.43 μmol/L
Chloride			
Early gestation	Approximately equal to serum chloride	—	Approximately equal to serum chloride
Term	Generally 1-3 mEq/l lower than serum chloride	1	Generally 1-3 mmol/L lower than serum chloride
Creatinine			
Early gestation	0.8-1.1 mg/dl	88.4	70.7-97.2 μmol/L
Term	1.8-4.0 mg/dl (generally > 2 mg/dl)		159.1-353.6 μmol/L (generally > 176.8 μmol/L)
Estriol			
Early gestation	<10 μg/dl	0.035	<0.35 μmol/L
Term	>60 μg/dl		>2.1 μmol/L
Lecithin/sphingomyelin		1	
Early (immature)	<1:1	1	<1:1
Term (mature)	>2:1	1	>2:1
Osmolality			
Early gestation	Approximately equal to serum osmolality	1	Approximately equal to serum osmolality
Term	230-270 mOsm/l	1	<230-270 mmol/L
Pco₂			
Early gestation	33-55 mm Hg	0.133	4.39-7.32 kPa
Term	42-55 mm Hg (increases toward term)		5.59-7.32 kPa (increase toward term)
pH			
Early gestation	7.12-7.38	1	7.12-7.38
Term	6.91-7.43 (decreases toward term)		6.91-7.43
Protein, total			
Early gestation	0.60 ± 0.24 g/dl	10	6.0 ± 2.4 g/L
Term	0.26 ± 0.19 g/dl		2.6 ± 1.9 g/L
Sodium			
Early gestation	Approximately equal to serum sodium	—	Approximately equal to serum sodium
Term	7-10 mEq/l lower than serum sodium	1	7-10 mmol/L lower than serium sodium
Staining, cytologic			
Oil red O			Stained fraction
Early gestation	<10%	0.01	<0.1
Term	>50%		>0.5
Nile blue sulfate			Stained fraction
Early gestation	0	0.01	0
Term	>20%		>0.2
Urea			
Early gestation	18.0 ± 5.9 mg/dl	0.166	2.99 ± 0.98 mmol/L
Term	30.3 ± 11.4 mg/dl		5.03 ± 1.89 mmol/L
Uric acid			
Early gestation	3.72 ± 0.96 mg/dl	0.059	0.22 ± 0.06 mmol/L
Term	9.90 ± 2.23 mg/dl		0.58 ± 0.13 mmol/L
Volume			
Early gestation	450-1200 ml	0.001	0.45-1.2 L
Term	500-1400 ml (increases toward term)		0.5-1.4 L (increases toward term)

Table A-8
Cerebrospinal fluid

Component	Typical reference intervals		
	Conventional units	Factor	Recommended SI units
Albumin	10-30 mg/dl	10	100-300 mg/L
Calcium	2.1-2.7 mEq/l	0.5	1.05-1.35 mmol/L
Cell count	0-5 cells/μl	10^6	$0\text{-}5 \times 10^6/L$
Chloride			
Adult	118-132 mEq/l	1	118-132 mmol/L
Glucose	50-80 mg/dl	0.055	2.75-4.40 mmol/L
Lactate dehydrogenase (LDH)	Approximately 10% of serum level	—	Activity fraction: approximately 0.1 of serum level
Protein			
Total CSF	15-45 mg/dl	10	150-450 mg/L
Ventricular fluid	5-15 mg/dl		50-150 mg/L
Protein electrophoresis			Fraction
Prealbumin	2-7%	0.01	0.02-0.07
Albumin	56-76%		0.56-0.76
Alpha-1 globulin	2-7%		0.02-0.07
Alpha-2 globulin	4-12%		0.04-0.12
Beta globulin	8-18%		0.08-0.18
Gamma globulin	3-12%		0.03-0.12
Xanthochromia	Negative	—	Negative

Table A-9
Miscellaneous

Component	Specimen	Typical reference intervals		
		Conventional units	Factor	Recommended SI units
Bile, qualitative	Random stool	Negative in adults	—	Negative in adults
		Positive in children	—	Positive in children
Chloride	Sweat	4-60 mEq/l	1	4-60 mmol/L
Clearances	Serum and urine (timed)			
Creatinine, endogenous		115 ± 20 ml/min	0.0167	1.92 ± 0.33 ml/s
Diodrast		600-720 ml/min		10.02-12.02 ml/s
Inulin		100-150 ml/min		1.67-2.51 ml/s
PAH		600-750 ml/min		10.02-12.53 ml/s
Diagnex blue (tubeless gastric analysis)	Urine	Free acid present	—	Free acid present
Fat	Stool, 72 hr			
Total fat		<5 g/24 hr	0.01	<5 g/24 h
				Mass fraction
		10-25% of dry matter	0.01	0.1-0.24 of dry matter
Neutral fat		1-5% of dry matter	0.01	0.01-0.05 of dry matter
Free fatty acids		5-13% of dry matter	0.01	0.05-0.13 of dry matter
Combined fatty acids		5-15% of dry matter	0.01	0.05-0.15 of dry matter
Nitrogen, total	Stool, 24 hr			Mass fraction
		10% of intake	0.01	0.1 of intake
		1-2 g/24 hr	0.071	0.071-0.142 mol/24 h
Sodium	Sweat	10-80 mEq/l	1	10-80 mmol/L
Trypsin activity	Random, fresh stool	Positive (2+ to 4+)	—	Positive (2+ to 4+)
Thyroid ^{131}I uptake		7.5-25% in 6 hr	0.01	Fraction uptake: 0.075-0.25 in 6 h
Urobilinogen				
Qualitative	Random stool	Positive	—	Positive
Quantitative	Stool, 24 hr	40-200 mg/24 hr	0.00169	0.068-0.34 mmol/24 h
		80-280 Ehrlich units/24 hr		

Table A-10
Selected pediatric reference values

S*-Acid phosphatase
Newborn: 7.4-19.4 U/L
2-13 yrs: 6.4-15.2 U/L

S-Aldolase
Newborn: to 4 × adult value
Child: to 2 × adult value

S-Alkaline phosphatase
Newborn: 40-300 U/L
Child: 60-270 U/L

S-Alpha fetoprotein
Newborn: up to 100 mg/L
2 weeks: undetectable

S-Amylase
Newborn: little, if any, amylase activity
1 year: adult values

S-Aspartate aminotransferase
Newborn: 16-74 U/L
1-3 yrs: 6-30 U/L

S-Bilirubin
	Pre-term	Full-term
Newborn:		
24 h	17.1-102.8 μmol/L (10-60 mg/L)	34.2-102.8 μmol/L (20-60 mg/L)
48 h	102.8-137.0 μmol/L (60-80 mg/L)	102.8-119.9 μmol/L (60-70 mg/L)
3-5 d	171.0-266.5 μmol/L (100-150 mg/L)	68.6-205.2 μmol/L (40-120 mg/L)

S-Calcium
Pre-term, first week: 1.5-2.5 mmol/L (60-100 mg/L)
Full-term, first week: 1.75-3.00 mmol/L (70-120 mg/L)
1-2 yrs: 2.5-3.0 mmol/L (100-120 mg/L)
2-16 yrs: 2.25-2.88 mmol/L (90-115 mg/L)

U*-Catecholamines
	Norepinephrine	Epinephrine
1 yr:	29.5-86.8 nmol/d (5.4-15.9 μg/d)	0.6-25.4 nmol/d (0.1-4.3 μg/d)
1-5 yrs:	44.2-168.1 nmol/d (8.1-30.8 μg/d)	4.7-53.8 nmol/d (0.8-9.1 μg/d)
6-15 yrs:	103.7-388.1 nmol/d (19.0-71.1 μg/d)	7.7-62.1 nmol/d (1.3-10.5 μg/d)
>15 yrs:	188.8-474.8 nmol/d (34.4-87.0 μg/d)	20.7-78.0 nmol/d (3.5-13.2 μg/d)

U-Chloride
Infant: 1.7-8.5 mmol/d
Child: 17-34 mmol/d

S-Cholesterol
Cord blood: 1.2-2.5 mmol/L (460-980 mg/L)
1-2 yrs: 1.8-4.9 mmol/L (700-1900 mg/L)
2-16 yrs: 3.5-6.5 mmol/L (1350-2500 mg/L)

U-Cortisol (free)
4 mos-10 yrs: 2-27 μg/d   5.5-74.5 nmol/d
11-20 yrs: 0.7-55 μg/d   1.9-151.8 nmol/d

S-Creatine kinase
Newborn: 3 × adult values
3 wks-3 mos: 1.5 × adult values
>1 yr: at adult values

S-Creatinine
Upper reference value:
Up to 5 yrs: 44 μmol/L (5.0 mg/L)
Up to 6 yrs: 53 μmol/L (6.0 mg/L)
Up to 7 yrs: 62 μmol/L (7.0 mg/L)
Up to 8 yrs: 70 μmol/L (8.0 mg/L)
Up to 9 yrs: 79 μmol/L (9.0 mg/L)
Up to 10 yrs: 88 μmol/L (10.0 mg/L)
>10 yrs: 106 μmol/L (12.0 mg/L)

S-Estradiol
0-2 yrs:	0-7 pg/ml	0-24 pmol/L
2-4 yrs:	0-7 pg/ml	0-24 pmol/L
4-6 yrs:	0-14 pg/ml	0-49 pmol/L
6-8 yrs:	0-10 pg/ml	0-35 pmol/L
8-10 yrs:	0-100 pg/ml	0-347 pmol/L
10-12 yrs:	0-100 pg/ml	0-347 pmol/L
12-14 yrs:	0-100 pg/ml	0-347 pmol/L
14-16 yrs:	7-105 pg/ml	24-364 pmol/L
16-25 yrs:	7-320 pg/ml	24-1110 pmol/L

Fecal fat
Pre-term newborn: up to 40% excreted
Full-term newborn: up to 20% excreted
3 mos-1 yr: up to 15% excreted
1 yr: up to 8.5% excreted

P-Nonesterified fatty acids
Newborn: 0-1845 mmol/L
4 mos-10 yrs: 300-1100 mmol/L

S-Glucose
Pre-term newborn: 1.2-3.6 mmol/L (200-656 mg/L)
Full-term newborn: 1.1-6.0 mmol/L (200-1100 mg/L)
Child: 3.3-5.8 mmol/L (600-1050 mg/L)

Information based on Meites, S. (ed.): Pediatric Clinical Chemistry. Washington, D.C., 1977, American Association for Clinical Chemistry.
*S, Serum; U, Urine.

Continued.

Table A-10
Selected pediatric reference values—cont'd

S-γ-Glutamyltransferase
Premature newborn:	56-233 U/L
Newborn-3 wks:	10-103 U/L
3 wks-3 mos:	4-111 U/L
1-5 yrs:	2-23 U/L
6-15 yrs:	2-23 U/L
16 yrs-adult:	2-35 U/L

S-Haptoglobin
Newborn:	detectable haptoglobin in only 10-20%
1 yr and older:	at adult values

S-Immunoglobulin IgG
0-5 wks:	7500-15,000 mg/L
6 mos:	1500-7000 mg/L
1 yr:	1400-10,300 mg/L
5 yrs:	3700-15,000 mg/L
10 yrs:	4400-15,500 mg/L

S-Immunoglobulin IgA
0-5 wks:	none
6 mos:	200-1300 mg/L
1 yr:	200-1300 mg/L
5 yrs:	300-2000 mg/L
10 yrs:	500-2300 mg/L

S-Immunoglobulin IgM
0-5 wks:	less than 200 mg/L
6 mos:	300-600 mg/L
1 yr:	300-1600 mg/L
5 yrs:	200-2200 mg/L
10 yrs:	300-1700 mg/L

Inulin clearance
<1 mo:	29-88 ml/min per 1.73 m^2 of body surface
1-6 mos:	40-112 ml/min per 1.73 m^2 of body surface
6-12 mos:	62-121 ml/min per 1.73 m^2 of body surface
>1 yr:	78-164 ml/min per 1.73 m^2 of body surface

U-17 Ketosteroids
0-3 days:	0-0.5 mg/d
1-3 yrs:	<2.0 mg/d
3-6 yrs:	0.5-3.0 mg/d
6-9 yrs:	0.8-4.0 mg/d
10-12 yrs:	male: 0.7-6.0 mg/d
	female: 0.7-5.0 mg/d
Adolescent:	male: 3-15 mg/d
	female: 3-12 mg/d

S-Lactate dehydrogenase
1-3 days:	up to 2 × adult values

S-Phosphorus (inorganic)

	Pre-term	Full-term
Newborn:	1.8-2.6 mmol/L (56.0-80.0 mg/L)	1.6-2.5 mmol/L (50.0-78.0 mg/L)
6-10 days:	2.0-3.8 mmol/L (61-117 mg/L)	1.6-2.9 mmol/L (49-89 mg/L)
4 mos:	1.6-2.6 mmol/L (48-81 mg/L)	
1 yr:	1.25-2.1 mmol/L (39-60 mg/L)	
2-16 yrs:	0.9-1.5 mmol/L (26-50 mg/L)	

S-Potassium
Pre-term newborn:	4.5-7.2 mmol/L
Full-term newborn:	5.0-7.7 mmol/L
2 d-2 wks:	4.0-6.4 mmol/L
2 wks-3 mos:	4.0-6.2 mmol/L
3 mos-1 yr:	3.7-5.6 mmol/L
1-16 yrs:	3.6-5.2 mmol/L

S-Thyroxine
1-3 days:	142-296 nmol/l (11-23 μg/dl)
1 wk-1 mo:	116-232 nmol/L (9-18 μg/dl)
1-4 mos:	97-212 nmol/L (7.5-16.5 μg/dl)
4-12 mos:	71-187 nmol/L (5.5-14.5 μg/dl)
1-6 yrs:	71-174 nmol/L (5.5-13.5 μg/dl)
6-10 yrs:	64-161 nmol/L (5.0-12.5 μg/dl)

S-Testosterone

Age	Male	Female
0-2 yrs:	0.14-1.28 nmol/L	0.24-0.62 nmol/L
2-4 yrs:	0.17-5.55 nmol/L	0.24-0.69 nmol/L
4-6 yrs:	0.28-1.39 nmol/L	0.35-0.69 nmol/L
6-8 yrs:	0.21-9.72 nmol/L	0.52-1.04 nmol/L
8-10 yrs:	0.31-1.74 nmol/L	0.69-1.39 nmol/L
10-12 yrs:	0.29-10.06 nmol/L	0.69-1.74 nmol/L
12-14 yrs:	0.17-26.37 nmol/L	1.04-2.43 nmol/L
14-16 yrs:	3.12-19.43 nmol/L	1.21-3.30 nmol/L
16-18 yrs:	9.02-25.33 nmol/L	1.39-3.30 nmol/L
18-20 yrs:	13.88-24.98 nmol/L	1.39-3.30 nmol/L
20-25 yrs:	11.80-38.86 nmol/L	1.39-3.30 nmol/L

DESIRABLE WEIGHTS

Table B-1
1983 Metropolitan height and weight tables*

Men			
Height	**Small frame**	**Medium frame**	**Large frame**
5'2"	128-134	131-141	138-150
5'3"	130-136	133-143	140-153
5'4"	132-138	135-145	142-156
5'5"	134-140	137-148	144-160
5'6"	136-142	139-151	146-164
5'7"	138-145	142-154	149-168
5'8"	140-148	145-157	152-172
5'9"	142-151	148-160	155-176
5'10"	144-154	151-163	158-180
5'11"	146-157	154-166	161-184
6'0"	149-160	157-170	164-188
6'1"	152-164	160-174	168-192
6'2"	155-168	164-178	172-197
6'3"	158-172	167-182	176-202
6'4"	162-176	171-187	181-207

Women			
Height	**Small frame**	**Medium frame**	**Large frame**
4'10"	102-111	109-121	118-131
4'11"	103-113	111-123	120-134
5'0"	104-115	113-126	122-137
5'1"	106-118	115-129	125-140
5'2"	108-121	118-132	128-143
5'3"	111-124	121-135	131-147
5'4"	114-127	124-138	134-151
5'5"	117-130	127-141	137-155
5'6"	120-133	130-144	140-159
5'7"	123-136	133-147	143-163
5'8"	126-139	133-150	146-167
5'9"	129-142	139-153	149-170
5'10"	132-145	142-156	152-173
5'11"	135-148	145-159	155-176
6'0"	138-151	148-162	158-179

*Weight in pounds at ages 29-59 years according to build. In shoes and 3 pounds of indoor clothing for women and 5 pounds for men. (Sources: Society of Actuaries, Build Study, 1979, Chicago, 1980, Society of Actuaries and Association of Life Insurance Medical Directors of America, Metropolitan Life Insurance Co., N.Y., 1983.)

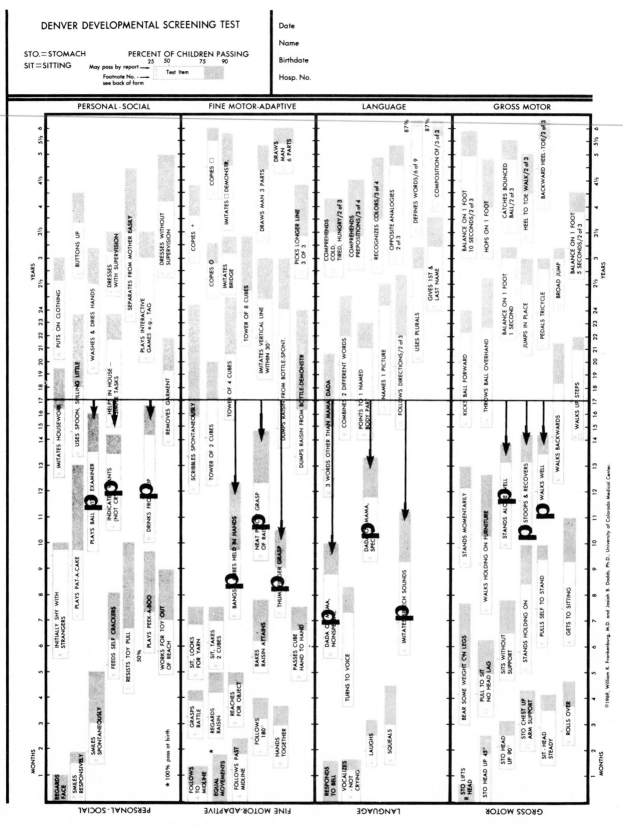

Fig. C-2

A, Denver Developmental Screening Test (DDST). NOTE: P indicates those 12 items used in the abbreviated testing procedure to identify children with suspect test results who require full DDST.

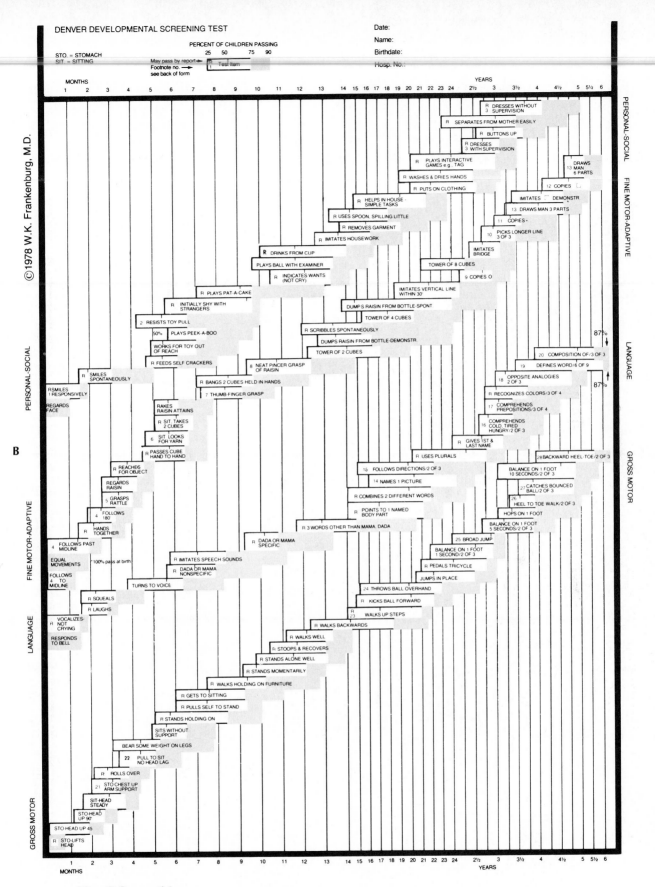

Fig. C-2, cont'd

B, DDST revised (DDST-R). Resembling a growth curve, this form places items at lowest age level starting at bottom left and progresses upward to right with increasing age. (**A** and **B,** from Frankenburg, W.K., Sciarillo, W., and Burgess, D.: The newly abbreviated and revised Denver Developmental Screening Test, J. Pediatr. **99**(6):995, 1981.)

Continued.

DATE

NAME

DIRECTIONS   BIRTHDATE

HOSP. NO.

1. Try to get child to smile by smiling, talking or waving to him. Do not touch him.
2. When child is playing with toy, pull it away from him. Pass if he resists.
3. Child does not have to be able to tie shoes or button in the back.
4. Move yarn slowly in an arc from one side to the other, about 6" above child's face. Pass if eyes follow 90° to midline. (Past midline; 180°)
5. Pass if child grasps rattle when it is touched to the backs or tips of fingers.
6. Pass if child continues to look where yarn disappeared or tries to see where it went. Yarn should be dropped quickly from sight from tester's hand without arm movement.
7. Pass if child picks up raisin with any part of thumb and a finger.
8. Pass if child picks up raisin with the ends of thumb and index finger using an over hand approach.

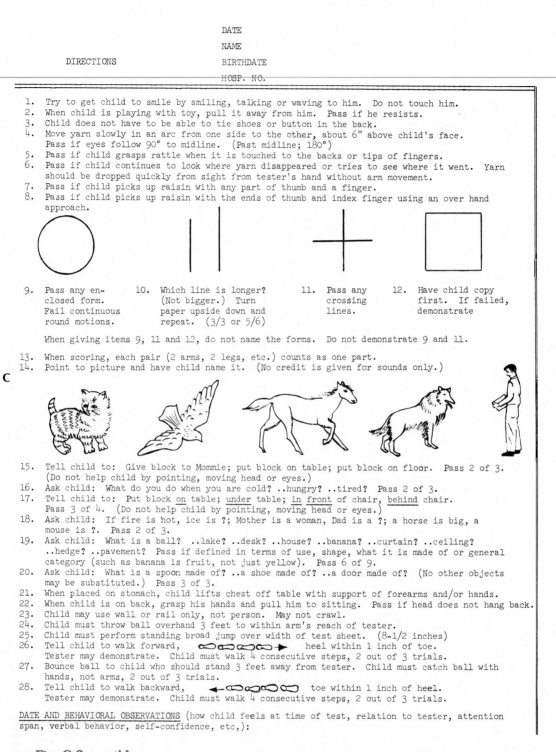

9. Pass any en-closed form. Fail continuous round motions.
10. Which line is longer? (Not bigger.) Turn paper upside down and repeat. (3/3 or 5/6)
11. Pass any crossing lines.
12. Have child copy first. If failed, demonstrate

When giving items 9, 11 and 12, do not name the forms. Do not demonstrate 9 and 11.

13. When scoring, each pair (2 arms, 2 legs, etc.) counts as one part.
14. Point to picture and have child name it. (No credit is given for sounds only.)

C

15. Tell child to: Give block to Mommie; put block on table; put block on floor. Pass 2 of 3. (Do not help child by pointing, moving head or eyes.)
16. Ask child: What do you do when you are cold? ..hungry? ..tired? Pass 2 of 3.
17. Tell child to: Put block on table; under table; in front of chair, behind chair. Pass 3 of 4. (Do not help child by pointing, moving head or eyes.)
18. Ask child: If fire is hot, ice is ?; Mother is a woman, Dad is a ?; a horse is big, a mouse is ?. Pass 2 of 3.
19. Ask child: What is a ball? ..lake? ..desk? ..house? ..banana? ..curtain? ..ceiling? ..hedge? ..pavement? Pass if defined in terms of use, shape, what it is made of or general category (such as banana is fruit, not just yellow). Pass 6 of 9.
20. Ask child: What is a spoon made of? ..a shoe made of? ..a door made of? (No other objects may be substituted.) Pass 3 of 3.
21. When placed on stomach, child lifts chest off table with support of forearms and/or hands.
22. When child is on back, grasp his hands and pull him to sitting. Pass if head does not hang back.
23. Child may use wall or rail only, not person. May not crawl.
24. Child must throw ball overhand 3 feet to within arm's reach of tester.
25. Child must perform standing broad jump over width of test sheet. (8-1/2 inches)
26. Tell child to walk forward, ⟨footprints⟩→ heel within 1 inch of toe. Tester may demonstrate. Child must walk 4 consecutive steps, 2 out of 3 trials.
27. Bounce ball to child who should stand 3 feet away from tester. Child must catch ball with hands, not arms, 2 out of 3 trials.
28. Tell child to walk backward, ←⟨footprints⟩ toe within 1 inch of heel. Tester may demonstrate. Child must walk 4 consecutive steps, 2 out of 3 trials.

DATE AND BEHAVIORAL OBSERVATIONS (how child feels at time of test, relation to tester, attention span, verbal behavior, self-confidence, etc,):

Fig. C-2, cont'd
C, Directions for numbered items on testing form. (**C** from Frankenburg, W.K., and Dobbs, J.B., University of Colorado Medical Center, 1969.)

DENVER ARTICULATION SCREENING EXAM
for children 2 1/2 to 6 years of age

Instructions: Have child repeat each word after
you. Circle the underlined sounds that he pro-
nounces correctly. Total correct sounds is the
Raw Score. Use charts on reverse side to score
results.

NAME

HOSP. NO.

ADDRESS

A

Date: _____ Child's Age:_____ Examiner: _____ Raw Score:_____
Percentile:_____ Intelligibility:_____ Result:_____

1. table   6. zipper   11. sock   16. wagon   21. leaf
2. shirt   7. grapes   12. vacuum   17. gum   22. carrot
3. door   8. flag   13. yarn   18. house
4. trunk   9. thumb   14. mother   19. pencil
5. jumping   10. toothbrush   15. twinkle   20. fish

Intelligibility: (circle one)   1. Easy to understand   3. Not understandable
                                 2. Understandable 1/2   4. Can't evaluate
                                        the time.

Comments:

Date: _____ Child's Age:_____ Examiner:_____ Raw Score _____
Percentile:_____ Intelligibility:_____ Result:_____

1. table   6. zipper   11. sock   16. wagon   21. leaf
2. shirt   7. grapes   12. vacuum   17. gum   22. carrot
3. door   8. flag   13. yarn   18. house
4. trunk   9. thumb   14. mother   19. pencil
5. jumping   10. toothbrush   15. twinkle   20. fish

Intelligibility: (circle one)   1. Easy to understand   3. Not understandable
                                 2. Understandable 1/2   4. Can't evaluate
                                        the time.

Comments:

Date: _____ Child's Age: _____ Examiner:_____ Raw Score_____
Percentile: _____ Intelligibility:_____ Result:_____

1. table   6. zipper   11. sock   16. wagon   21. leaf
2. shirt   7. grapes   12. vacuum   17. gum   22. carrot
3. door   8. flag   13. yarn   18. house
4. trunk   9. thumb   14. mother   19. pencil
5. jumping   10. toothbrush   15. twinkle   20. fish

Intelligibility: (circle one)   1. Easy to understand   3. Not understandable
                                 2. Understandable 1/2   4. Can't evaluate
                                        the time.

Fig. C-3
A, Denver Articulation Screening Examination for children 2½ to 6 years of age. (**A,** From
Drumwright, A.F., University of Colorado Medical Center, 1971.)   *Continued.*

To score DASE words: Note Raw Score for child's performance. Match raw score line (extreme left of chart) with column representing child's age (to the closest previous age group). Where raw score line and age column meet number in that square denotes percentile rank of child's performance when compared to other children that age. Percentiles above heavy line are ABNORMAL percentiles, below heavy line are NORMAL.

PERCENTILE RANK

Raw Score	2.5 yr.	3.0	3.5	4.0	4.5	5.0	5.5	6 years
2	1							
3	2							
4	5							
5	9							
6	16							
7	23							
8	31	2						
9	37	4	1					
10	42	6	2					
11	48	7	4					
12	54	9	6	1	1			
13	58	12	9	2	3	1	1	
14	62	17	11	5	4	2	2	
15	68	23	15	9	5	3	2	
16	75	31	19	12	5	4	3	
17	79	38	25	15	6	6	4	
18	83	46	31	19	8	7	4	
19	86	51	38	24	10	9	5	1
20	89	58	45	30	12	11	7	3
21	92	65	52	36	15	15	9	4
22	94	72	58	43	18	19	12	5
23	96	77	63	50	22	24	15	7
24	97	82	70	58	29	29	20	15
25	99	87	78	66	36	34	26	17
26	99	91	84	75	46	43	34	24
27		94	89	82	57	54	44	34
28		96	94	88	70	68	59	47
29		98	98	94	84	84	77	68
30		100	100	100	100	100	100	100

B

To Score intelligibility:

	NORMAL	ABNORMAL
2 1/2 years	Understandable 1/2 the time, or, "easy"	Not Understandable
3 years and older	Easy to understand	Understandable 1/2 time Not understandable

Test Result: 1. NORMAL on Dase and Intelligibility = NORMAL

2. ABNORMAL on Dase and/or Intelligibility = ABNORMAL

* If abnormal on initial screening rescreen within 2 weeks. If abnormal again child should be referred for complete speech evaluation.

Fig. C-3, cont'd
B, Percentile rank.

GLOSSARY

abatement Decrease in intensity of a pain or other symptom.

abdominal regions Surface divisions of the abdomen into nine or four sections.

abdominal zones Surface division of the abdomen into three sections: (1) the epigastric zone above the transpyloric plane, (2) the hypogastric zone below the transtubercular plane, and (3) the umbilical zone situated between the epigastric and hypogastric zones.

abduction Movement away from the axial line (for a limb) or the median plane (for the digits).

abreaction Release of painful emotion through recall or repressed memories, objective of freudian method of psychoanalysis.

abscess Circumscribed collection of necrotic cellular debris, white blood cells, and microorganisms demarcated by inflamed tissue.

abulia Loss or deficiency in ability to make decisions or to act on decisions; may occur in depression (absence of will power).

accommodation Reflex alteration of the refractory power of the lens of the eye during the viewing of objects at varying distance from the retina. The shape of the lens is changed as a result of the degree of contraction of the ciliary muscle. A blurred image on the retina evokes the brainstem reflex, which is mediated via parasympathetic fibers in cranial nerve III (oculomotor). Change in lens shape occurs equally in both eyes. When the focus is on a near object, accommodation is accompanied by convergence of the eyes and constriction of the pupils.

achalasia Failure of smooth muscle of the gastrointestinal tract to relax; particularly significant for the cardiac sphincter. The condition results from congenital absence of parasympathetic elements of Auerbach's plexus.

achondroplasia Disturbance in cartilage development.

acini Small, saclike dilatations found in various glands.

acromegaly Chronic disease caused by hypersecretion of growth hormone; characterized by overgrowth of the small parts.

acrophobia Abnormal fear of heights.

acute Severe symptoms, usually of rapid onset and of short duration.

adaptation The reduction of pupillary diameter size (constriction) to increased ambient light level and the widening of pupillary size to decreased ambient light level.

adduction Movement toward the axial line (for a limb) or the median plane (for the digits).

adenoid Resembling a gland; hypertrophy of the adenoid tissue situated in the pharynx; sometimes called pharyngeal tonsil.

adenoma Tumor consisting of glandular cells.

adhesion A fibrotic band or structure that joins two surfaces that are normally separated.

adiposis Excessive accumulation of adipose (lipoid) tissue; obesity or corpulence; fatty infiltration of an organ or tissue.

affect A mood or inner feeling; disturbances in affect are seen in most psychiatric illnesses.

afferent Conduction toward the center or controlling structure, i.e., the afferent nerve conducts impulses to the central nervous system, and the dendrite conducts impulses to the neuronal body.

afterload The load against which a muscle contracts. When used in reference to the heart, afterload is approximately the arterial pressure. An increase in afterload reduces the stroke volume.

ageusia Loss of the sensation of taste or the ability to discriminate sweet, sour, salty, and bitter tastes.

agitation Restlessness; inability to concentrate or remain motionless.

agnosia Inability to discriminate sensory stimuli. *Acoustic or auditory agnosia:* impaired ability to recognize familiar sounds. *Tactile agnosia:* impaired ability to recognize familiar objects by touch or feel. *Visual agnosia:* impaired ability to recognize familiar objects by sight. *Somatagnosia:* disturbance in recognition of body parts.

agonist (1) Prime mover; a muscle opposed in action by another muscle, the antagonist, i.e., the flexor of the arm (the biceps) and the extensor of the arm (the triceps). (2) A neurotransmitter, hormone, immune complex, or drug that competes for receptors and produces similar (same direction) effects as the substance normal to those receptors.

agoraphobia Marked fear of public places.

akinesia Delay or slowness in beginning and carrying through voluntary motor movements and sudden or unexpected stops in motion. Akinesia is a sign of extrapyramidal disease and is often seen in Parkinson's disease.

akinesthesia Inability to sense movement.

alienation Inability to identify with family, peer group, society, or culture; associated with schizophrenia.

alopecia Loss of hair to baldness.

Alzheimer's disease Progressive condition of atrophy of the brain and degeneration of the neurons that usually occurs in persons over 40 years of age. Histologic changes include the presence of neurofibrillary tangles and extraneuronal senile plaques containing amyloid. The EEG alpha rhythm is reduced. Behavioral changes may progress from mild cognitive defects to dementia.

amaurosis Blindness without perceptible disease of the visual structures.

amnestic syndrome Short- and long-term impairment of memory as a result of a specific organic factor.

amyotonia Lack of tone of the musculature of the body.

amyotrophy Wasting or atrophy of muscle tissue.

analgesia Loss of sensation; used particularly to denote relief of pain without loss of consciousness.

anarthria Loss of articulation.

anesthesia Loss of sensation.

aneurysm Dilatation of an artery.

angina pectoris Pain—substernal or radiating to the left arm, neck, or jaw; frequently correlated with myocardial ischemia.

angioma Benign tumor consisting of blood vessels or lymphatic vessels.

anisocoria Unequal dilatation of the pupils.

ankylosis Rigidity and consolidation of a joint.

anorexia Loss of appetite.

anosmia Inability to smell.

anosognosia Lack of insight or loss of ability to recognize one's disease.

antrum Cavity or chamber.

anuria Absence of excretion of urine.

anxiety Motor tension, autonomic hyperactivity, apprehension, or hyperattentiveness.

anxiety syndrome Anxiety of at least 1 month's duration.

apathy Lack of interest and blunting of affect in conditions that would normally stimulate interest or elicit feeling.

aphakia Absence of the lens of the eye; may be congenital or a result of surgery.

aphasia Dysfunction or loss of the ability to express thoughts by speech, writing, symbols, or signs. *Fluent aphasia:* ability to produce words but with frequent errors in the appropriate choice of words or in the creation of words. *Nonfluent aphasia:* inability to produce words, either in spoken or written form.

aphonia Inability to produce laryngeal voice sounds.

aplasia Failure of cellular formation or development of an organ or tissue or the cellular products from an organ or tissue, as an impairment in blood formation.

apnea Cessation of breathing in the end expiratory position.

apneustic breathing Respiration characterized by a sustained inspiratory phase interrupted by brief expirations.

apraxia Impairment of the ability to carry out purposeful movement (although muscle and sensory apparatus are intact), as an inability to draw or construct forms of two or three dimensions.

aqueous humor Fluid secreted in the ciliary body and found in the anterior and posterior chambers of the eye.

arcus senilis Gray to white opaque ring surrounding the cornea, generally seen in individuals older than 50 years of age, caused by lipoid position.

arrhythmia Any deviation from the normal pace of the heart.

arterial pressure The force exerted by the blood against the arterial walls. Blood pressure is measured in millimeters of mercury above sea level. The contraction of the heart results in a pulsatile ejection of the blood, resulting in variation of the pressure from a systolic peak of about 120 mm Hg at maximum left ventricular stroke output and a minimum *diastolic pressure* of about 80 mm Hg. The *pulse pressure* is equal to the difference between systolic and diastolic pressure. Mean arterial pressure MAP may be calculated by the following formula:

$$MAP = \text{Diastolic pressure} + \frac{\text{Pulse pressure}}{3}$$

arteriosclerosis Hardening (sclerosis) and thickening of the walls of arterioles.

arthritis Inflammation of a joint.

arthropathy General term for disease in a joint.

ascites The accumulation of free fluid within the abdominal cavity.

asterixis Liver flap, flapping tremor, or wrist flapping as a result of a sudden relaxation of wrist extensors; appears in hepatic failure with the occurence of metabolic encephalopathy.

asthenia Weakness; loss of strength or energy.

asthma Proxysmal dyspnea (wheezing) resulting from obstruction of the bronchi or spasm of smooth muscle.

astigmatism Irregularity of the spherical curve of the cornea such that light rays cannot be focused in a point on the retina. Astigmatism is corrected with contact lenses or eyeglasses ground to compensate for the defect.

astrocytoma Tumor composed of astrocytes. Astrocytoma is the most common tumor of the central nervous system.

asystole Cardiac standstill or arrest.

ataxia Impairment of coordination of muscular activity.

atelectasis Incomplete expansion of a lung compromised since birth; collapse of the adult lung.

atheroma Necrosis of a fibrous plaque of the arterial wall with degenerated lipid, seen in atherosclerosis.

atherosclerosis Type of arteriosclerosis characterized by deposits (atheromas) of cholesterol, lipoid material, and lipophages in the walls of large arteries and arterioles.

athetosis Slow, sustained, involuntary large amplitude muscle movements that are sinuous, writhing, or squirming in character.

atony Without normal tone or resistance to stretching.

atopy Predisposition to allergy.

atresia Congenital absence or closure of a tubular structure or orifice.

atrophy Wasting; decrease in the size of a cell, tissue, organ, or body part.

aura Premonitory sensation, generally applied to sensations preceeding epileptiform convulsions.

auscultation Examination made by listening, usually through the stethoscope.

autism Behavioral lack of responsiveness to other persons and defects in language skills; develops within the first 30 months of age.

AV block Impairment of impulse conduction from the atria to the ventricles.

azotemia Elevated serum concentration of nonprotein nitrogen substances, primarily urea.

Babinski's sign Reflex elicited by tactile stimulation of the lateral aspect of the sole and manifested by dorsiflexion and fanning of the toes. This sign is found in upper motor neuron (pyramidal tract) lesions. The sign is normal in infants less than 18 months of age.

Baker's cyst Swelling in the popliteal space resulting from herniation of the synovial membrane of the knee.

balanitis Inflammation of the glans penis.

ballismus Sudden flailing movements of the limbs; *hemiballismus* is the term for the condition affecting only one side of the body.

ballottement A palpation technique used to assess a floating object; fluid-filled tissue is pushed toward the examining hand so that the object will float against the examining fingers.

baragnosis Inability to perceive differences in weight pressure.

basophilia An abnormal increase in the basophilic leukocytosis.

Battle's sign Bluish discoloration along the course of the posterior auricular artery, with ecchymosis first appearing near the tip of the mastoid process; associated with basal skull fracture.

bigeminy Ventricular bigeminy is a pattern of arrhythmia consisting of coupled ventricular beats; alternating QRS complexes are ventricular premature depolarizations.

Bitot's spots White or light gray areas of keratinized epithelium on the conjunctiva seen in vitamin A deficiency.

blepharospasm Tonic spasm of the orbicularis oculi muscle.

blind spot The site of penetration of the optic nerve in the retina in which no light-sensitive receptors are found.

blister Vesicle; localized collection of fluid in the epidermis that separates and raises the horny upper layers.

blocking or thought deprivation Sudden pause in the train of thought caused by unconscious emotional conflict.

borborygmus Audible bowel sounds, generally caused by gas propulsion through the intestine.

bradycardia Slower than normal heart rate (<50 beats per minute).

bronchiectasis Chronic dilatation of one or more bronchi.

bronchitis Inflammation of one or more bronchi; condition may be chronic or acute.

bronchophony The sound of the voice as heard with abnormally increased clarity and intensity through the stethoscope over the lung parenchyma.

bruit Murmur (blowing sound) heard over peripheral vessels.

buccal Pertaining to the cheek.

bullous Characterized by vesicles (blisters) usually 2 cm or more in diameter.

bursa Sac or saclike cavity filled with fluid and located in sites where friction would otherwise develop, as in a joint or over a bony prominence.

bursitis Inflammation of a bursa.

cachexia Marked malnutrition.

calcinosis Abnormal deposition of calcium salts as nodules in muscles, tendons, and skin.

calculus Stone, abnormal concretion of chemicals, especially in the renal and biliary systems.

callus (1) Localized thickening of the horny layer of the epidermis resulting from hyperplasia. (2) Formation of cartilage and bone at a fracture site.

calor Localized increase in temperature; heat; classic sign of inflammation.

caries Decay of the calcified protein of teeth.

carpal tunnel syndrome Entrapment of the median nerve in the carpal tunnel resulting in paresthesias, pain, and muscle weakness.

caruncle Small elevation of tissue.

cataract Opacity of the lens of the eye or its capsule.

catatonic behavior Motor anomalies not accompanied by organic disease.

catatonic excitement Purposeless excited movement without apparent stimuli.

catatonic negativism Resistance to movement to both verbal instruction and physical attempts to move.

catatonic posturing Voluntary assumption of a bizarre or inappropriate posture; may be maintained for a long period of time.

catatonic rigidity Rigid posture in spite of physical efforts to be moved.

catatonic stupor Decreased response to environment; may appear to be unaware of environment.

catatonic waxy flexibility Body posture and limbs remain in positions in which placed; limbs feel like pliable wax to the examiner.

chalazion Sebaceous cyst on the eyelid formed by distention of a meibomian gland with secretion.

cholangitis Inflammation of the bile ducts.

cholelithiasis Presence of calculi in the bile ducts or gallbladder.

cholesteatoma Cystlike mass common to the middle ear and mastoid region characterized by outer layer of stratified squamous epithelium filled with desquamating debris, including cholesterol; generally associated with chronic infection.

chorea Rapid, brief, involuntary, asymmetric movements worsened by emotional stress; improve or disappear during sleep.

chorionic Pertaining to the chorion, a fetal membrane composed of trophoblast that forms the fetal portion of the placenta.

chronic obstructive pulmonary disease (COPD) General term for disease involving airway obstruction, such as chronic bronchitis, emphysema, or asthma.

Chvostek's sign Spasm of the facial muscle evoked by tapping branches of the facial nerve; may be caused by hypocalcemia or hypomagnesemia.

circumstantiality Interruption in the stream of thought caused by excessive associations of an idea reaching the conscious level. Circumstantiality is characterized by digression and extraneous thinking, which serve to avoid emotionally charged areas.

cirrhosis Disease characterized by destruction of liver parenchyma. The liver is characterized by fibrous tissue and yellow-tan nodules.

clanging Speech in which sounds govern word choice; may consist of rhyming or punning; most often observed in schizophrenia and manic individuals.

cleft palate Developmental defect or failure to fuse of the soft palate, hard palate, and the lip. This is the most common developmental defect of the head and neck.

clonus Rapid rhythmic alteration between contraction and relaxation of muscles, induced by stretching the muscle; may result in alternate flexion and extension.

clubbing Proliferation of soft tissue of terminal phalanges, generally associated with relative hypoxia of peripheral tissues, loss of the angle between the skin and nail base, and sponginess of the nail base.

coarctation A tightening or compression of the walls of a vessel, producing a narrowed lumen.

colic Acute abdominal pain associated with smooth muscle contraction of the gastrointestinal tract.

colitis Inflammation of the colon.

coma Deep unconsciousness from which the individual cannot be aroused, even by painful stimuli. *Comatose:* the condition of being affected by coma.

comedo Papule; hyperkeratotic thickening of the duct of a sebaceous gland with retention of sebum, associated with acne.

complex Emotionally charged attitudes and ideas that are unconscious and influence the behavior of the individual, such as an Oedipus complex.

compulsion behaviors Stereotyped behaviors resulting from obsessions.

condyloma Hyperkeratotic exophytic lesions of stratified squamous epithelium; develops as small, elevated, soft nodules that enlarge and coalesce to become cauliflower-like excrescences.

confabulation Fabrication of facts or events in response to questions about situations that are not recalled because of memory impairment.

consensual Reflex reaction in one pupil mimicking that occurring in the other, which is being stimulated.

consolidation Process in which liquid or solid replacement of lung parenchyma as exudate from an inflammatory condition is amassed.

constipation Infrequent or difficult evacuation of feces; often associated with drying and hardening of the stool.

contralateral On the opposite side.

contusion Bruise.

conversion Coordinated medial movement of the eyes in fixing on a near object.

conversion disorder Loss of or alteration in physical functioning suggesting a physical disorder. The symptom allows the individual to avoid some activity that is noxious to him or to get support from the environment that otherwise might not be possible. The symptom can be related in time to a psychological conflict or need.

convulsion Series of involuntary muscle contractions.

Cooper's ligaments Suspensory ligaments of the breast.

corneal limbus The edge of the cornea where it meets the sclera.

cor pulmonale Disease of the heart as a result of pulmonary disease; right heart hypertrophy and right ventricular failure resulting from pulmonary hypertension.

cramp Involuntary, painful skeletal muscle contraction.

crepitation, crepitus A dry, crackline sound in (1) the lung, when air passes through abnormally accumulated moisture; (2) the joints, when dry synovial surfaces rub together; and (3) the skin, when air is present subdermally.

cretinism Disease caused by congenital lack of thyroid hormone; characterized by retarded physical and mental development, deafness, dystrophy of bones and soft tissue and abnormally low concentrations of thyroid hormones.

crisis Sudden change in the course of a disease.

Crohn's disease Inflammatory process that involves the full thickness of the bowel wall and may be associated with mucosal ulcers and cyst abscesses. Bowel obstruction and fistula formation are common complications.

Cullen's sign Bluish coloration in the umbilical region associated with intraperitoneal bleeding.

Curling's ulcer Ulcer of the fundus and body of the stomach associated with stress accompanying extensive burn injuries.

cyanosis Dusky blue color imparted to skin when the hemoglobin saturation is less than 75% to 85% or PaO_2 is less than 50 mm Hg.

cyclothymic disorder Periods with some depressive and manic behavior over 2 years but not of sufficient severity or duration to be defined as major depressive or manic episodes; may have normal behavior between episodes.

cyst Collection of fluid surrounded by a membrane.

cystocele Herniation of the urinary bladder into the anterior vaginal wall.

dacryadenitis Inflammation of a lacrimal gland.

dacryocystitis Inflammation of the lacrimal sac.

decidua The endometrium during pregnancy that is shed in the postpartum period.

déjà vu A sensation of familiarity with a person, place, or activity during a first encounter; a feeling of "having been there before."

delirium Clouded state of consciousness, reduction in clarity of awareness of environment accompanied by a reduced capacity to shift, focus, and sustain attention to environmental stimuli.

delusion A false belief, improbable in nature; not influenced by contrary experience nor related to the cultural and educational background of the client.

dementia Loss of cognitive abilities of sufficient magnitude to interfere with social or occupational functioning; memory impairment and impairment of abstract thinking or impaired judgment or other disturbance of higher cortical function.

depersonalization Loss of the sense of personal reality or identity; withdrawal and isolation result from disappointments or unbearable sufferings that make one a witness to personal experiences rather than a participant.

depigmentation Loss of pigment, usually of melanin.

depression Term used to define (1) a mood, (2) a syndrome, and (3) an illness. The mood of depression is described as dejection and lowering of functional activity; it is a normal experience that may be incurred in response to frustration and loss. The syndrome of depression includes a depressed mood in combination with one or more of the following symptoms: inability to concentrate, anorexia, weight loss, and suicidal ideas. The illness of depression is characterized by the syndrome of depression but lasts longer. Functional impairment may include inability to carry on daily activities, particularly work.

derealization Feelings that the world around one is not real; generally associated with depersonalization.

dereistic thinking Illogical thought processes.

dermographia Abnormal skin sensitivity, so that firm stroking with a dull instrument or light scratching results in a wheal surrounded by a red flare; may be caused by allergy.

desquamation Scaling, shedding of epithelial tissue.

dextrocardia A rare condition in which the position of the heart is reversed and lies on the right side of the chest.

diarrhea Increased frequency and liquid content of fecal evacuation.

diastasis recti abdominis Separation of the rectus muscles of the abdominal wall; may occur in pregnancy.

dicrotic pulse Presence of two sphygmographic or polygraphic elevations to one beat of the pulse.

diopter Refractive power of a lens with a focal distance of 1 meter; a unit of measure of refractive power.

diplopia Double vision; perception of two images for a single object.

disease Abnormality of structure or function that has a single pathogenic mechanism and a predictable course.

disorientation Lack of awareness as to time, place, or person.

diverticulitis Usually refers to inflammation of colonic diverticula.

diverticulum Pouch or sac created by herniation of mucosal lining of a hollow organ (bladder or gastrointestinal tract) through a defect in the muscular wall.

dullness Decreased resonance on percussion.

dysarthria Difficulty in articulating single sounds or phonemes of speech. Individual letters: *f, r, g*; labials—sounds produced with the lips: *b, m, v* (cranial nerve [CN] VII); gutterals—sounds produced in the throat (CN X); linguals—sounds produced with the tongue; *l, t, n* (CN XII).

dysbasia Difficulty in walking, especially from neurological causes.

dyschezia Difficulty in passing stool; pain associated with defecation.

dyscoria Congenital abnormality in the shape of the pupil.

dysdiadochokinesia Impairment in the ability to stop a movement and to institute the opposite movement, such as pronation to supination.

dysesthesia Impairment of any sensation, particularly of touch.

dysgeusia Impairment or perversion of the sense of taste.

dyskinesia Difficulty of movement.

dyslexia Disturbance in understanding the written word; difficulty in reading.

dysmenorrhea Painful menstruation.

dyspareunia Difficult or painful sexual intercourse in women.

dyspepsia Impairment of the ability to digest food; especially, discomfort after eating a meal.

dysphagia Difficult or painful swallowing.

dysphasia Disturbance in speech evidenced by lack of coordination and failure to express words in proper order.

dysphonia puberum Difficulty in controlling laryngeal speech sounds that occurs as the larynx enlarges in puberty.

dysphoria Restlessness, agitation, malaise.

dysplasia Disorder in the size, shape, or organization of adult cells.

dyspnea Difficult or labored respiration. *Paroxysmal nocturnal dyspnea:* respiratory distress related to posture, especially noted when reclining at night.

dysprosody Difficulty in speech in which inflection, pronunciation, pitch, and rhythm are impaired.

dystrophy Disorder in which muscle wasting, atrophy, occurs.

dysuria Difficulty or painful urination.

ecchymosis A flat, round or irregular, blue or purplish lesion of the skin or mucous membranes resulting from intradermal or submucous hemorrhage.

echolalia Repetition by a client of words addressed to him; may also be the echo of his own thoughts; generally a sign of schizophrenia and organic mental disorders.

ectopic Abnormally located.

ectropion Eversion, or turning outward, of an edge, as of the eyelid.

eczema Superficial inflammatory process of the epidermis associated with redness, itching, weeping, and crusting; of multiple cause.

edema Abnormal increase in the quantity of interstitial fluid.

efferent Carrying from the center to the periphery.

egophony Voice sound of a nasal (telephone-like or bleating) quality, heard through the stethoscope; often defined by asking the client to say "ee," which sounds like "ay."

ejection sounds High-pitched, clicking sounds produced by the forceful opening of a diseased aortic or pulmonic valve heard soon after the first heart sound (S).

elation Elevation of mood, emotional excitement; may be temporary response to fortuitous event in a normal individual. Elation is the characteristic mood of mania and also is observed in some schizophrenics.

embolism Sudden obstruction of an artery by a clot or other foreign substance.

emphysema Refers to entrapment of air within tissue either interstitial or pulmonary. *Pulmonary emphysema:* also called chronic obstructive pulmonary disease (COPD) results from permanent dilatation or enlargement of the passages peripheral to the terminal bronchiole, which causes *increased resistance to airflow. Interstitial emphysema:* the presence of air in the subcutaneous tissue mediastinum or connective tissue of the lung resulting from air leakage through a damaged portion of the respiratory passages or alveoli; may result in swelling of tissue or a distinctive crackling sound called crepitation.

empyema Collection of purulent exudate in a body cavity or hollow organ.

encephalitis Inflammation of the cerebrum, cerebellum, or brainstem.

endometriosis Presence of endometrial stroma and glands in ectopic locations such as the ovaries, pelvic peritoneum, or colon.

encephalopathy A general designation for any cerebral disorder.

encopresis Repeated voluntary or involuntary defecation of normal or near normal feces into inappropriate places.

enophthalmos Recession of the globe of the eye into the orbit.

enteritis Inflammation of the small intestine.

enterocele Herniation of intestinal contents.

entropion Inversion, or turning inward of an edge, as of the eyelid.

enuresis Involuntary urination during sleep.

epilepsy Paroxysmal disturbances in brain function characterized by loss of consciousness, motor or sensory impairment, and disturbance of emotions or thought processes.

epiphora Abnormal tearing of the eyes.

epispadias Congenital anomaly in which the urethra opens on the dorsum of the penis.

epistaxis Bleeding or hemorrhage from the nose.

epulis Tumor of the gingiva.

erectile tissue Tissue capable of becoming rigid and elevated.

eructation Act of belching or bringing up gas (air) from the stomach.

erythema Dilatation of capillaries resulting in redness of the skin.

esophagitis Inflammation of the esophagus; may be caused by gastric reflux, corrosive chemicals, or infectious agents.

eversion A turning outward or inside out.

exanthem General eruption of the skin accompanied by fever.

exophthalmos (proptosis) Abnormal protrusion of the globe of the eye.

extrasystole Premature contraction.

extravasation Escape of blood or infused substance in extravascular tissue.

facies Term used to indicate the expression of the facial structures or the surface of a structure. *Adenoid f.:* open mouth, dull expression. *Elfin f.:* short, upturned nose, wide mouth, widely spaced eyes, full cheeks; associated with hypercalcemia and mental retardation. *F. hepatica:* sallow complexion, yellow conjunctiva. *F. hippocratic:* pinched expression of face, sunken eyes, hollow cheeks and temples, lax lips, and leaden complexion associated with debilitating illness. *Leontine f.:* deep folds, lionlike pattern. *Marshall Hall's f.:* disproportion of forehead to head seen in hydrocephalus. *Parkinson's f.:* masklike, infrequent blinking.

faint Temporary loss of consciousness may result from generalized lack of oxygen or glucose to the brain; may be associated with stress.

fasciculation Rapid, fine, twitching movements resulting from contraction of a fasciculus (bundle of muscle fibers) served by one anterior horn cell; usually does not cause movement of a joint.

febrile Characterized by fever.

festination Involuntary tendency to accelerate the speed of walking; occurs in paralysis agitans.

fever Pyrexia; elevation of the body temperature above normal for a given individual.

fiberoptics Transmission of an image along flexible bundles of coated glass or plastic fiber having special optical properties.

fibrillation Fine, continuous twitching caused by contraction of a single muscle or group of fibers.

flaccid Relaxed, without tone, flabby.

flatulence Excessive amount of gas in the gastrointestinal tract.

flight of ideas Nearly continuous flow of rapid speech with abrupt changes from topic to topic. Flight of ideas is most frequently observed in organic mental disorders, schizophrenia, psychotic disorders, and as a reaction to stress.

fremitus Palpable vibration.

friction rub A crackling, grating sound, heard through the stethoscope when two inflamed, roughened surfaces rub together.

FUO Abbreviation for fever of unknown origin.

fusiform Spindle or cigar shaped.

gallop rhythm Heart rate characterized by three sounds in the presence of tachycardia.

gangrene Necrosis of body tissue associated with ischemia.

gastritis Inflammation of the mucosa of the stomach.

gingivitis Inflammation of the papillary and marginal gingiva.

glabrous Smooth, free of hair.

glaucoma Diseases resulting in increased intraocular pressure. *Angle closure glaucoma:* blockage of the overflow channels for aqueous humor by the iris; results in an acute increase in pressure and pain. *Open angle glaucoma (simple or chronic glaucoma):* degeneration of the outflow channel, trabecular network on Schlemm's canal.

glomus jugulare Globus tympanicum tumor; tumor of the jugular bulb in the floor of the middle ear; may result in hearing loss, sense of fullness, and tinnitus; often seen as a bulging, reddish purple mass through the tympanic membrane.

glossitis Inflammation of the tongue.

goiter Increase in size of the thyroid gland.

gout Disease caused by deposition of crystals of monosodium urate; characterized by a disorder in purine metabolism and associated with exacerbations of arthritis of a single joint.

guilt Painful feeling caused by having transgressed personal or social ethical standards.

gumma Neoplasm composed of soft, gummy tissue resembling granulation tissue; may occur in tertiary syphilis or in tuberculosis.

gynecomastia Hypertrophy of breast tissue in a male subject.

habitus Body type, characteristic of the form of the body. *Asthenic:* slender body type, narrow thorax, internal organ at lower position than other body types. *Hypersthenic:* large, thick body type, with broad deep thorax; body organs in a higher position than other body types. *Hyposthenic:* intermediate body type.

hallucination Perception for which no external stimuli can be ascertained; an endogenous experience in an individual whose sensorium is clear. *Simple hallucination:* simple perception, such as seeing light. *Complex hallucination:* more detailed experience, such as seeing a figure or person.

Heberden's nodes or nodules Small, hard nodules of the terminal interphalangeal joints associated with osteoarthritis.

helix The superior and posterior free margin of the ear.

hemangioma Benign tumor made up of blood vessels; may be capillary or cavernous.

hemarthrosis Hemorrhage into a joint.

hematemesis Vomitus containing blood.

hematoma Localized collection of blood resulting from rupture of a blood vessel.

hematuria Presence of blood in the urine.

hemiballismus Involuntary, coarse, unilateral movements of limbs.

hemiplegia Paralysis involving one side of the body, generally an arm or a leg and sometimes the face, usually resulting from an abnormality of the corticospinal tract of the contralateral side.

hemolytic Pertaining to the release of hemoglobin from red blood cells.

hemophilia Genetic predisposition to bleed more than normal because of a deficiency of the clotting factors.

hemoptysis Spitting or coughing up of blood from the respiratory tract.

hemorrhoid Dilatation of a part of the venous hemorrhoidal plexus in the mucosal membrane of the rectum. Dilatation may occur as a result of increased hydrostatic pressure in the venous system, as in pregnancy, resulting from disease causing portal hypertension and straining at stool. *Internal hemorrhoid:* varicosity of superior or middle hemorrhoidal veins below the anal mucosa; may result in bleeding. *External hemorrhoids:* varicosity of the inferior hemorrhoidal vein under the anal skin; may cause pain and swelling around the anal sphincter, as well as itching and bleeding.

hernia Abnormal protrusion of an organ or tissue through an opening. *Incarcerated hernia:* protrusion of abdominal contents through a weakness in the abdominal wall, so that the contents cannot be returned to the abdominal cavity. *Inguinal hernia: direct*—protrusion of abdominal contents through a weakness in the abdominal musculature, region of Hesselbach's triangle; *indirect*—protrusion through an internal inguinal ring hernia descending beside the spermatic cord. *Scrotal hernia:* protrusion (generally indirect) of abdominal contents into the scrotal sac. *Strangulated hernia:* hernia in which the blood supply to the protruded tissue is obstructed.

herpes Any inflammatory skin disease caused by herpesvirus (a large group of intranuclear double-stranded DNA viruses capable of establishing a latent infection many years after a primary infection). *Cytomegalovirus:* causes cytomegalic inclusion disease. *Epstein-Barr virus:* causes infectious mononucleosis. *Herpes simplex type 1:* causes fever blister and keratoconjunctivitis. *Herpes simplex type 2:* causes venereal disease. *Herpes zoster:* causes shingles. *Varicella:* causes chickenpox.

hirsutism Excessive hairiness, especially in females.

hordeolum Inflammation of a sebaceous gland of the eyelid; sty.

hyaline Glasslike, as of casts in the urine.

hydrocele Circumscribed collection of fluid, particularly in the scrotum.

hydrocephalus Distention of the cerebral ventricular system from excessive production of cerebrospinal fluid or obstruction of the outflow channels.

hygroma Cystic space, bursa, or sac distended with fluid.

hyperesthesia Abnormally increased sensitivity of the skin or another sense organ.

hyperpigmentation An excess of pigment in tissue.

hyperplasia Cellular overgrowth.

hyperpnea Increase in the depth of respiration with or without an increase in rate.

hyperpyrexia Marked elevation of temperature, usually above 105.8° F (41° C).

hyperreflexia Increased amplitude of muscle contraction to evoked reflex.

hypersplenism Enlargement of the spleen associated with a reduction in red blood cells.

hypertension Persistent elevation of blood pressure.

hyperthermia Abnormally elevated body temperature.

hypertonia Increased resistance of muscle tissue to passive stretching.

hypertrichosis Excessive hairiness, especially in females.

hypertrophy Increase in size of a tissue or organ.

hyperventilation Increase in rate and depth of respiration.

hyphema Blood in the anterior chamber of the eye.

hypochondriasis Unrealistic interpretation of physical signs or sensations as abnormal; preoccupation with the fear or belief of having a serious disease.

hypochromic Abnormally decreased color; used to describe anemias in which the amount of hemoglobin in red blood cells is deficient.

hypoesthesia Abnormally decreased sensitivity of the skin or another sense organ.

hypoglossal Below the tongue.

hypopyon Purulent material in the anterior chamber of the eye.

hyposmia Partial loss of the sense of smell.

hypospadias A developmental anomaly in which the urethra opens on the underside of the penis.

icteric Jaundiced.

illusion Perception based on actual external stimulus with misinterpretation or distortion of the event.

impetigo Skin infection caused by staphylococcal or streptococcal organisms. The typical lesion is an eroded, ruptured vesicle covered by an amber crust.

incontinence Failure of control of excretory functions.

infarction Obstruction of circulation followed by ischemic necrosis.

inflammation Localized protective condition associated with vascular dilatation, exudation of plasma, and leukocytes. Clinical signs include redness, swelling, pain, heat, and limitation of function.

intellectualization A defense mechanism that consists of ruminating about philosophical or theoretical ideas or engaging in scholarly activities that serves to constrain instinctual drives. Intellectualization constitutes an interruption of the stream of thought.

ipsilateral On the same side.

iritis Inflammation of the iris.

jaundice Accumulation of bilirubin to serum concentration greater than 2 mg/dl; produces yellow to yellow-green to bronze color of skin, accompanied by itching.

Jolly test Recurrent stimulation of motor muscles. A positive response includes increasingly weaker muscle contraction, associated with myasthenia gravis.

keratitis Inflammation of the cornea.

koilonychia Spoon-shaped nail surface with thin nail, frequently associated with iron deficiency anemia.

Koplik's spots Small white spots on the buccal mucosa that appear in the prodromal stage of measles.

kraurosis vulvae Atrophic condition of the vulva with edema of the surface dermis with underlying inflammation.

Kussmaul respiration Rapid and deep respiratory cycles resulting from stimulation of the medullary respiratory center in metabolic acidosis, associated with pH less than 7.2 in diabetic ketoacidosis.

kwashiorkor Protein-calorie malnutrition; generalized pitting edema, ascites, inhibition of growth, skin rash, ulcers, anorexia, diarrhea, liver enlargement.

kyphoscoliosis Deformity of the spine characterized by curvature in lateral (scoliosis) and anteroposterior (kyphosis) planes.

kyphosis Increased posterior convexity of the spine (humpback).

labile Readily altered, unstable.

lamella Small sheet or leaf.

lassitude Feeling of weakness or exhaustion.

lethargy Condition of drowsiness.

leukopenia Abnormal diminution of leukocytes.

leukoplakia A disease appearing as white, thickened patches on mucous membranes.

leukorrhea White discharge from the vagina.

linea nigra Pigmentation of the linea alba, the tendinous median line on the anterior abdominal wall, during pregnancy.

lipofuscin Brown, granular pigment found in the lysosomes, nerve cells, muscle, heart, and liver in elderly persons.

lordosis. Anterior concavity of the lumbar spine (swayback, saddle back).

luxation Dislocation.

lymphadenitis Inflammation of one or more lymph nodes.

lymphadenopathy Disease of the lymph nodes.

lymphadenosis Hypertrophy or proliferation of lymphatic tissue.

lymphedema Edema caused by accumulation of lymph; may result from pathological condition of lymph ducts or nodes.

lymphoma Neoplastic disorder of lymphatic tissue.

lysis Gradual return to normal following a disease; generally refers to a fever.

macula Small spot on the skin that differs in color from the surrounding tissue and is not elevated.

malaise Feeling of general discomfort or uneasiness.

malignant Tending to become progressively worse and life threatening, especially a disease or tumor.

malingering Simulation of illness.

manic episode Period of behavior characterized by predominantly elevated, expansive, or irritable mood with a duration of at least 1 week. Behaviors that may accompany the elated feeling are increase in activity, restlessness, talkativeness, flight of ideas, feeling that thoughts are racing, grandiosity, decreased sleep time, short attention span, buying sprees, sexual indiscretion, inappropriate laughing, joking, or punning.

marasmus Malnutrition caused by inadequate intake of all nutrients; atrophy of muscles, growth retardation.

master two-step tests Clinical exercise stress test in which subject repeatedly climbs and descends a two-step stair with 9-inch risers for 1½ minutes. Test is meant to reveal subclinical coronary artery disease.

mastitis Inflammation of breast tissue.

meibomian glands Sebaceous glands found in the tarsal plates of the eyelid.

melanocyte A cell that produces melanin.

melanoma Malignant neoplasm of melanocytes.

melasma Circumscribed hyperpigmentation of the skin, especially the forehead, cheeks, chin, and lips in the presence of normal levels of melanocyte stimulating hormone (MSH). The "mask of pregnancy" is thought to be a result of progesterone effects.

melena Dark-colored stools that may be black or tarry stained with partially digested blood.

menorrhagia Excessive menstruation.

metaplasia Change of cell type as in the presence of squamous cells in the respiratory tract of chronic smokers, replacing columnar epithelium.

metrorrhagia Irregular uterine bleeding.

microcephaly Head circumference measuring less than three standard deviations below the mean for age and sex.

micrognathia Underdevelopment of the jaw.

migraine Paroxysmal headache, frequently unilateral.

miosis Abnormal contractions of the pupils.

mitral regurgitation Backward flow of blood from the left ventricle to left atrium associated with incompetent mitral valve caused by congenital defects, mitral calcification, papillary muscle rupture, ventricular aneurysm, or bacterial endocarditis. Early in the disease, fatigue and exertional dyspnea may occur, and failure of the right side of the heart may occur with progression of the disease. Auscultation signs include a holosystolic murmur and S_3 gallop. The heart is increased in size.

mitral stenosis Fibrosis and thickening of the cusps of the mitral valve with narrowing of the aperture between the left atrium and ventricle, which is usually seen in the aftermath of rheumatic heart disease. Auscultation reveals accentuated S_1. After the second sound, S_2, an opening snap is heard.

mitral valve prolapse Eversion of the valve cusps of the mitral valve during ventricular systole. Severity is related to the amount of regurgitation or auscultation. A midsystolic click is heard.

Montgomery's glands Small, sebaceous glands located on the areola.

morning sickness Nausea and vomiting associated with the period from the fith or sixth week of pregnancy to the fourteenth to sixteenth week. The cause is unknown.

mumps Viral infection involving the parotid gland.

murmur Blowing sound caused by turbulence of blood flow, heard through the stethoscope over the heart or the great vessels.

mydriasis Extreme dilatation of the pupil resulting from paralysis of the oculomotor muscles or the effect of a drug.

myoclonus Jerking movement of one or more limbs or the trunk caused by muscle contractions.

myopathy Disease of the muscles.

myxedema Hypothyroidism. Hypometabolism is present, and nonpitting edema results from the presence of hydrated mucopolysaccharides in connective tissue.

myringitis Inflammation of the tympanic membrane usually resulting from infection.

nabothian follicles Cystlike formations on the mucosa of the uterine cervix resulting from an accumulation of retained secretion in occluded glands.

nausea Feeling that emesis is impending.

neologism Newly coined word; meaningless word often uttered by a psychotic client.

nephritis Inflammation of the kidney.

nephrocalcinosis Condition in which there is precipitation of calcium salts in the tubules and parenchyma of the kidney.

nephrolithiasis Condition of renal calculi.

neuralgia Pain associated with the course of a nerve.

neurosis Psychiatric term for an emotional problem thought to be related to unresolved conflict; differs from a psychosis in that hallucinations, delusions, and illusions generally do not occur.

nevus Well-demarcated malformation of the skin, such as an area of pigmentation or a mole.

night blindness Slow adjustment from bright to dim light.

nociceptive Painful response of reflex evoked by a noxious stimulus.

nocturia Excessive urination at night.

nuchal Pertaining to the nape of the neck.

nullipara Woman who has not given birth to a viable offspring.

nystagmus Involuntary, rhythmic motion of the eye; may be horizontal, vertical, rotary, or mixed.

obsession Persistent, upsetting preoccupation with an idea that morbidly dominates the mind.

obstipation Severe constipation.

oligomenorrhea Decreased frequency of menstruation with an interval of 38 to 90 days.

oligospermia Less than 20 million spermatozoa per milliliter of semen.

oliguria Abnormally decreased urine secretion (<400 ml/24 hours).

omphalocele Congenital umbilical hernia.

onychia Inflammation of the matrix of the nail.

onycholysis Distal separation of the nails from the nail bed.

opisthotonos Hyperextension of the neck and marked flexion of hips and legs.

orthopnea Dyspnea relieved by sitting upright.

orthostatic (postural) hypotension Lowering blood pressure that occurs on rising to an erect position.

otalgia Earache.

Paget's disease Condition characterized by excoriating or scaling lesion of the nipple, extending from an intraductal carcinoma of the breast.

palpate Examination conducted by feeling or touching the object to be evaluated.

palpebra Eyelid.

palpitation Subjective awareness of the pulsations of the heart and arteries.

papilledema Edema of the optic papilla.

papule Elevated lesion of the skin with a diameter less than 5 mm.

paraesthesia Abnormal or perverted sensation; may include burning, itching, pain, or the feeling of electric shock.

paresis Slight or incomplete paralysis; weakness.

paronychia Inflammation and infection of the folds of tissue surrounding a fingernail.

parosmia Perversion of the sense of smell; olfactory hallucinations.

passive-aggressive personality disorder Resistance to demands for adequate performance in occupational or social settings. Resistance may take the form of "forgetfulness," intentional inefficiency, stubbornness, dawdling, or procrastination.

pediculosis Infestation with lice.

percussion Examination conducted by listening to reverberation of tissue after striking the surface with short, sharp blows.

peristalsis Wave of contraction moving along a muscular tube, particularly the gastrointestinal tract.

petechiae Very small, flat, purple-to-red skin or mucous membrane lesions caused by submucous or intradermal hemorrhage.

phimosis difficulty in retraction of the foreskin of the penis.

phobia Persistent and exaggerated fear of a particular object or situation.

phoria Mild weakness of the extraocular muscle(s). *Esophoria:* inward deviation of the eye(s). *Exophoria:* outward deviation of the eye(s).

photalgia Painful sensation in eye following exposure to light.

photophobia Abnormal intolerance of light.

pica Repeated consumption of nonnutritive substance for at least 1 month.

pinguecula Thickened, yellowish area of the cornea, a common degenerative condition.

pityriasis Skin disease characterized by the formation of fine, branny scales. *P. alba:* chronic patchy scaling and hypopigmentation of facial skin. *P. rosea:* acute inflammatory disease with oval, tan eruptions of scales in skin cleavage lines. *P. rubra polans:* chronic inflammatory skin condition with pink scales, macules, and papules.

plantar wart Infection with human wart virus characterized by a wart on the sole of the foot.

-plegia Complete paralysis. *Diplegia:* paralysis of both upper or lower limbs. *Hemiplegia:* paralysis of one side of the body. *Paraplegia:* paralysis of both legs and the lower part of the body. *Quadraplegia:* paralysis of all four limbs.

plethora Pertaining to a red, florid complexion.

pleural effusion Fluid of any kind in the pleural cavity.

pleurisy Pain accompanying pleural inflammation.

polycythemia Abnormal increase in the number of red blood cells.

polydipsia Excessive thirst.

polymenorrhea Abnormally frequent menstruation.

polyphagia Excessive ingestion of food.

polyuria Increased urinary excretion.

Poupart's ligament the inguinal ligament; the fibrous band that runs from the anterior superior iliac spine to the pubic spine.

prepuce Foreskin.

presbycusis Sensorineural hearing loss that develops as a part of the aging process.

presbyopia Reduced capacity of the lens of the eye to accommodate, which develops with advancing age.

perseveration An interruption in the stream of thought characterized by multiple repetitions of a word or phrase.

priapism Prolonged erection of the penis.

proctitis Inflammation of the rectal mucosa.

proctoscopy Examination of the rectum with a short cylindrical instrument called a proctoscope.

prodromal Sign or symptom indicating the onset of a disease.

progeria Manifestation of aging occurring in childhood.

prognathism Protrusion of the jaw.

prognosis Expected outcome of a pathological condition.

pronation (1) Assumption of the prone position; (2) turning the forearm so the palm is posterior; or (3) eversion and abduction of the foot.

proprioceptive sensation Muscle and joint sensations of position in space.

prostatitis Acute or chronic inflammation of the prostate gland, generally in conjunction with cystitis and urethritis. Symptoms: low back and perineal pain, fever, urinary frequency, and dysuria.

pruritus Itching.

psoriasis Papulosquamous dermatosis; characteristic lesion is bright red macule, papule, or plaque covered with silver scales.

psychasthenia Neurosis characterized by depersonalization, delusions, fear, and feelings of inadequacy.

psychogenic amnesia Sudden inability to recall important personal information that cannot be explained by normal forgetfulness.

psychosis Psychiatric term for a mental disorder associated with thought disorders, pathological perception (delusions, hallucinations), or extremes of affect.

pterygium Abnormal triangular thickening of the bulbar conjunctiva on the cornea, with the apex toward the pupil.

ptosis Drooping of the eyelid.

pulse Palpable rhythmical expansion of the artery.

purpura Small hemorrhage, less than a centimeter in diameter.

pustule Elevation of skin containing purulent exudate filled with neutrophils.

pyemia general septicemia marked by fever, chills, and abscesses.

pyorrhea Purulent inflammation of the gums.

pyrexia Fever; elevation of the body temperature above normal for a given individual.

pyrosis Heartburn.

pyuria Presence of pus in the urine.

quinsy Peritonsillar abscess.

rale Discrete, noncontinuous sound resembling fine crackling, radio static, or hairs being rubbed together, heard through the stethoscope; generally produced by air bubbling through an exudate.

rectocele Herniation of the rectum into the vagina.

regurgitation Reversal of the flow of a substance through a vessel, such as blood flow in the wrong direction or the return of food to the mouth without vomiting.

retinal exudates Cotton wool exudates are white, opaque areas seen in the retina in ophthalmoscopic examination; white, soft, fluffy exudates are microinfarctions of the retinal nerve and represent swollen axon cylinders referred to as cytoid bodies. Soft exudates occur in hypertension, collagen vascular disease, and diabetes mellitus. Hard exudates are true exudates that are yellowish and are in faint clusters or dense masses. These exudates are composed of serum lipids and fat-laden macrophages. Hard exudates occur primarily in diabetes mellitus and severe hypertension.

retraction Condition of being drawn back.

rhinorrhea Excessive, thin nasal secretion.

rhonchus Wheezing or snoring sound produced by airflow across a partially constricted air passage. *Sibilant rhonchus:* wheeze produced in a small air passage. *Sonorous rhonchus:* wheeze produced in a large air passage.

rigor Common term for shivering accompanying a chill or for muscle rigidity accompanying depletion of adenosine triphosphate, as in death (rigor mortis).

salpingitis Inflammation of the fallopian tubes as a result of infection. Leukorrhea, adnexal tenderness, abdominal pain, and fever may be present.

schizophrenic disorder Condition characterized by delusions, hallucinations, or incoherence with flat or inappropriate affect or disorganized behavior. Behavior has deteriorated from a previous level of functioning with regard to work, social relations, or self-care. *Disorganized schizophrenia:* a type of schizophrenia in which there is frequent incoherence, inappropriate affect, but no delusions. *Catatonic schizophrenia:* a type of schizophrenia characterized by any of the following: (1) catatonic stupor reduction in reactivity to environment, spontaneous movements, and mutism; (2) catatonic negativism (resistance to instructions or movement); (3) catatonic rigidity (maintenance of rigid posture even against attempts to move the client); (4) catatonic excitement (excited motor activity not influenced by external stimuli); (5) catatonic posturing (inappropriate or bizarre posturing). *Paranoid schizophrenia:* a type of schizophrenia characterized by persecutory delusions, grandiose delusions, delusional jealousy, or hallucinations with persecutory or grandiose content.

sciatica Pain, weakness, and/or paresthesias, associated with the course of the sciatic nerve: posterior aspect of the thigh, posterolateral and anterolateral aspects of the leg into the foot.

scoliosis Lateral deviation of the spine.

scotoma An islandlike blind gap in the visual field.

sebaceous Pertaining to or secreting sebum, an oily secretion composed of fat and epithelial debris.

sebaceous cyst Retention of the fatty secretion of the sebaceous gland.

sentinel node Also called Virchow's node; enlarged supraclavicular node that may be the indicator of abdominal carcinoma.

sign Objective evidence of disease that is perceptible to the examiner.

simian crease Single transverse crease on the palm; found in 70% of those who have Down's syndrome.

sleep terror (pavor nocturnus) Repeated experience of abrupt awakening from sleep in a state of anxiety or panic, generally occurring in stages 3 and 4 and in the time place of 30 to 200 minutes after the onset of sleep.

somatic Pertaining to the body.

somesthesia Sensation of touch-pressure, temperature, pain, and joint position.

somnambulism (sleep walking) Sleep disorder characterized by repeated acts of rising from bed during sleep and walking for a few minutes to a half hour, generally occurring in stages 3 and 4 and in the time phase of 30 to 200 minutes after the onset of sleep.

sordes Materia alba; undigested food bacteria encrusting the lips and teeth.

spasm Involuntary sudden contraction of a muscle or a group of muscles accompanied by pain and interference with function.

spastic Rigid; characterized by muscle spasm.

steatorrhea Abnormal increase of fat in the feces.

stereognosis Discrimination of objects by the sense of touch.

stereotypy Interruption in the stream of thought consisting of persistent repetition of a word or phrase.

sthenic Sturdy or strong; active.

stomatitis Inflammation of the mouth.

strabismus Disparity in the anteroposterior axes of the eyes; the optic axes cannot be directed to the same object because of lack of muscular coordination.

stress incontinence Involuntary urination incurred on straining, coughing, or lifting.

striae gravidarum Atrophic, pinkish or purplish scarlike lesions observed on the breasts, thighs, abdomen, and buttocks during pregnancy; lesions later become silvery white.

stridor Harsh, high-pitched respiratory sound heard in respiratory obstruction.

stupor Decreased responsiveness; partial unconsciousness.

succussion Procedure involving shaking an individual to demonstrate fluid in a hollow cavity.

symptom Subjective perception of a client of an alteration of bodily or mental function from basal conditions; change perceived by the individual.

syncope Fainting; temporary unconsciousness.

syndrome Recognized pattern of signs and symptoms.

tachycardia Rapid heart rate (>100 beats per minute). *Atrial flutter:* rapid, regular, uniform atrial contraction caused by AV block; ventricular rhythm varies with the degree of AV block. *Atrial tachycardia:* arrhythmia caused by the atria; rapid, regular beat of the entire heart. *Ventricular tachycardia:* arrhythmia caused by the ventricles; rapid, relatively regular heartbeat.

tachypnea Rapid respiratory rate.

telangiectasis Localized group of dilated capillaries.

tenesmus Uncomfortable straining; particularly, unsuccessful attempts at defecation or urination.

thrill Palpable murmur; vibration accompanying turbulence in the heart or the great vessels.

tic Sudden, short contractions of a muscle or group of muscles, always causing movement of affected part.

tinnitus Sensation of noise in the ear caused by abnormal stimulation of the auditory apparatus or its afferent pathways; may be described as ringing, buzzing, swishing, roaring, blowing, or whistling.

tophus Deposits of monosodium urate, seen in gout.

transient ischemic attack Occlusion of central nervous system vessel resulting in a focal neurological disturbance.

tremor Involuntary, somewhat rhythmic, oscillatory quivering of muscles, caused by alternate contraction of opposing groups of muscles. *Cerebellar tremor:* occurs during intentional movement, becoming more pronounced near end of the movement; associated with lesions of the dentate nucleus. *Coarse tremor:* slow rate and large amplitude movements. *Essential (familial) tremor:* begins usually around age 50 with fine tremors of the hands; aggravated by intentional movement; commonly affects head, jaws, lips, or voice. *Fine tremor:* rapid (10 to 20 oscillations per second) and low amplitude movements, usually in the fingers and hands. *Moderate tremor:* medium rate and medium amplitude movements. *Passive tremor:* present at rest, may improve during intentional movement; for example, pill-rolling tremor or Parkinson's disease. *Physiological tremor:* experienced by healthy people in fatigue, cold, and stress. *Toxic tremor:* caused by endogenous (thyrotoxicosis, uremia) or exogenous toxins (alcohol, drugs).

trimester A period of 13 weeks.

trophoblast The peripheral cells of the blastocyst that attach the fertilized ovum to the uterine wall and become the placenta and the membranes.

tropia Permanent deviation of the axis of an eye.

Trousseau's sign Elicitation of carpopedal spasm by compression of the upper arm with a tourniquet or blood pressure cuff. The sign is associated with hypocalcemic tetany.

tympany Drumlike note produced by percussion, generally over a gas-filled region.

ulcer Indentation of the surface of tissue or an organ resulting from the sloughing of necrotic, inflamed tissue.

undulant Wavelike variations, particularly as in fever and diurnal circadian fluctuations.

urticaria Rash characterized by wheals.

uveitis Inflammation of the middle, pigmented layer and vascular coat of the eye: iris, ciliary body, and choroid.

valgus Angulation of an extremity toward the midline. *Genu valgum:* condition in which knees are abnormally close together; knock-knee.

varicocele Distention of the veins of the spermatic cord.

varicose Dilated, particularly a vein.

varus Angulation of an extremity away from the midline. *Genu varum:* condition in which knees are abnormally separated; bowleg.

verbigeration (polyphasia) Repetition of meaningless words or phrases.

verruca Lobulated elevation of the epidermis thought to be caused by papillomavirus.

vertigo Illusion of movement, with imagined rotation of one's self (subjective vertigo) or of one's surroundings (objective vertigo).

vesicle Blister, elevation caused by separation of the epidermis by serous fluid or pus.

Virchow's node See sentinel node.

vitiligo Skin affliction characterized by patches of depigmented skin caused by destruction of melanocytes associated with autoimmune disorders.

whispered pectoriloquy Increased resonance of the whispered voice as heard through the stethoscope.

xerostomia Dryness of the mouth resulting from decreased production of saliva.

xiphisternum Xiphoid process of the sternum.

INDEX